D0203640

The American Psychiatric Publishing

# Textbook of Forensic Psychiatry

The American Psychiatric Publishing

# Textbook of Forensic Psychiatry

Edited by

Robert I. Simon, M.D.

Liza H. Gold, M.D.

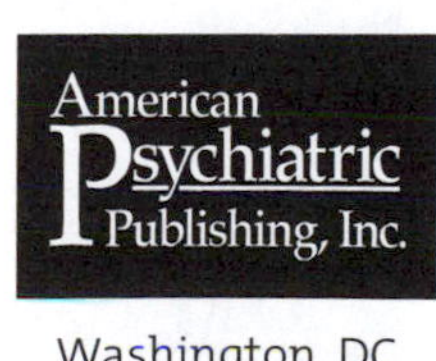


Washington, DC
London, England

**Note:** The authors have worked to ensure that all information in this book is accurate at the time of publication and consistent with general psychiatric and medical standards, and that information concerning drug dosages, schedules, and routes of administration is accurate at the time of publication and consistent with standards set by the U.S. Food and Drug Administration and the general medical community. As medical research and practice continue to advance, however, therapeutic standards may change. Moreover, specific situations may require a specific therapeutic response not included in this book. For these reasons and because human and mechanical errors sometimes occur, we recommend that readers follow the advice of physicians directly involved in their care or the care of a member of their family.

Books published by American Psychiatric Publishing, Inc., represent the views and opinions of the individual authors and do not necessarily represent the policies and opinions of APPI or the American Psychiatric Association.



Manufactured in the United States of America on acid-free paper
08 07 06 05 04 5 4 3 2 1
First Edition



Typeset in Adobe's Palatino and The Mix

American Psychiatric Publishing, Inc.
1000 Wilson Boulevard
Arlington, VA 22209-3901
www.appi.org

**Library of Congress Cataloging-in-Publication Data**
The American Psychiatric Publishing textbook of forensic psychiatry / edited by Robert I. Simon, Liza H. Gold.
p. ; cm.
Includes bibliographical references and index.
ISBN 1-58562-087-4 (alk. paper)
1. Forensic psychiatry. 2. Forensic psychiatry—United States. I. Title: Textbook of forensic psychiatry. II. Simon, Robert I. III. Gold, Liza H., 1958–
RA1151.A47 2004
614'.15—dc22

2003069699

**British Library Cataloguing in Publication Data**
A CIP record is available from the British Library.

*To my grandsons Justin and Nicholas Simon.*
R.I.S.

*To my parents, M. Eliot Gold and Susan Gold.*
*L.H.G.*

*Read not to contradict and confute,*
*nor to believe and take for granted,*
*nor to find talk and discourse,*
*but to weigh and consider.*

Francis Bacon, "Of Studies"
*Essays* (1625)

# Contents

## PART II
## Civil Litigation

## PART III
## Issues in Criminal Justice



## PART IV
## Special Topics

# Contributors

**Peter Ash, M.D.**
Director, Psychiatry and Law Service, and Associate Professor, Department of Psychiatry and Behavioral Sciences, Emory University, Atlanta, Georgia

**F. William Black, Ph.D.**
Professor of Psychiatry and Neurology and Director, Neuropsychology Laboratory, Tulane University Health Sciences Center, New Orleans, Louisiana

**Daniel Brown, Ph.D.**
Assistant Clinical Professor of Psychology, Harvard Medical School, Boston, Massachusetts

**Vladmir Coric, M.D.**
Assistant Clinical Professor, Department of Psychiatry, Yale University School of Medicine, New Haven, Connecticut

**Albert M. Drukteinis, M.D., J.D.**
Adjunct Associate Professor of Psychiatry, Dartmouth Medical School; Director of New England Psychodiagnostics, Manchester, New Hampshire

**Joel A. Dvoskin, Ph.D., A.B.P.P.**
Clinical Assistant Professor, University of Arizona Health Sciences Center, Tucson, Arizona

**Alan R. Felthous, M.D.**
Professor of Clinical Psychiatry and Director of Forensic Psychiatry Service, Department of Psychiatry, Southern Illinois University School of Medicine, Springfield; Professor, Southern Illinois University School of Law, Carbondale; Medical Director, Chester Mental Health Center, Chester, Illinois; Clinical Professor, Department of Psychiatry, St. Louis University School of Medicine, St. Louis, Missouri

**Marvin Firestone, M.D., J.D.**
Private practice, San Mateo, California

**Joan B. Gerbasi, M.D., J.D.**
Assistant Clinical Professor of Psychiatry, Division of Forensic Psychiatry, Department of Psychiatry, University of California, Davis, School of Medicine, Sacramento, California

**Liza H. Gold, M.D.**
Clinical Associate Professor, Program in Psychiatry and Law, Georgetown University School of Medicine, Washington, D.C.

**Robert P. Granacher Jr., M.D.**
Clinical Professor of Psychiatry, University of Kentucky College of Medicine; President, Lexington Forensic Institute, Lexington, Kentucky

**Thomas G. Gutheil, M.D.**
Professor of Psychiatry and Co-Director, Program in Psychiatry and the Law, Massachusetts Mental Health Center, Harvard Medical School, Boston, Massachusetts; Past President, American Academy of Psychiatry and the Law

**H.W. LeBourgeois III, M.D.**
Forensic Psychiatry Fellow, Division of Law and Psychiatry, Department of Psychiatry, University of Massachusetts Medical School, Worcester, Massachusetts

**Jeffrey L. Metzner, M.D.**
Clinical Professor of Psychiatry, University of Colorado Health Sciences Center, Denver, Colorado

**Donald J. Meyer, M.D.**
Senior Associate, Program in Psychiatry and Law at Massachusetts Mental Health Center; Associate Director, Forensic Psychiatry, Beth Israel Deaconess Medical Center; Assistant Clinical Professor of Psychiatry, Harvard Medical School, Boston, Massachusetts

**Douglas Mossman, M.D.**
Professor and Director, Division of Forensic Psychiatry, Wright State University School of Medicine; Adjunct Professor, University of Dayton School of Law, Dayton, Ohio

**Stephen Noffsinger, M.D.**
Assistant Professor of Psychiatry, University Hospitals of Cleveland/Case Western Reserve University, Cleveland, Ohio

**Debra A. Pinals, M.D.**
Director, Forensic Psychiatry Training and Forensic Evaluation Services; Associate Professor of Psychiatry, Law and Psychiatry Program, Department of Psychiatry, University of Massachusetts Medical School, Worcester, Massachusetts

**Marilyn Price, M.D.**
Director, The Law and Behavioral Health Program at Butler Hospital; Assistant Clinical Professor, Department of Psychiatry and Human Behavior, Brown University School of Medicine, Providence, Rhode Island

**Phillip J. Resnick, M.D.**
Professor of Psychiatry, University Hospitals of Cleveland/Case Western Reserve University, Cleveland, Ohio

**J. Adrienne Roth, Ph.D.**
Clinical Director of Research and Training, Connecticut Department of Mental Health and Addiction Services, Forensic Division; Clinical Faculty, Department of Psychiatry, Yale University School of Medicine, New Haven, Connecticut

**Robert L. Sadoff, M.D.**
Clinical Professor of Psychiatry and Director, Center for Studies in Social-Legal Psychiatry, University of Pennsylvania School of Medicine, Philadelphia, Pennsylvania

**Daniel W. Shuman, J.D.**
Professor of Law, Dedman School of Law, Southern Methodist University, Dallas, Texas

**Robert I. Simon, M.D.**
Clinical Professor of Psychiatry and Director, Program in Psychiatry and Law, Georgetown University School of Medicine, Washington, D.C.; Chairman, Department of Psychiatry, Suburban Hospital, Bethesda, Maryland

**Ralph Slovenko, J.D., Ph.D.**
Professor of Law and Psychiatry, Wayne State University Law School, Detroit, Michigan

**John W. Thompson Jr., M.D.**
Vice-Chairman, Department of Psychiatry and Neurology, and Director, Division of Forensic Neuropsychiatry, Tulane University School of Medicine, New Orleans, Louisiana

**Robert Weinstock, M.D.**
Clinical Professor of Psychiatry and Director, Forensic Psychiatry Fellowship Program, University of California, Los Angeles, California

**Robert M. Wettstein, M.D.**
Clinical Professor of Psychiatry, Department of Psychiatry, University of Pittsburgh School of Medicine, Pittsburgh, Pennsylvania

**Howard Zonana, M.D.**
Professor of Psychiatry and Director, Law and Psychiatry Division, Department of Psychiatry, Yale University School of Medicine; Clinical Professor (Adjunct), Yale Law School, New Haven, Connecticut

# Preface

The preacher in Ecclesiastes tells us, "of making books there is no end." Today, the publishing business is huge, the flood of books endless. Yet textbooks of forensic psychiatry are still rare. The textbooks that do exist are the province of the forensic specialist. To our knowledge, no textbook of forensic psychiatry has been written primarily for the general clinician.

Forensic psychiatry has developed as a subspecialty only recently. Despite its new subspecialty status, general clinicians still perform the bulk of forensic assessment. This has changed little over the last 150 years. Isaac Ray, in his landmark book *A Treatise on the Medical Jurisprudence of Insanity*, published in 1838, drew no distinction between the general psychiatrist and the forensic psychiatrist. They were one and the same. Nevertheless, Ray urged his colleagues to familiarize themselves with the skills that distinguished the clinician from the expert witness:

> It cannot be too strongly impressed upon our minds that the duty of an expert is very different from those which ordinarily occupy our attention, and requires a kind of knowledge, and a style of reflection, not indispensable to their tolerably creditable performance. [Clinical and diagnostic skills] will render him [the clinician] but indifferent service on the witness stand. There, he will feel the need of other resources than these, and fortunate will he be, if he do *[sic]* not learn his deficiency before he has exposed it. (Isaac Ray, "Hints to the Medical Witness in Questions of Insanity." *American Journal of Insanity,* Vol. VIII, no. 1, p. 55)

Many areas of psychiatry require specialized knowledge. Child and adolescent psychiatry, addiction psychiatry, and geriatric psychiatry are formal subspecialties in which general clinicians receive training. Residencies have required courses and both required and elective rotations in these complex areas of practice. Competent general clinicians are able on the basis of this training to evaluate, manage, and treat patients who fall into these categories.

In contrast, clinicians often receive little or no formal training in forensic psychiatry unless they pursue fellowships. Clinicians aware of their lack of training often are afraid to take forensic cases. They may avoid forensic practice entirely, and suffer undue anxiety when their participation becomes unavoidable. Others are unaware of the need for at least some training to navigate often-perilous legal waters. When forensically naive clinicians become involved in cases, as Isaac Ray noted, they often recognize too late that they do not have the skills needed to provide competent services. Their foray into forensic psychiatry often ends prematurely.

As in any other subspecialty of medicine or psychiatry, general practitioners are encouraged to have some training and knowledge and to practice within their expertise. They are also encouraged to recognize the limits of their expertise and to refer complicated cases to specialists. General internists provide diagnostic evaluation and treatment for any number of diseases and conditions. When these cases become complicated or severe, internists refer these patients to cardiologists, pulmonologists, and other specialists for further evaluation and treatment.

We hope to move general clinicians toward a similar standard of practice in respect to forensic psychiatry. This textbook is not intended to turn the general clinician into a forensic specialist. Rather, we hope to provide the basic information that general clinicians need to discharge forensic obligations, whether required or voluntarily, in a competent manner. We also want to help them recognize that certain areas of forensic practice, once identified, generally require the skills of a forensic specialist. In such cases, we encourage them to refer to forensic specialists or obtain consultation.

In this spirit, we take great pride in presenting to the general clinician this collection of outstanding authorities in forensic psychiatry. Not to exclude the specialist, we believe the knowledge and information contained in this book will also assist the most experienced forensic practitioner. Forensic specialists can always learn from the experiences of their colleagues. These chapters provide both general clinicians and forensic specialists with concise reviews and practice guidelines that will expand their level of expertise in this exciting and challenging specialty.

The law is foreign terrain for both the general clinician and the forensic specialist. One must learn the map of the landscape in order to negotiate this terrain safely. We hope that the combined knowledge and experience regarding forensic assessments presented in this book will help guide the clinician to a positive, rewarding experience in forensic practice.

## Acknowledgments

The idea for a textbook of forensic psychiatry came from Robert E. Hales, M.D., M.B.A., Editor-in-Chief of American Psychiatric Publishing, Inc. His capacity for generating innovative ideas seems limitless. We owe him and APPI our gratitude for their unfailing support for this important book project.

Many thanks to Ms. Tina Coltri-Marshall, to Ms. Lucinda Clark-Cramer, and to Ms. Polly Brody for their valuable assistance in providing essential help in the day-to-day production of this book. We want to express our special appreciation to Ian J. Nyden, Ph.D., for his excellent skills in reviewing and editing and his consistent encouragement. Dr. Gold (and Dr. Simon) would like to thank Alix and Joshua Nyden for their patience.

We gratefully acknowledge our chapter authors for their outstanding contributions. They bore with grace our editorial comments. The collaborative spirit was very gratifying.

Robert I. Simon, M.D.
Liza H. Gold, M.D.

# Foreword

Robert L. Sadoff, M.D.

Forensic psychiatry has become a recognized subspecialty in the practice of psychiatry. The practice of forensic psychiatry dates back many years. In the nineteenth century, individuals with mental disorders were considered to be "alienated" from themselves and from society. "Alienists," individuals who examined and treated the mentally ill, also provided testimony in legal cases involving defense or prosecution claims of mental disorders. More recently, forensic psychiatry has again begun to assume a more prominent role in the practice of medicine and psychiatry.

The trend in forensic psychiatry is for increasing expertise through education and fellowship training. Psychiatric residency programs today offer more courses in psychiatry and law than ever before. Some forensic training programs existed prior to the 1960s. However, such programs were not formally organized until after the founding of the American Academy of Psychiatry and the Law (AAPL), the first professional organization of forensic psychiatrists, in 1969. Since that time, more than 30 accredited forensic psychiatric fellowships have been developed. Board certification first became available in the 1970s through the American Board of Forensic Psychiatry. In 1992, subspecialty board certification became available through the American Board of Psychiatry and Neurology. To take the forensic subspecialty board examination, psychiatrists must already be board-certified in general psychiatry and complete a 1-year accredited fellowship.

Forensic psychiatry has become increasingly subspecialized to the point that many general forensic psychiatrists prefer to refer cases to colleagues who have expertise in the various forensic subspecialties. Board certification has increased the number of highly qualified experts in the field. Almost 2,500 psychiatrists are members of AAPL, and many of them work exclusively in the field of law and psychiatry. Increasingly, lawyers seek experienced forensic psychiatrists to conduct clinical assessments and then testify when necessary.

Nevertheless, general psychiatrists without subspecialty board certification or formal training in forensic psychiatry conduct most forensic psychiatric examinations. General psychiatrists also give the majority of forensic psychiatric testimony. The general clinician has been drawn into the courtroom as an expert for various reasons. The rise of HMOs and insurance controlled treatment has created economic pressures that have made other areas of psychiatric practice, such as forensic psychiatry, more appealing. Although the general psychiatrist may become more involved in civil or administrative cases than in criminal ones, the publicity that often accompanies high-profile forensic cases has also on occasion drawn practitioners to this subspecialty field. Finally, many attorneys prefer to retain academicians or general clinicians who have not specialized in forensic psychiatry. These attorneys are concerned about the "hired gun" label when utilizing the services of psychiatrists who have testified in hundreds of cases. They prefer someone with extensive clinical experience who has not been labeled as a forensic specialist.

This textbook is therefore both important and timely. It is geared to the general clinician working in psychiatry who may become involved in any of the fascinating aspects of forensic psychiatry. Once psychiatrists become known to attorneys as effective expert witnesses, they may be called on to participate in a number of future cases. Clinicians interested in developing an effective and successful forensic practice should have a basic understanding of the legal system and the role of the clinician in forensic cases.

General psychiatrists who increase the amount of time they devote to forensic psychiatry should not believe that by doing so they are giving up the clinical practice of psychiatry. The term *clinician* has at times created some confusion in respect to forensic subspecialists in that "clinical practice" is often used erroneously as a synonym for the practice of providing treatment to patients. This distinction is important and at times may be critical. When the term is used by attorneys, questions about "clinical practice" are often a means of discrediting experts by implying that they are not "real" doctors. Attorneys may also hope to bar the admission of the experts' testimony because in some states experts are prohibited from testifying if a certain percentage of their practice is not "clinical."

All forensic psychiatrists are clinical psychiatrists. All assessments, examinations, and review of medical and clinical records are included in the practice of clinical psychiatry. Not all forensic specialists have treatment practices (although most do). The approach taken by the editors of this textbook and the contributing authors is especially gratifying in that they have recognized that a good forensic psychiatrist first needs to be a good clinician. The authors of these chapters are acknowledged clinical as well as forensic experts.

The general practicing psychiatric clinician who enters the legal arena will find this textbook a "must read." However, experienced forensic psychiatrists will also find that this volume contains a great deal of useful information. The ethics associated with forensic psychiatry differ in significant ways from those associated with general psychiatry. These differences require changes in general practice when one is conducting forensic rather than clinical evaluations. Psychiatrists may find that the laws governing the insanity defense vary from state to state and from federal law. Duty to warn and other statutory laws may also vary from one state to another. Even experienced forensic psychiatrists often find it challenging to navigate these complex ethical and legal waters.

This textbook covers substantive issues in forensic psychiatry that are required knowledge for the general practitioner and experienced forensic psychiatrist. It contains information that is valuable both academically and practically. Each chapter provides practical guidelines to help clinicians structure their approach to each subject as well as suggested readings for those who want to further explore a given subject. Psychiatrists who wish to expand their knowledge and their practices to include the exciting and still developing field of forensic psychiatry are well advised to thoroughly acquaint themselves with this book's pages.

# PART I

# Introduction to Forensic Psychiatry

CHAPTER 1

# Rediscovering Forensic Psychiatry

Liza H. Gold, M.D.

> Plus ça change, plus c'est la même chose.
> [The more things change, the more they remain the same.]
>
> *Alphonse Karr (1849)*

## Introduction

Forensic psychiatry has become an acknowledged and respected psychiatric subspecialty in recent decades. Increasing numbers of general psychiatrists are practicing forensic psychiatry, primarily as an adjunct to clinical practice. The membership of the American Academy of Psychiatry and the Law (AAPL) has increased by nearly 50% in the past decade, from about 1,500 in 1992 to more than 2,200 in 2002 (Binder 2002). At present, approximately 45 forensic fellowship programs offer specialized training in the United States and Canada, and most positions in these programs are filled (AAPL 2002).

AAPL, the first professional organization of forensic psychiatrists, was founded with only 10 members in 1969. A few fellowships in forensic psychiatry were offered as early as 1965, but interest in such training was almost nonexistent in the 1960s and 1970s (Rappeport 1999). The American Board of Medical Specialties and the American Psychiatric Association officially recognized forensic psychiatry as a subspecialty in 1992 (Prentice 1995; Rappeport 1999). Social forces, including the impact of managed care on the practice of psychiatry, have played a role in stimulating interest in this subspecialty practice (Binder 2002; Rappeport 1999).

Although it appears to be a "new" area of practice, psychiatrists establishing forensic practices have in fact only rediscovered their professional roots. The field of psychiatry, arguably the first subspecialty of medicine[1] (Grob 1994), developed in the first decades of the nineteenth century. Forensic psychiatric practice played an important but underrecognized role in its development. The relationship of insanity and the law was a recognized branch of the growing nineteenth-century interest in medical jurisprudence, the practice of medicine in relation to the law, before clinical psychiatry fully evolved. The first "mad-doctors" or psychiatrists[2] were asylum doctors. They combined their interest and experience in mental disorders with the traditions of medical jurisprudence and considered forensic practice an integral part of their professional role. Once launched, forensic psychiatry quickly became an influential component of American medicolegal practice (Mohr 1997). Thus, forensic psychiatry helped the field of clinical psychiatry establish its professional identity.

The process by which medicine came to dominate the discourse concerning mental illness has engendered debate and controversy among historians and sociologists of science and medicine (Scull 1981a). These controversies revolve around the validity of internal and external historiography. Internal (or Whiggish) histories of medicine demonstrate the progressive advancement of objective knowledge and humanitarian contributions of practice, often without reference to any external social factors (Smith 1981). Critics of this approach point out that conceptions of disease and responses to it unquestionably show the imprint of our particular culture (Starr 1982). In contrast, some historians have focused primarily on the external forces that drove professionalization. Indeed, sociologists use the example of doctors to illustrate the developing prominence of the professional middle class. These interpretations are weakened by their indifference to the content of medical knowledge (Eigen 1991).

---

[1]The practice of surgery, already well established, evolved from a different historical tradition and not as a subspecialty of medicine.

[2]The term "mad-doctor" now carries a pejorative connotation, but it was once the standard English expression for those medical men who sought to make a living from the treatment of the mentally disordered. The term most commonly used in the nineteenth century was "alienist." The modern term "psychiatrist" originated in Germany and did not come into widespread use until the last third of the nineteenth century. The term "psychiatrist" was not generally preferred by the profession itself until the twentieth century (Scull et al. 1996).

This discussion will not attempt to resolve the historical and sociological debates that have characterized the history of psychiatry. Some historians have in fact acknowledged that the once-fashionable distinction between the external and internal histories of medicine and science is not productive (Scull et al. 1996). The development of psychiatry cannot be understood entirely as an internal process related to scientific advancement. It also cannot be fully understood by interpretations that evaluate only external social forces such as the desire for professional aggrandizement.

A variety of factors contributed to the emergence of psychiatry as a professional activity (Mohr 1997; Starr 1982). The rise of experts in madness and the development of a separate field of medicine devoted to the evaluation and treatment of the insane was a complex phenomenon related to the needs of an increasingly sophisticated, industrialized society (Eigen and Andoll 1986; Grob 1994). This chapter reviews the intimate association between the early development of organized psychiatry and forensic practice.[3] This association was an integral part of the professional identity of early specialists in mental disorders, and has implications for modern psychiatrists seeking a deeper understanding of forensic psychiatry.

## Development of Forensic Psychiatry

### Historical Vignette

In 1840, Edward Oxford was tried for firing a pistol at Queen Victoria. He pled not guilty by reason of insanity. At the beginning of the trial, the chief justice was adamant that no witness, including medical witnesses, could give an opinion on whether Oxford was insane, as this was the ultimate issue before the court. By the end of the trial, the medical witnesses were giving such opinions without objection by the prosecution or the judges (Freemon 2001). During the trial, the court questioned one medical witness, Dr. Hodgkin, about the basis of his opinion regarding Oxford's insanity.

[3]This discussion initially will consider developments in both England and the United States and then focus on the professional organization of psychiatry in the United States alone. Through the nineteenth century, English and American lawyers and psychiatrists closely followed cases on both sides of the Atlantic; key English decisions were sometimes cited in America. Much United States practice developed as an offshoot of English law (Smith 1981).

Question by the Court: Do you conceive that this is really a medical question at all, which has been put to you?

Hodgkin: I do. I think medical men have more means of forming an opinion on that subject than other persons.

Q: Why could not any person form an opinion, from the circumstances which have been referred to, whether a person was sane or insane?

H: Because it seems to require a careful comparison of particular cases, more likely to be looked to by medical men, who are especially experienced in cases of unsoundness of mind.

Q: What is the limit of responsibility [for criminal behavior] a medical man would draw?

H: That is a very difficult point. It is scarcely a medical question.

("Review of the Trials of Oxford and M'cNaughten" 1851, cited in Freemon 2001, p. 369)

## The Arrival of the Psychiatric Witness

The testimony in the Oxford case cited in the vignette above demonstrates that by 1840, a professional identity based on expertise in the evaluation of insanity existed. This development was new to the nineteenth century. Before that time, the legal profession had seen little need for advice on legal issues pertaining to insanity (Eigen 1991, 1995; Eigen and Andoll 1986; Maeder 1985; Mohr 1993, 1997; Robinson 1996).[4] Beliefs about mental disturbance were deeply rooted in common culture, and courts did not believe that medical specialists were needed to identify insanity or its causes (Eigen 1995). Cases that might involve psychiatric testimony, such as invalidating a will or a contract because of lunacy[5] or negating criminal responsibility, were considered social, not medical, issues. The prevailing definitions and criteria for legal cases were operationally related to the matter in question: whether the supposed lunatic appreciated his true relationship to the legatees, whether he understood

---

[4]Information regarding the role of psychiatric witnesses is based on historical records involving cases in which the insanity defense was invoked or in which testamentary capacity was challenged. Of these types of cases, the best studied are those involving the insanity defense (Eigen 1995; Mohr 1993).

[5]Terms such as "lunatic," "the deranged," "the distracted," "madmen," and "the insane" were used interchangeably to refer to individuals with mental disorders. In the eighteenth and nineteenth centuries, these were not considered pejorative terms. The use of these terms in this discussion reflects this historical tradition and is not meant to convey any negative meaning or implication.

the terms of a contract and appeared able to exercise due care in transactions, and whether or not he knew his act was right or wrong (Mohr 1997).

The insanity defense did not arouse much medical attention before about 1800 (Smith 1981). Indeed, medical testimony was a rarity at such trials before the early nineteenth century. For example, in 1724, Edward Arnold was tried for the attempted murder of Lord Onslow. Arnold's attorney attempted to prove that Arnold was insane, but no physician was called to testify. The trial of Earl Ferrers in 1760 included, for the first time, the testimony of a "mad-doctor." Dr. John Monro, physician to Bethlem Hospital,[6] provided testimony regarding Ferrers's uncle, who had been Monro's patient, and to the symptoms of insanity in general. Monro had never examined Ferrers (Eigen 1995; Freemon 2001; Maeder 1985). Only a few other cases recorded testimony of medical witnesses. Most defendants were unlikely to be able to afford the services of a physician. Therefore, they would be unlikely to be able to produce a physician who had provided treatment prior to the offense as a medical witness at the time of trial.[7]

By the mid-1800s, however, medical witnesses came to constitute a regular feature of insanity prosecutions, indicating that a professional special expertise was acknowledged by the courts. In the latter half of the eighteenth century, the relative frequency with which lunatics appeared in the dock at the Old Bailey, London's central criminal court, increased (Walker 1968), as did participation of medical witnesses in their trials. In 1760, mad-doctors appeared in only 1 in 10 insanity trials. Beginning in 1760 with the Ferrers case, and ending with the trial of Daniel M'Naghten[8] in 1843, 43% of the cases that came before the Old

---

[6]Dr. Monro was the second in a dynasty of famous Monros who served as superintendents of Bethlem Hospital. The first of the Monro family, James Monro, was medical director from 1728 to 1752. A member of the Monro family occupied this position until 1833.

[7]Only individuals who were well-to-do, such as Lord Ferrers, or a member of a community that looked after its own could produce physician testimony. An example of the latter category is provided by the Society for Visiting the Sick and Charitable Deeds, an organization established by the London Sephardic Jewish community. This group employed a doctor who appeared two or three times at the Old Bailey on behalf of Jews accused of shoplifting (Walker 1968).

[8]There are at least 16 variants of the spelling of the name M'Naghten (see Maeder 1985). This discussion arbitrarily uses the spelling that follows the convention adopted by the *American Journal of Psychiatry.*

Bailey offered evidence regarding the prisoner's mental state. By 1840 specialists in insanity testified in almost half of all insanity cases concerned with a property offense, and almost 90% of trials involving personal assault[9] (Eigen 1991, 1995; Eigen and Andoll 1986; Freemon 2001; Robinson 1996). As Eigen (1991) noted, "Such a dramatic increase in participation suggests that by the time of the M'Naghten trial, the specialist in forensic psychiatry had arrived" (p. 452).

## The Basis of Forensic Expertise: The Development of Clinical Psychiatry

The increased role of physicians in the courts coincided with the development of clinical psychiatry, as demonstrated by the shift in the content of the physician's testimony in the early decades of the 1800s. Before 1825, almost half of the medical witnesses in insanity trials were testifying about friends or former patients and did little more than legitimate the layman's testimony. Their acquaintance with the defendant predated the crime, and the eventual courtroom testimony was a consequence of a social or professional encounter that had already occurred.

In contrast, by the 1820s, the medical witness was likely to be an asylum physician or jail surgeon who, similar to the practice of modern experts, provided a more formal diagnosis in the course of "investigation" of the accused's sanity. Over half of all known post-1825 relationships between medical witness and defendant began after the crime, either while the defendant was in detention awaiting trial or while he or she was confined in a madhouse. This expert testified on the basis of "specialized knowledge" and not personal familiarity with the defendant. These medical witnesses claimed that their sustained familiarity with the mentally ill provided them with a level of professional insight into insanity not shared by the casual or lay observer, or even the general medical practitioner (Eigen 1991; Eigen and Andoll 1986).

---

[9]In the 1700s, England applied the death penalty to a wide range of personal and property offenses. The English legal system developed a series of escapes from execution, one of which was a plea of insanity (Eigen 1995; Walker 1968). Many of the defense medical witnesses in these trials were well known for their opposition to the death penalty. One of the witnesses in the Oxford trial frankly admitted that his opposition to capital punishment biased his opinion concerning the presence or absence of insanity (Freemon 2001).

## The Asylum Movement and Moral Treatment

The medical expert's specialized knowledge was a direct result of the development of the asylum in the early nineteenth century. The physicians associated with these institutions claimed that their study and treatment of large numbers of patients provided them with a special expertise in matters pertaining to insanity. General physicians who offered testimony in the eighteenth century might see one or two cases of mental derangement a year. In contrast, asylum physicians could cite a wealth of experiences in treatment and case management. The more experience in treatment, the more credible the opinion. Even general practitioners began to defer in court to those specialists with greater numbers of patients (Eigen 1991, 1995; Eigen and Andoll 1986; Freemon 2001).

References to "madhouses" in England can be traced back to the seventeenth century, and perhaps before. Most, like Bethlem Hospital in London,[10] had their origin as religious or municipal charities (Scull et al 1996). Institutionalization of the insane in the colonies first appeared in the eighteenth century.[11] Until the close of the eighteenth century, however, madhouses were not primarily medical institutions; their goals were custodial rather than remedial (Walker 1968). In England and in the United States, families or local communities were responsible for providing care for the insane (Grob 1994; Walker 1968). Only the most dangerous or violent individuals were institutionalized, generally in jails.

The asylums of the nineteenth century were a new phenomenon. Their origins lay in the rationalism and optimism of the Age of Enlightenment. This eighteenth-century philosophy posited that although man was corrupt and imperfect, this was not his natural state. The belief that men could better themselves, and that society was responsible for assisting its more imperfect members to assist themselves, led to humanistic and progressive social movements. Naturalistic and secular ways of explaining human behavior replaced mystical or divine explanations. The successes in astronomy and physics, the rapid strides made in technology, and the struggles for political democracy in the United States, France, and England were practical proofs of the validity of the belief that man could control his environment and improve his life on earth (Barton 1987; Dain 1964; Grob 1994).

---

[10]Bethlem, originally Bethlehem Hospital, was established in 1247 by the order of St. Mary of Bethlehem and began admitting lunatics around 1400. In 1547, King Henry VIII took Bethlem away from the religious orders and made it a hospital for indigent lunatics.

[11]The first hospital devoted exclusively to the care of the mentally ill in colonial America was the Public Hospital for the Insane, opened in 1773 in Williamsburg, Virginia.

Explanations of insanity, which had previously been considered a demonstration of divine intervention or punishment, also began to reflect a rational, humanistic view. By the mid–eighteenth century, madness came to be viewed as a pathological condition that could be treated (McGovern 1985; Mohr 1997; Grob 1994). In 1758, Dr. William Battie declared in his *Treatise on Madness* that insanity was as manageable and curable as other disorders.[12]

By the latter part of the eighteenth century, medical interest in insanity was on the upswing (Scull 1981b). Phrenology, considered the first science of the brain, served as a vital theoretical mediation of this change. This new "science" provided a clear physiological explanation of the brain's operations that was basic to psychiatry during the first four decades of the nineteenth century. Phrenology proposed that the brain was composed of discrete anatomical organs, each of which was associated with certain functions, emotions, or behavioral traits. This concept explained mental organization and could account for both normal and abnormal mental function. It also provided a physical basis for the development of medical theories of insanity and the specialty of psychiatry (Coliazzi 1989; Cooter 1981; Dain 1964; Scull 1981b).

Doctors developed medical models of madness that connected the brain and other organs to mental disturbances. Common medical treatments of insanity had been based on traditional theories of humoral imbalances, the mainstay of medical theory and treatment for centuries. If mental illness resulted from a physical disease that involved lesions of the brain, it could be treated similarly to any other somatic disorder. The goal of such treatment was the restoration of balance through standard interventions such as bloodletting, blistering, and purging (Grob 1994).

Many, however, felt that standard medical treatment left something to be desired. Physicians and lay people alike began to call for more humane and humanistic treatment of the insane. At the end of the eighteenth and the start of the nineteenth century a method of treatment was developed that promised new hope in treating this seemingly incurable affliction.

In 1801, Philippe Pinel published his *Traité médico-philosophique sur l'aliénation mentale,* illustrating his success at curing the insane through a pro-

---

[12]Battie was the first English physician of status to make treatment of the mad his primary concern and the first to give clinical instruction on insanity and deliver lectures on mental diseases. He was one of the very few psychiatrists to become president of the Royal College of Physicians of London. With John Monro as his opposite number at Bethlem Hospital, Battie became the leading "mad-doctor" of the day (Hunter and MacAlpine 1982; Scull 1981b; Walker 1968).

gram he called "traitement moral."[13] This treatment emphasized social/ psychological interventions. Pinel concluded that a carefully constructed social environment could help bring the emotions under control better than medical treatment or mechanical restraints. He amassed empirical evidence about his effective moral treatment of the insane and promoted a reformed asylum milieu using innovative management techniques (Porter 1997). Pinel's ideas on the treatment of insanity were translated quickly into multiple languages and spread rapidly. An English translation of *Traité* was published in 1806 and was widely known in America.

William Tuke in England independently came to conclusions similar to those of Pinel. Tuke put his theories in practice by founding the York Retreat in 1792. Tuke's philosophy of treatment was based on creating attractive surroundings in which patients were treated like family or guests. The goal of moral treatment was to provide humane care and to demonstrate that the mad could learn to control themselves and their behaviors. Tuke emphasized kindness and compassion in the care of the insane. Mechanical restraints, intimidation, and bloodletting were not permitted. In contrast to the York Retreat, "Bethlem Hospital... appeared as a kind of medieval hell" (Porter 1997, p. 497). Tuke's theories and practices were widely disseminated by Samuel Tuke's publication of *Description of the Retreat* in 1813, which spread news of the Tukes's work at the York Retreat to both sides of the Atlantic (McGovern 1985; Porter 1997). Vincenzio Chiarugi in Italy and Benjamin Rush in the United States also played roles in modifying theory and practice associated with moral treatment (Barton 1987; Dain 1964).

This form of treatment lent itself well to the newly developing theories regarding the etiology of madness. In addition to somatic etiologies, physicians came to believe that the majority of cases of mental disease resulted from degenerate behavior or the pressures of an increasingly industrialized society. Degenerate behavior was typically considered to be that which departed from normative Victorian, Protestant, and bourgeois standards held both in England and in the United States (Smith 1981). Causal factors related to behavior or social problems included intemperance, masturbation, overwork, domestic difficulties, excessive ambitions, faulty education, personal disappointments, marital problems, excessive religious enthusiasm, jealousy, and pride (Grob 1994).

---

[13]The adjective "moral," as in moral treatment or moral insanity, began with the French. In the original sense of the word, "moral" was used not in contradistinction to "immoral" but in contrast to "intellectual" or "rational" (Mohr 1997). However, the English use of the term "moral treatment" or "moral insanity" came to refer to both affective forms of insanity and insanity related to immoral behaviors.

Moral therapy assumed that confinement in a well-ordered institution was an indispensable part of the treatment of insanity. The work of Pinel, Tuke, and others led to the conclusion that recovery from mental derangement, particularly those disorders with "moral" causes, was not only possible but probable. The effects of improper behavioral patterns or a deficient social environment could be corrected by exposure to a judicious mix of medical and moral treatment. Once the individual was in a regulated environment, natural restorative elements could act upon the deranged mind, leading to a reversal of mental disturbances. In addition, an authoritative regimen could be employed in ways that persuaded patients to internalize the behavior and values of normal society and thus promote recovery (Grob 1994).

By the end of the eighteenth century, multiple social factors had made the traditional and informal methods of caring for the mentally ill less effective.[14] The Enlightenment faith that long-standing problems could be solved by purposeful human intervention based on a combination of intellectual and scientific approaches resulted in the concept of using institutions to help solve social problems (Grob 1994). The humanitarian spirit of reform combined with medical theory resulted in the founding of insane asylums in the United States and England. The "new" asylums were promoted as progressive institutions and the only effective and humane site for treatment of insanity (Porter 1997). After 1800, systematic provision began to be made for segregating the insane into specialized institutions (Scull et al. 1996).

The earliest American asylums for the treatment of the insane opened in the 1810s and 1820s and were modeled on the work of Pinel and Tuke (McGovern 1985). The early asylums were often founded with the aid of citizen philanthropy. During the second quarter of the nineteenth century, responsibility for the care and treatment of the insane slowly fell under the jurisdiction of asylums established and administered by the states.[15] From 1825 to 1865, the number of asylums in the United States grew from 9 to 62. Most of these were state supported. Indeed, mental asy-

---

[14]These included significant growth of the population and a proportionate increase in the numbers of the mentally ill, urbanization, industrialization, and the decentralization of families (Grob 1994).

[15]In the United States, no one contributed more to the growth of institutions for the mentally ill than Dorothea Dix, one of the great social reformers in American history. Her social and political activism is credited with being responsible for the building of 32 mental hospitals. It was she who most influenced the policy of state responsibility for the care of the mentally ill (Barton 1987; Grob 1994).

lums were among the greatest public works of the nineteenth century, consuming huge amounts of public money from the 1820s through the end of the century (Dain 1964; Grob 1994; Mohr 1997).

Most nineteenth-century physicians accepted the precepts of moral treatment, which did not involve somatic theory. Nevertheless, they maintained that insanity was ultimately rooted in the organism, particularly the brain. Moral therapy therefore needed to be incorporated within a medical model and prescribed in conjunction with conventional medical therapeutics (Porter 1997). Physicians who espoused moral treatment were generally unwilling to apply it without the use of common remedies such as bleeding, purging and blistering, and drugs such as opium and morphine, tonics, and cathartics (Grob 1994). The ability of physicians to apply both moral and medical theory to the treatment of the insane led in large part to their ascendancy to positions of authority within the asylum system.

The general medical profession and informed physicians increasingly acknowledged these physicians as experts in matters pertaining to insanity. They demonstrated their faith in the skills and opinions of these specialists by sending patients to the asylums, adopting their views when testifying in court cases, and reading their articles published in medical journals. The popular press had also gradually accepted the special role of asylum doctors. Newspapers and popular journals published excerpts from their annual reports, described activities at the hospitals, and urged the building of more asylums (Dain 1964; McGovern 1985).

Worcester State Hospital in Massachusetts, opened in 1833, typified the institutions of this period. Unlike existing asylums, Worcester State admitted relatively large numbers of patients. Under the leadership of the physician Samuel B. Woodward, its first superintendent, it quickly acquired a national reputation. The hospital was structured to maximize contemporary moral and medical treatment. Between 1833 and 1845, Woodward reported that the number of recoveries of recent cases (insane for a year or less) averaged between 82% and 91%. The hospital seemed to prove that insanity could be cured with prompt medical and moral treatment. Woodward himself soon became widely regarded as the most established authority in the treatment of mental disorders (Barton 1987; Grob 1994; Scull 1981b).

## Partial Insanity

The confinement and isolation of the mentally ill created opportunities for the accumulation of observations of patient behavior and symptoms. This led to new descriptions and classification of illness. Before the eighteenth century, deranged reason was considered the sine qua non of all cases of insanity, regardless of what other manifestations were present. Psychiatrists began developing theories, which introduced a large number of gradations and variations of sanity (or insanity).[16] These began to replace older, sharper distinctions between persons who were clearly deranged on the one hand and those who were merely troubled on the other. Toward the end of the eighteenth century, physicians specializing in mental illness accepted the concept that people could be "partially" insane, that is, not totally irrational. The theories of the French clinicians such as Pinel and Jean Etienne Esquirol were highly influential in the development of theories of partial insanity.

James Cowles Prichard was the first to use the term "moral insanity," in his book *A Treatise on Insanity and Other Disorders Affecting the Mind* (1835), to identify one of the forms of insanity described by Pinel. Prichard defined moral insanity as a form of mental disorder "consisting in a morbid perversion of feelings, affections and active powers, without an illusion or erroneous conviction impressed upon the understanding: it sometimes coexists with an apparently unimpaired state of the intellectual faculties" (p. 20). He argued that although the disorder was difficult to diagnose with certainty, observation, as well as the authority of Pinel and Esquirol, proved that this illness did exist (Coliazzi 1989; Dain 1964; Dain and Carlson 1962; Eigen 1991; Maeder 1985; Mohr 1997; Porter 1997; Smith 1981).

Physicians postulated that moral insanity, like other forms of insanity, resulted from a localized physical change in the brain. In his testimony in the Oxford trial, Dr. Hodgkin called Oxford's form of insanity "a lesion of the will." Physicians and medical authors in the early nineteenth century, including Prichard, frequently used the word "lesion" in discussing mental illness. This word evoked the spirit of the new empirically based clinical medicine institutionalized in France. In using this term in connection with partial insanity, Prichard explicitly proposed an organic etiology for this newly defined form of insanity.[17] Phrenological

---

[16]Through such observations general paresis, epilepsy, and "idiotism" were recognized as distinct disorders. Kraepelin's classification of psychiatric disorders, which provided the framework for modern psychiatric nosology, was the culmination of a century of descriptive clinical psychiatry accumulated through asylum admissions.

[17]Except for a few cases in which autopsies revealed the presence of a brain tumor or other gross abnormality, the link between the brain and madness remained (and to a great degree still remains) a mystery. These references to lesions generally lacked empirical support, and acceptance of their presence rested on faith rather than observation. The development of clinical medicine based on pathology nevertheless gave rise to a new confidence that empirical methods would systematically uncover the physical causes of mental illness (Grob 1994; Smith 1981).

theories also had no difficulty embracing the concept that the moral faculties might be deranged while those of the reason remained intact (Dain and Carlson 1962).

Before the 1830s, the concept of partial or moral insanity had encountered relatively little opposition in the United States. In the decade following the appearance of Prichard's work, moral insanity became an important and controversial issue in American psychiatry. Moral insanity served as a catchall for many forms of mental illness in which intellectual powers seemed to remain partially or completely intact. The concept of such a disorder was not unanimously accepted, and the medical debate regarding its existence continued throughout the century. Nevertheless, by the 1840s most physicians prominent in the treatment of the mentally ill had accepted to at least some extent the existence of moral or partial insanity (Rosenberg 1968).

The concept of moral insanity opened the door to a forensic role for psychiatrists. Until the early nineteenth century, madness was considered to be a visible and obvious form of behavior. By the midpoint of the nineteenth century, certain forms of insanity were argued to be more hidden and subtle afflictions. The accurate detection of these disorders required professional skill and experience. A form of insanity that produced no impairment in understanding or cognition was beyond the realm of the lay observer and even of the general physician. Diagnoses of partial insanity, such as delusions, monomania, and moral insanity, cast doubt on the layman's ability to discern sanity from purposeful and seemingly rational behavior (Eigen 1991; Robinson 1996). The second quarter of the nineteenth century witnessed a sixfold increase in medical participation in insanity trials at the Old Bailey. Half of all medical witnesses who appeared in these trials employed a form of partial insanity to support their diagnosis of insanity (Eigen 1991).

The Hadfield case (1800) was the first to introduce into the courts the concept of a partial insanity that was beyond the knowledge of the ordinary citizens of the jury. James Hadfield was indicted for high treason for attempting to kill George III in 1800. In this case, Hadfield's partial insanity was said to involve mental derangement limited to the formation of delusions (Freemon 2001). His counsel, the well-known jurist Thomas Erskine, argued that Hadfield's delusional thinking affected only part of his mind. He was able to demonstrate that Hadfield's delusions developed after Hadfield had sustained head injuries during the course of military service. Erskine obtained the testimony of an eminent author in the field of insanity, who stated that Hadfield's head wound could result in a form of insanity that might spare the rational powers and be evident only in particular subjects

(Freemon 2001; Robinson 1996).[18] Hadfield was found not guilty and sent to Bethlem Hospital.[19]

Successful defenses of insanity had been a regular feature of Old Bailey trials for at least 60 years (Walker 1968). The Hadfield case, however, made clear that the ordinary perceptions of the courts or of laymen could not provide conclusive evidence of a defendant's sanity. A form of partial insanity that could not be appreciated by ordinary people required the introduction of witnesses with special expertise in the recognition of this hidden condition. Only trained experts could identify the individual who was insane in a partial way, or only with regard to certain subjects (Freemon 2001). Professional insight required daily scrutiny and comparison of large numbers of like cases. Only in asylums and prisons were the deranged subject to close inspection and repeated observations (Eigen 1991). Thus, asylum doctors naturally stepped into a forensic role.

## The Field of Medical Jurisprudence

By the early decades of the nineteenth century, legal issues were increasingly likely to involve medical expertise and testimony. The field of medical jurisprudence, defined as the interaction between those who possessed medical knowledge and those who exercised legal authority, predated clinical psychiatry (Mohr 1993). The practice of medical jurisprudence included issues relating to criminal justice, public health, and the functions of public medical examiners and coroners. Doctors had provided testimony regarding cause of death, wounds, poisoning, and other matters (including signs of witchcraft) for centuries. The new specialty of psychiatry, however, helped propel the field of medical jurisprudence to greater levels of prominence in the early nineteenth century.

---

[18]Dr. Alexander Crichton, author of *An Inquiry into the Nature and Origins of Mental Derangement,* published 2 years earlier in 1798, examined Hadfield the night before the trial. Dr. Crichton later became physician to Tsar Alexander I of Russia.

[19]Until this time, acquitted lunatics were either sent to jail or released to the custody of their family, depending on what seemed appropriate to the court. Hadfield's case prompted passage of the Criminal Lunatics Act of 1800. This act created an automatic process whereby the court could order an individual who was acquitted on the grounds of insanity "to be kept in strict custody, in such place and in such manner as to the court shall seem fit, until His Majesty's pleasure be known" (Walker 1968, p. 78). While in Bethlem, Hadfield killed another patient by knocking him over a bench. Several years later, he escaped and reached Dover before he was recaptured. Hadfield died in Bethlem in 1841 after 40 years of confinement, at the age of 69 (Maeder 1985; Walker 1968).

From the outset, the field of medical jurisprudence included the role of the doctor in matters relating to the adjudication of insanity and competence. Psychiatrists became more interested and involved in this aspect of medical jurisprudence as asylums and asylum psychiatry developed. Forensic psychiatry provided a public means for these new clinicians to reinforce their claims to specialized expertise in the diagnosis and treatment of the insane, especially in regard to moral insanity. Historically, the mad-doctor in court had never been very far from challenges to claims of expert knowledge. The fact that the new specialists in madness were medically qualified enabled them to fit into the forensic witness role established by the traditions of medical jurisprudence occupied by physicians in European courts since at least the sixteenth century (Eigen 1991). The medical qualifications of psychiatrists allowed them to draw on these traditions, conferring a certain status to their participation in legal proceedings.

The spirit of Enlightenment and reform included a commitment on the part of physicians to help improve society. Many physicians believed that training in medical jurisprudence would enhance the public contribution of physicians by helping them achieve a working relationship with lawyers, judges, and legislators. During the first half of the nineteenth century, medical schools endorsed the concept that medical jurisprudence should be an essential aspect of professional training for America's future physicians. The first formal chair in medical jurisprudence was created in Edinburgh in 1807; in the United States, it occurred at Columbia in 1813 (Mohr 1993). Most American medical schools had faculty chairs in medical jurisprudence by 1840. Virtually every lecturer in every course on medical jurisprudence addressed the subject of insanity.

Medical literature related to jurisprudential issues, including mental disorders, multiplied dramatically between 1820 and 1850. Almost all comprehensive publications dealing with the subject included a detailed discussion of legal issues relating to insanity. Of this literature, the most influential was the work of T.R. Beck, a professor of medical jurisprudence at Western Medical College in Albany, New York. Beck wrote the first American text on the subject, *Elements of Medical Jurisprudence,* published in 1823. *Elements* was an attempt to summarize the issues that had concerned the great medicolegalists since the Middle Ages. This two-volume work was reprinted in 12 editions through 1860 and became the most frequently cited medicolegal text in American court cases (Mohr 1993). Beck emphasized the importance of the role of the medical expert in legal cases. "It need hardly be suggested that in many instances, a legal decision depends on the testimony of medical witnesses" (Beck 1823, Vol. 1, p. vii).

Although not a psychiatrist, Beck stressed the primary role of insanity in the field of medical jurisprudence. His work led him to become president of the Board of the Utica State Asylum of New York, thus demonstrating the close connection between these two developing branches of medicine. In 1841, Beck wrote, "[T]he nature of insanity as excusing from the responsibility of criminal acts was one of the two primary subjects in legal medicine" (Mohr 1993, p. 122). The first volume of Beck's *Elements* contained a chapter entitled "Mental Alienation" that specifically covered those aspects of the subject relevant to civil and criminal cases. These included the symptoms that constituted a state of insanity; the problems of identifying feigned and concealed insanity; the legal rules governing insanity in court proceedings; the various types of mental impairment short of insanity; monomania and partial insanity; and the state of mind necessary to make a valid will (Mohr 1993). This chapter defined the next two centuries of the history of forensic psychiatry in the United States.

## Psychiatrists, Moral Insanity, and Medical Jurisprudence

The medical community regarded itself as an integral part of the program of human and social improvement. Most medical jurisprudents believed that they could help society deal with the troubling and difficult problems posed by mental illness, and many felt it was their social duty to so (Mohr 1993; Robinson 1996). The new specialists in mental disorders took the same position. The increasing number of texts on the causes and treatments of moral insanity was accompanied by an increasing number of texts devoted to the medical jurisprudence of insanity. Both typically urged the medical community to recognize the existence of moral and partial insanity and to provide medical testimony regarding this and other mental illnesses as their social duty.

Benjamin Rush provides the earliest example of the psychiatric specialist who believed a physician's social duty demanded legal involvement, and whose theories included a belief in partial insanity. Rush was highly influential in the development of the field of psychiatry. He advocated more humane treatment of the insane as well as the use of most of the remedies commonly used in the eighteenth century, such as bloodletting, restraint, and stimulation of terror as shock therapy (Dain 1964). Rush also believed that certain insane persons suffered primarily from affective or volitional impairment and, although mentally disordered, demonstrated no impairment in their ability to reason (Dain 1964; Porter 1997). He called this disorder "moral derangement," which he defined as "that state of mind in which the passions act involuntarily through the instrumentality of the will, without any disease in the understanding" (Rush 1811, p. 380).

Rush encouraged all physicians to develop stronger medicolegal skills and stated it was their social responsibility to do so:

> They entertain very limited views of medicine who suppose its objects and duties are confined exclusively to the knowledge and cure of diseases. Our science was intended to render other services to society. It was designed to extend its benefits to the protection of property and life, and to detect fraud and guilt in many of their forms. This honour has been conferred upon it by the bench and the bar, in all civilized countries both in ancient and modern times. That part of our science, which qualifies us to discharge these important civil duties, has been called medical jurisprudence. (Rush 1811, p. 363)

In 1810, Rush urged his medical students to obtain a strong grounding in the medical jurisprudence of insanity. He explicitly connected the concept of moral insanity to medical jurisprudence and discussed in detail "those states of the mind which should incapacitate a man to dispose of his property, to bear witness in a court of justice, and exempt him from punishment for the commission of what are called crimes by the laws of our country" (Rush 1811, pp. 365–366).[20]

John Haslam's *Medical Jurisprudence as It Relates to Insanity* (1817) was the first major work specifically calling for the use of medical experts in cases involving insanity on the basis of their expertise in diagnosing and treating the insane. Haslam occupied a position at the forefront of the mad-doctoring trade as the resident apothecary of Bethlem[21] (Scull et al. 1996). His book was reprinted in the first major compilation on medical jurisprudence to appear under an American imprint, *Tracts on Medical Jurisprudence* by Thomas Cooper, published in Philadelphia in 1819.

In some instances, Haslam stated, an individual's insanity is evident and demonstrable without the need for the testimony of a medical practitioner. However, he argued, many insane people can conduct them-

---

[20]Rush concluded the lecture by stating that the only objection to the use of medical knowledge for legal reasons might be that such testimony could result in the "more certain and general" conviction for several offenses punishable by death. The solution to this problem, he stated, was "sure and infallible"; he went on to call for the abolishment of the punishment of death in all cases including murder (p. 393).

[21]Haslam was dismissed from his position in 1816 as a result of a Parliamentary investigation into conditions at Bethlem (Scull et al. 1996).

selves with propriety and appear perfectly reasonable, and "ordinary persons have been much deceived" by such appearances:

> Is the person accused, of insane mind?...In those cases where the prisoner is so bereft of his reason, that any twelve men would not entertain a different opinion, where numerous evidences appear to testify to repeated acts of insanity, which are so manifest that they cannot be otherwise interpreted; and where he has been confined and treated for this malady, the physician will have an easy duty to perform: but it is in cases which appear to be involved in difficulty, where the disorder, although existing and directing the actions, is not so ostensibly developed that the medical evidence become important, and capable by sagacity, experience and truth, of explaining and characterizing the state of the person's intellect. (Haslam 1817, pp. 2–3)

Cases of partial insanity, Haslam observed, involved considerable doubt about the person's state of mind. He insisted that medical specialists were uniquely qualified to detect such forms of madness, and were certainly more skilled in their diagnosis than the general populace because of their asylum experience (Eigen and Andoll 1986). "Patient enquiry, daily communication with deranged persons and attentive observation of their habits, confer the means of judging on medical practitioners, and more especially on those, who have for a series of years, solely confined their practice to this department of the profession" (Haslam 1817, pp. 7–8). Haslam also pointed out that unlike the lay observer, the trained observer could identify those attempting to escape responsibility by feigning madness (Eigen 1991).

Isaac Ray is associated with the development of forensic psychiatry more than any other nineteenth-century physician. Ray's *A Treatise on the Medical Jurisprudence of Insanity,* published in 1838, resulted in gaining him an international reputation, the first such widespread recognition for an American physician. Notably, Ray came to forensic psychiatry through medical jurisprudence, rather than vice versa. At the time he wrote the *Treatise,* Ray was 31 and a general practitioner in Maine with no particular experience in treating the insane.[22] In many ways, Ray epitomized the type of physician attracted to medical jurisprudence during the first half of the nineteenth century. He was strongly influenced by French medicine, committed to the scientific method, and op-

---

[22]After publication of the *Treatise,* Ray became the administrator at the Maine Insane Asylum in Augusta from 1841 to 1845 and then administrator of Butler Hospital for the Insane in Providence, Rhode Island, from 1845 to 1866 (Hughes 1982; McGovern 1985).

timistic about the treatment of insanity and the future role of medical experts in court proceedings.

Ray's *Treatise* was the most comprehensive and systematic English presentation of the nineteenth-century understanding of insanity in the context of litigation (Mohr 1997). Ray drew on the work of authors such as Haslam, Pinel, and Prichard. He laid out the various types of mental disorders postulated by experts through 1837 and described the ways in which enlightened courts should deal with each type. The first edition of Ray's book was followed a year later by two reprintings, one in London and the other in Edinburgh. The second edition appeared in 1844, and three more revised editions followed in 1853, 1860, and 1871. The *Treatise* became the standard text on the subject throughout the nineteenth century and established Ray as a leading authority in this field. His work was quoted extensively by the defense in the M'Naghten trial in 1843, and it was cited again more than a century later by Judge David Bazelon in his decision in *Durham v. United States* (1954; Robinson 1996).

Like Rush and other adherents of medical jurisprudence, Ray believed that medical practitioners were obligated to address the legal status of the insane and to educate the courts and the public. He believed that the public had a claim on such services from physicians, especially those who occupied official positions.

> The frequency with which questions of insanity are now raised in courts of justice, has rendered it a very common duty for those who are engaged in our department of the healing art, to give their testimony in the capacity of experts....I see no reason why [this duty] should be evaded, upon any other ground, than interference with other engagements, but many reasons why it should be cheerfully and intelligently performed. (Ray 1851, pp. 53–54)

Ray also held that insanity was a physical disease (Cooter 1981; Dain 1964; Hughes 1982; Scull 1981b). He believed that the clinical features of insanity were the result of pathological changes in the brain. Ray, a vocal advocate of phrenology, accepted the existence of subtle and varying grades of insanity based on his belief in the existence of discrete faculties and propensities in cerebral tissue. He became the foremost American proponent of the concept that impairment of the will or the emotions could occur in the absence of impaired cognition or rationality. "That the insane mind is not entirely deprived of this power of moral discernment, but on many subjects is perfectly rational, and displays the exercise of a sound and well balanced mind, is one of those facts now so well established, that to question it would only betray the height of ignorance and presumption" (Ray 1838, p. 32).

Ray criticized American courts for retaining concepts of insanity based solely on derangement of reason, which he considered narrow and outdated (Mohr 1997). "Few, probably, whose attention has not been particularly directed to the subject, are aware how far the condition of the law relative to insanity is behind the present state of our knowledge concerning that disease" (Ray 1838, p. vii). He believed that fewer citizens would have to suffer punishments for actions they could not willfully control or reasonably understand, if the courts and the public could be educated up to the levels of understanding that the experts in mental illness had attained.

Ray became an ardent and capable defender of the special standing of experienced clinicians in adjudicative settings in which questions of mental health were at issue. Most "experts," he observed, were general practitioners who saw insane patients only rarely and who were unfamiliar with the current literature. Determinations regarding insanity, particularly moral insanity, required a deeper understanding of mental disorders that could only be gained through familiarity with a large number of patients. "Cases of doubtful mental condition are not those whose true character can be discerned at a glance. The delicate shades of disorder can only be recognized by one who has closely studied the operations of the healthy mind, and is familiar with that broad, debatable ground that lies between unquestionable sanity, and unquestionable insanity" (Ray 1851, p. 55).

Ray (1838) considered the physicians who manage "lunatic asylums and retreats for the insane" (p. 58) uniquely qualified to provide such testimony and "peculiarly competent for this high duty" (p. 57):

> It is not enough, that the standing of the medical witness is deservedly high in his profession, unless it is founded on extraordinary knowledge and skill relative to the particular disease, insanity.... An enlightened and conscientious jury...will be satisfied with nothing less than the opinions of those, who have possessed unusual opportunities for studying the character and conduct of the insane, and have the qualities of mind necessary to enable them to profit by their observations. (Ray 1838, pp. 58–59)

## Clinical Psychiatry and the Expert Witness

Fortunately, Ray noted, a class of physicians especially equipped to offer sound opinions on insanity was available. These early psychiatrists usually served in mental hospitals as superintendents, assistant superintendents, and visiting physicians, and exercised a virtual monopoly over the therapeutic care of the insane (Dain 1964). By the 1840s, the branch of medicine concerned with mental illness had developed into a recognized specialty associated with asylums. The number of asylum superintendents and physicians probably never exceeded 200, and for much of the time before 1865, there were fewer than 100. Nevertheless, by midcentury, the expertise of these new specialists in the diagnosis and treatment of insanity, although not universally accepted, was widely acknowledged.

The increasing use of psychiatric witnesses seems to have been more court-inspired than professionally generated (Eigen 1991). Scientific advances, social and political reforms, and the optimistic outlook bequeathed by the Enlightenment resulted in the increased reliance of courts and legislatures on medical witnesses and scientific authorities (Robinson 1996). Problems seldom arose in cases where defendants were obviously irrational, demented, or hallucinatory. In contrast, courts found cases where defendants claimed moral or partial insanity highly problematic. The identification of these more subtle forms of insanity and their implications for legal responsibility required specialized knowledge beyond that of the layman or the general physician. More and more, especially in high-profile trials, medical witnesses were authors, lecturers, and asylum superintendents (Eigen 1991).

Although Ray is the nineteenth-century psychiatrist most closely associated with forensic practice, many of the preeminent asylum psychiatrists regularly provided expert witness services to the courts. These physicians took for granted that providing expert testimony was part of the new specialized practice of psychiatry. The most difficult cases were often referred to established experts for evaluation and testimony. Their sustained, professional association and clinical experience with the insane spoke directly to the common law's requirement of the specialized knowledge required to form an expert opinion (Eigen 1991). As a result, then, as now, certain "mad-doctors" became celebrated for their courtroom testimony, their treatises on forensic psychiatry (Porter 1997), and their theories regarding partial insanity.

That the two roles were both compatible and congruent was widely accepted and indeed encouraged, as demonstrated by the careers of the leaders in this new field. In 1844, the first medical specialty organization in the United States, the Association of Medical Superintendents of American Institutions for the Insane (AMSAII), was founded by 13 of these specialists.[23] Ten additional members joined when the Associa-

---

[23]The American organization was preceded by an English organization. In 1841, the Association of Medical Officers of Asylums and Hospitals for the Insane was founded in England. This professional organization ultimately became the Royal Medico-Psychological Association and, in 1971, the Royal College of Psychiatrists.

tion convened for its second meeting in 1846 (Barton 1987; Grob 1994). These men played key roles in shaping early American psychiatry. Ray, one of the founding members, served as vice-president from 1851 to 1855 and as president from 1855 to 1859. Other founding members included Samuel Woodward, the first president of the organization and the superintendent of Worcester State Asylum; Luther V. Bell, the superintendent of McLean Asylum; Pliny Earle, superintendent of the Bloomingdale Asylum in New York; and Amariah Brigham of the Hartford Retreat and then the Utica State Asylum (Barton 1987). Many had been strongly influenced by phrenology and its somatic implications (Cooter 1981; Dain 1964; Hughes 1982; Scull 1981b). All endorsed the concept of partial or moral insanity (Dain and Carlson 1962).

The professional identity of these early specialists in mental disorders included the practice of medical jurisprudence in relation to insanity (Dain 1964; McGovern 1985). At its first meeting, all the members of the group agreed that the jurisprudence of insanity was one of five primary subjects that needed to be addressed by the organization (Medical Association 1845). The asylum psychiatrists did not differentiate between the roles of clinician and expert witness. Providing expert testimony based on their specialized expertise was part of this new specialty practice.

Members of AMSAII testified regularly in the courts. For example, in 1846, Dr. Amariah Brigham served as the prime witness and personal consultant for former New York State governor William H. Seward in Seward's use of the insanity plea in the defense of two murderers, Wyatt and Freeman[24] (Spiegel and Spiegel 1998). Brigham helped Seward prepare his defense by sending him several books. These included Prichard's *A Treatise on Insanity and Other Disorders Affecting the Mind*; Esquirol's *Mental Maladies, A Treatise on Insanity*; Samuel Tuke's *Description of the York Retreat*; and Isaac Ray's *Treatise on the Medical Jurisprudence of Insanity*. Brigham also provided dramatic testimony.[25]

---

[24]Although Seward lost both of these publicized cases, they helped establish his fame as a jury lawyer and a legal expert on the jurisprudence of insanity. Seward eventually served as a New York state senator, the governor of New York, and a U.S. senator. In 1860, Seward was appointed secretary of state by Abraham Lincoln after losing the nomination for president to him (Spiegel and Spiegel 1998).

[25]During his testimony, Brigham pointed at a man sitting in court and was proven correct when he declared that he, Brigham, recognized him to be deranged and insane simply from his looks. In a letter to his wife, Seward said that "Brigham was wonderful" on the witness stand (Spiegel and Spiegel 1998, p. 240).

Luther V. Bell also regularly provided forensic testimony. In 1843, he testified for the defense in the case of Abner Rogers. Rogers was tried for murdering the warden of the prison in which he was already incarcerated and pled insanity (Ray 1873). In 1857, Bell was consulted by the defense in a case before the Eighth Circuit Court in Illinois. The defendant, accused of murder, claimed that an overdose of chloroform during a surgical procedure resulted in damage to his brain. He was acquitted on the grounds of insanity and sent to the Illinois State Asylum. The prosecutor in this case was Abraham Lincoln (Spiegel and Suskind 1997).

Other lesser-known superintendents and asylum physicians provided statements and testimony to the courts. In 1845, Dr. Allan, described by Isaac Ray as "the worthy superintendent of the Kentucky Lunatic Asylum" (Ray 1873, p. 237), provided testimony in an attempt to prevent the execution of a convicted murderer who had unsuccessfully pled insanity. J.H. Worthington, superintendent of Friends' Asylum for the Insane in Philadelphia, and S. Preston Jones, assistant physician of the Pennsylvania Hospital for the Insane, addressed the court to the same end in the case of a convicted murderer who pled insanity on the basis of a history of epilepsy (Ray 1873). In 1866, Dr. Nichols, superintendent of the Government Hospital for the Insane, now known as St. Elizabeths Hospital, provided testimony in the successful defense of Mary Harris, a woman acquitted on the basis of insanity of the murder of her former lover. Dr. Lee, assistant physician at the Worcester State Hospital, provided testimony in 1848 regarding insanity in a case involving a contested contract (Ray 1848).

These specialists also testified in testamentary cases. In the highly publicized Parish will case of 1856, Amariah Brigham testified that the late testator was sane. Samuel Woodward, Isaac Ray, and Luther Bell provided opinions that he was insane (Dain 1964; Mohr 1993; Zilboorg 1944). Lesser-known asylum physicians also provided testimony in cases involving contested wills. In the Angell will case, Dr. Tyler, associated with McLean Asylum, provided an opinion concurring with Dr. Isaac Ray that a testatrix was insane when she wrote her will and codicils (Ray 1873). In 1847, Drs. Woodward, Brigham, and Bell (as well as Isaac Ray) testified in the Oliver Smith will case (Ray 1848).

The interest in and importance of forensic practice was reflected in the content of the *American Journal of Insanity*,[26] AMSAII's official publi-

---

[26]In 1922, when the American Medico-Psychological Association changed its name to the American Psychiatric Association, it changed the name of its journal from the *American Journal of Insanity* to the *American Journal of Psychiatry*.

cation. Amariah Brigham founded and published the journal in 1844 some months before the founding of AMSAII. It quickly became the representative journal of the association. It acquired a broad audience in the United States and Britain and gained a reputation as the most authoritative American periodical dealing with insanity (Dain 1964; Grob 1994). The Journal was the first periodical in English devoted exclusively to issues regarding "psychological medicine" (Bunker 1944, p. 196).

The early years of the *American Journal of Insanity* demonstrate that a forensic identity was an integral aspect of the new profession of psychiatry. The medicolegal orientation of the editors is unmistakable. The forensic activities of the journal's first editor, Amariah Brigham, have already been reviewed. Even more notably, upon Brigham's death in 1849, T.R. Beck became the journal's second editor and served in that capacity from 1850 to 1854. Beck, the author of *Elements of Medical Jurisprudence* (1823), was not a psychiatric specialist but an expert in medical jurisprudence.

From its inception, the *American Journal of Insanity* frequently published papers on the relationship between psychiatry and the law. Authors often expressed indignation with the fact that nonspecialists served so frequently as expert witnesses on mental illness (Stokes 1855). The first volume (1844–1845) contained an article entitled "Medical Jurisprudence of Insanity," by C.B. Coventry (1845), professor of medical jurisprudence at Geneva College and a member of the Board of Managers of Utica State Asylum.[27] Coventry discussed the M'Naghten rules, which had been formulated the previous year. He stated regretfully that the 15 English jurists failed to take into consideration the existence of moral insanity. Coventry implicitly indicated that the M'Naghten rules disregarded the fundamental principles of clinical psychiatry.

The first volume of the *American Journal of Insanity* also contained case histories involving the medical jurisprudence of insanity (pp. 75-77); an article by Samuel Woodward (1845) entitled "Homicidal Impulse"; book reviews of two new texts on the subject of the medical jurisprudence of insanity (pp. 281–283, 370–372); and a detailed review of the trial of Abner Rogers, which extensively quoted the testimony of Drs. Bell, Woodward, and Ray (Coventry 1845, pp. 258-274).

In the first 10 years of publication, from 1844 to 1854, authors and editors publicized, reviewed, and commented on significant trials. T.R. Beck provided comments on the case of Lord Ferrers ("Case of Lord Fer-

[27]Coventry, along with Amariah Brigham, also provided testimony in Seward's unsuccessful defense in the Wyatt and Freeman trials.

rers 1845"). Many issues included reviews of books on medical jurisprudence and forensic medicine. The cases of Oxford and M'Naghten were reviewed in detail ("Review of the Trials of Oxford and M'cNaughten" 1851). Cases of contested wills and the capacity to enter a contract (Ray 1848; "A Will Contested" 1848) were also discussed. In an 1851 article entitled "Hints to the Medical Witness in Questions of Insanity," Ray gave practical advice to psychiatrists serving as experts.[28]

Indeed, during the first three or four decades of its publication, almost every issue of the *American Journal of Insanity* contained a discussion of medicolegal principles or an account of court proceedings in a criminal case in which a plea of insanity had been entered or in which AMSAII's members testified (Bunker 1944). Many of these were discussed in detail. The percentage of the forensic articles in these years was significantly higher than that represented by forensic articles in the present *American Journal of Psychiatry.*

## Backlash Against Forensic Psychiatry

The Oxford trial marked a turning point in the role of expert psychiatric witnesses (Freemon 2001). The influence of specialists and theories of partial insanity was at its height. In 1840, Edward Oxford, age 18, was charged with high treason for shooting at Queen Victoria and Prince Albert while they rode in their carriage. Five physicians testified at Oxford's trial. All five testified they believed Oxford to be insane. Two had treated members of Oxford's family, but three were of the new class of expert.[29] These three specialists interviewed Oxford the night before the trial. They invoked their clinical credentials in the treatment of large numbers of patients to support their opinions (Freemon 2001; Moran 1986). Two testified that Oxford's form of insanity was labeled "a lesion of the will" and made reference to French authors such as Esquirol on the subject (Eigen 1991; Free-

---

[28]This article raised many of the issues that experts still face today, including the influence of adversarial bias, the unscientific nature of cross examination, legal trick questions that seem surprisingly familiar to modern experts, and the need to maintain composure on the witness stand.

[29]One expert, John Conolly, was the author of *An Inquiry Concerning the Indications of Insanity* (1830) and the physician in charge of Hanwell Lunatic Asylum in Middlesex. Conolly testified in many insanity trials and developed a reputation as a "hired gun" who would testify that a person who suffered virtually any form of mental dysfunction, no matter how slight, was insane (Freemon 2001).

mon 2001). Oxford was found not guilty on the grounds of insanity.[30]

The next highly publicized trial involving the testimony of experts in an insanity defense resulted in a backlash against psychiatric testimony. In 1843, Daniel M'Naghten was tried for murdering Edward Drummond, Sir Robert Peel's private secretary. M'Naghten's trial involved nine medical witnesses.[31] All concurred that M'Naghten's acts were the result of delusion. The principal medical expert was Edward Thomas Monro, the fourth generation of the Bethlem Monro's. The majority of witnesses gave their opinions after having seen M'Naghten for only a few minutes. Two of these witnesses had not interviewed M'Naghten at all (Maeder 1985; Walker 1968). Isaac Ray was the expert in absentia. His *Treatise* was quoted extensively by defense counsel (Robinson 1996). The prosecution offered no medical evidence at all. The chief justice stopped the trial after hearing the testimony of the experts, and the jury found M'Naghten not guilty on the grounds of insanity. M'Naghten was sent to Bethlem Hospital (Maeder 1985; Walker 1968).[32]

The verdict resulted in an outpouring of resentment.[33] The success of M'Naghten's defense, the judges' direction that the jury find M'Naghten not guilty by reason of insanity, the role that medical texts and witnesses played, and fears that insanity and a lack of responsibility would become confused all contributed to the indignation and outrage the trial provoked. The House of Lords asked the judges of England to clarify points of law raised by the trial by posing five questions. The answers to these questions, which became known as the M'Naghten Rules (1844), addressed the increasingly controversial role of medical experts and the legal definition of insanity.

---

[30]Oxford was committed to Bethlem Hospital and spent the next 27 years in confinement. Most people who interviewed him thought he was sane. Oxford was among the first patients transferred to the new Broadmoor Criminal Lunatic Asylum when it opened in 1864. In 1867, a discharge warrant was issued on the condition that he leave the country and never return. Then 45 years old, Oxford boarded a ship for Melbourne, Australia, and nothing more is known about him (Freemon 2001; Maeder 1985).

[31]Two witnesses were physicians to the Royal Lunatic Asylum in Glasgow; two other witnesses had written books on madness (Freemon 2001).

[32]M'Naghten was also one of the first male patients transferred to the Broadmoor Criminal Lunatic Asylum when it opened in 1864. He died there of tuberculosis in 1865 at age 52.

[33]Queen Victoria herself was indignant at M'Naghten's acquittal. She reportedly commented that she did not believe anyone who wanted to murder a conservative prime minister could be insane (Maeder 1985).

The M'Naghten Rules defined the legal standard of insanity as the inability to distinguish right from wrong. This formula scotched the psychiatric claim for the recognition of disorders of partial insanity without disordered cognition (Porter 1997).[34] The M'Naghten Rules guided the Anglo-American law of insanity for the next century. By 1900, they had been adopted in England, throughout the British Empire, and in almost every American state (Freemon 2001; Maeder 1985; Smith 1981).

In the United States, the 1845 murder trial of Abner Rogers in Massachusetts aroused similar public prejudice against the plea of insanity. The defense attorneys claimed that Rogers was insane and committed the act as a result of his disease. The prosecution explicitly relied on the M'Naghten Rules and insisted that even if Rogers was insane (which they doubted), he was still responsible. The prison physician testified that Rogers was feigning insanity. The judge was sympathetic to a defense of insanity as testified to by three experts: Bell, Woodward, and Ray. The judge stated, "The opinions of professional men on a question of this description are competent evidence, and in many cases are entitled to great consideration and respect" (Coventry 1845). Rogers was found not guilty on the grounds of insanity and sent to Worcester State Asylum, where he came under Woodward's care.[35] Many felt justice had not been well served by this verdict.

A similar backlash occurred in response to the increasing role of psychiatric experts in cases involving wills. Ultimately, the public's concern regarding the power of these specialists to overturn wills through retroactive rulings of testamentary incompetence resulted in litigation in some states curtailing such testimony (Mohr 1993, 1997). The popular feeling against such medical testimony was expressed by one judge in an 1857 trial of a man accused of poisoning his wife. After hearing testimony regarding the insanity of the defendant, the judge sided with the prosecution. He said to the jury, "Experts in madness! Mad doctors! Gentlemen, I will read you the evidence of these medical witnesses—these 'experts in madness'—and if you can make sane evidence out of

---

[34]As might be expected, Ray and other leading psychiatrists criticized the M'Naghten Rules as psychologically unsound. Ray stated that the mental impairment of the insane is indicated by their feelings of freedom from the obligation of the law, not by their failure to recognize the illegality of the act. Ray felt it was absurd to expect the insane to act "reasonably" while delusional (Payne and Luthe 1980).

[35]"After some months of confinement, while at chapel, he [Rogers] begged to leave the room as it was 'full of dead bodies.' His request not being heeded, he bolted head first through the window, fell fourteen feet, and died the next day" (Ray 1873, p. 220).

what they say, do so; but I confess it's more than I can do" (quoted in Smith 1981, p. 136).

## Separation of Clinical and Forensic Psychiatry

The insanity plea and the public role of psychiatry became a matter of dispute (Porter 1997) and increasing criticism. The psychiatric experts acknowledged that judges, jurors, and the public in general had developed a growing distrust of the value and honesty of expert testimony (Mohr 1993). In 1845, AMSAII's president, Samuel Woodward, observed: "It cannot be denied that there is a suspicion abroad in the community, that these new views of medical jurisprudence tend to prostrate the ends of justice, by disturbing the settled principles of criminal law" (Woodward 1845, pp. 323–324). By midcentury, the medical jurisprudence of insanity had resulted in the development of serious credibility problems for those who claimed expertise in the subject of insanity.

Through the second half of the nineteenth century, the forensic practice of psychiatry became less popular. Practicing physicians were increasingly battered by medicolegal interactions. The pressures discouraging the practice of forensic psychiatry included the effects of courtroom testimony on clinical reputations; internal dissension regarding the concepts of moral insanity; criticism of asylums and asylum medicine; challenges from the new field of neurology[36]; and accusations that asylum psychiatrists were primarily administrative and custodial rather than clinical specialists (Grob 1994; McGovern 1985; Mohr 1993; Smith 1981).

The sociopolitical backlash against the new view of insanity and the physicians who propounded this view in their courtroom testimony was reflected in a steady stream of articles, essays, and lectures. These reminded both professionals and lay citizens that the issue of insanity had become a nightmare in the courts that reflected poorly on medical experts involved in such cases. "Insanity had shifted from an area in which physicians were humane heroes to one in which they were unjustly imprisoning the innocent in asylums and making excuses for guilty criminals" (Mohr 1993, p. 248). The first generation of psychiatrists, the founders and early members of AMSAII, and especially Isaac Ray, continued to promote a forensic role for psychiatrists. By midcen-

---

[36]The trial of Charles Guiteau in 1881 for the assassination of President James Garfield, the most celebrated American insanity trial of the nineteenth century, established the expertise of neurologists in matters pertaining to mental disorders (Rosenberg 1968).

tury, however, evidence mounted that physicians were consciously avoiding involvement with legal situations (Mohr 1993).

As behaviorism and psychoanalysis became the dominant schools of psychological thought in the twentieth century, the legal concept of insanity became increasingly separated from the basic and clinical medical sciences. Neither of these new psychological disciplines placed an especially high premium on neurological modes of inquiry and explanation (Robinson 1996). Freud himself believed that psychoanalytic principles should be applied very cautiously (if at all) in legal proceedings (Goldstein 1983). In 1923, William Alanson White, the superintendent of St. Elizabeths Hospital in Washington, D.C., an ardent defender of psychoanalysis and the foremost forensic psychiatrist in the county, contended that insanity was a legal term with no medical meaning (Quen 1983). The integral role of the medical jurisprudence of insanity to the practice of clinical psychiatry was lost.

## M'Naghten Revisited: The Hinckley Trial

The debates that began in the mid–nineteenth century regarding the role of psychiatric experts in the courts have not been resolved. More than a century after M'Naghten, public outrage over the verdict in the John Hinckley trial led to another reexamination and redefinition of the laws governing criminal responsibility. In 1982 John Hinckley was found not guilty by reason of insanity of all charges stemming from an attempted assassination of President Ronald Reagan. As in the M'Naghten case, the public's interpretation of the verdict was that Hinckley had gotten away with his crimes. Although committed to a mental hospital, Hinckley theoretically could have been declared well and released the next day.[37] The ensuing debates, which included calls for abolition of the insanity plea, ultimately resulted in the Insanity Defense Reform Act of 1984 (Maeder 1985), just as the M'Naghten case resulted in a redefinition of the laws of insanity in the nineteenth century.

The medical profession, including the specialty of psychiatry, took a hard look at its role in legal proceedings in the wake of the Hinckley trial. The eminent psychiatrist Alan Stone noted the increased interest in forensic practice but questioned the scientific and ethical basis of psychiatrists' participation in legal proceedings (Stone 1984). The American Medical Association (AMA) took an even more extreme position. Its

---

[37]Hinckley was committed to St. Elizabeths Hospital in Washington, D.C., where he remains confined.

Committee on Medicolegal Problems drafted a special report on the subject bluntly declaring that "the special defense of insanity of should be abolished" ("Insanity Defense in Criminal Trials" 1984). Despite pleas for moderation from the presidents of the American Bar Association and the American Psychiatric Association, the AMA's House of Delegates voted in 1983 to accept its committee's report (Mohr 1993).

## Conclusion

Now, as in the nineteenth century, the role of psychiatry in the law remains controversial. The response of the psychiatric and medical community to the public outrage over the Hinckley verdict demonstrated that the practice of forensic psychiatry still presents some of the same challenges that it did 150 years ago. Despite these problems, psychiatrists are again becoming aware that the forensic practice of psychiatry can be professionally rewarding. An understanding of the origins of forensic psychiatry and its close relationship with clinical practice facilitates understanding the role of the expert witness and how expert psychiatric testimony can assist the court.

Some of the difficulties involved in providing expert services to the courts have remained the same over the last century and a half. In 1851, Isaac Ray warned that an expert "must make up his mind to have his sentiments travestied and sneered at, his motives impugned, and pitfalls dug in his path" (pp. 66–67). In 1994, another prominent forensic psychiatrist observed, "No professional undergoes more intense scrutiny than the psychiatrist who testifies in court." He warned that it takes courage to undergo what amounts to a "crucifixion by criticism." Nevertheless, this author draws the same conclusions as did Benjamin Rush, Isaac Ray, and other psychiatrists for whom the practice of forensic psychiatry was a social and professional obligation. "A life spent serving justice is a life well spent" (Resnick 1994, p. 39).

Psychiatrists interested in rediscovering their forensic "roots" should therefore heed the words of Isaac Ray. As noted in the preface to this volume, Ray warned that "[i]t cannot be too strongly impressed upon our minds that the duty of an expert is very different from those which ordinarily occupy our attention, and requires a kind of knowledge, and a style of reflection, not indispensable to their tolerably creditable performance" (Ray 1851, p. 55). Ray advised clinicians to acquire skills beyond those of clinical practice before entering the courtroom. This suggestion is as relevant today as it was when first made 150 years ago. The subsequent chapters in this book will enable clinicians to explore and develop the skills of forensic psychiatry.

## Key Points

- The field of forensic psychiatry developed in conjunction with the specialty of clinical psychiatry.
- The participation of psychiatrists in litigation has historically been initiated by parties within the legal system.
- The legal system asks psychiatrists to provide forensic services to educate the court in matters that are beyond the knowledge of the layperson.
- The ability to provide expert opinions and testimony has historically been based on special knowledge and expertise derived from clinical practice.
- Although forensic psychiatry developed simultaneously with and as an important adjunct to the practice of clinical psychiatry, it is derived from a different tradition. Thus, the practice of forensic psychiatry requires skills that differ from those associated with clinical practice.

## Practice Guidelines

1. Be aware of the significant differences between the practice of clinical and forensic psychiatry.
2. Obtain appropriate forensic training to provide the courts with quality expert services.
3. Be prepared for challenges to your professional reputation and opinions, no matter how extensive your clinical experience or forensic skills.
4. Remain humble: the trier of fact ultimately settles the matter in dispute. The expert's testimony is one part of a larger picture, seen in its entirety only by the court.

## References

American Academy of Psychiatry and the Law: Available at: www.aapl.org. Accessed December 14, 2002.

Barton WE: The History and Influence of the American Psychiatric Association. Washington, DC, American Psychiatric Press, 1987

Beck TR: Elements of Medical Jurisprudence. Albany, Webster's & Skinner's, 1823

Binder R: Liability for the psychiatrist expert witness. Am J Psychiatry 159:1819–1825, 2002

Bunker HA: Psychiatric literature, in One Hundred Years of American Psychiatry. Edited by Hall JK, Zilboorg G, Bunker HA. New York, Columbia University Press, 1944, pp 195–271

Case of Lord Ferrers. American Journal of Insanity 2:188-189, 1845

Coliazzi J: Homicidal Insanity, 1800–1985. Tuscaloosa, University of Alabama Press, 1989

Cooter R: Phrenology and British alienists, ca 1825–1845, in Madhouses, Mad-Doctors and Madmen: The Social History of Psychiatry in the Victorian Era. Edited by Scull A. Philadelphia, University of Pennsylvania Press, 1981, pp 58–104

Coventry CB: Medical jurisprudence of insanity. American Journal of Insanity 1:258–274, 1845

Dain N: Concepts of Insanity in the United States, 1789–1865. New Brunswick, NJ, Rutgers University Press, 1964

Dain N, Carlson ET: Moral insanity in the United States, 1835–1866. Am J Psychiatry 118:795–801, 1962

Durham v United States, 214 F.2d 862 (1954)

Eigen JP: Mad-doctors in the dock: forensic psychiatry's early claims to expert knowledge. Trans Stud Coll Physicians Phila 13:445–462, 1991

Eigen JP: Witnessing Insanity: Madness and Mad-Doctors in the English Court. New Haven, CT, Yale University Press, 1995

Eigen JP, Andoll G: From mad-doctor to forensic witness: the evolution of early English court psychiatry. Int J Law Psychiatry 9:159–169, 1986

Freemon FR: The origin of the medical expert witness: the insanity of Edward Oxford. J Leg Med 22:349–373, 2001

Goldstein RL: Sigmund Freud: forensic psychiatrist. Bull Am Acad Psychiatry Law 11:273–277, 1983

Grob GN: The Mad Among Us: A History of the Care of America's Mentally Ill. New York, Free Press, 1994

Haslam J: Medical Jurisprudence as It Relates to Insanity According to the Law of England. London, C Hunter, 1817

Hughes JS: In the Law's Darkness: Insanity and the Medical-Legal Career of Isaac Ray, 1807–1881. Ann Arbor, MI, University Microfilms International, 1982

Hunter R, MacAlpine I: Three Hundred Years of Psychiatry, 1535–1860. Hartsdale, NY, Carlisle Publishing, 1982

Insanity defense in criminal trials and limitation of psychiatric testimony. Report of the Board of Trustees. JAMA 251(22):2967–2981, 1984

Maeder T: Crime and Madness: The Origins and Evolution of the Insanity Defense. New York, Harper & Row, 1985

McGovern C: Masters of Madness: Social Origins of the American Psychiatric Profession. Hanover, NH, University Press of New England, 1985

Medical Association. Meeting of the Association of the Medical Superintendents of American Institutions for the Insane. American Journal of Insanity 1:253–258, 1845

Mohr JC: Doctors and the Law: Medical Jurisprudence in Nineteenth-Century America. Baltimore, MD, Johns Hopkins University Press, 1993

Mohr JC: The origins of forensic psychiatry in the United States and the great nineteenth century crisis over the adjudication of wills. J Am Acad Psychiatry Law 25:273–284, 1997

Moran R: The punitive uses of the insanity defense: the trial for treason of Edward Oxford (1840). Int J Law Psychiatry 9:171–190, 1986

Payne H, Luthe R: Isaac Ray and forensic psychiatry in the United States. Forensic Sci Int 15:115–127, 1980

Porter R: The Greatest Benefit to Mankind: A Medical History of Humanity. New York, WW Norton, 1997

Prentice SE: A history of subspecialization in forensic psychiatry. Bull Am Acad Psychiatry Law 23:195–203, 1995

Prichard JC: A Treatise on Insanity and Other Disorders Affecting the Mind (1835). New York, Arno Press, 1973

Quen JM: Isaac Ray and the development of American psychiatry and the law. Psychiatr Clin North Am 6:527–537, 1983

Rappeport JR: Thirty years and still growing. J Am Acad Psychiatry Law 27:273–277, 1999

Ray I: A Treatise of the Medical Jurisprudence of Insanity (1838). Birmingham, AL, Gryphon Press, 1989

Ray I: A contract sought to be avoided on the ground of insanity. American Journal of Insanity 5:79–94, 1848

Ray I: Hints to the medical witness in questions of insanity. American Journal of Insanity 8:53–67, 1851

Ray I: Contributions to Mental Pathology (1873). Delmar, NY, Scholars' Facsimiles & Reprints, 1973

Resnick PJ: Guidelines for courtroom testimony, in Principles and Practice of Forensic Psychiatry. Edited by Rosner R. New York, Chapman & Hall, 1994, pp 34–40

Review of the trials of Oxford and McNaughten, with an account of their present condition. American Journal of Insanity 7:317–358, 1851

Robinson DN: Wild Beasts and Idle Humours: The Insanity Defense From Antiquity to the Present. Cambridge, MA, Harvard University Press, 1996

Rosenberg CE: The Trial of the Assassin Guiteau: Psychiatry and Law in the Gilded Age. Chicago, IL, University of Chicago Press, 1968

Rush B: On the study of medical jurisprudence, in Sixteen Introductory Lectures by Rush B (1811). Oceanside, NY, Dabor Science Publications, 1977, pp 363–395

Scull A: Introduction, in Madhouses, Mad-Doctors and Madmen: The Social History of Psychiatry in the Victorian Era. Edited by Scull A. Philadelphia, University of Pennsylvania Press, 1981a, pp 1–3

Scull A: The social history of psychiatry in the Victorian era, in Madhouses, Mad-Doctors and Madmen: The Social History of Psychiatry in the Victorian Era. Edited by Scull A. Philadelphia, University of Pennsylvania Press, 1981b, pp 5–32

Scull A, MacKenzie C, Hervey N: Masters of Bedlam: The Transformation of the Mad-Doctoring Trade. Princeton, NJ, Princeton University Press, 1996

Smith R: Trial by Medicine: Insanity and Responsibility in Victorian Trials. Edinburgh, Edinburgh University Press, 1981

Spiegel AD, Spiegel MB: The insanity plea in early nineteenth century America. J Community Health 23:227–247, 1998

Spiegel AD, Suskind PB: Chloroform-induced insanity defense confounds lawyer Lincoln. History of Psychiatry 8:487–500, 1997

Starr P: The Social Transformation of American Medicine. New York, Basic Books, 1982

Stokes WH: On a court of medical experts in cases of insanity. American Journal of Insanity 10:112–122, 1855

Stone AA: The ethical boundaries of forensic psychiatry: a view from the ivory tower. Bull Am Acad Psychiatry Law 12:209–219, 1984

Walker N: Crime and Insanity in England, Vol 1. Edinburgh, Edinburgh University Press, 1968

A will contested on the ground of the insanity of one of the attesting witnesses. American Journal of Insanity 4:226–246, 1848

Woodward S: Homicidal impulse. American Journal of Insanity 1:323–326, 1845

Zilboorg G: Legal aspect of psychiatry, in One Hundred Years of American Psychiatry. Edited by Hall JK, Zilboorg G, Bunker HA. New York, Columbia University Press, 1944, pp 507–588

## Suggested Readings

Dain N: Concepts of Insanity in the United States, 1789–1865. New Brunswick, NJ, Rutgers University Press, 1964

Freemon FR: The origin of the medical expert witness: the insanity of Edward Oxford. J Leg Med 22:349–373, 2001

Grob GN: The Mad Among Us: A History of the Care of America's Mentally Ill. New York, Free Press, 1994

Mohr JC: Doctors and the Law: Medical Jurisprudence in Nineteenth-Century America. Baltimore, MD, Johns Hopkins University Press, 1993

Ray I: A Treatise of the Medical Jurisprudence of Insanity (1838). Birmingham, AL, Gryphon Press, 1989

Ray I: Hints to the medical witness in questions of insanity. American Journal of Insanity 8:53–67, 1851

Robinson DN: Wild Beasts and Idle Humours: The Insanity Defense From Antiquity to the Present. Cambridge, MA, Harvard University Press, 1996

Scull A (ed): Madhouses, Mad-Doctors and Madmen: The Social History of Psychiatry in the Victorian Era. Philadelphia, University of Pennsylvania Press, 1981

Walker N: Crime and Insanity in England, Vol 1. Edinburgh, Edinburgh University Press, 1968

CHAPTER 2

# Introduction to the Legal System

Daniel W. Shuman, J.D.

## Introduction

The practice of good clinical psychiatry is the foundation of good forensic psychiatry. However, psychiatrists who bring only good clinical psychiatry to the courtroom are often frustrated by their forensic experiences. Psychiatrists are asked to play a very different role in the courtroom than in their professional world outside the courtroom, and the settings in which these roles are played out are shaped by different values. Moving between these worlds successfully and effectively requires a mastery of the different rules that apply in each setting and an understanding of the different values that apply in each domain. For example, although confidentiality is the hallmark of effective clinical psychiatry, presentation to the court of the results of a forensic examination is premised on the absence of confidentiality. Successful forensic psychiatrists understand these different rules and values, even if they do not always agree with them.

In this chapter, I examine some of the fundamental differences in clinical and forensic psychiatric practice and the implications of these differences. I begin with a discussion of the differences in the mechanics of consent and the related notion of autonomy in clinical and forensic psychiatric relationships, then proceed to examine the role of truth in the realms of clinical and forensic psychiatry. The legal system's choice of the adversary process in the search for truth is explored, as well as the implications of this process in the use of expert witnesses. Understanding these differences is necessary to appreciate how forensic practice and clinical practice differ, as well as to understand what the legal system expects of forensic psychiatrists and why.

## Consent and Autonomy in Clinical and Forensic Psychiatry

One of the most profound differences in clinical and forensic psychiatric practice is the role of consent. Consent is a prerequisite to psychiatric treatment (at least in private practice settings), and private practice patients are free to leave treatment at any time for any reason without penalty. Treatment rendered in the absence of effective consent is unlawful as well as unethical. The foundation of the relationship between forensic psychiatrists and the litigants they evaluate is different. Although a forensic examination should not occur in the absence of consent, consent operates differently than in the clinical setting. A criminal defendant who asserts an insanity defense must submit to an examination by the state's expert, without input into that expert's selection or evaluation methods, or be precluded from presenting expert evidence in support of an insanity defense (*Henry v. State* 1991). A personal injury plaintiff who seeks to recover damages for emotional distress will not be permitted to refuse to be examined by the defendant's expert and still maintain that damage claim, again without input into the defendant's expert's selection or evaluation methods (*Newell v. Engel* 1994). Litigants who place their mental condition at issue may not withhold consent to a psychiatric examination by an opponent's expert without penalty, nor do they have the option available to a private practice patient to refuse a particular diagnostic test or technique. Forensic relationships rest on a fundamentally different foundation than do private practice treatment relationships.

Consent is grounded in concerns with personal autonomy. Clinicians typically hold their patients' autonomy in high regard and seek to avoid exercising control over their patients' lives. One of the common goals of treatment is to assist patients in taking responsibility for their own decisions. However, in the litigation setting psychiatric expert witnesses often wield significant power over litigants. For example, litigants understand that a court-ordered examiner's report about the best interest of the child whose custody is at issue is likely to have a significant impact on the decision-maker (Champagne et al. 2001). Psychiatrists serving as expert witnesses exercise power over other people, power that psychiatrists treating private practice patients seek to avoid.

Clinical psychiatrists try to help their patients get better, provide them with evaluation and treatment, and avoid actions that are likely to harm them (American Psychiatric Association 2001). The goal of the forensic psychiatrist is not to provide beneficial treatment but to acquire and communicate information. Forensic psychiatrists are ethically obligated to avoid causing unnecessary harm, for example, by protecting the confidentiality of communications that are not relevant to the issue before the court (Appelbaum 1990). However, it is the duty of the forensic psychiatrist to gather and communicate accurate, relevant information to the court even if it will cause harm to a litigant (American Academy of Psychiatry and the Law 1995).

Consider a personal injury case in which the examining psychiatrist concludes that the plaintiff's current mental distress was not caused by the defendant's wrongdoing but resulted from a prior injury. The psychiatrist knows that the impoverished plaintiff has no health insurance. However, the obligation of the forensic psychiatrist is to provide an accurate assessment of the cause of the current emotional distress without regard to its impact on the plaintiff's ability to obtain mental health care. It is not the psychiatrist's duty to find a solution that will enable the plaintiff to obtain mental health care or other necessary support. Similarly, a psychiatrist who undertakes an examination for competence to be executed is obligated to provide accurate information to the court about whether the prisoner's "mental illness prevents him from comprehending the reasons for the penalty or its implications" (*Ford v. Wainwright* 1986, p. 399), without regard to the harm that a finding of competence to be executed will cause the prisoner.

The role of truth in clinical versus forensic psychiatry is another important distinction that helps to explain what the courts expect of psychiatric expert witnesses. Although ascertaining historical truth may not be the goal of clinical psychiatry, truth or accuracy does clearly matter to the practice of psychiatry in some contexts, for example, in determining the efficacy of sertraline in treating posttraumatic stress disorder (Davidson et al. 2001). These types of questions of truth or accuracy in psychiatry can be studied through controlled scientific studies, and an answer can be reached with a high degree of confidence. In contrast, the legal system is inherently limited in its ability to validate truth in individual cases through techniques such as controlled scientific studies. It is simply not possible to conduct randomized, double-blind studies to determine, for example, whether the person who authored a will some years ago, who is now deceased, had "sufficient mental capacity to know the nature and extent of his property and the natural objects of his bounty and to formulate a rational scheme of distribution" (*In re* Estate of Herbert 1996). Everything that takes place in life is not recorded on videotape, and the ability to reconstruct legally relevant past events with any degree of confidence will be determined to a large extent by happenstance (Simon and Shuman 2002).

This does not imply that accuracy is unimportant to the law, only that its subject matter imposes inherent limits on the nature of the inquiry. Common sense tells us that accuracy or truth matters to the law. Convicting the wrong person does not make society safer and risks undermining society's confidence in the criminal law, in addition to the horror of imprisoning an innocent person. Wrongly finding a psychiatrist liable for malpractice confuses everyone in the profession about how they are expected to behave, imposes unnecessary costs on psychiatrists and their patients, and erroneously maligns a professional's reputation.

But, as commonsensical as truth may seem as a goal of the legal system, careful consideration reveals that truth is not its only goal. Rule 102 of the Federal Rules of Evidence, which articulates the goals of the rules of evidence that govern admissibility at trial, illustrates some of the other goals:

> These rules shall be construed to secure fairness in the administration, elimination of unjustifiable expense and delay, and promotion of growth and development of the law of evidence to the end that the truth may be ascertained and proceedings justly determined.

The rule articulates the goal of ascertaining truth as well as eliminating "unjustifiable expense and delay" and stipulates that "proceedings [be] justly determined." Closer analysis reveals how these goals may compete in individual cases.

The adage "justice delayed is justice denied" reflects an understanding that justice is tied to the passage of time. "Memories fade and witnesses die," both of which interfere with the ability to achieve accuracy in the face of significant delays. Criminal defendants must be convicted or released, deserving civil plaintiffs compensated, and unjustly accused civil defendants exonerated—all in a timely manner if justice is to be done (Shuman 2000). Yet we also know that careful investigation takes time, and in some instances the passage of substantial time may bring about the discovery of new evidence or investigational techniques (such as the DNA techniques now resulting in the exculpation of some convicted rapists) (Shuman and McCall Smith 2000). Thus, the avoidance of unnecessary delay and the search for truth may exert conflicting legal demands.

The rules of evidence also recognize that courts must balance expense and the discovery of truth. Courts are public entities beholden to legislative bodies that face competing fiscal demands. A court's time must be managed with an awareness of these demands. Accordingly, the pursuit of truth must be tempered by fiscal responsibility. Litigants are also faced with fiscal limitations on expenditures. In a legal dispute over a $50,000 claim, it is not economical for a party to spend more than that amount to prevail. It may not be reasonable for a party to pay an expert to do everything that could be done to reach an accurate result. Thus, containing expense and attaining truth may exert conflicting demands.

Truth and justice, goals of the rules of evidence that are commonly regarded as synchronous, may also conflict. A civilized society would regard the use of evidence obtained through torture as unjust, even if it produced a truthful result. Similarly, discovering inculpatory information from a criminal defendant by leading him or her to believe that the forensic psychiatric examination was for the purpose of treatment would be regarded as unjust. For this reason psychiatrists are obligated to clarify with the litigants the purpose of the examination and to provide the names of the persons to whom the findings will be disclosed (Shuman 1993).

Apart from the ways in which justice, delay, and expense may conflict with obtaining truth in litigation, there are other competing demands on the legal system's search for truth. The attempt to foster certain therapeutic relationships (physician-, psychologist-, and psychotherapist-patient) with a relational privilege limits the ability of courts to compel disclosure of confidential communications cloaked by those privileges. Thus, relational privileges may also limit the discovery of truth in litigation (Shuman and Weiner 1987). Peer review privileges that encourage health care facilities to learn from errors to reduce morbidity and mortality may also limit litigants' access to relevant evidence (Tex. Occ. Code § 160.007 2002). In addition, rape shield laws that seek to protect victims of sexual assault by placing their prior sexual history off limits may limit access to relevant evidence (Fed. R. Evid. 412; Gold, in press).

Within this pragmatic framework of competing demands, the adversary system seeks to achieve truth by placing the responsibility for its discovery in the hands of those who have the greatest interest in the outcome, that is, the parties. That approach to the discovery of truth contrasts starkly with the methods of science and accounts for much frustration on the part of experts schooled in the methods of scientific investigation. "The adversarial model assumes we are more likely to uncover the truth about a contested event as the result of the efforts of the parties who have a self-interest in the discovery of proof and exposing the frailties of an opponent's proof than from the efforts of a judge charged only with an official duty to investigate the case" (Shuman 2001, p. 269). This model also embodies constitutional norms ensuring that litigants have the opportunity to tell their story and confront their opponents. Proponents of the adversary system understand the use of the word "adversary" in this context to have a positive meaning, and successful forensic psychiatrists learn not to take personally the demands of a zealous advocate.

The decision to use an adversary system that relies heavily on amateur lay decision-makers—jurors—has profound implications for the use of experts. Expert witnesses are permitted to testify on issues that a fact finder would otherwise lack the capacity to assess competently. Moreover, experts are neither independent agents nor directors of the adversary system. The parties employ their own experts in our legal system. This use of partisan experts whose believability is judged by laypersons has created a schism within the legal system about how to scrutinize the admissibility of experts.

> To understand how the law addresses claims of expertise...requires an understanding of two very different ideals about trials which vie for dominance in the U.S. judicial system. These two ideals, represented by the traditional adversarial approach and the gatekeeper approach, reflect two different ways of accommodating the tension among core values at stake in the dispute resolution process—accuracy, fairness, efficiency, consistency, and accessibility. (Shuman 2001, p. 268)

The search for truth takes place in the larger context of a democratic society in which tensions between demands for scientific accuracy and popular decision making color the use of experts. Raising the threshold for the admissibility of experts limits democratic decision making, whereas lowering the threshold limits the ability to protect jurors from unreliable claims of expertise. In *Daubert v. Merrell Dow Pharmaceuticals, Inc.* (1993), the Supreme Court wrestled with these tensions in its articulation of the standard for the admissibility of scientific evidence under the Federal Rules of Evidence. Addressing these tensions, the Court discussed the differences in the pursuit of truth in the courtroom and the laboratory:

> Petitioners...suggest that recognition of a screening role for the judge that allows for the exclusion of "invalid" evidence will sanction a stifling and repressive scientific orthodoxy and will be inimical to the search for truth....It is true that open debate is an essential part of both legal and scientific analyses. Yet there are important differences between the quest for truth in the courtroom and the quest for truth in the

> laboratory. Scientific conclusions are subject to perpetual revision. Law, on the other hand, must resolve disputes finally and quickly. The scientific project is advanced by broad and wide-ranging consideration of a multitude of hypotheses, for those that are incorrect will eventually be shown to be so, and that in itself is an advance. Conjectures that are probably wrong are of little use, however, in the project of reaching a quick, final, and binding legal judgment—often of great consequence—about a particular set of events in the past. We recognize that, in practice, a gatekeeping role for the judge, no matter how flexible, inevitably on occasion will prevent the jury from learning of authentic insights and innovations. That, nevertheless, is the balance that is struck by Rules of Evidence designed not for the exhaustive search for cosmic understanding but for the particularized resolution of legal disputes. (*Daubert v. Merrell Dow Pharmaceuticals, Inc.* 1993, pp. 596–597)

Recognizing that the adversary system is "designed not for the exhaustive search for cosmic understanding but for the particularized resolution of legal disputes" highlights the tension between truth and considerations of fairness and justice.

Considerations of fairness and justice also speak strongly to the issue of *process*. Process concerns are addressed in the due process clause contained in the Fifth Amendment to the Constitution (applicable to federal governmental action) and the Fourteenth Amendment to the Constitution (applicable to state governmental action). Due process has two important but different constitutional meanings—substantive due process and procedural due process. *Substantive due process* refers to the power of the courts to declare legislation unconstitutional because it does not reasonably advance a legitimate governmental goal. For example, in *Kansas v. Hendricks* (1997, p. 352) the U.S. Supreme Court heard and rejected a substantive due process challenge to Kansas's statutory scheme for civil commitment of a dangerous sex offender who had a mental abnormality. The act defined *mental abnormality* as a "congenital or acquired condition affecting the emotional or volitional capacity which predisposes the person to commit sexually violent offenses in a degree constituting such person a menace to the health and safety of others."

> Kansas argues that the act's definition of "mental abnormality" satisfies "substantive" due process requirements. We agree. Although freedom from physical restraint "has always been at the core of the liberty protected by the Due Process Clause from arbitrary governmental action," ...that liberty interest is not absolute. The Court has recognized that an individual's constitutionally protected interest in avoiding physical restraint may be overridden even in the civil context." (*Kansas v. Hendricks* 1997, p. 356)

Forensic psychiatrists can provide assistance in efforts to understand the impact of legislation on behavior in assessments of substantive due process claims.

*Procedural due process* refers to limitations on the process used by the government to deprive a citizen of life, liberty, or property. The hallmark of procedural due process is a meaningful opportunity to be heard. Thus, for example, the U.S. Supreme Court's decision in *Ake v. Oklahoma* (1985), recognizing an indigent defendant's right to expert assistance in presenting an insanity defense, was grounded in procedural due process:

> This Court has long recognized that when a State brings its judicial power to bear on an indigent defendant in a criminal proceeding, it must take steps to assure that the defendant has a fair opportunity to present his defense. This elementary principle, grounded in significant part on the Fourteenth Amendment's due process guarantee of fundamental fairness, derives from the belief that justice cannot be equal where, simply as a result of his poverty, a defendant is denied the opportunity to participate meaningfully in a judicial proceeding in which his liberty is at stake....without the assistance of a psychiatrist to conduct a professional examination on issues relevant to the defense, to help determine whether the insanity defense is viable, to present testimony, and to assist in preparing the cross-examination of a State's psychiatric witnesses, the risk of an inaccurate resolution of sanity issues is extremely high. With such assistance, the defendant is fairly able to present at least enough information to the jury, in a meaningful manner, as to permit it to make a sensible determination....We therefore hold that when a defendant demonstrates to the trial judge that his sanity at the time of the offense is to be a significant factor at trial, the State must, at a minimum, assure the defendant access to a competent psychiatrist who will conduct an appropriate examination and assist in evaluation, preparation, and presentation of the defense. (*Ake v. Oklahoma* 1985, p. 83)

Forensic psychiatrists may assist in implementing this right of procedural due process or assessing the impact of its denial.

Process considerations also serve other purposes beyond a fair opportunity to present a claim or defense. Because there are not enough law enforcement personnel to force the law on the citizenry, voluntary compliance with the law is at the heart of a successful democratic system of government. Process considerations are thought to play an important role in the public's confidence in and compliance with the rule of law. "The adversarial model also assumes that the parties' participation in the investigation and telling of their story, and the use of a decision maker who is independent of the investigation of the case, will enhance support of the judicial system and confidence in its decisions" (Shuman 2001, p. 269).

These demands on the legal system have important implications for the role of the actors in the adversary system. Most psychiatrists who testify as experts do so as retained experts at the behest of one of the parties to litigation (Cecil and Willgang 1992). Although courts have the power to appoint experts to serve the court in a neutral role, that power is rarely exercised outside of a narrow category of cases such as child custody determinations (Champagne et al. 2001).

The role of retained expert also has important implications for the rules that govern psychiatrists' conduct. Unlike the treating psychiatrist, whose communications with a patient are governed by the psychiatrist-patient privilege (or its equivalent), a forensic psychiatrist's communications with a litigant whose attorney retained him or her are governed by the attorney-client privilege. Communications between a litigant and a psychiatrist functioning in a forensic role are privileged only to the extent that they assist in the fulfillment of the attorney's role. Thus, a forensic relationship initiated by the litigant rather than the litigant's attorney will not be cloaked by the attorney-client privilege or the psychotherapist-patient privilege. The forensic psychiatrist's duty of confidentiality (e.g., the duty to maintain confidences and the competing duty to warn third persons or report child abuse) is also modified by the forensic role, although there is little statutory or case law that clarifies the full scope of these differences.

Although the psychiatrist's employment in a litigation context is determined by an advocate, the forensic psychiatrist is ethically obligated to exercise independent judgment (American Academy of Psychiatry and the Law 1995). Thus, successful forensic psychiatric practice demands a seemingly impossible balance between advocacy and objectivity (Shuman and Greenberg 2003). Moreover, unlike lay witnesses, whose existence and numbers are typically fixed at the time of the incident at issue (e.g., the eyewitnesses to a collision), potential expert witnesses typically constitute a much larger pool, and this results in pressure to conform to the advocate's demands. As an illustration, in 1999 there were 1,310 psychiatrists certified in the subspecialty of forensic psychiatry by the American Board of Psychiatry and Neurology, from among whom attorneys might choose a board-certified forensic psychiatrist. The number of practicing forensic psychiatrists who are not board-certified further expands the pool of potential experts. Attorneys may therefore "audition" a large group of experts and employ only the expert who is most supportive of their case.

Striking a balance between objectivity and advocacy is made all the more difficult by the manner in which experts contribute to the trial process. Although the psychiatrist expert may contribute to the advocate's decision about the issues that will be relevant in the case (e.g., by reporting that an insanity defense cannot be supported but suggesting psychiatric grounds for mitigation of capital punishment), neither the issue before the court nor the questions asked of the expert are decided by the expert. Experts are not asked on the stand if there is anything else they would like to say. Their input at trial is ultimately in the form of a question-and-answer colloquy in which the attorney asks the questions, the expert gives the answers, and nonresponsive answers may be stricken from the record with an accompanying judicial scolding.

The practice of good forensic psychiatry is much more than the practice of good clinical psychiatry in the courtroom. It requires the psychiatrist to dwell in an environment with rules and values that are often at odds with the values that dominate the psychiatrist's clinical domain. Yet, it also demands that the psychiatrist not abandon professional judgment. It is no small feat to balance these demands.

## Irreconcilable Differences Between Therapeutic and Forensic Practice

Therapeutic and forensic practice are distinct; however, a psychiatrist may be asked to perform both functions on behalf of a patient-litigant. For example, a psychiatrist who has treated a patient following a complaint of workplace sexual harassment may be asked to testify as a treating expert about the patient's treatment and prognosis and as a forensic expert about the cause of the emotional problems from which the plaintiff claims to suffer. These functions are inconsistent and should not be simultaneously performed on behalf of a patient-litigant (Strasburger et al. 1997). Failure to maintain these role boundaries threatens the efficacy of therapy and accuracy of the judicial process.

> [P]sychiatrists may appropriately testify as treating experts (subject to privilege, confidentiality, and qualifications) without risk of conflict on matters of: the reported history as provided by the patient; mental status; the clinical diagnosis; the care provided to the patient and the patient's response to it; the patient's prognosis; the mood, cognitions, or behavior of the patient; and any other relevant statements that the patient made in treatment. These matters, presented in the manner of descriptive "occurrences" and not psycholegal opinions, do not raise issues of judgment, foundation, or historical truth. Therapists do not ordinarily have the requisite data base to testify appropriately about psycholegal issues of causation (i.e., the relationship of a specific act to claimant's current condition) or capacity (i.e., the relationship of diagnosis or mental status to legally defined standards of functional capacity). These matters raise problems of judgment, foundation, and historical truth which are problematic for treating experts. (Greenberg and Shuman 1997, p. 56)

The potential harm of the therapeutic-forensic role conflict cannot be obviated by the patient-litigant's consent because its consequences not only involve the particular patient-litigant but affect the interests of the judicial system in the discovery of truth as well. These irreconcilable conflicts and the harm they portend are explained by examining four fundamental differences in the therapeutic and forensic roles.

The first fundamental difference is that the *goals* of the therapeutic and forensic relationship fundamentally and irreconcilably differ. Whereas the goal of the therapeutic relationship is to help the patient, the goal of the forensic relationship is to provide information to the legal system. A treating psychiatrist who seeks to serve the informational demands of the legal system as a forensic expert compromises treatment, and a treating psychiatrist testifying as a forensic expert who seeks to serve the therapeutic interests of the patient compromises the informational demands of the legal system.

The second fundamental difference in the therapeutic and forensic roles is that the role of *truth* differs fundamentally and irreconcilably in the forensic versus the therapeutic relationship. Courts seek to realize truth, albeit pragmatically. Thus, forensic psychiatrists are expected to use multiple independent sources of information to validate a litigant's claims and the information provided in support of them. "[T]he goal of therapy is not archeology" (American Psychological Association 1998, p. 936). In therapy, narrative truth matters more than historical truth. The use of multiple independent sources of information to validate a patient's claims in therapy is uncommon and presents a threat to confidentiality. Treating psychiatrists do not and cannot expect to acquire information about the truth of information asserted by their patients to the level of confidence that the legal system expects of forensic psychiatrists. Treating psychiatrists who cross these boundaries by testifying as forensic experts and assume that they have discovered historical truths about their patients are often incredulous when cross-examined with persuasive evidence to the contrary that was not available to them as a therapist.

The third fundamental difference in the therapeutic and forensic roles is *judgment*. An important characteristic of a good treating psychiatrist is being nonjudgmental, to assist in developing a positive, trusting therapist-patient alliance. In contrast, a good forensic psychiatrist, operating in an environment fraught with incentives for secondary gain, is judgmental and skeptical about the claims of the person being evaluated. If the psychiatrist has not occupied a position of trust, acting judgmentally toward the patient-litigant may cause legal harm but not emotional harm. However, if the psychiatrist has developed a trusting therapist-patient alliance, a judgmental forensic assessment risks serious emotional harm to the patient, whereas a nonjudgmental forensic assessment risks harm to the legal process.

The fourth fundamental difference in the therapeutic versus the forensic role is how society addresses the *reliability* of the psychiatrist's methods and procedures. Society takes a laissez-faire attitude toward psychotherapeutic techniques. Licensed mental health professionals are permitted to offer, and a competent adult patient is permitted to consent to, the use of a particular talk therapy without scientific proof of its efficacy. For example, analysts are not required to present rigorous scientific proof to the government or their patients that psychoanalysis is an effective form of treatment as a condition of its use. The judicial system is not so trusting. Legal rules governing the admissibility of experts permit the legal system to demand proof of the reliability of the procedures employed by psychiatrists who are providing expert testimony that is not demanded of treating psychiatrists.

It is appropriate for forensic psychiatrists to treat patients and for treating psychiatrists to serve as forensic experts. However, it is not appropriate for a psychiatrist to occupy both roles on behalf of a particular patient-litigant. Mixing these roles portends negative outcomes in both domains. Learning to resist this temptation is an important lesson for psychiatrists who hope to provide both clinical and forensic services.

## What the Law Demands of the Forensic Psychiatrist

The law's approach to the admissibility of expert testimony is characterized by a preference for lay testimony. Particularly in jury trials, the law expects the parties to present the testimony of lay witnesses to describe their firsthand sensory impressions of relevant events to the jurors; it expects jurors to draw inferences from the data or reach opinions based on the data to apply to the ultimate issue(s) in the case. However, the law recognizes that lay witnesses and lay jurors lack the capacity to understand and apply specialized knowledge. It has therefore acknowledged a specific role for expert witnesses in the litigation process, to fill the gaps in understanding that would result if only lay testimony were provided.

Courts protective of juries once demanded that juries had to be incapable of resolving an issue without expert assistance before considering the admission of an expert's testimony on that issue. That standard has been liberalized in most jurisdictions to admit expert testimony that would be helpful to the jurors even if they could conceivably resolve the issue without expert testimony. The liberalized standard of helpfulness is, however, still demanding. Consider a sexual assault prosecution in which the defendant claims that the complainant consented to sexual relations. A psychiatrist's testimony that the complainant is being truthful when she says she was sexually assaulted would be rejected as intruding on the jury's province without providing useful assistance to the jury (*State v. Bressman* 1984). Conversely, expert psychiatric testimony describing and applying scientific research about common characteristics of victims of sexual assault is more likely to be regarded as meeting the helpfulness requirement (*State v. Allewalt* 1986).

The law subjects all testimony—lay and expert—to two levels of scrutiny; however, this scrutiny is more explicit in the case of expert witnesses. First, the judge must determine that the witness is legally competent to testify. Second, the fact finder (the jury if the case is being tried in the presence of a jury; otherwise, the judge) must determine the weight to assign the witnesses' testimony in its deliberations. All witnesses are subject to the legal competence requirement. Thus, for example, if a witness (lay or expert) refuses to take an oath or affirmation "calculated to awaken the witness' conscience and impress the witness' mind with the duty to [testify truthfully]" (Fed. R. Evid. 603), the witness would not be legally competent to testify.

There are two additional legal competence requirements for expert witnesses. First, because experts such as psychiatrists rest their claims of expertise, in whole or in part, on the collective research and experience of their profession, they must prove that they have the appropriate qualifications to claim membership in the relevant branch of that profession. In a psychiatric malpractice case alleging inappropriate drug prescriptions leading to a fatal drug overdose, legal competence would demand not only proof of general psychiatric education and training but also specialized training and experience in psychopharmacology.

Second, because experts such as psychiatrists rest their claims of expertise, in whole or in part, on the accuracy of the methods and procedures they use, they must prove that good grounds exist to support the reliability of these methods and procedures. Competing legal tests emphasize general professional acceptance of the techniques versus independent scientific testing demonstrating the reliability of the technique (Shuman 1994). The older test, which arose in a federal court of appeals decision in *Frye v. United States* (1923), turned to the scientific community from which a new scientific method emerged to ask about its general acceptance. Although *Frye* has been replaced in the federal courts and many state courts, it still remains the relevant test for the admissibility of new scientific evidence in many states.

In 1993, the U.S. Supreme Court concluded that in federal court *Frye* did not survive the promulgation of the Federal Rules of Evidence in 1974. The Court's decision in *Daubert v. Merrell Dow Pharmaceuticals, Inc.* (1993) substituted a pragmatic test grounded in Karl Popper's conceptualization of falsifiability as the hallmark of the scientific enterprise. That test asks the trial judge to consider, among other factors, whether the technique or theory had been or could be tested, whether it had been subjected to professional scrutiny through peer review and publication, whether it yielded an acceptable rate of error, and whether it had been accepted in the relevant scientific community. Ultimately, the rigor applied to the admissibility determination may turn on who is scrutinizing the proffered testimony as much as the standard that is applied. To satisfy the most demanding threshold standard of scrutiny, to prepare for rigorous cross-examination, and to satisfy professional ethical requirements, forensic psychiatrists should assume that the most demanding scientific standards that their professional colleagues use will apply, and hence they should only present information derived from demonstrably reliable methods and procedures (Shuman and Sales 2001).

Psychiatrists who act as expert witnesses bring expertise acquired outside of the legal controversy to information generated within the legal controversy. Another set of legal rules (Fed. R. Evid. 702 and 703) addresses the information (basis) to which the forensic psychiatrist's expert knowledge is applied. Courts must determine whether the opinion is based on information that is sufficiently reliable. The courts' concern with the reliability of the information on which the expert relies for the factual basis of an opinion is illustrated by the following judicial observation:

> As late as 1980, Texas law disallowed admission of expert opinions based solely on hearsay evidence, mainly because this basis for the expert's testimony was not considered sufficiently trustworthy.... The Court's adoption of the Rules, however...allowed an expert to base opinion testimony entirely on inadmissible evidence, but the concern for the trustworthiness of the underlying basis for the expert's opinion did not evaporate. Instead, Rule 703 requires that if an expert intends to base an opinion solely on hearsay evidence, that it must be *of a type* reasonably relied upon by experts in the particular field in forming opinions or inferences upon the subject. (*E.I. du Pont de Nemours & Co. v. Robinson* 1995, p. 463)

Once the psychiatric expert witness has formulated an opinion, the next legal threshold is the form in which that opinion may be expressed. The issue here that has been a source of controversy is the ultimate opinion rule. With their preference for lay jury decision making, common-law courts once assiduously excluded any expert testimony that touched on the ultimate legal issue the jury was being asked to address as an intrusion on the province of the jury. Ultimately, when the Federal Rules of Evidence were adopted in 1974, their drafters rejected the "ultimate issue rule" as a legal artifact that no longer served a useful purpose. Not only were there innumerable appeals attempting to sort out what the ultimate legal issues were in a particular case, but the ultimate issue rule assumed that jurors lacked the capacity to distinguish the expert's reasoning and conclusions. In addition, the drafters of the federal rules noted that other rules permitted the court to exclude confusing or unhelpful expert testimony (Fed. R. Evid. 403; Fed. R. Evid. 702). The states that adopted a version of the Federal Rules of Evidence followed suit and jettisoned rules that excluded expert testimony merely because it embraced an ultimate issue in the case. A decade later, however, the reaction to the John Hinckley not guilty by reason of insanity (NGRI) verdict led to a partial reintroduction of the ultimate issue rule in federal criminal trials:

> (b) No expert witness testifying with respect to the mental state or condition of a defendant in a criminal case may state an opinion or inference as to whether the defendant did or did not have the mental state or condition constituting an element of the crime charged or of a defense thereto. Such ultimate issues are matters for the trier of fact alone. (Fed. R. Evid. 704[b])

Thus, experts testifying to the defendant's mental state in an insanity defense in federal court are now restricted from testimony "that, at the time of the commission of the acts constituting the offense, the defendant, as a result of a severe mental disease or defect, was unable to appreciate the nature and quality or the wrongfulness of his acts" (18 U.S.C.S. § 17 [2002]).

This limitation on ultimate issue testimony by experts does not apply in federal civil cases or the vast majority of state courts that have not adopted this provision. In those instances not covered by Federal Rule of Evidence 704(b) or a state law equivalent, some advocate that forensic psychiatrists should not address the ultimate issue as a matter of ethics because such matters involve legal or moral issues on which they have no claim of expertise (Goldstein 1989). Although this is an admirable goal, the approach asks nonlawyers to take on a legal determination that the courts abandoned as impracticable. Moreover, the ethical response to ultimate issue testimony is frustrating for judges and lawyers and is an inadequate justification for a psychiatric expert witness to refuse a court order to answer a question.

A preferable approach is for psychiatrists "to testify or not testify about ultimate issues, based on their data rather than arbitrary rules" (Rogers and Shuman 2000, p. 48). In this approach, the expert is asked to ascertain whether there are good grounds based on the use of reliable methods and procedures to answer the question, without regard to whether it is an ultimate issue. Indeed, this approach is the test that psychiatrists providing expert opinions should apply to all issues they are asked to address. A decision as to whether the data provide a reliable basis for a response should guide the psychiatrists' responses to all questions. For example, if a psychiatrist is asked in a sexual assault prosecution whether the complainant's postevent behavior suggests that she consented to sexual relations with the defendant, the response ought not to turn on whether this is an ultimate issue in the case. Rather, it should turn on whether there are any validated procedures that permit a psychiatrist to make this postdiction with a high degree of reliability (Simon and Shuman 2002).

The legal and ethical rules that govern the behavior of psychiatrists functioning as expert witnesses are neither intuitive nor flexible. They impose a set of restrictions on the conduct of psychiatrists that attorneys use for the benefit of their clients and to the detriment of those who stand in the way of achieving their client's goals. Psychiatrists who choose to enter this forensic realm must, at their peril, master these unique legal rules.

## Conclusion

In the not so distant past, most psychiatrists, along with other physicians, diligently sought to avoid testifying in legal proceedings. That situation has changed for numerous reasons, including decreased reimbursement to physicians for patient care (as a result of managed care) and increased lucrative opportunities for forensic experts. Forensic psychiatry is a growth industry. Yet, the forensic world is not to be entered into casually. It is a subspecialty with a culture and a language foreign to most psychiatrists that is best learned through specialized education and training.

## Practice Guidelines

1. Obtain comprehensive education and training addressing the ethical guidelines and legal rules that govern the practice of forensic psychiatry before providing expert witness services or consultations.

2. Do not mix therapeutic and forensic roles.
3. Provide expert testimony only on questions for which your education, training, and experience provide specialized expertise.
4. Use methods and procedures whose reliability has been tested and proven according to the most demanding standards of the profession.
5. Offer opinions that are based on sufficient, reliable information.
6. Present your findings in a manner that permits the fact finder to follow your analysis.

## References

Ake v Oklahoma, 470 U.S. 68 (1985)

American Academy of Psychiatry and the Law: Ethical Guidelines for the Practice of Forensic Psychiatry. Bloomfield, CT, American Academy of Psychiatry and the Law, 1995

American Psychiatric Association: The Principles of Medical Ethics With Annotations Especially Applicable to Psychiatry, 2001 Edition. Washington, DC, American Psychiatric Association, 2001

American Psychological Association, Working Group on Investigation of Memories of Childhood Abuse: Final Conclusions of the American Psychological Association Working Group on Investigation of Memories of Childhood Abuse. Psychology, Public Policy, and Law 4:933–939, 1998

Appelbaum PS: The parable of the forensic psychiatrist: ethics and the problem of doing harm. Int J Law Psychiatry 13:249–259, 1990

Cecil JS, Willgang TE: Defining a role for court-appointed experts. FJC Directions 4:6–17, 1992

Champagne A, Easterling D, Shuman DW, et al: Are court-appointed experts the solution to the problem of expert testimony? Judicature 84:178–183, 2001

Daubert v Merrell Dow Pharmaceuticals, Inc, 509 U.S. 579 (1993)

Davidson J, Pearlstein T, Londborg P, et al: Efficacy of sertraline in preventing relapse of posttraumatic stress disorder: results of a 28-week double-blind, placebo-controlled study. Am J Psychiatry 158:1974–1981, 2001

E.I. du Pont de Nemours and Co v Robinson, 923 S.W.2d 549 (Tex. 1995)

Ford v Wainwright, 477 U.S. 399 (1986)

Frye v United States, 293 F. 1013 (D.C. Cir. 1923)

Gold LH: Sexual Harassment: Psychiatric Assessment in Employment Litigation. Washington, DC, American Psychiatric Publishing (in press)

Goldstein RL: The psychiatrist's guide to right and wrong: Part II: a systematic analysis of exculpatory delusions. Bull Am Acad Psychiatry Law 17:61–67, 1989

Greenberg SA, Shuman DW: Irreconcilable conflict between therapeutic and forensic roles. Professional Psychology: Research and Practice 28:50–57, 1997

Henry v State, 574 So.2s 66 (Fla. 1991)

In re Estate of Herbert, 1996 Haw. App. LEXIS 162

Kansas v Hendricks, 521 U.S. 346 (1997)

Newell v Engel, 899 P.2d 273 (Colo. App. 1994)

Rogers R, Shuman DW: Conducting Insanity Defense Evaluations, 2nd Edition. New York, Guilford, 2000

Shuman DW: The use of empathy in forensic examinations. Ethics Behavior 3:289–302, 1993

Shuman DW: Psychiatric and Psychological Evidence. Deerfield, IL, Clark Boardman Callaghan, 1994

Shuman DW: When time does not heal: understanding the importance of avoiding unnecessary delay in the resolution of tort cases. Psychology, Public Policy, and Law 6:880–897, 2000

Shuman DW: Expertise in law, medicine, and health care. J Health Polit Policy Law 26:267–290, 2001

Shuman DW, Greenberg SA: The expert witness, the adversary system, and the voice of reason: reconciling impartiality and advocacy. Professional Psychology: Research and Practice 34:219–224, 2003

Shuman DW, McCall Smith A: Justice and the Prosecution of Old Crimes: Balancing Legal, Psychological and Moral Considerations. Washington, DC, American Psychological Association, 2000

Shuman DW, Sales BD: Daubert's wager. Journal of Forensic Psychology Practice 1:69–77, 2001

Shuman DW, Weiner MF: The Psychotherapist-Patient Privilege: A Critical Examination. Springfield, IL, Charles C Thomas, 1987

Simon RI, Shuman DW: Retrospective Assessment of Mental States in Litigation: Predicting the Past. Washington, DC, American Psychiatric Publishing, 2002

State v Allewalt, 517 A.2d 741 (Md. 1986)

State v Bressman, 689 P.2d 901 (Kan. 1984)

Strasburger LH, Guthiel TH, Brodsky A: On wearing two hats: role conflict in serving as both psychotherapist and expert witness. Am J Psychiatry 154: 448–456, 1997

Tex. Occ. Code § 160.007 (2002) [18 U.S.C.S. § 17 (2002)]

## Suggested Readings

Greenberg SA, Shuman DW: Irreconcilable conflict between therapeutic and forensic roles. Professional Psychology: Research and Practice 28:50–57, 1997

Shuman DW: The use of empathy in forensic examinations. Ethics Behavior 3:289–302, 1993

Shuman DW: Psychiatric and Psychological Evidence. Deerfield, IL, Clark Boardman Callaghan, 1994

Shuman DW, Greenberg SA: The expert witness, the adversary system, and the voice of reason: reconciling impartiality and advocacy. Professional Psychology: Research and Practice 34:219–224, 2003

Simon RI, Shuman DW: Retrospective Assessment of Mental States in Litigation: Predicting the Past. Washington, DC, American Psychiatric Publishing, 2002

# CHAPTER 3

# Starting a Forensic Practice

Robert P. Granacher Jr., M.D.

## Introduction

Psychiatrists in the United States generally develop a forensic practice in one of two ways. They may complete a forensic psychiatry fellowship and enter forensic practice thereafter. More commonly, psychiatrists increasingly add forensic psychiatry to an established clinical practice. Less than a handful of American psychiatrists practice full-time forensic psychiatry. Most members of the American Academy of Psychiatry and the Law (AAPL) devote less than 20% of their practice to forensic matters (Tanay 2000). Regardless of how they get started, psychiatrists tend to organize their forensic practices in one of two ways. They either operate as solo practitioners with a small support staff or work within a larger multidisciplinary practice comprising a variety of professionals (e.g., psychiatrists, psychologists, nurses, social workers, and business managers). In this chapter I explore how to get started in both models, with emphasis on the more common solo practice model.

The psychiatrist developing a forensic practice should at all times bear in mind that forensic psychiatry is a business. An expert examination or consultation service is rendered, and a fee is generated for that service. This arrangement differs distinctly from the practice of clinical psychiatry. In a treatment setting, a doctor-patient relationship is established. A psychiatrist provides a medical service, and then the patient pays for that service out-of-pocket or generally through a third-party insurance plan. Critical differences between the clinical and forensic practice of psychiatry and the treatment practice of psychiatry are discussed in other chapters. In this chapter I review the distinctions between the business aspects of forensic and clinical psychiatry. The business elements of forensic psychiatric practice in a private-practice model are stressed.

## Clinical Vignettes

### The Novice Forensic Psychiatrist

Mary Neophyte, M.D., became frustrated in her efforts to develop a forensic psychiatry practice. Since completing her forensic fellowship 18 months earlier, she had been retained in only two forensic cases. She sought out her colleague, Jack Mentor, M.D., who practiced forensic psychiatry in her city for 20 years. She asked him to meet her for lunch to develop ideas for enhancing her forensic psychiatric practice.

Dr. Neophyte asked Dr. Mentor if he could explain why she was not getting more referrals. Dr. Mentor suggested that they review various aspects of her practice together to identify the problem. He asked her to give him a description of her practice model. Dr. Neophyte stated that she didn't have a specific model. He asked her if she had a particular skill or interest. She told him that she had specialized in psychiatric employment issues during her fellowship. However, Dr. Neophyte was unable to define her practice goals or describe how she hoped to develop referrals. Dr. Mentor asked her how many forensic case referrals she projected receiving in the upcoming year. She said that she hoped to receive referrals for or to complete two cases per month. She no longer saw this as realistic because she was receiving no referrals at all.

Dr. Mentor asked Dr. Neophyte how she had planned to introduce herself to the legal community and generate referrals. She said that she had sent an introduction letter to various legal practices and psychiatrists in the city. She had assumed that given her credentials, this would be sufficient to generate a steady stream of referrals. Dr. Mentor then asked how she had made herself visible to the legal or business community. Dr. Neophyte acknowledged that she had made no particular efforts to do so because she was busy with her current activities: her staff position at a local hospital, her attendance at medical society meetings, her part-time employment at a community mental health center, and her part-time teaching professorship at a local medical school.

Dr. Mentor then asked Dr. Neophyte to describe the mechanics of a referral to Dr. Neophyte's office. She said that attorneys who called would generally have to leave a message on her answering machine, although she had a receptionist/business manager. She would return the calls herself but often found it difficult to reach the attorney directly. Many times, she could only directly contact employees in the attorney's office who were not familiar with the case or the specific referral issue.

Dr. Mentor asked Dr. Neophyte to describe her usual procedure for conducting a forensic examination. She said that she would obtain as many medical records and legal records as possible in a case, review them thoroughly, and then personally examine the plaintiff or defendant. She always took a complete history from the examinee, performed a face-to-face mental status examination, and then wrote a report. In the two cases she had completed, she obtained no psychological testing and performed no measures of effort. She did not determine whether malingering or symptom magnification was an issue and felt no need to obtain laboratory studies or imaging studies. Dr. Mentor asked Dr. Neophyte if she had developed a relationship with a psychologist, a neuropsychologist, or radiological physicians should she need their services for more complex cases. She said she had not done so and didn't see the need for such relationships. At the conclusion of their lunch, Dr. Mentor suggested that Dr. Neophyte meet with him at his office in a week, and they scheduled an appointment. He told her that he would then provide her with a structured format for enhancing her forensic psychiatric practice.

## Adding a Forensic Component to an Existing Practice

Charles Granite, M.D., had practiced general psychiatry for about 12 years. He was in practice with two other psychiatrists, one psychologist, one social worker, and one nurse. He developed an interest in forensic psychiatry and wanted to add a forensic component to his existing practice. His psychiatric partners supported this goal, although they themselves were not interested in practicing forensic psychiatry. Dr. Granite was unsure how to develop a forensic practice within his clinical practice model. He called Jack Mentor, M.D., a local successful forensic psychiatrist, for advice. Dr. Mentor suggested that they meet to discuss Dr. Granite's existing practice and his goals.

At the meeting, Dr. Granite provided Dr. Mentor with a short business plan that his accountant had helped him develop. His psychiatric partners had requested that he do so before they approved his pursuit of forensic psychiatry to assess the impact on the clinical practice. Dr. Granite had also developed a mission statement for his practice that identified his primary interest as assessment of psychiatric injury claims in personal injury litigation. However, he could not define a strategic plan for how he intended to achieve his vision for a practice with a forensic psychiatry component. He was also concerned about managing the referral and examination process within the existing treatment model of his group practice.

Over the next few months, Dr. Granite and Dr. Mentor met regularly. Together they developed a structured format for adding a forensic psychiatry component to Dr. Granite's existing practice. They identified techniques and strategies to reduce the impact of providing forensic assessments on the existing treatment practice and Dr. Granite's partners. The psychologist within the practice could not provide forensic testing services, so Dr. Granite developed a consultation relationship with another psychologist in his medical building. Over a 2- to 3-year period, with Dr. Mentor's advice, Dr. Granite was able to successfully add a strong forensic component to his psychiatric practice without stressing the practice relationships. He was also able to maintain a strong clinical practice and enhance his treatment skills.

## Planning the Practice

The four major components involved in planning any business, including a forensic psychiatry practice, are the mission, vision, core values, and strategies. Table 3–1 defines the relationship of the individual psychiatrist to each of these components.

All businesses should begin with a *mission statement*. This is a statement of the overall philosophy of the practice and the driving force, or heartbeat, of the practice. The mission statement can consist of a few sentences that concisely state the forensic psychiatrist's purpose. It should be short and pithy so that everyone in the psychiatry practice can easily remember it and bear it in mind at all times. An example of such a statement might be, "The mission of the ABC Forensic Psychiatry Practice is to provide state-of-the-art forensic analysis of personal injury cases that may have produced psychological harm."

A succinctly articulated mission statement enhances the likelihood of meeting the mission of the forensic psychiatry business. Many businesses of all kinds begin without a mission statement and tend to evolve in an unpredictable fashion. For psychiatrists planning to practice forensic psychiatry, a well-articulated mission statement helps all the people working toward the goal to function as a cohesive group. A mission statement is also of great value to solo practitioners, because they lack the checks and balances provided by peers to keep the practice goals on course.

The *vision statement* of a forensic psychiatry practice describes how the practice will proceed from point A to point B as it seeks to fulfill the mission of the practice. It is the description of where the practice is heading, as guided by the mission statement. The vision statement resembles the mission statement in that it is expressed in as few sentences as possible and is sufficiently short and easy to understand so that the psychiatrist is able to remember it. Using the aforementioned mission statement as a guide, the vision statement for planning a forensic practice might be, "The ABC Forensic Psychiatry Practice will be recognized as the region's leading provider of personal injury forensic psychiatric assessments."

**TABLE 3–1.** Planning the forensic practice

| | |
|---|---|
| **Mission** | Why you are here |
| **Vision** | Where you are going |
| **Core values** | How you will practice |
| **Strategies** | How you will accomplish the mission and vision |

The *core values* should express in simple terms the ethics and values (the business culture) that will be used to guide the mission and vision of the practice. Like the mission statement and the vision statement, a core values statement should be succinct, to the point, and clearly expressed. A core values statement of the hypothetical ABC forensic psychiatric practice might be, "The ABC Forensic Psychiatry Practice will embrace the core values of honesty and objectivity when providing forensic psychiatric examinations. Examinations will be conducted with integrity, compassion, and excellence."

The strategic portion of planning the forensic practice follows development of the mission statement, vision statement, and core values statement. The *strategies* describe how the mission and vision of the practice will be accomplished. There are two components to developing strategies: strategic thinking and then strategic planning. In general, strategy is the *what* of the process, while operations are the *how* (Robert 1993). Strategic thinking creates the vision of the future forensic psychiatric practice and clarifies the future strategic profile of the practice. Strategic thinking results in shaping the framework for the strategic and operational plans.

Developing a vision of the future forensic psychiatric practice around a visual picture of the anticipated practice yields much better results than focusing on complex documents, numbers, and jargon. Even many large corporations rarely have a clear strategic vision. Kim and Mauborgne (2002) believe this stems from defects in the strategic-planning process itself. Whether the psychiatrist commits the strategic plan to writing or not, the language used should provide visual images that convey meaning to others, as well as the psychiatrist. One of the best ways to do this is to go into the field and actually talk to prospective customers. These customers include lawyers, judges, and staff of corporations, insurance companies, and workers' compensation management companies.

The forensic psychiatrist should review the strategic plan to find physical indicators that enable practitioners to analyze situations and make decisions. These might be written in a tabular fashion so that all persons participating in the development of the forensic practice can read the document and understand the vision of the strategic plan. At a minimum, thinking about the following physical indicators is important in developing a cohesive plan (Granacher 2001):

- Services offered by the practice and types of cases to be evaluated
- Human resources and skills that the practice will need to obtain
- Customers (lawyers, institutions, courts, businesses, etc.) to be served

- Forensic psychiatry competitors in the region
- Vendors who will supply the practice (such as those supplying psychological services, laboratory services, or brain imaging)
- Legal market segment in which the practice will compete (e.g., personal injury, criminal, workers' compensation, employment law)
- Budget for monies intended to capitalize the practice
- Facilities and physical plant needed to provide these services

As the strategic plan is developed, the psychiatrist must remember to think also in the null. For instance, important questions to ask in the negative include

- Which forensic psychiatric services will not be offered?
- Which customer groups will not be served?
- Which forensic areas or areas of litigation support will not be sought?
- In which geographic areas will the practice not compete?

These questions help the psychiatrist visualize the limits of the strategic vision.

The strategic plan should be proactively developed within the skill set and philosophy of the individual psychiatrist and not directed toward a target forensic psychiatric practice or competitor. One dangerous form of thinking is to focus on other practices and attempt to either mimic those practices or compete directly with a particular forensic practice. Instead, psychiatrists should focus on their vision as articulated earlier in this chapter and develop the practice according to that vision.

## Developing the Business Plan

New businesses should begin with a business plan. The forensic psychiatrist does not need a master's degree in business administration to develop and implement a business plan. The main factors of success when developing a business plan for forensic psychiatry are flexibility in design and adaptation to changing trends within the business practice of forensic psychiatry. If you lack sufficient experience or skill to prepare a plan, your accountant or business consultant can assist you. Table 3–2 outlines a standard model for organization of the business plan.

Although a written plan is not required, and many psychiatrists may choose not to complete a plan, a properly constructed and occasionally revised business plan can be an important tool in developing the forensic psychiatric practice, particularly in the case of the solo practitioner. Even if a written plan is not developed, reviewing the elements of Table 3–2

**TABLE 3–2.** Elements of the business plan

1. Cover page
2. Contents page
3. Executive summary
4. Business background: structure and organization
5. Analysis of strengths, weaknesses, opportunities, and threats
6. The market(s) and marketing strategies
7. Strategies for production and human resources
8. Profit performance
9. Financial projections (business model)
10. Exit strategy

will help the solo practitioner to envision a cognitive map of the future practice. As discussed earlier, solo practice does not provide professional feedback or checks and balances. This review can forestall significant scotomas leading to serious business lapses.

The development of a business plan requires a business model even if the model is cognitive rather than written. The term *business model* first came into widespread use after development of the personal computer and spreadsheet software (Magretta 2002). A spreadsheet allows psychiatrists to ask *what-if* questions about the critical assumptions on which the practice will depend. Although it is not required, a spreadsheet enables the practitioner to model the future business behavior under different circumstances. For instance, what if clients are more price-sensitive in a particular city than you thought? With a few keystrokes on the computer, you can model how a change would play out in every aspect of the practice.

The main business model can be thought of as a subsection or component of the business plan. If you choose to develop a spreadsheet model, it would fit most accurately into the portion of the business plan dealing with financial projections and profit performance.

A business plan need not be long. A good business plan for a novice forensic psychiatry practitioner can be 8–10 pages long. It should include a cover page outlining the name of the practice, a contents page to guide the reader through the document, and a brief executive summary. The business plan should also contain a description of an exit strategy, a key element that is often neglected. Psychiatrists should clearly explain how they would leave the practice should it fail or require dissolution.

All parts of the business plan should be synthesized and distilled into an executive summary. Most financial planners, bankers, and other providers will read only the executive summary; therefore, it should describe

- The purpose of the business plan and the specific forensic psychiatric services to be provided to clients.
- The market potential for forensic psychiatric services in the practitioner's geographic area.
- The services that will be provided, in language that a businessperson can understand.
- The major financial projections for the practice for the next 3 years.
- How the practice will be marketed, what management skills are available from other members of the practice, and whether it is a multipractitioner model.

The rest of the business plan should be developed in some detail. The section on structure and organization should describe

- History and background of the individual forensic psychiatrist (if a solo practitioner) or those within the group or academic practice (if a group practice).
- Forensic services the psychiatrist will provide in a solo practice model
- Economics of forensic psychiatry within the practitioner's geographic area.
- Practice trends.
- Potential legal, ethical, or professional problems and how they will be handled if they arise.

The next section of the business plan should analyze both the psychiatrist's strengths and weaknesses or lack of skills relevant to the practice of forensic psychiatry. As stated previously, psychiatrists should be aware of the areas of practice they will not pursue. This decision may be informed by an honest assessment of the skills and training of the individual psychiatrist. Special opportunities in the geographic area should be addressed. For instance, psychiatrists who have skills in the evaluation of employment issues should emphasize this as a strength in a geographic area that has no similarly experienced practitioner. Threats should also be identified. For example, recent changes in the regulatory climate of workers' compensation in a particular jurisdiction should be outlined if the practice intends to pursue workers' compensation as an area of development.

Psychiatrists devising a business plan should also describe strategies for key areas such as production and human resources. How will the forensic psychiatrist produce personal injury assessments and provide testimony within the context of an ongoing treatment practice with demands on the practitioner to admit and discharge patients from the hospital? The human resources available to support the psychiatrist in the endeavor of forensic psychiatry should be carefully delineated. Any obvious vulnerabilities relating to support services should be explained in detail, particularly if the psychiatrist is practicing solo.

Last, the business plan should clearly state financial projections. The first-year projection of target revenue should be stated, and some attempt should be made to determine the break-even point for the practice. Obviously, treatment revenue will be comingled with forensic revenue. The capital needed to start the practice, if necessary, should be specifically stated, and a budget for the funds should be outlined. If the capital is to be borrowed, the business plan should describe how repayment will be made. Cash flow should be projected by month for the first year and in subsequent years, if necessary, until a positive cash flow is maintained. Thereafter, projections should be made annually. Projections beyond 3–5 years are unnecessary, however, because they are likely to be unrealistic and inaccurate.

## Developing Strategy and Tactics for Starting a Forensic Practice

Psychiatrists who add a forensic psychiatric practice to a treatment practice should carefully analyze how to balance the two disciplines. The *maintenance of dynamic stability* in a business is a process of continual but relatively small changes that involve the reconfiguration of existing practices and business models rather than the creation of new ones (Abrahamson 2000). Dynamic instability could result from attempting to combine the two types of practice without careful consideration. Psychiatrists should plan to gradually add an increasing amount of forensic work to their clinical practices. The risk of creating instability is lower for the solo practitioner but higher for the psychiatrist merging a forensic practice into a clinical group practice. Colleagues may develop resistance to change, which can produce instability in both the interpersonal and business dynamics of the practice.

Combining the two types of psychiatric practice involves developing both strategy and tactics. *Strategy* may be conceptualized as the art of planning or method. *Tactics* are the art of employing available means to accomplish an end. The tactics of forensic psychiatry are the day-to-day behaviors and tasks that lead to successful practice. These tactics can be introduced at any point within the overall business model or business plan. This in turn will help maintain stability and not overly stress the practice. The following subsections review tactics and strategies that may be helpful in starting a forensic practice.

### *Providing Direct Contact With Potential Clients*

When first developing a forensic psychiatric practice, psychiatrists should consider the value of direct human contact with potential clients, especially if practicing alone. Telephone routing systems, answering services, and voice mail may be appropriate for a retail business. However, the complex interactions and communications necessary in forensic psychiatry best lend themselves to having a person available to answer calls and provide information to the potential client. People generally prefer speaking to a human being rather than voice mail or a computer system. The loss of business in a forensic psychiatric practice as a result of voice mail is substantial. In addition, the use of mechanical answering systems removes the opportunity for the forensic psychiatrist to develop an early relationship with the potential client.

### *Maintaining Internet Web Sites*

An individual who answers the phone for the psychiatrist should be trained to provide as much aid as possible to the caller. Posting information on an Internet Web site may make the communication of such information even more efficient and effective. When a potential client calls, if the employee cannot answer all questions and the psychiatrist is unavailable, the client can be referred to the Web site. This can also increase productivity, because it will decrease the amount of time the psychiatrist has to spend on nonpaying, time-consuming clerical functions. Thus, a Web site may be a particularly cost-effective tool for the solo practitioner.

A few years ago, use of an Internet Web site by a forensic psychiatrist was considered controversial. Today, most juries are highly familiar with Web sites. A Web site is clearly a form of advertising; however, it is also a very effective form of communication and can be an integral part of the forensic psychiatric business. For example, the psychiatrist's forensic Web site can contain the types of examinations offered, a description of the office location and directions, and an abbreviated curriculum vitae. Other information about the technical or philosophical aspects of the practice can be placed on the site so that they can be downloaded by clients or prospective clients. Many lawyers still wish to use psychiatrists' Web sites to discredit them at trial. Therefore, it is recommended that the Web site be conservative, accurate, and not embellished.

## *Using an Evidence-Based Medical Model for Forensic Evaluations*

Forensic psychiatrists should rely on an objective, evidence-based medical model. When lawyers use psychiatrists to provide expert testimony in court, the lawyers want the jury or fact finder to understand that psychiatrists are medical doctors. Lawyers are interested in the psychiatrists' medical skills, not their legal or forensic knowledge. The medical model relies on an evidence-based treatment system to provide quality clinical services to patients. The same practice should be pursued within forensic psychiatry to enhance the objectivity and honesty of forensic testimony.

Practicing evidence-based, medical-model psychiatry will best demonstrate both medical and forensic skills. Whenever possible, forensic psychiatrists should quantify the mental status examination. The face-to-face mental status examination is the sine qua non of the psychiatric examination. However, triers of fact also assume that a portion of this examination will be quantified in a standardized fashion. This may include, for instance, the measurement of reading skill, intellectual capacity, organic mental dysfunction by neuropsychological assessment, and psychopathology by instruments such as the Minnesota Multiphasic Personality Inventory–2 (MMPI-2) (Pope et al. 2000). In cases in which such issues become a focus of litigation, consultation with a psychologist will probably be required for proper quantification. The use of structural and functional brain imaging may be required in cases involving potential functional or organic brain injury, such as traumatic brain injury, toxic torts, or perinatal birth injury. In addition, when appropriate, the psychiatrist should perform or arrange for a neurological examination when evaluating claims of cognitive disorders or brain injury.

Forensic psychiatry also encompasses special skills that are not used within the treatment models of psychiatry. Bradford and Glancy (2000) noted that forensic psychiatrists have gained the respect of their peers and the public at large by developing some unique skills that separate them from their treatment-oriented colleagues. For example, forensic psychiatrists often have additional training in the evaluation of deception as it relates to the malingering of mental illness. This evaluation should also be evidence-based. The forensic evaluation should always consider whether an evaluee is malingering. Gutheil and Simon (2002) noted that failure to consider malingering constitutes substandard practice for the forensic psychiatrist (see Chapter 19: "Malingering," this volume).

## *Using Technology*

Psychiatrists developing a forensic psychiatric practice should also use widely available technology to increase productivity, efficiency, and accuracy in written reports. For example, reports generated by word-processing programs permit crisp editing and the production of a visually attractive product. Such programs also allow psychiatrists to retain templates that can be used repeatedly when appropriate. Use of templates will reduce time and improve the quality of reports and make the production less burdensome both for the psychiatrist and the psychiatrist's staff.

In addition, software now available enables the forensic psychiatric practice to maintain a client list, schedule examinations on-line, and immediately generate contractual letters at the time the examination is scheduled. These tools can significantly reduce demands on time, especially for the solo practitioner. Psychiatrists should consider centralized computer scheduling, run by the person who serves as the liaison between the forensic practice and the users of services. This may serve to reduce scheduling errors. Computer scheduling will enable the psychiatrist to print the entire upcoming week's schedule each Friday and have easy access to it at all times. In a group practice, a copy of the schedule can be made available to all the staff, enhancing communication and efficiency.

## *Working With Staff to Enhance the Business Process*

Forensic psychiatrists can implement a number of practices that use support staff to enhance the business process. For instance, even if the practice consists only of a psychiatrist and one employee, meeting weekly with the staff to review upcoming forensic examinations will be both practical and efficient. Psychiatrists should develop the habit of requesting that the client provide the medical and legal records of the examinee well before the examination. These records then can be reviewed by the psychiatrist, or a psychologist and other staff members if in a group practice, and a format can be developed in the weekly meetings for the particular examination. This meeting can also provide an opportunity to develop strategies for future forensic examinations based on the medicolegal questions at issue. The need for psychological testing or brain imaging can be determined and scheduled if indicated.

Productivity is enhanced by the secondary improvement in internal communication of the practice that occurs as a result of weekly meetings. This meeting can provide a regular opportunity to review upcoming trials, depositions, and other important forensic matters that may require the collection of data or further review of records. This weekly review assists the psychiatrist with practice organization and improves foresight. Finally, when the examinee arrives at the office, all parties involved in the evaluation, from the receptionist to the psychiatrist, will fully be aware of what is needed. This will help ensure that the evaluation process goes as smoothly as possible for the examinee and the staff.

## *Establishing Clear Fee Policies*

Some psychiatrists establishing a forensic psychiatric practice are uncomfortable with managing financial issues. However, financial arrangements in clinical and forensic psychiatry differ, and so they must be addressed for a forensic practice to succeed as a business. Psychiatrists should be sure to have clear written contracts with clients. This prevents professional or ethical lapses. Once the examinee is scheduled for examination, a contractual letter should be forwarded immediately to the retaining attorney. This letter should state the date of the examination, the cost for the examination, and when payment is expected. Any additional services, such as deposition or courtroom testimony, should also be documented in such letters and forwarded to the attorney.

In forensic psychiatry, the practice of obtaining a retainer fee or prepayment of estimated costs is both advisable and ethical. Prepayment ensures that no perception of contingency fee arrangements exists and facilitates honesty and objectivity in the examination. Acceptance of the retainer fee seals the contractual arrangement and thus allows the psychiatrist unlimited objective latitude. This becomes particularly important when the psychiatrist's opinion is not helpful to the retaining attorney. In such cases, financial arrangements will not become an issue, and the psychiatrist will be paid for his or her time.

## *Facilitating the Evaluation Process*

Psychiatrists should think about how to make the forensic examination as user-friendly as possible, both for the psychiatrist's client and for the examinee. For example, they should consider sending a short list of instructions to the retaining attorney who can forward them to the examinee prior to the evaluation. This letter should contain directions to the office, instructions on use of medications prior to testing, the estimated length of the examination, the necessity of a good night's sleep, and a proscription against substance abuse. Examinees rarely are told that a psychiatric examination may last all day, and they may become understandably distressed when they find that out at the time of the examination. Providing this and other relevant information may decrease the stress associated with a litigation-related psychiatric evaluation and thus enhance the quality of the data obtained from the examinee.

### *Communicating Effectively*

Poor communication is the Achilles' heel of a developing forensic psychiatry practice. Forensic psychiatrists who cannot communicate effectively both orally and in writing might not succeed in forensic practice. Many psychiatrists find that regardless of the depth of their scientific knowledge and medical expertise, they cannot effectively communicate their findings in a medicolegal forum. Medical school and psychiatric residency generally do not emphasize communication skills.

The role of the forensic psychiatrist is to educate the court. Testimony is in fact a method of teaching and providing information to people who must make decisions about the legal matters at hand. Forensic psychiatrists should therefore learn to clearly teach their opinions. The more skillfully expert witnesses can explain their opinions, either verbally or in writing, the more likely the trier of fact will understand the point of their testimony. The most efficient method of improving and maintaining communication skills is the continual teaching of others. Whenever possible, forensic psychiatrists should improve these skills by teaching medical colleagues, lawyers, or judges. The ability to communicate orally is fundamental to the success of a forensic practice. Forensic psychiatrists should therefore be certain to develop good oral communication skills. If communication skills are poor, psychiatrists should consider obtaining a skills coach.

Plain talk, which avoids the use of complicated scientific terms or psychiatric jargon, is the best style of communication when speaking to a trier of fact. President Lincoln's Gettysburg Address, one of the best examples of a short speech with elegant language provided in a straightforward fashion, is instructive. This speech contains a preponderance of nouns and verbs rather than adjectives and adverbs. It contains abstract principles such as liberty and equality, but it focuses on concrete benefits of those principles to the audience. The speech was given not as a lecture but as a kind of conversation (Griffin 2001).

Psychiatric testimony can be given in the same manner. People communicate with each other in narratives or stories. This same method of communication is best when testifying to laypeople. The expert should strive to engage the audience. The educational level of the average juror in the United States is that of a high school graduate or less. The language style of Harvard, Stanford, or Johns Hopkins may sound pretentious and therefore not be well received. Moreover, nonverbal communication is a significant factor in testimony. It is not just what one says but how one says it (Mandel 2000). If the message is not heard, the testimony will not be received. Speaking in a monotone, communicating without enthusiasm, and moving in a stiff manner with little animation may ensure that the listener will dismiss the testimony.

Psychiatrists delivering testimony should make direct eye contact with the trier of fact, whether judge or jury. In our culture, eye contact opens the channel of communication between people, establishes and builds rapport, and enhances credibility. Psychiatrists who deliver testimony with darting eyes or while looking at the ceiling, constantly reviewing notes, and avoiding eye contact with the trier of fact may only be apprehensive or have poor communication skills. However, juries may perceive them as lacking credibility, characterize their testimony as arrogant or sloppy, and reject their opinions. A significant portion of testimony today is taken by videotaped deposition. Psychiatrists giving testimony by videotape should make certain to look directly into the camera lens often. This will ensure direct eye contact with jurors watching a video monitor in court.

Forensic psychiatrists should also be conscious of the quality of their written reports. The writing of reports is fundamental to successful practice. Reports that are poorly written, digress excessively, do not answer questions at hand, and contain poorly connected logic or sloppy writing are not likely to help a psychiatrist's reputation or garner more referrals. Reports should contain subject headings to guide the reader. Introductory paragraphs describing the nature and purpose of a mental status examination, psychological testing, brain imaging, or neurological examination will also assist the reader. Reports of psychological testing should contain a brief description of each test, followed by the evidence-based numerical data. If brain imaging has been obtained, a brief description of the nature of a magnetic resonance imaging (MRI) or positron emission tomography (PET) scan is generally appreciated by lawyers and other readers of forensic reports.

## *Maintaining a Clinical Practice*

A few psychiatrists in the United States practice solely as forensic psychiatrists and do not provide any treatment services. This may be an effective strategy for certain highly visible psychiatrists with national reputations. However, it is not recommended for everyone who initiates a forensic psychiatric practice. Lack of skill in clinical psychiatry may severely limit the business opportunities for the forensic psychiatrist at the local and regional level. Lawyers are generally suspicious of forensic psychiatrists with limited treatment skills. Recent tort reforms can result in limiting the types of referrals psychiatrists receive. In some jurisdictions, such as Ohio, a psychiatrist who does not devote at least 50% of practice time to treatment and medical consultation cannot testify in a medical malpractice case (Oh. Stat. Rev. 1980). Moreover, legal claims concerning civil rights violations in state hospitals or jails may also involve the evaluation of treatment provided.

Lawyers want a medical expert, not a pseudo-lawyer. They generally seek a skilled clinical psychiatrist who is also, secondarily, a skilled forensic specialist. Forensic psychiatry therefore requires that psychiatric and medical skills be honed to the highest level. Even experienced clinicians find that their knowledge and skills become degraded if they stop treating patients. Information such as advances in general medical science, treatment planning, psychopharmacology, the interaction of medical diseases with psychiatric illnesses, and multiple pathological states that may affect mental status require a treatment focus to maintain skill levels. Providing active treatment and obtaining continuing education in patient-centered psychiatry ensures continual enhancement of these skills.

### *Using Ethical Marketing*

The practice of forensic psychiatry is a business, which, like any other business, requires marketing. Some forms of marketing are unseemly, such as advertising on a billboard or running advertisements on television similar to those used by hair transplant surgeons or personal injury attorneys. In addition, advertising of this nature tends to portray the forensic psychiatrist as an advocate or shill rather than an impartial examiner. Such advertisements, without doubt, would show up in the courtroom during cross-examination. Some psychiatrists publish their name in "expert witness networks" as a way of marketing. This practice is unwise and suggests that the psychiatrist is a hired gun. Nevertheless, ethical marketing of forensic psychiatry is possible.

Psychiatrists interested in building their practices through marketing should remember that they themselves are the advertisement. Every testimony is an audition. The opposing lawyer and the lawyer client will note the psychiatrist's skill, polish, teaching style, and clarity of opinion (or lack thereof). Psychiatrists should therefore dress conservatively, display professional competence and self-respect, and communicate effectively. Clear, concise, honest, and objective reports and testimony are forensic psychiatrists' best marketing tools. Psychiatrists should be certain to provide understandable opinions based on medical evidence, consistent with *Daubert* rules (*Daubert v. Merrell Dow Pharmaceuticals, Inc.* 1993).

Forensic psychiatrists should consider developing specialty areas of interest within forensic practice, and they should market their specialized skills. Novice forensic psychiatrists should establish a credible track record within an area of forensic practice. If, for instance, the focus of the practice is employment issues, the psychiatrist will need to establish credibility in areas such as violence prediction in the workplace, workers' compensation, workplace sexual harassment, workplace age discrimination, and the like.

Attorneys also specialize and have specialty professional organizations, meetings, journals, and newsletters. Psychiatrists interested in practicing in a particular area can make themselves visible and network with these select groups. For example, psychiatrists interested in criminal evaluations may want to offer pro bono services to legal aid groups or work part-time at a jail clinic or inpatient forensic unit. These patients will generally have attorneys who need forensic services. Psychiatrists interested in employment litigation may want to publish articles on forensic issues in litigation attorneys' newsletters or journals or arrange to speak at a meeting of such attorneys. These activities will provide opportunities to create contacts and build relationships with potential referral sources by demonstrating clinical and teaching skills without engaging in unseemly or unethical advertising.

## Defining Critical Success Factors

Critical success factors are the metrics used to determine how the practice is performing. Four common critical success factors in any business providing services are 1) client satisfaction, 2) stewardship of resources, 3) strategic growth, and 4) people. In a large company, client satisfaction usually is measured by some form of survey. This is generally not feasible within a solo forensic psychiatric practice or even a small-group forensic psychiatric practice. In these models, some indirect measure of client satisfaction must be undertaken.

Psychiatrists in small-group or solo practices may choose to keep a log of complaints about quality and timeliness of reports and a list of clients who fail to send return business. A yearly review of these metrics provides a database for analysis. If a pattern emerges, clients can be contacted to determine if they had complaints or concerns about the services provided. Psychiatrists can then adjust their practices to correct these problems. However, the psychiatrist must guard against advocacy bias resulting from the desire to obtain repeat business. Evaluation results that do not meet the goals of the retaining attorney must be reported with the same vigor as more favorable results. Psychiatrists who do so may lose repeat business but will in the long term enhance their practices by gaining respect as fair and objective evaluators. Psychiatrists can also maintain their reputations for objectivity by striving for balance and performing evaluations for both plaintiffs and defendants.

Proper stewardship of resources will enable the practice to grow financially. The strategic growth of the practice will depend on increasing a steady supply of forensic referrals. Success breeds success. Forensic psychiatrists who improve their evaluation and testimony skills and follow the practice recommendations provided in this chapter and summarized at the end will generally find that their practice will grow. Psychiatrists who note flat or declining growth in their practices should consider what is deterring referrals. They should evaluate whether clients have been satisfied, whether sufficient technology has been added to the practice to improve efficiency and reduce cost, and whether they are providing top-quality forensic psychiatric evaluations and reports.

Last, psychiatrists should remember that support staff are critical to success. Employing more staff than needed is a poor stewardship of resources (Wiley 2002). However, the forensic psychiatrist should not be performing tasks that can be completed by unlicensed personnel at a lower hourly rate than the psychiatrist. If the psychiatrist feels constantly rushed but doesn't see as many examinees as time allows, more help may be required. Client complaints about long waits for reports may point to an overworked staff or a poorly performing staff member. This may also indicate the need for the solo psychiatrist to add staff.

## Conclusion

Forensic psychiatry is not a team sport. Rather, it resembles cross-country running. The runner can glide along with the rest of the pack and become indistinguishable, or separate himself or herself from the pack through effort and skill. If the novice forensic psychiatrist strives for excellence, the marketing aspects will take care of themselves by word of mouth among lawyers and by expert witness reporting services used by lawyers. Starting a forensic practice is similar in many respects to starting any other kind of business. However, the critical factors in its success are the clinical skills and integrity of the forensic psychiatrist.

## Key Points

- Although a business plan is not mandatory to the development of a forensic psychiatric practice, as with any good business, it is an important component to consider.

- The primary value of a business plan to solo practitioners is that it forces them to engage in a structured review of how to achieve the vision for the practice.
- Lack of specific tactics produces more risk for a larger practice than for a solo practice. Because there are many more variables involved in group practice than solo practice, more structure is required than in the solo practice to ensure the achievement of business goals.
- The forensic expert should strive to develop sophisticated written and oral communication skills.
- The marketing of a forensic psychiatric practice will take care of itself if the forensic psychiatrist produces a superior work product, maintains honesty and objectivity at all times, provides a balance in forensic evaluations, and develops visibility in the legal and business communities.

## Practice Guidelines

1. Provide human interaction to schedule medicolegal clients.
2. Interact frequently with the legal and business communities.
3. Practice an objective, evidence-based medical model.
4. Embrace technology to improve efficiency.
5. Produce coherent, user-friendly reports.
6. Use clear, written contracts with clients.
7. Provide clear instructions to examinees.
8. Consider posting an Internet Web site.
9. Conduct weekly reviews with staff of future evaluations.
10. Constantly hone communication and teaching skills.
11. Keep clinical skills at a high level.
12. Review the budget and practice performance regularly.

## References

Abrahamson E: Change without pain. Harvard Business Review 78(4):75–79, 2000

Bradford JMW, Glancy G: Commentary on "insuring that forensic psychiatry thrives as a medical specialty in the 21st century." J Am Acad Psychiatry Law 28:20–22, 2000

Daubert v Merrell Dow Pharmaceuticals, Inc, 509 U.S. 579 (1993)

Granacher RP: The business aspects of forensic psychiatry. J Am Acad Psychiatry Law 29:216–224, 2001

Griffin J: How to Say It From the Heart. Paramus, NJ, Prentice-Hall, 2001

Gutheil TG, Simon RI: Mastering Forensic Psychiatric Practice: Advanced Strategies for the Expert Witness. Washington, DC, American Psychiatric Publishing, 2002

Kim WC, Mauborgne R: Charting your company's future. Harvard Business Review 80(6):77–83, 2002

Magretta J: Why business models matter. Harvard Business Review 80(5):86–92, 2002

Mandel S: Effective Presentation Skills, 3rd Edition. Menlo Park, CA, Crisp Learning, 2000

Oh. Stat. Rev., Rule 601 (D) (1980)

Pope HS, Butcher JN, Seelen J: The MMPI, MMPI-2, and MMPI-A in Court: A Practical Guide for Expert Witnesses and Attorneys, 2nd Edition. Washington, DC, American Psychological Association, 2000

Robert M: Strategy Pure and Simple: How Winning CEOs Outthink Their Competition. New York, McGraw-Hill, 1993, pp 27–28, 181–212

Tanay E: Letter. J Am Acad Psychiatry Law 28:113–115, 2000

Wiley MJ: Is your practice staffed correctly? Med Econ 79(12):66–73, 2002

## Suggested Readings

Berger SH: Establishing a Forensic Psychiatric Practice: A Practical Guide. New York, WW Norton, 1997

Granacher RP: The business aspects of forensic psychiatry. J Am Acad Psychiatry Law 29:216–224, 2001

Gutheil TG, Simon RI: Mastering Forensic Psychiatric Practice: Advanced Strategies for the Expert Witness. Washington, DC, American Psychiatric Publishing, 2002

# CHAPTER 4

# The Expert Witness

Thomas G. Gutheil, M.D.

## Introduction

*Cross-examining attorney:* Doctor, in your writings you have described the expert's "role." Are you admitting that you are faking your testimony?

*Psychiatric expert witness* [baffled]: I'm sorry, I don't understand the question.

*Attorney:* You repeatedly refer to the expert's "role," do you not?

*Expert* [catching on]: I see the problem! I'm not describing a role like that of an actor playing a part in a drama. I am describing the particular role function that an expert witness plays in the court system. I'm also indicating that your expert, who is also the plaintiff's treater, is in a role function incompatible with being an expert witness.

Every psychiatrist is expected to have some basic expertise in the field of psychiatry. Does that mean that every psychiatrist who ends up in a courtroom is consequently an expert witness? As the above excerpt from an actual trial suggests, the answer is "no," as "expert witness" is the name of a particular role function within the legal system. Although this chapter is specifically aimed at the psychiatric expert witness, the basic principles apply to experts in all fields of endeavor who might be called into court to play that role.

The role of expert witness most closely resembles a consultation coupled with teaching. The psychiatrist provides a consult to the attor-

---

I thank Robert Simon, M.D., members of the Program in Psychiatry and the Law, and James T. Hilliard, Esq., for useful comments.

ney, who draws on the psychiatrist's clinical knowledge to contribute to the psychiatric aspects of the legal case; the focus is on legal issues in legal—not clinical—contexts. In practical terms this means that forensic psychiatrists must become acclimatized to a system of thought composed of rules, assumptions about human nature, and basic philosophies often profoundly different from their own. Moreover, when you enter the legal system, you play by their rules. This telegraphs the fact that often the task of the forensic psychiatrist is best understood as a translation process, bridging two disparate realms of discourse: psychiatry and law.

The consultation also draws on the witness' skills as a teacher. First, the witness teaches the lawyer the relevant psychiatry in the case. Later, if the case goes to trial, he or she teaches the jury. Obviously both these teaching procedures require different approaches, imagery, and even vocabulary to be accomplished effectively in the respective contexts.

A second implication of the role of expert witness is that the forensic psychiatrist remains at heart a skilled and knowledgeable clinician even when translating data and concepts into those other realms. To function as an expert witness, the testifier need not be a forensic psychiatrist (though often such witnesses do have forensic training); what is required at a minimum is familiarity with the legal issues and context of the case, the ability to formulate a forensically relevant opinion, and the ability to testify usefully and to withstand cross-examination. All these qualities require that old standby—practice—and collaboration with the retaining attorney.

A *fact witness* is someone called into court to describe the observations of the five senses as they relate to a case; thus, the questions asked of that type of witness are variations on a theme, "What did you see (hear, smell, etc.)?" When a treating clinician is called to court to testify (as a fact witness) about a patient, the content of the testimony usually consists of direct observations of the patient and closely adherent concepts, such as diagnoses that the clinician reached or identification of the patient's behavior as a particular symptom or syndrome.

In contrast, an *expert witness,* after being qualified by the court, is entitled by that role to go beyond his or her own direct observations to draw inferences and express opinions based on the observations of others (such as medical records, other documents, and treaters or other witnesses) and to draw conclusions from those sources—conclusions that have legal significance, as the following vignettes will show.

Note that expert witnesses should be governed in their work by the ethical principles of honesty and striving for objectivity (American Academy of Psychiatry and Law 1995; see also Chapter 5: "Ethics in

Forensic Psychiatry," this volume). *Honesty* as used here is another aspect of truth telling, regardless of whether one is under oath at the time. *Striving for objectivity* refers to the efforts made by the expert to minimize bias factors that may derive from a host of sources.

Finally, psychiatrists usually enter the role of expert in two major ways. First, an attorney may ask you to serve that role because of a recommendation from a colleague or friend, your reputation, an article you wrote on the key subject, or another reason specific to you. This text is designed to make that transition easier and more effective.

Second, you may decide on your own to step into this challenging field. Textbooks (see the references and suggested readings at the end of this chapter), courses, and fellowships are available to help you with your basic knowledge and skills in this new role.

## Clinical Vignettes

### Vignette 1

A patient on suicide watch on an inpatient unit screams something then unexpectedly hurls himself through a window and dies from the fall. The family brings a malpractice suit against the treating psychiatrist, claiming that the suicide precautions were inadequate and that this inadequacy caused the suicide to be successful.

A different psychiatrist who happened to be passing nearby at the critical moment is called as a fact witness to tell the court what the man screamed, what his demeanor was, and who else was nearby. Here, the psychiatrist—though professionally trained in the field—is a bystander to the action and testifies as fact witness only on the data from her five senses.

The treating psychiatrist, now a defendant in the suit, is called as a fact witness to describe what the patient told her and her diagnoses, treatment plan, and observations of the patient, as well as what precautions she had instituted.

Yet another psychiatrist, not associated with the treatment team or hospital, is called by the plaintiff's attorney as an expert witness to testify regarding the "standard of care." The standard of care is usually defined as something like, "the care rendered by the average reasonable or prudent practitioner in similar circumstances"; the expert must be familiar with the exact wording of the standard for that jurisdiction. The standard of care in a malpractice context is the benchmark against which a particular patient's treatment is measured to determine whether the care was negligent—a conclusion drawn from all the data in the case. A comparable expert may be retained by the defense attorney to testify about how the care did not fall below that standard. The two experts between them, in an adversarial proceeding, lay out for the jury the strengths and weaknesses of the malpractice case. The jury ultimately decides whether or not the care provided was up to the standard.

## Vignette 2[1]

Dr. J helped Mrs. S leave her husband, whom she had described in treatment as abusive. In the subsequent custody battle following the divorce, Mrs. S's attorney asks for "a brief note on the therapy" to aid custody-related legal proceedings. Dr. J's note mentions the stress on Mrs. S. of child raising, her use of occasional diazepam for anxiety and to control excess alcohol use, and her efforts to leave a "sadomasochistic" relationship with her husband, labeled "a classic abuser." An unexpected subpoena designates Dr. J as "an expert," and during his "expert" deposition (examination under oath), the attorney reveals that his letter ("expert report") is interpreted as calling Mrs. S an inadequate mother, an abuser of alcohol and prescription drugs, and someone into "heavy S&M" paraphernalia. The attorney also notes that the husband is called a classic abuser without an examination. Much is made of an ethics code from the American Academy of Psychiatry and Law, an organization about which Dr. J has never heard. Dr. J's reaction is: "That isn't what I meant at all!"

Here Dr. J failed to grasp the basic paradigm shift involved in his now functioning in the expert witness role. There are a number of reasons why treaters in general should not serve as experts; these reasons are extensively explored elsewhere (Strasburger et al. 1997; see also Chapter 2: "Introduction to the Legal System," this volume). The most critical differences between treater and expert are that the clinician works only for the patient's welfare and the expert witness works for the truth, even if that might cause harm to the "examinee" (not "patient"); the expert warns the examinee about the lack of confidentiality in the examination and the need for objectivity under oath, come what may; and the empathic bond of treater with patient, so necessary for clinical work, would constitute a bias to the expert's forensically necessary objectivity.

Note also that the legal system may grasp for ethical standards from areas that the actual witness does not know. A consultation with a more experienced forensic psychiatrist might have averted some of these difficulties.

---

[1]Modified from Gutheil and Hilliard 2001.

## Vignette 3

A forensic psychiatrist had testified several years earlier in the trial of an alleged gangster as to his incompetence to be sentenced (a legal standard); on the basis of an extensive database and direct interview, the expert had offered the opinion for the subject's attorney that the subject was incompetent.

Years later in the context of an additional charge against the alleged gangster, the prosecution claimed to be calling the expert as a fact witness to certain data. The prosecutor played wiretapped tape recordings of the alleged gangster's recent conversations with family members and asked for the former expert's "reaction" to them. The former expert, now supposedly functioning as a fact witness, commented that the man sounded tired (data from the senses). The prosecutor pressed for more detailed responses. Sensing that the prosecutor was duplicitously seeking an essentially expert opinion (under fact witness guise) about the mental condition of the alleged gangster, the expert replied that such an opinion would ethically require a present expert evaluation of the total clinical picture, medical records, tests, and so on—and that no fact witness could provide such an opinion. The prosecutor left disappointed.

Here the contrast and tension between expert and fact roles constituted the crux of the psychiatrist's dilemma. The psychiatrist's challenge was to keep the narrow fact witness role clearly in mind despite having previously served in the expert role, despite the temptation to give an expert's view again, and despite the attorney's attempt to distort that role. As implied, an expert's role sometimes means protecting the truth from attorneys.

## Vignette 4

A novice expert witness observed that early in her career she felt extremely triumphant when the case was won by the side retaining her and extremely crestfallen when that side lost. A senior forensic consultant pointed out that, although this was a common early reaction, it constituted a form of bias by linking expert to outcome. In reality, he indicated, a case may be won or lost on a number of determinants including jury demographics; opening statements; the nature, appearance, and demeanor of plaintiff, defendant, attorneys, or judge; and the simple facts of the case itself. The pitfall created by a personal investment in case outcome was the danger of slanting testimony to achieve a particular result; the attorneys win or lose, the expert just testifies. The novice expert felt relieved from excess pressure and worked toward a more realistic and dispassionate emotional position consistent with greater objectivity.

## The Expert Witness Role

The expert witness role differs in significant ways from that of the treating clinician.

### Two Fundamental Forensic Questions

#### *Source of the Consultation*

The first question an expert witness must ask is, For whom am I working? The treater works unambiguously for the patient and the patient's welfare. The expert witness, in contrast, works for the retaining person or agency. The latter is both the employer that gives the expert standing to present an opinion and a source of potential bias.

#### *Scope of the Consultation*

The second question for the expert witness is, What, if any, is the psychiatric aspect of this case? or What is the forensic psychiatric question I am being asked to answer? This question may be more difficult to answer than it first appears. Some attorneys are regrettably unclear regarding the nature of psychiatry and what a forensic consultation can reasonably provide. Attorneys may want psychiatrists to fulfill certain roles, such as those of lie detector, illness curer, mind reader, or mind changer, that lie outside the purview of even modern psychiatry.

### The Issue of Bias

The bias issue is a vital element of expert witness work. Although no expert is bias-free in all circumstances, the expert's job description includes recognizing and overcoming any bias that may exist or arise. If the bias is insurmountable—for example, the defendant is a relative—the expert should not accept the case. Vignette 4 describes the bias aspects of feeling that you win the case as an expert. On the popular Las Vegas–based television show *CSI: Crime Scene Investigation,* the lead character, Dr. Grissom, commented, "Courts are like dice: they have no memory. What works this time may not work next time." Different contextual factors in the courtroom will similarly vary, and comparable expert testimony may be persuasive in one court and not the next.

What is the origin of bias? Working with an attorney may lead to liking or identifying with that attorney (or, for that matter, hating and being unable to identify with the attorney); these natural feelings may tempt experts to slant their assessments for (or against) the attorney's position in the case (Gutheil and Simon 2002).

Money may serve as a bias, and perhaps the most critical one: the attorney who retained you wants to use you, and you want to make a living and be retained again. These facts may create pressures to slant testimony—pressures the ethical expert must resist. The extreme proponent of this bias is the pejoratively labeled "hired gun." The hired gun sells testimony—is willing to say whatever the attorney wants for the fee—rather than charging for the time it takes to perform the expert tasks.

Sometimes expert witnesses may be retained directly by the court or judge. This neutral position tends somewhat to decrease the intensely adversarial nature of the process, but fierce cross-examination by one side or the other is likely inescapable and should be prepared for.

## The Expert's Database

The novice expert often falls into the misperception that the clinical interview of the plaintiff or defendant or the current medical records are all that one needs to assess. Instead, in many cases the database on which the opinion is based should extend beyond the immediate context. The term *database* refers to the totality of materials—records, legal documents, police and witness reports, and so forth—that are reviewed by the expert in assessing a case (Gutheil 1998b).

The database may include interviews of litigants and, sometimes, psychological testing. Some useful guidelines for these examinations are provided by Simon and Wettstein (1997). Perhaps the most important step in these interviews is to provide the examinee with warnings (Gutheil 1998b) that distinguish the forensic proceeding, which takes place in an adversarial context, from the more familiar clinical interview, which is devoted to a patient's welfare. The examinee should be warned about the nonconfidentiality of the interview; the unpredictable, not necessarily favorable, effect of its conclusions; the freedom of the examinee to take breaks and to refrain from answering questions; and the freedom to consult with an attorney as desired.

There are, of course, exceptions. A defendant's competence to stand trial is based almost entirely on a here-and-now, present-state examination (see Chapter 7: "The Forensic Examination and Report," this volume), but the expert is usually obligated, as noted, to review comprehensively many data sources, depending on the nature of the case, such as past medical, school, and military records; legal documents such as deposition transcripts, interrogatories, and affidavits; witness and police reports; and similar materials. In addition, the expert should compare these items one with another to seek inconsistencies, contradictions, or corroborations that may emerge from such comparative processes.

The expert should insist on obtaining all relevant data. Regrettably, an occasional attorney will withhold even critical data for reasons of cost, expediency, or venality; alternatively, shortcuts, such as a deposition or record summary instead of the whole document, will be offered. These maneuvers should be resisted and, if continued, may serve as grounds to withdraw from the case, as such maneuvers compromise the expert's necessarily comprehensive view of the case.

## The Opinion

The development of the preliminary opinion about the merits of the case is the "go–no go" pivot point. After careful review of the entire database, the expert must decide whether—from a forensic psychiatric viewpoint—the case has merit for the retaining side. This may be a black-and-white issue or one of shades of gray. With strict candor, the expert shares that opinion in all its complexity with the retaining attorney. The attorney now makes an independent decision as to whether that expert can help the case. If not, the parties part in a friendly manner. If so, the expert may or may not write a report about the opinion, may or may not be deposed (examined under oath) by the opposing attorney or attorneys, and may or may not actually testify in court. This last task depends on the host of vicissitudes to which cases are subject, such as varying jurisdictional rules, attorney strategies, and successful challenges to the admissibility of the opinion, settlement, dismissal, mistrial, summary judgment, and the like.

In "gray-zone" cases the expert and attorney may have to negotiate the extent, limits, and boundaries of the expert's opinions. This is the art of forensic work (Gutheil and Simon 2002). The expert often walks a tightrope between maintaining flexibility as to phrasing and emphasis and altering substantive aspects of the opinion under attorney pressures (Gutheil and Simon 1999; Gutheil et al. 2001). Probably no guiding factor is as critical here as actual experience.

This negotiation is especially common regarding expert reports, which provide a durable record of the expert's opinion and may be used at trial to assert a point or to challenge or impeach the report's author. Attempts by the retaining attorney to alter substantive elements of the report must be resisted. Changes in wording (e.g., to match precisely statutory language) can usually be accepted but may have to be acknowledged on cross-examination.

Note that not all experts are chosen with the goal of ultimately testifying. The "consulting expert" may play several behind-the-scenes roles such as guiding the attorney's literature search, identifying impeaching data about the other side's expert opinion, and aiding in jury selection. For various reasons (Strasburger et al. 1997), the consulting expert should usually not move into the testifying role.

## Qualification

Although any psychiatrist with adequate training and experience may demonstrate expertise in treatment, consultation, lectures, or articles, an expert witness is essentially defined by being so qualified by a court. One might informally say that an expert is anyone whom the court qualifies as an expert (Gutheil 1998b). Support for this broad statement may be drawn from the fact that residents in training may be qualified as expert witnesses for hospital-based commitment hearings (though, of course, the functional role of supplying the court with observed data more closely resembles that of fact witness).

Qualification of an expert is a stage in court proceedings in which the attorney who retained the expert reviews before the court the expert's general and specific credentials and experiences that suit the expert to render opinions in this particular case. After such review, the attorney formally or informally proffers the witness as an expert to the court. The attorney for the other side of the case may accept the witness, argue about accepting the witness, ask the witness questions to probe his or her credentials further, challenge the suitability of the witness or of the witness's methodology as in the next section, and so on. The opposing attorney's approach just described is termed "voir dire" (loosely translated, "see what [the expert] will say"). The judge rules on the matter, and the expert either becomes or does not become an expert witness.

## New Expert Thresholds

Forensic psychiatrists and courts have both been troubled by the arrival in courtroom testimony of what has been called "junk science" (Gutheil and Bursztajn 2003). This term refers to expert opinions that are based on specious, idiosyncratic, or unsupported testimony that does not draw on current scientific evidence but instead appears to flow from the expert's wish to persuade the jury, willy-nilly, about the point at issue.

An important series of decisions by the U.S. Supreme Court—*Daubert v. Merrell Dow Pharmaceuticals, Inc.* (1993), *General Electric Co. v. Joiner* (1997), and *Kumho Tire Co. Ltd. v. Carmichael* (1999)—coupled with the Federal Rules of Evidence that govern federal courts, have addressed the thresholds for admissibility of expert testimony in the federal court system; a number of state courts have also adopted the general principles involved. The first such case, *Daubert v. Merrill Dow Pharmaceuticals, Inc.* (1993), designated trial judges as screeners (called "gatekeepers") of expert testimony before it is presented to the jury; the later two cases, *General Electric Co. v. Joiner* (1997) and *Kumho Tire Co. Ltd. v. Carmichael* (1999), essentially refined the details. The requirements of the cases gave rise to the possibility of "*Daubert* hearings": preliminary hearings before the judge to determine whether the expert's testimony met the essential criteria of relevance and reliability. That is, the expert's opinion had to be based on science relevant to the case at hand, and the methodology used to reach the opinion had to be based on reliable science. The court suggested some criteria for reliability such as established professional opinion, peer-reviewed literature, known error rates, and the like (*Daubert v. Merrell Dow Pharmaceuticals, Inc.* 1993). Although not constituting a definitive checklist, these criteria may be useful for the expert to keep in mind in preparation of an opinion.

In this series of cases, in addition to defining the practice for federal courts, the Supreme Court has set the conceptual bar for expert testimony and provided some guidance as to what level of support the expert's opinion must have before it is presented to any court. Experts are thus advised to be clear about their methodology in presenting an opinion.

## Standard for Opinions

The expert expresses opinions to "a reasonable [degree of] medical certainty" (Rappeport 1985). This legal term does not mean "certainty" in its common usage. Rather, what the expert expresses as an opinion must be true "more likely than not" in many jurisdictions (though this standard should be checked for your jurisdiction). Although "more likely than not" is the common phrasing, it may be expressed as "reasonable psychiatric (or psychological) certainty," "reasonable medical probability," or similar phrasings. The meanings are similar, but the expert should consult with the retaining attorney to clarify the local standard and its exact wording.

The expert's testimonial threshold (standard for testimony) of reasonable medical certainty should be distinguished from the standard of proof that a judge or jury must reach to render a verdict. Depending on jurisdiction, the standard may be "preponderance of the evidence," "clear and convincing evidence," or "beyond a reasonable doubt." Thus, the jury is operating at a different, and legally driven, threshold from that of the expert.

As earlier noted, the third standard relevant to expert witness practice is the standard expressed in the criteria for the issue; for example, the standard for competence to stand trial. These criteria are usually established by legal statutes but may be formed in case law, the ultimate decision in a relevant legal case.

## Common Pitfalls in Expert Witness Practice

Even experienced expert witnesses are vulnerable to the narcissistic pitfall of feeling that the case is in their hands, to win or lose at will, or that they are somehow the center of the case. In reality, operating in a foreign environment such as the courtroom (Gutheil 1998a), experts are lucky to be able to shape even their own testimony, as admissibility considerations, vigorous cross-examination with attempts to distort that opinion, and the limitations of the attorneys on both sides may conspire to make the expert's goal—teaching the jury something useful about the psychiatric aspects of the case—frustratingly incomplete.

The true position of the expert was beautifully captured by Robert Simon (personal communication, December 1998), who noted that "the expert witness is a hood ornament on the vehicle of litigation, not the engine." Accepting this image should inspire proper expert humility.

A related pitfall is the illusion of control. Although an expert may use skill, training, and experience to provide a clear, data-based, and persuasive opinion in direct testimony, much of what happens in the courtroom beyond that point, including the jury's ultimate decision, is quite outside the expert's control. This reality limitation must be accepted if one wishes to work within the court system.

Beginning experts may encounter the "clinical pitfall" as well. Confronted with a strange setting in court, the novice expert may retreat to the belief that familiar clinical considerations will apply to this new world: that the court has a therapeutic purpose or intent; that the welfare of the patient, party, or examinee is paramount in everyone's mind; and that being helpful to a victim or a mentally ill person is the shared goal.

None of these principles apply. The legal system operates on time-honored precedents aimed at a perception of fairness and is not driven by primary clinical concerns such as doing no harm, even to ill persons. Furthermore, instead of operating as current clinicians do in an alliance-based collaborative team approach, the law operates within an adversarial system whose representatives attempt, in essence, to thwart—not aid—each other.

Perhaps the most subtle and challenging pitfall for the beginner is the failure to understand the fundamental and profound difference between the attorney's appropriate and unconflicted partisanship in a case—an essential element of the adversary model—and the expert's needed nonpartisan objectivity. Put another way, the attorney advocates for the retaining party and advocates energetically for that side to win the case. The expert, having painstakingly formed an opinion, advocates only for that opinion and energetically attempts, within the limits of courtroom rules, to prevent that opinion from being inappropriately distorted, misrepresented, or obscured by cross-examination.

A clinician usually functions by scheduling various clinical activities, from patient appointments to Grand Rounds, in a regular and systematic manner. This may make the legal system's quite irregular approach confusing and demoralizing to the beginner. Beyond the classic "hurry up and wait" rhythm of the courtroom, the novice expert must learn to expect last-minute postponements, continuances, precipitous calls into court on short notice, and other manifestations of chaos theory.

## Out-of-State Practice and Its Vicissitudes

As part of a multifocal effort to thwart "hired gun" testimony, in which out-of-state experts are viewed as coming into a state and testifying as to the standard of care to which local doctors must be held, some states and the American Medical Association have taken steps aimed at containing or controlling hired-gun practice. Some states demand that the expert be licensed in the state of testimony or that the expert have spent a specified percentage of time in defined clinical practice. In a curious move, the American Medical Association has taken the position that forensic work is the practice of medicine, with the apparent aim of permitting control of expert testimony through peer review or board of registration complaints (Zonana 1999). This organizational decision, of course, does not resolve the ethical, legal, or clinical dilemmas of an expert being considered a (treating) clinician (Simon and Shuman 1999; Strasburger et al. 1997). In the same time frame, ethics complaints and attempted civil suits against experts have increased.

## Conclusion

Despite its many pitfalls and the inherent challenge of shifting paradigms from a treatment context, the role of expert witness presents many opportunities both to teach and to assist the legal system. The intellectual stimulation of attempting to translate among differing realms of discourse also provides great reward. When the task is properly and ethically undertaken, the expert witness can make a significant contribution to this specialized area of psychiatric practice.

## Key Points

- The expert witness draws conclusions from the database; the fact witness reports on data from the five senses.
- The first forensic question is, For whom am I working?
- The second forensic question is, What is the forensic psychiatric question I am being asked to answer?
- The expert is qualified by the court to give testimony that is reasonable and reliable.
- The expert's opinion is given to reasonable medical certainty.
- The novice expert witness may encounter pitfalls of narcissism, illusions of control, clinical reasoning, and complexities of expert advocacy. Similar to countertransference, these should be countered.

## Practice Guidelines

1. Understand the meaning of the expert's role functions in the legal system.
2. Thoroughly review the database, and request missing pieces from the attorney.
3. Derive an opinion supportable by the evidence in the database; this may mean telling the retaining attorney that you cannot support the case. Be morally, financially, and psychologically prepared to turn down a case that has no merit.
4. Strive to overcome bias, or failing this, pass on the case. The overarching principles of honesty and striving for objectivity should govern the process.
5. In gray-zone cases, negotiate with the attorney about the limits and boundaries of the opinion, permitting flexibility but resisting attorney pressures for substantive changes.
6. Do not, with some exceptions, serve as expert witness for your own patients. In rare cases—geographic unavailability of other clinicians or unique training or knowledge—you may be drafted into the expert role, though this may alter the treatment relationship.
7. Accept and prepare for the chaotic time lines of the legal system.

## References

American Academy of Psychiatry and the Law: Ethical Guidelines for the Practice of Forensic Psychiatry. Bloomfield, CT, American Academy of Psychiatry and the Law, 1995

Daubert v Merrell Dow Pharmaceuticals, Inc, 509 U.S. 579 (1993)

General Electric Co v Joiner, 522 U.S. 136 (1997)
Gutheil TG: The Psychiatrist in Court: A Survival Guide. Washington, DC, American Psychiatric Press, 1998a
Gutheil TG: The Psychiatrist as Expert Witness. Washington, DC, American Psychiatric Publishing, 1998b
Gutheil TG, Bursztajn H: Avoiding *ipse dixit* mislabeling: post *Daubert* approaches to expert clinical opinions. J Am Acad Psychiatry Law 31(2):205–210, 2003
Gutheil TG, Hilliard JT: The treating psychiatrist thrust into the expert role. Psychiatr Serv 52:1526–1527, 2001
Gutheil TG, Simon RI: Attorneys' pressures on the expert witness: early warning sings of endangered honesty, objectivity and fair compensation. J Am Acad Psychiatry Law 27:546–553, 1999
Gutheil TG, Simon RI: Mastering Forensic Psychiatric Practice: Advanced Strategies for the Expert Witness, Washington, DC, American Psychiatric Publishing, 2002
Gutheil TG, Commons ML, Miller PM: Withholding, seducing and threatening: a pilot study of further attorney pressures on expert witnesses. J Am Acad Psychiatry Law 29:336–339, 2001
Kumho Tire Co, Ltd v Carmichael, 119 S. Ct. 1167 (1999)
Rappeport JR: Reasonable medical certainty. Bull Am Acad Psychiatry Law 13: 5–15, 1985
Simon RI, Shuman DW: Conducting forensic examinations on the road: are you practicing your profession without a license? J Am Acad Psychiatry Law 27:75–82, 1999
Simon RI, Wettstein RM: Toward the development of guidelines for the conduct of forensic psychiatric examinations. J Am Acad Psychiatry Law 25:17–30, 1997
Strasburger LH, Gutheil TG, Brodsky A: On wearing two hats: role conflict in serving as both psychotherapist and expert witness. Am J Psychiatry 154: 448–456, 1997
Zonana H: Medical director's report. Newsletter of the American Academy of Psychiatry and the Law 24:3–4, 1999

## Suggested Readings

Berger S: Establishing a Forensic Psychiatric Practice. New York, WW Norton, 1997
Babitsky S, Mangravitti JJ: How to Excel During Cross-Examination: Techniques for Experts That Work. Falmouth, MA, SEAK, 1997
Brodsky SL: Testifying in Court: Guidelines and Maxims for the Expert Witness. Washington, DC, American Psychological Association, 1991
Gutheil TG: The Psychiatrist in Court: A Survival Guide. Washington, DC, American Psychiatric Press, 1998
Gutheil TG: The Psychiatrist as Expert Witness. Washington, DC, American Psychiatric Press, 1998
Gutheil TG: The psychiatric expert witness. Psychiatric Times 19(April): 37–39, 2002

Gutheil TG, Simon RI: Mastering Forensic Psychiatric Practice: Advanced Strategies for the Expert Witness. Washington, DC, American Psychiatric Publishing, 2002

Feder HA: Succeeding as an Expert Witness. Glenwood Springs, CO, Tageh Press, 1993

Malligan W: Expert Witnesses: Direct and Cross Examination. New York, Wiley, 1987

Melton GB, Petrilla J, Poythress NG, et al (eds): Psychological Evaluations for the Courts: A Handbook for Mental Health Professionals and Lawyers, 3rd Edition. New York, Guilford, 1997

Poynter D: The Expert Witness Handbook: Tips and Techniques for the Litigation Consultant, 2nd Edition. Santa Barbara, CA, Para, 1997

CHAPTER 5

# Ethics in Forensic Psychiatry

Robert Weinstock, M.D.

Liza H. Gold, M.D.

## Introduction

Forensic psychiatrists function at the interface of psychiatry and the law, two disciplines based on different ethical values. These differences may at times create challenging dilemmas in forensic practice. The majority of forensic cases lend themselves to noncontroversial ethical solutions. Nevertheless, complex problems may arise, particularly when practitioners are unfamiliar with basic forensic ethical principles and guidelines.

Clinical psychiatrists beginning forensic practice, as well those more experienced in forensic psychiatry, can easily fall into some common ethical pitfalls. Ethical violations, even when inadvertent, can compromise the psychiatrist's credibility in court and his or her professional reputation. They can even lead to sanctions against the practitioner by medical licensing boards and professional organizations. Thus, clinicians interested in the challenge of practicing forensic psychiatry should consider familiarity with forensic ethics an essential part of their knowledge base. This chapter reviews the sometimes conflicting forensic, clinical, and legal ethical principles that clinicians may encounter in forensic cases.

## Forensic Ethics: Bases and Analysis

Different levels of ethical values and imperatives can be found in any professional field. Those unconcerned with ethical analysis may operate from a basis of "minimalist" ethics, which refers to the practice of merely figuring out how to stay out of trouble (Weinstock 1997). Such individuals are satisfied to know enough to avoid ethical sanctions. The fact that one has avoided ethical sanctions, however, does not mean that well-reasoned ethical judgments have been made or that a chosen course of action is the best one. Most professionals want to go beyond this minimum level of effort; they try to practice from a basis of aspirational ethics (Dyer 1988; Weinstock 1997). This involves performing an informed analysis with some level of sophistication to determine the most appropriate and ethical course of action in a complex situation.

The development of ethical frameworks specifically applicable to forensic psychiatry is a relatively new development. Stone (1984) was among the first to challenge forensic psychiatry to define the ethical basis of the field. Although not all of his concerns have been completely addressed, forensic psychiatry as a profession has gone a long way toward clarifying its ethical underpinnings.

A number of ethical frameworks for the practice of forensic psychiatry have been proposed. Appelbaum (1997) based his approach to forensic ethics on the principles of truth telling, respect for persons, and justice. Griffith (1998) proposed a narrative ethical framework in forensic evaluation that is sensitive to the issues of individuals who come from nondominant cultures. His approach took into account the power differential between dominant and minority social groups.

Candilis et al. (2001) developed a robust conception of professional integrity that integrated these approaches. They favored allowing forensic ethical principles to at times include the traditional role of medicine as a healing profession. In some circumstances, forensic psychiatrists could function in a more therapeutic role. For example, a psychiatrist may be asked to evaluate a severely medically ill patient's competence to make a decision to stop life-sustaining treatment. The psychiatrist might find the most appropriate approach involved working with the patient and family to help them communicate effectively and arrive at a decision acceptable to everybody concerned, as opposed to restricting the role solely to answering the legal question in an adversarial manner. In contrast, other forensic ethicists (Ciccone and Clements 2001) would conceptualize such an intervention as temporarily stepping out of the forensic role.

Some authors have emphasized that even though forensic and clinical ethics differ, medical principles still inform certain areas of forensic ethics. Weinstock et al. (1990), as well as Candilis et al. (2001), consider traditional medical values and ethics an important factor in balancing the forensic psychiatrist's conflicting ethical responsibilities. Weinstock (1998, 2001) concurred with Appelbaum's opinion that the forensic psychiatrist's primary duty is to the legal system. However, Weinstock believed this primary duty should be balanced against secondary duties, derived from medical ethics, such as that of nonmaleficence to an evaluee. In some circumstances this secondary duty can outweigh the primary duty and become the dominant consideration. For example, this secondary duty may result in refusal to participate in restoring a prisoner's competence to be executed or refusal to present aggravating circumstances to a jury considering a death penalty.

Ethical analysis of a problem requires clarification of the issue, the criteria to be employed in its analysis, and the differentiation of relevant ethical and nonethical issues, regardless of the ethical framework used. Gutheil et al. (1991) reduced ethical decisions into their component parts to arrive at actual practical decisions. They distinguished professional ethics, personal ethics (morals), and medical, legal, and policy factors. Through decision analysis, they identified ethical assumptions and biases and articulated relevant values. For example, some professionals hold the opinion that some actions (such as certain death penalty roles) violate professional ethics, even though professional organizations currently only prohibit participation in a legally authorized execution (narrowly defined). Psychiatrists may oppose certain actions because of personal views about the death penalty based on personal ethical (moral) grounds, a religious basis, or social policy considerations. Some may oppose the death penalty personally but have no problem with certain professional roles. Others may support the death penalty personally but believe certain roles are not proper for a physician. Such analyses clarify the bases for various assumptions and considerations and can help in arriving at the best ethical decision.

Rosner (1997) articulated a four-step model for the analysis of ethical issues similar to his model for the analysis of forensic psychiatric issues. He recommended that decision-makers first state the ethical issue, describe the criteria to be considered in analyzing the ethical issue, accumulate the relevant data, and then apply the data to the criteria for the ethical issue.

## Forensic Psychiatry, the Practice of Medicine, and Conflicting Ethical Duties

Such frameworks and analyses are essential to balance the conflicting duties and values that arise in the practice of forensic psychiatry. Ethical conflicts are not unique to forensic practice. All areas of psychiatric practice may at times raise problems that require balancing professional obligations. Any psychiatric role may involve competing responsibilities, with the potential to be a "double agent." For example, treating psychiatrists encounter such problems when the law requires them to place the welfare of society over that of an individual patient. Examples of such legal requirements include mandatory reporting of child abuse and Tarasoff warnings (Weinstock 1998). Society has made the decision that in such cases, the greater good is more important than the welfare of the individual. Nevertheless, these legal duties place treating psychiatrists in the position of potentially causing harm to their patients.

When forensic psychiatrists act as consultants to the legal system, they bring their medical skills to a system with values and priorities different from those of their own profession. The goal of clinical psychiatry is to help patients according to the principles and values of medicine. The goal of the law is to resolve disputes; truth and justice are its paramount priorities. The law may also serve to fulfill purposes such as retribution, deterrence, and rehabilitation, but in recent years, rehabilitation has had less priority. Although it is rarely required in clinical psychiatry, the legal system is willing to cause harm to an individual to achieve its goals.

Thus, at times, the practice of forensic psychiatry requires the balancing of conflicting duties and traditional medical values (Candilis 2001; Hundert 1990; Weinstock 1998, 2001; Weinstock et al. 1990). The psychiatrist's role in litigation is to assist the court in adjudicating legal issues. Forensic psychiatry is rooted in the clinical and ethical principles of medical practice and uses skills that were developed to help patients. However, the practices and ethics of the traditional doctor-patient relationship do not apply to forensic evaluations. No treatment relationship is established with the evaluee. The goal of the forensic evaluation is to form a legally relevant opinion, not to provide treatment.

Psychiatrists generally do not consider the provision of expert services and courtroom testimony to be the practice of medicine. Nevertheless, they should bear in mind that medical values and ethics are still relevant when they use their professional skills and knowledge to provide forensic services. In fact, some state medical boards, as well as the American Medical Association (AMA), have stated that forensic testimony does constitute the practice of medicine. The AMA considers courtroom testimony subject to peer review as well as state medical board action. Moreover, the AMA has indicated that it will assist medical organizations in disciplining physicians who testify falsely against their colleagues and will report its findings to state licensing boards (American Medical Association 2003b). Ethical violations, even in the provision of forensic services, may result in medical board sanctions (American Medical Association 2003a, 2003b, 2003d; Appelbaum 2001; Binder 2002; Simon and Shuman 1999; Weinstock and Garrick 1995).

## Professional Ethical Guidance

### Clinical Vignette

Dr. D was called by the district attorney (DA) and asked to perform a forensic evaluation on an individual in jail who had just been arrested for a serious crime. The DA said that he wanted the prisoner evaluated before he was arraigned and had a chance to talk to an attorney who might advise him not to cooperate. The DA told Dr. D that he could inform the evaluee of the purpose and lack of confidentiality of the evaluation. When Dr. D raised concerns about the ethics of an evaluation under such circumstances, the DA told him this procedure was legal in the jurisdiction and that other psychiatrists had conducted evaluations under these circumstances. Dr. D was not convinced but wanted to get future referrals, as he was just starting his forensic practice. What should Dr. D do?

Dr. D consulted his professional organizations' ethical guidelines. He found that the American Academy of Psychiatry and the Law (AAPL) and the American Psychiatric Association (APA) have specifically addressed this problem (AAPL 1995; American Psychiatric Association 2001a). Both organizations consider forensic evaluations of criminal defendants before access to or availability of legal counsel unethical. Defendants may not be in a position to give truly informed consent before consulting an attorney. They may not fully understand their situation or be aware that the psychiatrist retained by the DA may be biased in favor of the prosecution. Thus, AAPL and the APA consider a psychiatrist who conducts an evaluation under such circumstances to be in violation of professional ethics.

The guidelines allow that Dr. D could see the prisoner if Dr. D only intended to provide treatment. If treatment is needed, however, Dr. D should limit his interventions to the prisoner's immediate clinical needs and avoid discussion of details related to his state of mind at the time of the crime. After reviewing these guidelines, Dr. D contacted the DA, explained the ethical problem, and offered to conduct the evaluation after the prisoner had spoken to his attorney.

Psychiatrists may be asked to provide professional services that are legally ethical and permissible but may violate forensic ethical principles. Professional organizations have provided guidelines that address many of the common ethical dilemmas created by such conflicts and can help psychiatrists determine the most appropriate course of action. Anyone beginning a forensic practice should consider these guidelines required reading. Experienced forensic psychiatrists should also review them regularly.

AAPL (1995) has published ethical guidelines specifically for the practice of forensic psychiatry. The APA provides annotations to the AMA's *Principles of Medical Ethics* (American Psychiatric Association 2001a), many of which are relevant to forensic psychiatry. AAPL is currently revising its ethical guidelines in response to recent revisions to the AMA's *Principles of Medical Ethics* (American Medical Association 2003e) and ongoing revisions to the APA's annotations to the *Principles.* Many opinions of the APA ethics committee (American Psychiatric Association 2001b) also are relevant and involve forensic psychiatric issues.

Other organizations also have guidelines that may be relevant to forensic practice. Psychiatrists providing forensic services for children and adolescents should be familiar with the ethical guidelines of the American Academy of Child and Adolescent Psychiatry. The American Academy of Forensic Sciences (AAFS) has an ethical code that it enforces for its own members. The AAFS ethical code's main provisions forbid distortion of data and credentials (American Academy of Forensic Sciences 2002). Its Committee on Good Forensic Practice developed aspirational guidelines for good forensic practice.

Familiarity with professional ethical guidelines is more than academically useful. Most ethical issues that arise in forensic psychiatry fall within the APA's jurisdiction and thus are subject to the same procedure for enforcement or sanction as any other ethical violation. The APA enforces its ethics through its local district branches according to its own administrative process (American Psychiatric Association 2001a). If Dr. D had conducted the examination under the circumstances requested by the DA, despite professional ethical prohibitions, he might be subject to sanctions through his local APA district branch. If the forensic psychiatrist does not belong to the APA, state medical boards or equivalent organizations provide the only means of enforcement and can at times be especially punitive.

The AAPL guidelines are not necessarily subject to enforcement. AAPL refers complaints about ethical violations to the APA and relies on the APA's administrative process to address them. The APA will only sanction behavior that violates its own ethical standards. However, the ethical principle of refraining from an evaluation unless the prisoner has had access to counsel is included in the APA's annotations to the AMA's *Principles* (American Psychiatric Association 2001a). Thus, if Dr. D had examined the prisoner before the prisoner had an opportunity to consult an attorney in the hopes of getting future referrals, he would have violated both the APA and AAPL ethical guidelines.

Moreover, Dr. D would likely not have advanced his forensic career by violating his professional ethics. Failure to adhere to professional ethical guidelines may result in challenges to the admissibility of the expert's testimony. Legal scholars have recently suggested that serious ethical violations are "red flags" that should alert the court to closely examine the expert's reliability (Greenberg and Shuman 1997; Jansonius and Gould 1998). Such legal experts suggest that unexcused violations of a relevant professional ethical rule should result in a presumption in favor of exclusion of that testimony. It may be argued that the identification of ethical or other professional violations should speak to the weight rather than the admissibility of such testimony (R.I. Simon, personal communication, April 2000). Nevertheless, the degree to which examiners adhere to professional ethical guidelines will have some bearing on both the admissibility and the credibility of their testimony.

## Honesty and Striving for Objectivity

The ethical imperative to strive for honesty and objectivity in the forensic practice of psychiatry is the basis of the value, and ultimately the admissibility and credibility, of such testimony to the courts. Expert opinions, regardless of their technical expertise, can assist the court only when the fact finder can be assured that such opinions are honest and that the expert has tried to be objective.

### Clinical Vignette

Dr. A had been developing a professional relationship with a local defense attorney. At the attorney's request, Dr. A performed a forensic psychiatric evaluation on a criminal defendant. Dr. A reached an opinion that the evaluee had a delusional disorder and met the legal criteria for an insanity defense in the jurisdiction in question. He submitted a draft of his report for review to the attorney. The attorney suggested some changes in wording to make the opinion clearer, corrected a spelling error, and improved the grammar. The attorney also pointed out a minor factual inaccuracy regarding the defendant's past history. He asked Dr. A to alter his report to include these observations.

The attorney then asked Dr. A whether he could change his diagnosis to schizophrenia to strengthen the opinion. The attorney had read psychiatric literature that indicated unresolved debate regarding the validity of the diagnosis of delusional disorder. The defense attorney was concerned that the prosecution expert might characterize the delusions as merely obsessional fixed ideas in a paranoid personality. He believed a diagnosis of schizophrenia would be less vulnerable to challenge by the opposing expert and said he might not be able to use the report unless Dr. A changed the diagnosis. Although Dr. A acknowledged some diagnostic uncertainty, he still believed that delusional disorder was the appropriate diagnosis. Is it ethical to make the changes?

Dr. A told the defense attorney that he could make the minor changes as discussed but could not ethically change his diagnosis. The retaining attorney would need to decide whether or not to use Dr. A's report. Dr. A recognized that his desire for "repeat business" from the attorney was biasing him toward making the substantial change the attorney requested. However, Dr. A was familiar with the AAPL guidelines that stress that forensic psychiatrists are ethically obligated to provide honest assessments and strive for objectivity in their evaluations (AAPL 1995). He decided not to compromise his ethical integrity despite the risk that he might not get future business from this attorney. He also considered it might be best not to become involved in future cases with this attorney if the attorney would insist on Dr. A violating his professional ethics.

The psychiatrist's opinion may not be helpful to the retaining attorney's case. That does not mean that the psychiatrist should change an opinion that has been objectively and honestly provided. Psychiatrists can ethically accept changes in wording that correct factual inaccuracies and that help clarify the opinion so long as they do not change the opinion in any substantive way. They may also accept changes that address issues of law that were not addressed accurately or adequately in the original report. However, revising the diagnosis to strengthen the attorney's case would substantially change the psychiatrist's opinion. Thus, this change is not ethical. Even a change that only alters the emphasis or "spin" of the opinion would be dishonest and would represent a violation of the forensic ethical requirement of honesty (AAPL 1995; Diamond 1990). Attorneys who do not feel that an expert's honest opinion is of use to their clients are free to hire another expert.

In the past some psychiatrists (Pollack 1974) claimed that the ethical obligation of forensic psychiatrists was to be impartial and unbiased. Diamond (1959) argued that biases and desires to defend an opinion preclude the possibility that forensic psychiatrists could be truly impartial. AAPL's ethics committee recognized these practical realities and revised the current ethical guidelines (AAPL 1995) to require honesty and an effort to be objective, despite inevitable personal, professional, and adversarial biases.

The practical meaning of objectivity is a complex philosophical issue. Biases are inherent in all human endeavors. Absolute objectivity is not attainable regardless of approach or methodology. To further complicate matters, the "truth" is rarely black and white. Many perspectives can be equally valid. In the judicial system, the philosophical issues regarding objectivity and factual truth are managed, to some extent, by the use of differing standards of proof. Those used are chosen on the basis of the seriousness of the charge or offense in question. In science, these issues are addressed, at least in part, by use of the scientific method.

Legal and forensic ethics create conflict between attorneys and psychiatrists in this area perhaps more than any other and commonly create the type of problem confronted by Dr. A. Legal ethics require attorneys to be zealous advocates for their clients. Attorneys are expected to "spin" their clients' cases in any way possible, short of telling untruths and other legally unethical practices, to help them win. In contrast, experts are obligated to provide honest opinions to the court, having taken an oath to "tell the truth, the whole truth, and nothing but the truth," unlike attorneys. Experts may also be required to submit their reports under penalty of perjury.

The adversarial legal system provides numerous opportunities for increased partiality and decreased objectivity. Advocacy bias—that is, the pressure to conform opinions to assist the retaining attorney—is one such influence. The partisan nature of the legal system exposes forensic psychiatrists to the potential for both overt pressure and subtle bias to distort their opinions to the retaining attorney's benefit. This pressure may become stronger when the expert is retained repeatedly by the same attorney and becomes dependent on these referrals as a source of income. Nevertheless, forensic psychiatrists should adhere to their ethical obligations to perform an honest evaluation and be as objective as possible. They must not accept pressures to conform their opinions to the desires of the retaining attorney.

Other types of advocacy bias may also be difficult to avoid. Indeed, the *Ake* case (*Ake v. Oklahoma* 1985) implied that in some circumstances, advocacy by an expert was appropriate. In addition, human nature is such that avoiding advocacy for one's own opinion is difficult (Diamond 1959). Various models of honest advocacy have been proposed that address some of these conflicts (Diamond 1992; Gutheil 1998). These models advise that ethical problems should not arise so long as advocacy for the opinion is honest and based on objective facts.

Biases other than those related to advocacy can influence forensic psychiatric evaluations. On an interpersonal level, some evaluees are simply more likable than others. All professionals have personal opinions and biases on social issues that may arise in legal cases. Some favor punishing criminal defendants and protecting society; others see the defendants more as victims of social circumstances. Some sympathize in civil cases with people who have an impairment, regardless of cause; others are concerned with abuses of the legal system that can result in higher insurance premiums. Some psychiatrists allow biases based on their personal beliefs or morals to influence them to always testify in a certain way. For example, regardless of the facts in a specific case, such experts might testify for the prosecution or defense in a death penalty case based on their personal ethics regarding this controversial sentence.

Such biases do not preclude the ability to adhere to the ethical obligation to strive for objectivity. The influence of any type of bias on the ability to provide honest and objective testimony depends to a great extent on how that bias is defined and on the degree to which it is present. Personal preferences, attitudes, and professional biases ordinarily do not rise to a level that adversely influences expert opinions. Even the presence of significant bias regarding a particular case may not necessarily prove deleterious, provided the bias is recognized by the expert, who continues to strive for objectivity (Simon and Wettstein 1997).

Psychiatrists who do not adhere to this guideline may find that their failure to do so may have far-reaching consequences. The ethical directive for honesty and striving for objectivity recognizes that dishonest or biased testimony compromises the value of expert testimony. Psychiatrists who refuse to consider and address possible sources of bias are more vulnerable to challenges of the credibility of their testimony. Assessments that ignore or distort factual data or involve no attempt to obtain contrary data as a result of biasing influences are much easier to discredit in court and, thus, may ultimately harm the retaining attorney's client.

In addition, psychiatrists who do not provide honest testimony and strive for objectivity may undermine their personal reputations and credibility as well as the reputation and credibility of their profession. Finally, in failing to meet these ethical obligations, they also undermine the legal system by casting doubt on the usefulness and value of any expert testimony.

## The Problem of the Hired Gun

Discussions regarding the ethics of honesty and striving for objectivity inevitably turn to the widespread perceptions that expert testimony is inherently unethical. Psychiatrists, as well as other professionals who testify in court, are often referred to as "hired guns": individuals who provide testimony that reflects the opinions of those paying the experts' fees, regardless of the facts of the case. A computer search of court decisions that make or refer to derogatory statements concerning mental heath experts documented the perception among legal professionals that many such experts are unscrupulous (Mossman and Kapp 1998). A survey of forensic psychiatrists found they considered this perception the greatest ethical problem in forensic psychiatry (Weinstock 1986).

The existence of "the venal expert" has been described as "the bête noire of forensic work" (Gutheil and Simon 1999, p. 552). These practices are troublesome and difficult to control. Nevertheless, they "pose few ethical puzzles . . . they are obviously wrong" (Mossman 1994, p. 348). The unethical basis of the practice of "hired guns," whether for money or for a cause, is easily distinguished from the stance of honest advocacy (Diamond 1990).

Most psychiatrists strive to conform to ethical standards in the provision of professional services. The perception that all forensic psychiatrists are hired guns arises in part from the frequency with which legal cases present a "battle of the experts." Legitimate differences of opinion may result in two experts holding opposite opinions. Even in clinical psychiatry, experts often legitimately disagree. The adversarial system encourages the exaggeration of such differences, which can result in the appearance that the opinions of most experts are simply for sale.

## The Clinical Versus the Forensic Role

### Clinical Vignette

Dr. B has provided psychotherapy to Mr. J for several years for a diagnosis of anxiety disorder NOS [not otherwise specified]. Mr. J had been involved in a serious automobile accident by a negligent driver. Mr. J's anxiety symptoms increased significantly after the accident, although he did not meet all the diagnostic criteria for posttraumatic stress disorder (PTSD). Mr. J was too anxious to work for several months after the accident. He continued in psychotherapy but also required antianxiety medication to control his symptoms.

Mr. J filed a civil suit against the insured driver of the other vehicle. Mr. J's attorney suggested that Mr. J ask Dr. B to do a forensic evaluation and prepare a report. The attorney reasoned that Dr. B would make the best expert because he was already familiar with Mr. J's case. Mr. J raised concerns about his confidentiality. The attorney dismissed these concerns. He told Mr. J that because Mr. J had placed his mental state at issue in filing the suit, his treatment would not be protected by doctor-patient confidentiality. Thus, Dr. B might as well do the evaluation.

The attorney also told Mr. J that he was concerned that a forensic psychiatrist hired by the insurance company would write a report stating Mr. J did not have PTSD. He thought the opposing expert would emphasize that Mr. J had a preexisting anxiety disorder but say nothing about the severe exacerbation of the anxiety since the accident, as the opposing expert was known to have done this in other cases. The attorney believed that Dr. B, by virtue of his therapeutic relationship with Mr. J, would be more knowledgeable about his condition and write a more favorable report. Mr. J agreed with the attorney's reasoning and requested that Dr. B perform the forensic evaluation. He offered to pay Dr. B's usual forensic fees. What is the ethically appropriate thing for Dr. B to do?

Dr. B advised Mr. J to speak with his attorney about retaining another psychiatrist to perform a forensic evaluation and serve as his expert witness. Many of the ethical dilemmas faced by forensic psychiatrists arise from the conflict between the roles of clinician and expert witness. These two roles are incompatible in many ways. AAPL's ethical guidelines indicate that whenever possible, a treating psychiatrist should avoid occupying both forensic and treatment roles (AAPL 1995). Until the last decade or so, psychiatrists, like other physicians, routinely provided forensic testimony for their patients. At present, however, most forensic psychiatrists follow the AAPL's ethical recommendations to avoid the dual roles of treating clinician and expert witness if at all possible.

The ethical dilemmas that arise in trying to fill both roles simultaneously generally result from the differences in the goals and methods of law and psychiatry. The goals and values of medicine are paramount in clinical practice. Certainly, the therapeutic process occurs within clinicians' awareness of their secondary duties to society such as reporting child abuse and protecting the public. The law also places other constraints on clinical practice such as requiring confidentiality of psychiatric records in certain circumstances and prohibiting sexual relationships with patients. Nevertheless, the well-being of the patient is a clinician's primary consideration and responsibility.

In contrast, as Appelbaum (1990) has indicated, forensic psychiatrists are useful to the legal system only insofar as they can offer opinions that may potentially be harmful to the evaluee. Opinions that only benefited evaluees would not be of much assistance in the determination of justice and the resolution of disputes. Opinions that assist the legal system, however, may harm the evaluee, both psychologically and materially. When psychiatrists attempt to provide both clinical treatment and expert witness services, their obligation to assist the legal system usually comes into direct conflict with their obligation to avoid doing harm to the patient and to the therapeutic relationship.

Attorneys often believe that the best expert witness is the treating physician. They feel having the treating physician serve in both capacities makes the most efficient use of the most knowledgeable source of information and reduces the costs associated with retaining a separate expert. Patients themselves may resist bringing in another person and having to repeat what is often a painful story to someone they do not know. They may also see their therapists as their advocates who should come to their assistance by serving as their expert.

In medical specialties such as orthopedics and radiology, the treating clinician is indeed often the best expert witness. However, psychiatrists who attempt to occupy both roles simultaneously typically find that they cannot perform either role effectively (Greenberg and Shuman 1997; Strasburger et al. 1997).

Clinical and forensic evaluations emphasize different aspects of truth and causation. Although these aspects may overlap, they may not comfortably coexist. The process of psychotherapy involves searching for meaning rather than facts. This distinction is frequently referred to as "narrative truth" rather than "historical truth." Clinicians are trained to adopt a nonjudgmental position that allows these two versions of truth to be different. They credit the narrative truth as a representation of the patient's inner reality. Although they do not necessarily expect the narrative truth to be factually accurate, clinicians may not challenge even obviously distorted reports for therapeutic reasons. They withhold judgment, listen empathically, and attempt to help patients develop insight into their own biases, projections, and distortions.

In contrast, forensic evaluators must approach evaluations from a stance of appropriate skepticism and are expected to reach judgments and conclusions. Forensic examiners should not base their opinions on the examinee's subjective report alone and should, as far as possible, attempt to verify the examinee's report with collateral information. It can be both clinically inappropriate and ethically a breach of confidentiality for clinicians to attempt to gain information from outside sources. Forensic examiners have a limited time in which to formulate their opinions. The clinician, anticipating a long relationship with a patient, can wait for evidence of patterns of bias or distortion to become evident and can withhold final judgment.

When clinicians attempt to function as both therapist and expert, the therapy itself is altered. Patients who know that their clinicians will be testifying in court cannot help but be constrained in therapy. They may consciously or unconsciously edit their comments, either to lay the basis for their legal case or to avoid revealing information that might hurt their case should it come out in court. Reasonable therapeutic goals cannot be set and achieved under such circumstances.

The therapeutic relationship is also adversely affected and often irreparably damaged. The therapeutic alliance is the sine qua non of psychotherapy and is based on confidentiality. Patients must feel free to discuss anything and everything and feel confident that this information will be used to help them. Such confidentiality is not possible in a forensic evaluation. If the treating clinician becomes the expert witness, even with the patient's consent to the loss of privacy, information gathered under the previous clinical assumption of confidentiality will inevitably be used for legal purposes. As the AAPL (1995) ethical guidelines point out, it is usually impossible to restore the prior confidential relationship once the litigation is ended.

Other ethical conflicts arise when clinicians attempt to fulfill the forensic obligation to strive for objectivity. Psychiatrists ordinarily have some positive countertransference toward their patients. In addition, clinicians are supposed to maintain an appropriate professional clinical bias toward their patients. The fact that treating clinicians are ethically bound to work in their patients' interests lends itself to discrediting the objectivity of their testimony. Moreover, if the clinician's prognosis and treatment recommendations include long-term treatment, it may appear that the clinician stands to benefit financially from a judgment in the patient's favor. This can further add to the appearance of bias and personal interest. An effective cross-examination can expose all these potential biases, compromising the effectiveness of testimony.

Clinicians may agree to serve as their patients' experts with the best of intentions, believing that they can and should help their patients in their legal difficulties. However, they may inadvertently harm their patients both legally and clinically by occupying both roles. Their participation in the traumatic process of litigation can cause direct harm to their patients (Strasburger 1987, 1999; Strasburger et al. 1997). The damage to and possible loss of the therapeutic alliance and of confidentiality can harm patients. In addition, damage done by inadequate or ineffective testimony resulting from the therapist's inexperience with the legal system may be emotionally, financially, and personally costly.

Circumstances may exist that make separation of the clinical and forensic roles unavoidable (Miller 1990; Strasburger et al. 1997), but psychiatrists should endeavor to separate the treatment and evaluation roles whenever possible. Patients who put their mental status at issue in litigation waive the privilege of confidentiality. Their privacy will without doubt be compromised if the therapist's treatment notes are subpoenaed and the therapist is called as a fact witness. Nevertheless, the degree of therapeutic compromise involved when the therapist becomes a fact witness is often less than that associated with occupying both the roles of treating and expert psychiatrist. The separation of the roles often allows clinicians to help patients through the litigation process while preserving the therapeutic relationship.

## The Ethical Practice of Forensic Psychiatry

Despite the differences in clinical and forensic ethics and practice, many ethical principles overlap. For example, sexual relations, bullying, and deliberate rudeness and disrespect are unethical behavior in both clinical and forensic settings. Forensic psychiatrists, like clinical psychiatrists, are required to respect human dignity and autonomy (AAPL 1995; Weinstock 1992, 1995). However, the parameters of the overlapping issues or the ethical principles may be based on different values and sometimes result in differing ethical courses of action. The following discussion reviews issues that are familiar to clinical psychiatrists and highlights the different parameters and ethical bases in their application to forensic practice.

## Qualifications

Psychiatrists should provide forensic services only in areas in which they have expertise; that is, areas of actual knowledge and skills, training, and experience. Certain assessments, such as the evaluation of children, individuals from foreign cultures, or prisoners, may require special training and expertise (AAPL 1995). Forensic psychiatrists can claim the type of expertise that all general psychiatrists have in these areas. However, psychiatrists without special expertise or training should not indicate that they have such expertise, especially in cases in which this experience is central to the legal issue. In clinical practice, psychiatrists asked to treat a patient with a special need or problem outside their area of expertise would provide an appropriate referral. Similarly, if consulted in cases outside their areas of expertise, forensic psychiatrists would do best to direct the attorney to a colleague with the necessary experience.

## Confidentiality

Forensic psychiatrists are ethically obligated to maintain an evaluee's confidentiality, although the parameters of this obligation differ from those of clinical practice. Legal contexts and constraints automatically limit confidentiality. Psychiatrists may be required to write reports or provide courtroom testimony that would reveal material that in a clinical context would never be discussed outside the treatment setting. Forensic evaluees should be advised about the limits of confidentiality before beginning the evaluation. Psychiatrists have an affirmative obligation to make certain that these limitations are communicated clearly to the evaluee. A pro forma description without adequate explanation and discussion is not sufficient to fulfill this ethical obligation.

Within these parameters, forensic psychiatrists should restrict disclosures of information obtained during the performance of a forensic evaluation as far as possible. Information that is not relevant to the forensic evaluation should be considered confidential. For example, an evaluee may reveal information about his or her children unrelated to the legal issue in question. Such information should not be included in a report. In addition, any information not used in court should not later be discussed in public. For example, some cases attract media attention. Forensic psychiatrists should not disclose information that they obtained in the course of their evaluation that did not become public knowledge. Such disclosures are ethically inappropriate and may even result in legal liability (Appelbaum 2001; Binder 2002; Weinstock and Garrick 1995).

Forensic ethics also requires psychiatrists to take precautions to prevent confidential information from falling into the hands of unauthorized persons. Preserving confidentiality in treatment that occurs in the context of a legal system, such as in correctional settings, can be challenging. In such situations, psychiatrists should be clear about any limitations on the usual principles of confidentiality. They should be familiar with the institutional policies regarding confidentiality, and if no policy exists, they should clarify confidentiality issues with the institutional authorities and develop working guidelines to establish the extent and preservation of confidentiality within the institution (AAPL 1995).

Forensic psychiatrists hired by a party to a case and given privileged information are also obligated to maintain this information as confidential. Sometimes if the original evaluation was not privileged, a psychiatrist can be called by the other side and forced by a judge's ruling to testify. However, such information should not be shared voluntarily. Psychiatrists who have been retained by one side who then "switch sides" and reveal this information to the opposing party are committing an ethical violation. Unfortunately, some attorneys will try to take advantage of this ethical restriction. They may call an expert with no intention of retaining him and discuss a case briefly for the sole purpose of preventing the opposing side from having access to the services of that expert (Gutheil et al. 2001). Psychiatrists should be certain to clarify with a potential retaining attorney that any discussion is only a preliminary inquiry to avoid being disqualified from a case by this tactic (AAPL 1995).

## Consent

Obtaining informed consent is another ethical principle that applies in both clinical and forensic contexts but differs depending upon the context. For example, in clinical settings, psychiatrists must respect an individual's the right to refuse treatment. In the forensic setting, psychiatrists should also respect the individual's right to refuse treatment within the context of the jurisdiction's rules (AAPL 1995). Nevertheless, an evaluation may be court-ordered, and an evaluee's consent in such circumstances is not legally required. If the evaluee refuses to participate, the psychiatrist may still conduct the examination as far as possible without the evaluee's cooperation. (Under these circumstances, the evaluee should be advised that his refusal to participate will be noted in the psychiatrist's report or testimony.)

Psychiatrists should obtain the informed consent of the subject of a forensic evaluation whenever possible (AAPL 1995). In the forensic setting, this requires a detailed explanation clarifying the nature and purpose of the forensic evaluation and the psychiatrist's role. Evaluees should be clearly advised that although the forensic psychiatrist is a doctor, he or she will not be functioning as the evaluee's doctor. Psychiatrists should also clearly state for whom they are conducting the examination and what they will do with the information.

Ethical problems arise when forensic psychiatrists mislead the evaluee, even if unintentionally. The public is most familiar with the physician's role as a provider of medical care, and evaluees may not appreciate the differences between a doctor's clinical and forensic roles. For example, an evaluee may believe that a psychiatrist has been sent to provide clinical assistance when opposing counsel has in fact retained him or her. In such cases, information uncovered in the evaluation can be used against the evaluee. Psychiatrists who themselves cannot effectively separate treatment and forensic roles run the risk of inadvertently misleading both the evaluee and the court.

One explanation may not be sufficient. Even though a warning and explanation has already been given, psychiatrists should remain sensitive to the examinee's possible tendency to assume a traditional doctor-patient relationship. Evaluees easily slip into the perception that the interview is part of a developing treatment relationship, and so may need to be reminded during the evaluation of the purpose of the examination. Moreover, examiners may appear to be empathic and to be using the professional skills doctors use when performing a medical evaluation. Forensic psychiatrists therefore have a continuing obligation to monitor the evaluation for such "slippage." Psychiatrists should clarify their roles as many times as necessary before continuing the evaluation (AAPL 1995) and not take advantage of such slippage to obtain incriminating evidence.

Psychiatrists should document the consent as part of the initial part of the evaluation. A form explaining the purpose of the evaluation, the nature of the relationship with the examiner, and the limits of confidentiality can be provided for evaluees' review before the interview. At the very least, the explanation and consent should be documented in notes and the forensic report. Before the interview begins, the psychiatrist should review this information again with the evaluee and provide an opportunity for him or her to ask questions and receive clarification. If the evaluee refuses to consent, he or she should be referred to his or her attorney, unless a court has ordered the evaluation.

## Fees

### Clinical Vignette

Dr. C was called by an attorney to perform a forensic evaluation on one of his clients. The attorney stated that the client had an excellent civil case against a city and would prevail. The client had little money. The attorney said he had taken the case on a contingency basis and that he could not afford to lay out his own money to retain an expert. He stated that he had hired several other experts in other disciplines on a lien basis and that they would all be able to collect full forensic fees once the case was settled. The attorney wanted Dr. C to take the case on a lien. Dr. C expressed reservations about accepting the case on a lien basis. The attorney told him that the AMA considers liens ethical. Should Dr. C take the case on a lien basis?

Dr. C told the attorney that he would take the case if the attorney would pay his fees. The attorney refused, and Dr. C declined the case. Dr. C knew that a lien theoretically applies regardless of the case's outcome. He also knew that the AMA does consider it ethical to take a case or treat a patient on a lien (American Medical Assocation 2003d). An old opinion of the AMA Council on Ethical and Judicial Affairs still in effect says that in states "in which there are lien laws, a physician may file a lien as a means of assuring payment of his or her fee provided the fee is fixed in amount and not contingent on the amount of settlement of the patient's claim against a third party."

Nevertheless, in most instances, taking a forensic case on a lien basis is essentially the same as taking the case on a contingency basis. Plaintiffs who have no money will only be able to pay if they prevail in court. The AAPL guidelines (AAPL 1995) review some of the issues that arise frequently in regard to fees. Dr. C knew that the AAPL considers contingency fees unethical. Such a fee arrangement interferes with the ethical requirement to be honest and to strive for objectivity. Experts will not get paid unless the plaintiff wins and so are highly motivated to advocate for the plaintiff's case. Even if the expert can maintain objectivity under these circumstances, a contingency fee arrangement gives the appearance of having a personal interest in the outcome of the case, thus undermining the expert's credibility.

Attorneys can appropriately accept contingency fees, as their ethical obligation is to provide advocacy. A contingency fee does not compromise these ethics, and in many cases it reassures clients that the attorney will work as hard as possible to win the case, and such attorneys appropriately lay out money for expenses. It is ethical for the attorney to pay the psychiatrist's fees. These are recoverable if the case is won. If, as the attorney claimed, the client was sure to prevail, the attorney would not be taking a financial risk.

Accepting a retainer would present no problem and might be especially advisable in a case in which the attorney shows resistance to paying. In contrast to contingency fees, retainers are ethical. They do even more to help objectivity because the expert is paid in advance and is under no financial pressure to provide an opinion that satisfies the attorney.

## Death Penalty Cases

Death penalty cases present perhaps the most challenging personal and professional ethical dilemmas and, so, deserve some direct discussion. Efforts to facilitate cases in which the outcome may include the death penalty or to facilitate the sentence of death when already imposed present clear examples of ethical and moral conflict. Some psychiatrists consider such cases qualitatively different because of the seriousness of the issue. Others believe that evaluations in death penalty cases are no different from evaluations for much less severe offenses.

Not all aspects of such cases are controversial. For example, most forensic psychiatrists consider it ethically permissible to testify for either side in the early phases of a death penalty case. In contrast, psychiatric organizations have unambiguously deemed certain roles professionally unethical regardless of an individual psychiatrist's personal beliefs. For example, the APA and AAPL both prohibit participation in a legally authorized execution (AAPL 1995; American Psychiatric Association 2001a). This prohibition has generally been interpreted to include giving or supervising a lethal injection, determining death, and witnessing an execution as a physician unless specially requested by the prisoner. Although some consider this interpretation quite narrow, such prohibitions are not particularly controversial.

Other death penalty roles are the subject of significant controversy (Leong et al. 2000; Weinstock et al. 1991). For example, it may be ethically problematic to testify as to aggravating circumstances for the purpose of helping the prosecution get a death penalty verdict. Some psychiatrists believe it is unethical to perform a competence-to-be-executed evaluation, because if psychiatrists find that the individual is competent to be executed, they have generally removed the last obstacle to execution. However, professional organizations in the United States have not taken that position. If such evaluations were formally deemed unethical, it would never be possible for a psychiatrist to help find any individual incompetent to be executed. The AMA states that a physician should not determine competence to be executed but can provide information to be used in such a determination (American Medical Association 2000b). The AMA also states that physicians should not treat prisoners to restore competence to be executed, but treat them to restore competence only if a commutation order is issued before treatment begins (American Medical Association 2003c).

Regardless of professional ethics, in some cases personal ethics or morals may override professional ethical guidelines. For example, psychiatrists opposed to the death penalty may be willing to provide honest opinions in such cases, but only if they will assist the defendant (Weinstock et al. 1992). Others, such as the infamous "Dr. Death" in Texas, seem willing, in the sentencing phase of death penalty cases, to testify almost always that the convicted defendant presents an ongoing danger to society, a requirement in Texas for a sentence of death. He does so regardless of the facts of the case and of the professional censure he has received for his unethical professional behavior.

Opinions differ as to where professional ethical lines should be drawn in death penalty cases. Thus, psychiatrists should carefully consider both their personal beliefs and the professional ethics before becoming involved in such litigation. Some may believe that certain roles should be professionally unethical despite professional organizations not taking such a position. Bloche (1993) argues that ethical problems arise in death penalty assessments in which the professional's actions undermine the authority of medicine as a helping profession. Pellegrino (1993) believes physicians should never participate in certain state functions that clearly stand in direct opposition to the purposes of medicine and the public expectation of beneficence from physicians. In his opinion, the moral authority for medicine arises from the nature of the medical activity (helping, healing, and caring), which transcends social, political, and cultural whims.

Pellegrino, however, considers some double-agent roles permissible. Such roles allow the legal system the benefits of medical consultation even if the outcome is unfavorable to a defendant. For example, the outcome of providing treatment to help someone become competent to stand trial cannot be known beforehand. In contrast, Pellegrino views the treatment of an inmate for the purpose of rendering him competent to be executed essentially the moral equivalent of killing.

Foot (1990) presents similar arguments. She states that psychiatrists opposed to the death penalty should nevertheless participate honestly in these cases and not leave these assessments to death penalty advocates with a prosecutorial bias. She argues that any attempt to do good is not unethical, even if it ultimately causes the defendant harm. For that reason, psychiatrists performing honest assessments of death penalty defendants in the hopes of averting their death are not committing an ethical violation if they find such defendants competent to be executed.

## Conclusion

Forensic psychiatry ethics presents special challenges because of the conflicts that arise at the interface of law and psychiatry. The profession has provided guidelines for practitioners on how to function at this interface and how to balance conflicting principles and values. When questions arise that are not readily answered by professional guidelines, psychiatrists should consider consultation with more experienced practitioners, especially those with some expertise in ethics. It also is possible to raise questions in advance to an ethics committee in an especially difficult case.

Legal cases, however, move on a timeline that often results in the unexpected presentation of a problem that must be resolved without sufficient time to obtain adequate consultation. Psychiatrists should therefore be familiar with the ethical precepts of forensic and clinical psychiatry. This will prepare them to perform their own ethical analysis in problematic cases. They should be willing and able to attempt to weigh conflicting guidelines and values (Candilis et al. 2001; Hundert 1990; Weinstock 1998) in an effort to arrive at the most ethical course of action.

## Key Points

- Although in many respects clinical and forensic psychiatric ethics overlap, they also differ in significant ways.
- Legal ethics and psychiatric ethics are not equivalent.
- Professional organizations such as the American Psychiatric Association and American Academy of Psychiatry and the Law provide ethical guidelines that can provide guidance when ethical dilemmas in forensic psychiatry arise.
- Many of the ethical conflicts in the practice of forensic psychiatry arise from dual-agency situations, such as simultaneously attempting to function as treating clinician and expert witness.

## Practice Guidelines

1. Be familiar with the ethical guidelines provided by AAPL, the APA, and other professional organizations as they relate to clinical and forensic practice.

2. As far as possible, consider the ethical aspects of any potential forensic case before agreeing to participate, and attempt to withdraw from any case in which there is pressure to perform an unethical role.
3. Adhere to the ethical principles of honesty and striving for objectivity in all forensic cases.
4. Avoid occupying dual-agency roles whenever possible.
5. When in doubt regarding the ethics of a given situation, consult ethics committees or fellow professionals, especially experienced forensic psychiatrists with expertise in the ethics facets.

## References


Ake v Oklahoma, 470 U.S. 68, 105 S. Ct. 1087 (1985)

American Academy of Forensic Sciences: Code of Ethics. Colorado Springs, CO, American Academy of Forensic Sciences, 2002

American Academy of Psychiatry and the Law: Ethical Guidelines for the Practice of Forensic Psychiatry. Bloomfield, CT, American Academy of Psychiatry and the Law, 1995

American Medical Association: Council on Ethical and Judicial Affairs: Code of Medical Ethics: Current Opinions With Annotations 2002–2003, Chicago, IL, American Medical Association, 2002

American Medical Association: Board of Trustees, H-265.992, H-265.993, H-265.994, reaffirmed, 1999, 2000. Available at: http://www.ama-assn.org. Accessed January 12, 2003a.

American Medical Association: Council on Ethical and Judicial Affairs E-2.06. Available at: http://www.ama-assn.org. Accessed January 12, 2003b.

American Medical Association: Letter to the editor. New York Times, February 13, 2003c

American Medical Association: Opinions of the Council on Ethical and Judicial Affairs E-8.10. Available at: http://www.ama-assn.org. Accessed January 12, 2003d.

American Medical Association: Principles of Medical Ethics. Available at: http://www.ama-assn.org. Accessed January 12, 2003e.

American Psychiatric Association: Opinions of the Ethics Committee on the Principles of Medical Ethics, With Annotations Especially Applicable to Psychiatry. Washington, DC, American Psychiatric Association, 2001a

American Psychiatric Association: The Principles of Medical Ethics, With Annotations Especially Applicable to Psychiatry. Washington, DC, American Psychiatric Association, 2001b

Appelbaum PS: The parable of the forensic psychiatrist: ethics and the problem of doing harm. Int J Law Psychiatry 13:249–259, 1990

Appelbaum PS: A theory of ethics for forensic psychiatry. J Am Acad Psychiatry Law 25:233–247, 1997

Appelbaum PS: Law and psychiatry: liability for forensic evaluations: a word of caution. Psychiatr Serv 52:885–886, 2001

Binder R: Liability for the psychiatrist expert witness. Am J Psychiatry 159:1819–1825, 2002

Bloche MG: Psychiatry, capital punishment and the purpose of medicine. Int J Law Psychiatry 16:301–357, 1993

Candilis PL, Martinez R, Dorning C: Principles and narrative in forensic psychiatry: toward a robust view of professional role. J Am Acad Psychiatry Law 29:167–173, 2001

Ciccone JR, Clements C: Commentary: forensic psychiatry and ethics—the voyage continues. J Am Acad Psychiatry Law 29:174–179, 2001

Diamond BL: The fallacy of the impartial expert. Archives of Criminal Psychodynamics 3:221–236, 1959

Diamond BL: The psychiatrist expert witness: honest advocate or "hired gun"?, in Ethical Practice in Psychiatry and the Law. Edited by Rosner R, Weinstock R. New York, Plenum, 1990, pp 75–84

Diamond BL: The forensic psychiatrist: consultant versus activist in legal doctrine. Bull Am Acad Psychiatry Law 20:119–132, 1992

Dyer AR: Ethics and Psychiatry. Washington, DC, American Psychiatric Press, 1988

Foot P: Ethics and the death penalty: participation by forensic psychiatrists in capital trials, in Ethical Practice in Psychiatry and the Law. Edited by Rosner R, Weinstock R. New York, Plenum, 1990, pp 207–217

Greenberg SA, Shuman DW: Irreconcilable conflict between therapeutic and forensic roles. Professional Psychology: Research and Practice 28:5–57, 1997

Griffith EEH: Ethics in forensic psychiatry: a response to Stone and Appelbaum. J Am Acad Psychiatry 26:171–184, 1998

Gutheil TG: The Psychiatrist as Expert Witness. Washington, DC, American Psychiatric Press, 1998

Gutheil TG, Bursztajn H, Brodsky A, et al: Decision Making in Psychiatry and the Law. Baltimore, MD, Williams & Wilkins, 1991

Gutheil TG, Simon RI: Attorneys' pressures on the expert witness: early warning signs of endangered honesty, objectivity and fair compensation. J Am Acad Psychiatry Law 27:546–553, 1999

Gutheil TG, Simon RI, Hilliard JT: The phantom expert: unconsented use of an expert's name and/or testimony as a legal strategy. J Am Acad Psychiatry Law 29:313–318, 2001

Hundert EM: Competing medical and legal ethical values: balancing problems of the forensic psychiatrist, in Ethical Practice in Psychiatry and the Law. Edited by Rosner R, Weinstock R. New York, Plenum, 1990, pp 53–72

Jansonius JV, Gould AM: Expert witnesses in employment litigation. Baylor Law Review 50:267–331, 1998

Leong GB, Silva JA, Weinstock R, et al: Survey of forensic psychiatrists on evaluation and treatment of prisoners on death row. J Am Acad Psychiatry Law 28:427–432, 2000

Miller RD: Ethical issues involved in the dual role of treater and evaluator, in Ethical Practice in Psychiatry and the Law. Edited by Rosner R, Weinstock R. New York, Plenum, 1990, pp 129–150

Mossman D: Is expert psychiatric testimony fundamentally immoral? Int J Law Psychiatry 17:347–368, 1994

Mossman D, Kapp MB: "Courtroom Whores"?—or Why do attorneys call us? Findings from a survey on attorneys' use of mental health experts. J Am Acad Psychiatry Law 26:276, 1998

Pellegrino ED: Societal duty and moral complicity: the physician's dilemma of divided loyalty. Int J Law Psychiatry 16:371–391, 1993

Pollack S: Forensic Psychiatry in Criminal Law. Los Angeles, University of Southern California Press, 1974

Rosner R: Foundations of ethical practice in the forensic sciences. Journal of Forensic Sciences 42:1191–1194, 1997

Simon RI, Shuman DW: Conducting forensic examinations on the road: are you practicing your profession without license? J Am Acad Psychiatry Law 27: 75–82, 1999

Simon RI, Wettstein RM: Toward the development of guidelines for the conduct of forensic psychiatric examinations. J Am Acad Psychiatry Law 25:17–30, 1997

Stone AA: The ethics of forensic psychiatry: a view from the ivory tower, in Law, Psychiatry, and Morality. Washington, DC, American Psychiatric Press, 1984, pp 57–73

Strasburger LH: "Crudely, without any finesse": the defendant hears his psychiatric evaluation. Bull Am Acad Psychiatry Law 15:229–233, 1987

Strasburger LH: The litigant-patient: mental health consequences of civil litigation. J Am Acad Psychiatry Law 27:203–211, 1999

Strasburger LH, Gutheil TG, Brodsky A: On wearing two hats: role conflict in serving as both psychotherapist and expert witness. Am J Psychiatry 154: 448–456, 1997

Weinstock R: Ethical concerns expressed by forensic sciences. Journal of Forensic Sciences 31:596–602, 1986

Weinstock R: Opinions by AAPL's committee on ethics. Newsletter of the American Academy of Psychiatry and the Law 17:5–6, 1992

Weinstock R: AAPL's committee on ethics: additional opinions. Newsletter of the American Academy of Psychiatry and the Law 20:51, 1995

Weinstock R: Ethical practice in forensic science: an introduction. Journal of Forensic Sciences 42:1189–1190, 1997

Weinstock R: Comment on a theory of ethics for forensic psychiatry. J Am Acad Psychiatry Law 26:151–156, 1998

Weinstock R: Commentary: a broadened conception of forensic psychiatric ethics. J Am Acad Psychiatry Law 29:180–185, 2001

Weinstock R, Garrick T: Is liability possible for forensic psychiatrists? Bull Am Acad Psychiatry Law 23:183–193, 1995

Weinstock R, Leong GB, Silva JA: The role of traditional medical ethics in forensic psychiatry, in Ethical Practice in Psychiatry and the Law. Edited by Rosner R, Weinstock R. New York, Plenum, 1990, pp 31–51

Weinstock R, Leong GB, Silva JA: Opinions by AAPL forensic psychiatrists on controversial ethical guidelines: a survey. Bull Am Acad Psychiatry Law 19:237–248, 1991

Weinstock R, Leong GB, Silva JA: The death penalty and Bernard Diamond's approach to forensic psychiatry. Bull Am Acad Psychiatry Law 37:830–838, 1992

## Suggested Readings

Appelbaum PS: Ethics in evolution: the incompatibility of clinical and forensic functions. Am J Psychiatry 154:445–446, 1997

Appelbaum PS: Clarifying the ethics of clinical research: a path towards avoiding the therapeutic misconception. American Journal of Bioethics 2:22–23, 2002

Diamond BL: The Psychiatrist in the Courtroom: Selected Papers of Bernard L Diamond MD. New York, Analytic, 1994

Gutheil TG, Commons M, Miller PM: Withholding, seducing, and threatening: a pilot study of further attorney pressures on expert witnesses. J Am Acad Psychiatry Law 29:336–339, 2001

Halleck SL: The ethical dilemmas of forensic psychiatry: a utilitarian approach. Bull Am Acad Psychiatry Law 12:279–288, 1984

Rosner R (ed): Principles and Practice of Forensic Psychiatry, 2nd Edition. London, Arnold, 2003

Rosner R, Weinstock R (eds): Ethical Practice in Psychiatry and the Law. New York, Plenum, 1990

Stone AA: Law, Psychiatry, and Morality. Washington, DC, American Psychiatric Press, 1984

Stone AA: Revisiting the parable: truth without consequences. Int J Law Psychiatry 17:79–97, 1994

Weinstock R: Special article: ethics in forensic psychiatry—an annotated bibliography. Bull Am Acad Psychiatry Law 23:473–482, 1995

CHAPTER 6

# Psychiatric Diagnosis in Litigation

Robert I. Simon, M.D.

Liza H. Gold, M.D.

## Introduction

The drafters of the *Diagnostic and Statistical Manual of Mental Disorders* (DSM) have consistently expressed concerns about the use of the DSM in litigation. Nevertheless, the courts often rely on DSM diagnoses, and the use of the standard diagnostic nomenclature contained in the DSM continues unabated. DSM-IV (American Psychiatric Association 1994), and its text revision, DSM-IV-TR (American Psychiatric Association 2000), state, "When the DSM-IV categories, criteria, and textual descriptions are employed for forensic purposes, there are significant risks that diagnostic information will be misused or misunderstood. These dangers arise because of the imperfect fit between the questions of ultimate concern to the law and information contained in a clinical diagnosis" (American Psychiatric Association 2000, pp. xxxii–xxxiii). The information presumably conveyed by the diagnosis may not be the information sought by the courts. This imperfect fit sometimes results in attempts to fit square pegs into round holes and in both psychiatric and legal emphasis on diagnosis over assessment of function.

The concerns raised by the use of DSM in the courts are significant for both psychiatry and the law. The standards regarding the judicial determination of scientific reliability were set forth in the recent Supreme Court decisions of *Daubert v. Merrell Dow Pharmaceuticals, Inc.* (1993) and *Kumho Tire Co., Ltd. v. Carmichael* (1999). These decisions raise the question of whether DSM's formal system of categorization is sufficiently scientific to justify its admission in evidence. Federal courts have on occasion questioned the scientific reliability of a DSM diagnosis (*United States v. Torniero* 1983). Some courts and some psychiatric authorities have raised criticisms of the science, as well as the social and political influences underlying DSM diagnostic categories (Gold 2002). In these decisions, the Court conferred responsibility upon the trial judge to assess the relevance and reliability of all proffers of expert testimony involving scientific, technical, or other specialized knowledge in federal courts. Nevertheless, DSM diagnoses are generally accepted and relied on by the courts (Gold 2002; Shuman 1989).

The more significant question raised by the acceptance and reliance of the legal system on DSM is whether DSM diagnoses provide an adequate understanding of psychological states for forensic purposes. Legal determinations, whether civil or criminal, typically revolve around issues of impairment. A DSM diagnostic category is not directly relevant to such determinations. For example, in criminal matters, defendants acquitted through a "not guilty by reason of insanity" (NGRI) verdict are typically evaluated on the basis of their ability to distinguish right from wrong or to resist their impulses. Such verdicts are not rendered simply on the basis of whether defendants meet DSM criteria for certain diagnoses such as schizophrenia or bipolar disorder. Nor will specific diagnoses qualify a defendant for an NGRI verdict when others will not. In personal injury litigation, functional impairment is the critical issue for determining damages (Simon 2002). The legal question in such litigation is not whether the plaintiff has a psychiatric diagnosis but how the plaintiff's pre- and postincident conditions differ and whether that difference can be attributed to the defendant's wrongful conduct.

The use of DSM diagnoses in forensic settings can encourage misguided attempts to force diagnosis into legal criteria as a proxy for impairment. Diagnosis and impairment are not equivalent. No diagnosis carries specific information regarding level of impairment or information as to whether an impairment associated with that diagnosis is relevant to the legal issue under examination by the court. The use of categorical DSM diagnosis in litigation may result in missing the most important aspect of the forensic evaluation: the assessment of impairment. When categorical DSM diagnoses are used for purposes other than clinical treatment or research, misconceptions about the role and importance of these diagnoses result in the "imperfect fit" that concerned the framers of DSM. These misconceptions may be held both by the legal system and, at times, by psychiatrists providing forensic evaluations in litigation.

The legal system is rarely concerned with the imperfect fit between diagnosis and legal concerns. Attorneys and judges usually focus on the presence or absence of the diagnosis. Courts and attorneys may require psychiatrists to provide DSM diagnoses or insist that they do so. This, in turn, may lead psychiatrists to give undue importance to diagnosis in forensic evaluations and to miss the essential assessment of impairment in function. Even when a diagnosis is appropriate and accurate, the categorical nature of DSM's nosology is such that necessary dimensional information may be overlooked or misinterpreted. This text will address these issues by examining the use of the diagnosis of subthreshold posttraumatic stress syndrome (PTSD). Although discussed only in the context of personal injury litigation, the "imperfect fit" of categorical DSM diagnosis applies across the spectrum of civil and criminal litigation.

## Clinical Vignette

Ms. J, a 36-year-old chief financial officer of a large corporation, was returning home aboard a jet aircraft when it skidded off the runway in a snowstorm. The aircraft entered a bordering harbor and came to a stop in 5 feet of icy water. Ms. J was momentarily dazed when her head struck the seat in front of her. She was terrified that she would drown, as she had never learned to swim. She escaped the aircraft by sliding down an emergency chute and was able to walk ashore.

Ms. J twisted her ankle as she emerged from the water. She was taken to a local emergency room, where her examination showed an abrasion on her forehead and swelling of her left ankle but no serious injuries. After receiving appropriate treatment in the emergency room, she was released from the hospital. The accident occurred on a Friday night before a 3-day weekend. Ms. J returned to work on the following Tuesday.

One year later, Ms. J filed a personal injury suit against the airline, demanding $500,000 in damages. She claimed that negligence on the part of the airline caused physical and psychological injuries. Soon after she filed her suit, Ms. J was examined by a psychiatrist retained by her attorney. She reported that shortly following the accident, she experienced occasional nightmares of falling or drowning. She had daily recollections of the accident, psychological and physical reactivity to situations that reminded her of the accident, and difficulty in concentration. She denied insomnia, irritability, and depression. Ms. J reported that over the course of the subsequent year, her work function seemed to be particularly affected by the events. She stated that she began to have difficulty "staying focused" at work. Ms. J had difficulty managing a substantial increase in her workload. She claimed that her lack of concentration caused "a lot of serious mistakes," which resulted in her being passed over for promotion. Ms. J had not lost time from work.

Ms. J's work required frequent travel, which she had always enjoyed. After the accident, she developed significant anxiety related to flying. Her primary care physician prescribed a minor tranquilizer for use as needed for flying-related anxiety. She was able to fly, but she had to take medication to do so. Although this tranquilizer provided some relief, Ms. J was still uncomfortable whenever she traveled by plane. She claimed that both the stress of flying and the effects of the tranquilizer left her physically and emotionally depleted. She resisted her primary care physician's recommendation to seek psychological help. She feared reexperiencing the trauma and the worsening of her symptoms, stating, "I just want to forget it."

Ms. J continued to see some of her friends and her fiancé, but her plans to marry were placed on hold. The marriage plans had been interrupted once before the accident because of "storminess" in the relationship. Sexual intimacy had also waxed and waned throughout the relationship. Nevertheless, Ms. J reported that the relationship with her fiancé became more "troubled" and unstable following the accident. Ms. J's unwillingness to take vacations with her fiancé that would require flying led to discord and more frequent arguments. Her fiancé threatened to leave. In addition, although she maintained close relationships with some friends, Ms. J stated that she avoided casual friends who asked questions about the accident and the lawsuit.

Ms. J's history revealed that she was the only child of a troubled marriage. Her parents fought frequently. Her father was an alcoholic who was physically and verbally abusive to both Ms. J and her mother. Ms. J was an outstanding student in high school and college. At age 28, she married a much older business executive. The couple had no children. They were divorced after 2 years of marriage because of "incompatibility." Ms. J denied any history of significant psychological symptoms or treatment for a psychiatric condition. She had no significant medical problems and no history of drug or alcohol abuse.

The plaintiff's expert determined that Ms. J exhibited symptoms of subthreshold PTSD following the life-threatening airplane accident. She met only four of six minimal symptom criteria necessary for a DSM-IV diagnosis of PTSD and had only two of three criterion C symptoms: efforts to avoid thoughts, feelings, or conversations associated with the trauma and efforts to avoid activities, places, or people that arouse recollections of the trauma. In addition, she manifested only one of two criterion D symptoms: difficulty concentrating. This psychiatrist considered but rejected other DSM-IV diagnoses as incorrect, including generalized anxiety disorder, anxiety disorder not otherwise specified (NOS), and adjustment disorder, chronic. He considered but resisted the temptation to diagnose anxiety disorder NOS merely to gain the imprimatur of DSM-IV in court. The examiner made the diagnosis of subthreshold PTSD because the minimal DSM-IV symptom criteria for PTSD were not met.

The plaintiff's attorney was uncomfortable with the diagnosis of subthreshold PTSD. She expressed concern that the defense attorney would attack subthreshold PTSD as a suspect and incredible non-DSM diagnosis. The attorney was also concerned that the judge and jury would become confused and reject a diagnosis not found in DSM-IV. The examining expert experienced considerable pressure from the attorney to "consider the possibility of an official diagnosis." The expert did believe that Ms. J could be legitimately diagnosed as having PTSD on the basis of meeting clinical significance criteria: "The disturbance causes clinically significant distress or impairment in social, occupational, or other important areas of functioning" (criterion F in PTSD). Although this reasoning was clinically valid, the expert was certain that opposing counsel would accuse him of circumventing DSM-IV criteria by invoking "clinical significance criteria" to reach a diagnosis of PTSD. He anticipated the cross-examination: "Isn't it true, Doctor, that she does not meet the DSM-IV criteria for PTSD, does she? Let's go over each of the criteria," and so forth.

## Categorical and Dimensional Diagnosis

### General Issues

A *categorical* system of classification is most efficient when all members of a diagnostic class are homogeneous, when the boundary between classes is clear, and when the classes are mutually exclusive. Categorical classification assists clinicians by providing a pragmatic tool to facilitate diagnosis and to treat illnesses. In medical school, students are taught the principle of parsimony; that is, to think of a single disorder that can explain a patient's multiple symptoms. Throughout the history of medicine, there has been a continuing quest for a coherent classification of mental disorders. Many methodologies have been proposed, but little agreement has existed on which mental disorders to include and the best way to organize them (Sadler et al. 1994). During the nineteenth century, psychiatry began developing a categorical system of classification similar to that long favored by medical tradition.

In a categorical diagnostic system, the patient either meets the diagnostic criteria for a disorder or does not. For example, a brain tumor either is or is not present. In a pure categorical diagnosis, all the diagnostic criteria for the disorder must be met. DSM-IV recognizes the heterogeneity of clinical presentations by establishing polythetic criteria sets in which the individual may meet only a subset of diagnostic criteria from a longer list. For example, the diagnosis of borderline personality disorder can be made with only five of nine inclusion criteria. Unlike medical diagnoses, DSM-IV psychiatric diagnoses usually do not inform about the etiology and pathogenesis of a disorder.

Individuals with a specific diagnosis are often heterogeneous regarding the diagnostic criteria.

> In DSM-IV, there is no assumption that each category of mental disorder is a completely discrete entity with absolute boundaries dividing it from other mental disorders or from no mental disorder. There is also no assumption that all individuals described as having the same mental disorder are alike in all important ways. The clinician using DSM-IV should therefore consider that individuals sharing a diagnosis are likely to be heterogeneous even in regard to defining features of the diagnosis and that boundary cases will be difficult to diagnose in any but a probabilistic fashion. (American Psychiatric Association 2000, p. xxxi)

As a consequence, DSM-IV uses a modified categorical diagnostic system.

In a dimensional classification system, no discrete categories are present. Individuals are classified along a continuum. A dimensional system classifies clinical presentations based on quantitative or qualitative factors or attributes rather than establishing diagnostic categories. The dimensional system is most useful in describing conditions or levels of severity that are distributed continuously, without clear boundaries. For example, Axis V in DSM-IV, the Global Assessment of Functioning (GAF) Scale, is numerically coded from 0 to 100. Qualitative dimensional approaches found in DSM-IV include severity specifiers such as mild, moderate, and severe. Anxiety, depression, obsessions, and compulsions, formerly considered to fit into neat categorical diagnoses, are now recognized as spectrum disorders—a qualitative dimensional classification.

Categorical and dimensional diagnostic systems often coexist. For example, the diagnosis of a brain tumor is categorical (present or absent), but the extent and severity of the disease (staging) helps inform treatment decisions and prognosis. Rating scales for severity of illness, such as the Hamilton Rating Scale or the Brief Psychiatric Rating Scale, measure severity and change in an illness that is diagnosed categorically (Bogenschutz and Nurnberg 2000).

## Implications for Forensic Psychiatry

DSM-IV relies on a system of diagnosis that establishes categorical boundaries, using both inclusion and exclusion criteria. The categorical nature of DSM diagnoses can create problems for psychiatrists providing assessments in litigation. This categorical diagnostic model does not accommodate dimensional posttraumatic stress spectrum syndromes such as the subthreshold PTSD diagnosed in Ms. J's case (Kinzie and Goetz 1996). Mental conditions such as subthreshold PTSD, which exhibit symptoms that fall outside the DSM-IV diagnostic criteria, are thereby excluded. A dimensional system of diagnosis avoids categorical boundaries, permitting stress spectrum syndromes to be recognized along with associated impairments (Maser and Patterson 2002).

DSM-IV readily acknowledges the importance of dimensional diagnosis in increasing reliability while also communicating more clinical information. However, DSM-IV cautions that dimensional systems have serious limitations and have been less useful than categorical systems in clinical practice and in stimulating research. For example, dimensional systems lack agreement on the choice of operational dimensions for classification purposes. Moreover, numerical dimensions are less familiar to clinicians than is categorical description of mental disorders.

DSM-IV itself suggests a flexible approach to diagnosis. It fairly states the limitations of a categorical approach while at the same time providing cautionary warning about idiosyncratic use of diagnoses.

> The specific diagnostic criteria included in DSM-IV are meant to serve as guidelines to be informed by clinical judgment and are not meant to be used in a cookbook fashion. For example, the exercise of clinical judgment may justify giving a certain diagnosis to an individual even though the clinical presentation falls just short of meeting the full criteria for the diagnosis as long as the symptoms that are present are persistent and severe. On the other hand, lack of familiarity with DSM-IV or excessively flexible and idiosyncratic application of DSM-IV criteria or conventions substantially reduces its utility as a common language for communication. (American Psychiatric Association 2000, p. xxxii)

Diagnosis is relevant to the treatment instituted by clinicians to restore the plaintiff to his or her preaccident condition, but it does not play the same role in determining the plaintiff's right to compensation. For example, "pain and suffering" can exist in the absence of a mental disorder. Insisting on the provision of categorical diagnoses does not necessarily provide more useful information for the decision-makers or provide a useful incentive for litigants. In certain cases, dimensional diagnosis may permit consideration of spectral, subthreshold disorders that are more meaningfully associated with associated impairments. Categorical psychiatric diagnosis will remain an important feature of forensic practice. However, the imperfect fit between the use of diagnoses for clinical purposes and their use in litigation makes the prominent role played by categorical diagnoses in forensic settings problematic.

Lawyers, judges, and juries much prefer categorical diagnoses because of their seeming clarity. In litigation, decisions must be made at the time of trial. The assessment of an individual over time as occurs in clinical settings is a luxury not available to judicial decision-makers.

However, categorical diagnostic models exclude spectral conditions that fall outside preestablished inclusion criteria. Disorders classified prototypically and categorically, such as PTSD, have dimensions that complicate psychiatric diagnosis.

## Dimensional Diagnosis in Litigation: Subthreshold Posttraumatic Stress Disorder

Subthreshold PTSD is an example of a disorder with dimensional features that does not have official diagnostic recognition, yet clearly exists and frequently causes significant functional impairment. Subthreshold PTSD can be conceptualized as a dimensional entity that manifests categorical characteristics (defined symptoms causing impairment) and is a good example of such a model (Frank et al. 1998; Maser and Patterson 2002; Ruscio et al. 2002).

The diagnosis of PTSD may present clinically with significant variations from the prototype. Subthreshold PTSD, although not a formally recognized DSM diagnosis, has been recognized in the professional literature (Schützwohl and Maercker 1999; Stein et al. 1997). It is common in Vietnam veterans (Warshaw et al. 1993; Weiss et al. 1992) and is highly represented among sexual abuse survivors and in other traumatized persons (Blanchard et al. 1996; Carlier and Gersons 1995). The number of PTSD symptoms present generally correlates with the severity and chronicity of the disorder (Breslau and Davis 1992; Green et al. 1990; Marshall et al. 2001).

Subthreshold conditions in medicine and psychiatry are common and often cause significant impairment. For example, in medicine, a patient may have some, but not all, of the clinical symptoms necessary to make a diagnosis of migraine headache but is, nonetheless, debilitated by the pain. Subthreshold psychiatric conditions may not fit into categorical diagnostic classifications but also may be debilitating (Maser and Akiskal 2002). Subsyndromal symptoms of major depression can be disabling (Broadhead et al. 1990; Judd et al. 1998; Pincus et al. 2003). Subthreshold social phobia can be associated with severe limitations (Davidson et al. 1994; Schneier et al. 2002).

Subthreshold PTSD may be a longitudinal variant of full PTSD. Like most disorders, PTSD develops over time. Likewise, it may remit with or without treatment over time. A diagnosis of subthreshold PTSD may apply to persons who are newly diagnosed and to those in the process of recovery. Like full PTSD, however, the subthreshold variant may become chronic and persist for years (Moreau and Zisook 2002). Finally,

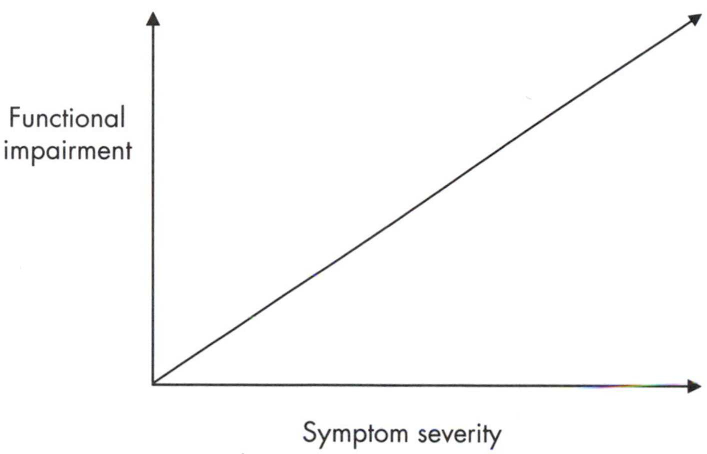


**FIGURE 6–1.** Hypothetical dimensional model of functional impairment and symptom severity.

across study groups, the percentage of participants meeting the DSM-IV reexperiencing criterion or the hyperarousal criterion is much greater than the percentage who meet the avoidance criterion. This implies that those who have genuine PTSD symptoms are often excluded from the diagnosis of PTSD because of the absence of the requisite three avoidant symptoms (Schützwohl and Maercker 1999).

Persons with subthreshold PTSD exhibit clinically significant levels of functional impairment associated with their symptoms. The accompanying schematic figures illustrate dimensional models of psychological trauma. In Figure 6–1, a one-to-one linear relationship between symptom severity and functional impairment is presented for heuristic purposes only. Although a correlation usually exists between symptom severity and functional impairment, rarely, if ever, is the correlation a one-to-one linear relationship (Mezzich and Sharfstein 1985). Figure 6–2 demonstrates possible categorical diagnoses that may occur on a dimensional axis of increasing severity of psychological trauma.

Research has demonstrated that persons with subthreshold PTSD report significantly more interference with work or education than do traumatized persons with fewer symptoms, though they report significantly less interference than persons with the full disorder (Stein et al. 1997). An examination of comorbidity, impairment, and suicidality in a cohort of adults with subthreshold PTSD found that impairment, number of comorbid disorders, rates of comorbid major depressive disorder, and

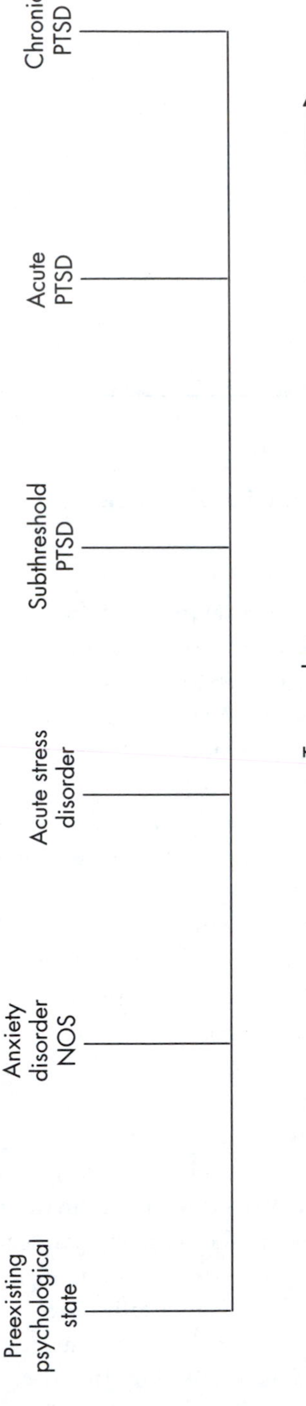


**FIGURE 6–2.** Categorical diagnoses on a dimensional axis of psychological trauma.

current suicidal ideation increased linearly and significantly with increasing number of subthreshold PTSD symptoms (Marshall et al. 2001). Such findings may be relevant when assessing damages in forensic evaluations.

In clinical practice, the fact that a patient's symptoms do not meet all the criteria of a diagnostic category may not be critically significant. Diagnosis in a clinical setting guides treatment. Treatment of a patient with all the symptom criteria of depression, social phobia, or PTSD, in most cases, will not differ significantly from treatment of a patient with a moderate to severe subthreshold form of the disorder. The threshold for treatment intervention generally is severity of symptoms or impairment in function, not whether every diagnostic criterion has been met. If treatment does differ, the clinician has the option over time to change treatment recommendations in response to the evolution or remission of the patient's disorder.

In contrast, in a forensic setting, the difference between a DSM diagnosis and no diagnosis, or between a DSM diagnosis and a non-DSM diagnosis, regardless of degree of impairment, may be significant. In the vignette, Ms. J's degree of functional impairment causally related to the accident, as indicated by a comparison of her pre- and postincident functioning, should be the most significant factor in the award of damages. However, the expert psychiatrist's diagnosis of subthreshold PTSD in the case of Ms. J demonstrates the problems that can arise between the legal system's desire for a categorical diagnosis and the dimensional presentation of a subthreshold syndrome.

## Plaintiff's Case

During trial, the plaintiff's expert testified that he relied on the psychiatric literature to make the diagnosis of chronic subthreshold PTSD. He pointed out the persistent decrements in Ms. J's quality of life following the airplane accident. The plaintiff's attorney elicited testimony from the expert about the professional literature support for the diagnosis of subthreshold PTSD and its association with clinically significant impairment in social and occupational functioning. The plaintiff's expert explained that PTSD is a spectrum or dimensional disorder rather than an all-or-none categorical diagnosis. He emphasized that "pain and suffering" also can exist in the absence of a DSM diagnosis of mental disorder. The attorney was convinced by this argument and felt she could successfully present it to the court.

In anticipation of the defense argument that DSM-IV is the "bible" for the diagnosis of mental illness, the plaintiff's attorney stated during closing arguments that DSM-IV is a work in progress. She directly quoted from DSM-IV:

> It must be noted that DSM-IV reflects a consensus about the classification and diagnoses of mental disorders derived at the time of initial publication. New knowledge generated by research or clinical experience will undoubtedly lead to an increased understanding of the disorders included in DSM-IV, to the identification of new disorders, and to the removal of some disorders in future classifications. The text and criteria sets included in DSM-IV will require reconsideration in light of evolving new information. (American Psychiatric Association 2000, p. xxxiii)

The attorney argued that since 1994, when DSM-IV was published, new research has recognized the existence and importance of subthreshold PTSD in causing functional impairments.

The plaintiff's attorney also quoted from the part of the "Cautionary Statement" in DSM-IV that warns, "These diagnostic criteria and the DSM-IV Classification of mental disorders reflect a consensus of current formulations of evolving knowledge in our field. They do not encompass, however, all the conditions for which people may be treated or that may be appropriate topics for research efforts" (American Psychiatric Association 2000, p. xxxvii). Finally, the plaintiff's attorney noted that the manual itself stated that it was not to be applied mechanically by untrained individuals in "cookbook fashion." She advised the jury, quoting from DSM, that the diagnostic criteria "are meant to be employed by individuals with appropriate clinical training and experience in diagnosis" (American Psychiatric Association 2000, p. xxxii). She pointed out the expert's qualifications and experience, again emphasizing that subthreshold PTSD is nonetheless PTSD with significant associated impairments. She reminded the jury of Ms. J's functional impairments resulting from her condition.

## Defense's Case

In an earlier proceeding, the defense attorney filed a motion *in limine* during a *Daubert* hearing to exclude a subsyndromal diagnosis as lacking credibility. The judge rejected the motion. During trial, on cross-examination, the defense attorney produced DSM-IV and pointedly asked the plaintiff's expert, "Doctor, isn't DSM-IV the bible of authoritative diagnosis that psychiatrists rely on in their clinical practice?" The expert responded that "DSM-IV is an official guide to psychiatric diagnosis but is not the last word. All patients with psychiatric conditions do not necessarily meet DSM-IV diagnostic criteria." The defense attorney then proceeded to demonstrate how the expert had departed from customary diagnostic practice to arrive at an idiosyncratic diagnosis that served the plaintiff's purpose in litigation. He produced an enlarged chart of the diagnostic criteria of PTSD and specifically challenged the expert on each symptom. The expert had to acknowledge that all the symptom criteria required for a diagnosis of PTSD had not been met.

The attorney then tried to get the plaintiff's expert to agree that when fewer PTSD symptoms are present, there is little or no functional impairment. The plaintiff's expert replied that this can be true in some instances but that persons with fewer PTSD symptoms may nevertheless have significant impairment based on comorbidity and predispositional factors. The defense attorney retorted, "Well, Doctor, didn't you just tell this jury that Ms. J did not have any prior psychiatric conditions? You also told the jury that she does not currently suffer from any psychiatric condition other than subthreshold PTSD, is that correct?" The plaintiff's expert conceded this point. The defense attorney continued, "Isn't it true, Doctor, that Ms. J did not seek treatment?" The expert testified that, although this is true, over half of those persons with PTSD or subthreshold PTSD do not seek professional help for their condition, in order to not reexperience the trauma and exacerbate their symptoms.

The defense expert testified that little or no functional impairment was actually caused by the airplane accident. He stated that the absence of treatment supported this conclusion. The defense expert testified that Ms. J's symptoms of anxiety and lack of concentration were related to work stress and preexisting difficulties in her relationship with the fiancé. In closing arguments, defense counsel used this testimony to support his arguments regarding lack of damages. He contested the claim that the litigant's subthreshold PTSD "causes clinically significant distress or impairment in social, occupational, or other areas of functioning." The defense attorney asserted that many individuals experience stress at work that causes suboptimal performance. He argued to the jury that many people fly who fear flying, often purchasing an alcoholic beverage to calm themselves. Moreover, the person alleging symptoms of PTSD or subthreshold PTSD has a duty to mitigate his or her symptoms by seeking treatment.

In closing arguments, the defense attorney attacked the diagnosis of subthreshold PTSD as a nonexistent "designer disorder" that was not recognized in DSM-IV. The defense attorney stated that DSM-IV is the psychiatric diagnostic authority, arguing to the jury that the diagnostic criteria be strictly interpreted. He also quoted from DSM-IV, citing the admonition concerning the "excessively flexible and idiosyncratic application of DSM-IV criteria" (American Psychiatric Association 2000,

p. xxxii). When a diagnosis of PTSD is made in the absence of meeting the diagnostic criteria, the defense attorney argued, the PTSD diagnosis is forced so that the plaintiff can provide an incident-specific trauma to establish proximate causation. In doing so, the attorney said, the plaintiff is attempting to exclude other, more likely causes of Ms. J's psychiatric condition.

The case was settled at the end of closing arguments for $50,000. The plaintiff's attorney was afraid that, although Ms. J appeared to make a favorable impression with the jury during her testimony, her avoidance of treatment coupled with an unofficial subthreshold diagnosis could lead to a defense verdict. Also, the jury appeared to have difficulty grasping subthreshold disorders. The defense attorney settled because of the plaintiff's continued work impairment and difficulties in her relationship with her fiancé following the accident. Monetary damages awarded by a jury might be considerable because of Ms. J's loss of promotion opportunity. Although these impairments could be ascribed to other causes, no work impairment was discovered before the accident.

## Psychiatric Diagnosis in Litigation: Square Pegs in Round Holes

DSM-IV, with its system of diagnostic categorization, attempts to encourage greater precision in communication among mental health practitioners. However, the problems of diagnostic categorization noted in the previous section reinforce the importance of DSM's admonition about its limitations as a vehicle to communicate with greater precision in the forensic setting (American Psychiatric Association 2000). The use of categorical DSM diagnosis risks encouraging legal decision-makers to attempt to fit diagnostic categories into legal categories for which they were not intended. If it cannot be assumed that all individuals described as having the same diagnosis are alike in important ways, then the likelihood that the use of a categorical diagnosis will encourage greater precision in communication in the forensic setting is diminished.

A dimensional model of psychological trauma informs the court much more effectively than categorical diagnosis about the relationship between the severity of symptomatology and the degree of functional impairment. Nevertheless, the use of dimensional diagnosis in litigation does not resolve all the problems created by the imperfect fit of psychiatric diagnoses in the law. Dimensional diagnoses have their own set of associated limitations. For example, the use of subthreshold diagnoses in court might allow psychiatrists to legitimize their pet diagnoses. Jurors not familiar with psychiatric diagnosis may have even greater difficulty understanding the significance of non-DSM-defined terms.

A dimensional diagnostic system may also be misleading in the specific and relevant assessment of functional impairment unless additional information is provided. For example, according to DSM-IV, the determination of the level of functional impairment is coded on Axis V by use of the GAF scale. Moderate impairment in either social or occupational functioning may provide similar GAF scores, but each is likely to have very different implications for compensation. A narrative assessment that explains the individual's specific areas of functional impairment to the trier of fact is required.

The use of the "not otherwise specified," or NOS, diagnostic categories of classification, which are designed to catch psychiatric symptom clusters that constitute atypical disorders, also does not resolve the problems of imperfect fit in litigation. For example, anxiety disorder NOS can be used for an individual with subsyndromal PTSD. In this instance, one of the PTSD-specific rating scales, such as the Clinician-Administered PTSD Scale, can complement the NOS diagnosis. However, forcing subsyndromal disorders into catchall NOS diagnoses substitutes a categorical but vague diagnosis for a dimensional diagnosis that could better inform the court about the relationship between symptom severity and functional impairment.

## Role of Psychiatric Diagnosis in Litigation

The categorical diagnostic system of DSM was not intended to be used as a tool for legal purposes, as DSM makes clear. Alternative dimensional models of diagnosis also do not fit neatly into legal considerations. If diagnoses do not address the needs of the legal system, why should they be used in court at all? The American Academy of Psychiatry and the Law defines forensic psychiatry as "[a] subspecialty of psychiatry in which scientific and clinical experience is applied to legal issues in legal contexts embracing civil, criminal, correctional or legislative matters" (American Academy of Psychiatry and the Law 1995, Preamble I). Thus, the objectives of forensic psychiatry are legal. In contrast, the objectives of medical evaluation are either treatment or research. In these contexts, diagnosis is essential.

The preeminent jurist Judge David Bazelon expressed similar concerns about expert witnesses testifying "in misleading and conclusory terms about the medical or psychiatric definitions of mental disease" (*United States v. Brawner* 1972). These legal and psychiatric authors have recognized that a diagnosis is a translation of thoughts, feelings, and behaviors that must then be translated back into thoughts, feelings, and behaviors by judges and jurors. Because any translation is necessarily imprecise, the authors understood the dangers of psychiatric and psychological testimony that takes the form of diagnostic conclusions rather than clinical descriptions. Legal experts have also suggested that the use of diagnostic labels be done away with in forensic settings (Schopp and Sturgis 1995).

Yet given the forensic allure of categorical diagnoses, use of diagnoses in forensic mental health evaluations is unlikely to disappear. Moreover, diagnoses are often threshold requirements needed to meet specific legal sanctions or determinations. These threshold requirements limit legally sanctioned excuses, entitlements, and curtailments of liberty to persons who suffer from mental illness. For example, in criminal law every legal test for criminal responsibility specifies that the legally relevant impairment must be the result of "mental disease or defect." Many standards for incompetence to stand trial, including those of the Model Penal Code, require that the defendant's limitations be the result of mental disorder. In civil law, the existence of a mental disorder may be necessary to establish that a party was incompetent to contract or unable to write a valid will (Halleck et al. 1992; Shuman 2002). In some cases, the law makes the presence of a mental disorder an element of a party's prima facie case or defense (Shuman, in press). Even when not specifically required by statute, both lawyers and forensic evaluators often think they must have a diagnosis for credibility.

Thus, DSM-IV seeks to warn about the risks of misunderstanding and misuse of psychiatric diagnoses for forensic purposes:

> In most situations, the clinical diagnosis of a DSM-IV mental disorder is not sufficient to establish the existence for legal purposes of a "mental disorder," "mental disability," "mental disease," or "mental defect." In determining whether an individual meets a specified legal standard (e.g., for competence, criminal responsibility, or disability), additional information is usually required beyond that contained in the DSM-IV diagnosis. (American Psychiatric Association 2000, p. xxxiii)

If psychiatrists and other mental health practitioners regularly testify to diagnostic categories without thorough explication of functional impairment, DSM's admonition about the risks of misunderstanding and misusing psychiatric diagnoses is unlikely to be appreciated by judges, lawyers, and jurors.

Nevertheless, despite all these limitations, diagnostic considerations can be relevant in forensic evaluations. Although not dispositive, some degree of association clearly exists between DSM diagnoses, impaired mental capacity, and impaired functioning. As noted, formal mental disorders are threshold requirements in a number of legal statutes. In general, mental disorders serve these threshold functions because they are believed to be meaningfully associated with diminished abilities or functional impairments. Even though a diagnosis does not specify the nature of this association in regard to a specific functional capacity or a specific legal standard, psychiatrists' assessment of a relevant impairment may be informed or guided by a psychiatric diagnosis. When mental disorder is a threshold requirement for certain legal determinations, the diagnostic requirement is meant to serve as a validator of the main legal contention that certain relevant impairments are present, and can do so (Halleck 1992).

In making a diagnosis, psychiatrists identify a range of possible symptoms. Evaluators may be directed by their own diagnostic assessment or by the earlier diagnostic impressions of others toward closer examination of those symptoms that are associated with the functional impairments and specific capacities that are legally relevant. Conversely, by identifying symptoms associated with a given illness, the use of diagnosis can serve as a restraint on ungrounded speculation regarding an individual's past mental status or degree of functional impairment. As a result of their specialized knowledge, psychiatrists providing forensic evaluations can draw reasonable connections between or refute unreasonable claims about symptoms associated with a diagnosis and impaired functions associated with those symptoms.

Use of diagnoses also allows psychiatrists to make knowledgeable observations about the longitudinal course of a disorder. This too may provide essential information regarding symptoms that may have affected relevant legal capacities. The identification of a chronic, episodic, or progressively deteriorating course of mental illness associated with various diagnostic categories provides forensic examiners with a framework for identifying the course of a particular individual's illness and the likelihood of symptoms creating functional impairments at a certain point in time. In addition, the natural history of a disorder often provides clues to the possible duration of such impairments. Such information may also be legally relevant.

Finally, the use of a diagnosis can serve as a point of reference that enhances the value and reliability of psychiatric testimony even though it may not be the determinative factor for the trier of fact. When a diagnosis is established, an extensive body of literature and research important in rendering legal determinations can be introduced to the court. The subject of the evaluation can be assessed in relation to others of the same diagnostic category aided by the cumulative experiences and research of the fields of psychiatry and psychology.

Making a diagnosis is only the beginning of any assessment, whether clinical or forensic. More information in addition to diagnosis must be gathered to understand the patient's psychological state and to devise and implement an appropriate treatment plan. For example, a diagnosis of major depression does not convey any specific information regarding a patient's risk of suicide. An individual with active suicidal ideation, a plan, means, and intent would be provided with vastly different treatment than an individual with no suicidal ideation, even though both may have the same categorical DSM diagnosis. Similarly, in forensic evaluations, the legal system's reliance on DSM should not lead psychiatrists to simply provide categorical diagnosis without further information. Evaluation of the relevant functional impairment or changes resulting from the mental disorder should be specific and explicit and, where appropriate, use a dimensional model of description.

## Conclusion

Psychiatrists and other mental health practitioners who offer expert testimony should take steps to prevent categorical diagnosis from casting a spell of certitude on the court. To do so involves appreciating and avoiding the misuse and misunderstanding of psychiatric diagnosis in forensic settings. Impairment, not diagnosis, is the central issue in most types of litigation. Subthreshold diagnosis, especially subthreshold PTSD, illustrates the significant differences between the application of DSM categorical diagnosis versus that of dimensional diagnosis in litigation. Dimensional diagnosis permits consideration of subsyndromal conditions and their associated impairments along a continuum of symptom severity rather than on all-or-none categorical terms.

The law's reliance on "official" DSM diagnosis, however, makes the use of a dimensional model problematic. Categorical DSM diagnoses are the clear preference for attorneys and the courts for judicial decision making. Nevertheless, "gray" medical and psychiatric conditions may not conform to preestablished "black-and-white" categorical diagnoses. Overreliance on categorical diagnoses in litigation can result in the use of diagnoses to convey or imply information that they were not designed to encompass.

Psychiatrists providing forensic evaluations and expert testimony should make certain that the law's emphasis on categorical diagnosis does not result in failure to specifically assess functional impairment. In assessing impairment, expert testimony should be couched in a qualitative or quantitative dimensional context that uses clinically based data, severity of illness assessments, and the pertinent psychiatric literature to help the fact finder assess the functional effect of the diagnosis.

## Key Points

- There is an "imperfect fit" between categorical DSM diagnosis and the legal process across the spectrum of civil and criminal litigation.
- Subthreshold diagnosis illustrates the significant differences between the application of DSM categorical diagnosis and dimensional diagnosis in litigation.
- Regardless of the legal system's desire or requirement for a formal DSM diagnosis, legal determinations often hinge on relevant impairment and not diagnostic category.
- No diagnosis implies any specific level of impairment.

## Practice Guidelines

1. Identify the necessity for inclusion or exclusion of psychiatric diagnosis in accordance with the relevant legal statute.
2. Identify the functional capacity directly relevant to the legal issue in question and evaluate functional impairment, if any.
3. Explain the relationship between the diagnosis and the relevant functional capacity. If an unreasonable or invalid inference of functional impairment is being made on the basis of any given diagnosis, explain the lack of correlation between or incorrect reasoning about the diagnosis and functional capacity in question.
4. Do not substitute the formulation of a DSM diagnosis for a careful forensic evaluation of the relevant functional capacity in question.
5. In assessing functional impairment, moderate impairment in either social or occupational functioning may provide similar dimensional GAF scores. However, each is likely to have different implications for compensation or eligibility for legal status. A narrative summary may be necessary that explains to the court the litigant's specific functional impairments.
6. Avoid forcing subsyndromal and other psychiatric conditions into catchall NOS diagnoses. This results in the substitution of an imprecise diagnosis for the provision of substantive information about the relationship between symptom severity and functional impairment.

## References

American Academy of Psychiatry and the Law: Ethics Guidelines for the Practice of Forensic Psychiatry. Bloomfield, CT, American Academy of Psychiatry and the Law, 1995

American Psychiatric Association: Diagnostic and Statistical Manual of Mental Disorders, 4th Edition. Washington, DC, American Psychiatric Association, 1994

American Psychiatric Association: Diagnostic and Statistical Manual of Mental Disorders, 4th Edition, Text Revision. Washington, DC, American Psychiatric Association, 2000

Blanchard EB, Hickling EJ, Barton KA, et al: One-year prospective follow-up of motor vehicle accident victims. Behav Res Ther 10:775–786, 1996

Bogenschutz MP, Nurnberg HG: Classification of mental disorders, in Comprehensive Textbook of Psychiatry/VII, 7th Edition. Edited by Sadock BJ, Sadock VA. Philadelphia, PA, Lippincott Williams & Wilkins, 2000, pp 824–839

Breslau N, Davis GC. Posttraumatic stress disorder in an urban population of young adults: risk factors for chronicity. Am J Psychiatry 149:671–675, 1992

Broadhead WE, Blazer DG, George LK, et al: Depression, disability days, and days lost from work in a prospective epidemiological survey. JAMA 264: 2524–2528, 1990

Carlier IVE, Gersons BPR: Partial posttraumatic stress disorder (PTSD): the issue of psychological scars and the occurrence of PTSD symptoms. J Nerv Ment Dis 183:107–109, 1995

Daubert v Merrell Dow Pharmaceuticals, Inc, 509 U.S. 579 (1993)

Davidson JRT, Hughes DC, George LK, et al: The boundary of social phobia: exploring the threshold. Arch Gen Psychiatry 51:975–983, 1994

Frank E, Lassano GB, Shear MK, et al: The spectrum model: a more coherent approach to the complexity of psychiatric symptomatology. CNS Spectrums 3:23–34, 1998

Gold LH: Psychiatric diagnoses and the retrospective assessment of mental states, in Retrospective Assessment of Mental States in Litigation: Predicting the Past. Edited by Simon RI, Shuman DW. Washington, DC, American Psychiatric Publishing, 2002, pp 335–367

Green BL, Grace MC, Lindy JD, et al: War stressors and symptom persistence in posttraumatic stress disorder. J Anxiety Disord 4:31–39, 1990

Halleck SL, Hoge SK, Miller RD, et al: The use of psychiatric diagnoses in the legal process: Task Force Report of the American Psychiatric Association. Bull Am Acad Psychiatry Law 20:481–499, 1992

Judd LL, Akiskal HS, Maser JD, et al: A prospective 12-year study of subsyndromal and syndromal depressive symptoms in unipolar major depressive disorders. Arch Gen Psychiatry 55:694–700, 1998

Kinzie JD, Goetz RR: A century of controversy surrounding posttraumatic stress-spectrum syndromes: the impact on DSM-III and DSM-IV. J Trauma Stress 9:159–179, 1996

Kumho Tire Co, Ltd v Carmichael, 526 U.S. 137 (1999)

Marshall R, Olfson E, Hellman F, et al: Comorbidity, impairment and suicidality in SPTSD. Am J Psychiatry 158:1467–1473, 2001

Maser JD, Akiskal HS (eds): Spectrum concepts in major mental disorders (entire issue). Psychiatr Clin North Am 25(4), 2002

Maser JD, Patterson T: Spectrum and nosology: implications for DSM-V. Psychiatr Clin North Am 25(4):855–886, 2002

Mezzich JE, Sharfstein SS: Severity of illness and diagnostic formulation: classifying patients for prospective payment systems. Hosp Community Psychiatry 36 (suppl 7):770–772, 1985

Moreau C, Zisook S: Rationale for posttraumatic stress disorder spectrum. Psychiatr Clin North Am 25(4):775–790, 2002

Pincus HA, McQueen LE, Elinson L: Subthreshold mental disorders: nosological and research recommendations, in Advancing DSM: Dilemmas in Psychiatric Diagnosis. Edited by Phillips KA, First MB, Pincus HA. Washington, DC, American Psychiatric Publishing, 2003, pp 129–144

Ruscio AM, Ruscio J, Keane TM: The latent structure of posttraumatic stress disorder: a taxometric investigation of reactions to extreme stress. J Abnorm Psychol 111:290–301, 2002

Sadler JZ, Wiggins OP, Schwartz MA (eds): Philosophical Perspectives on Psychiatric Diagnostic Classification. Baltimore, MD, Johns Hopkins University Press, 1994

Schneier FR, Blanco C, Antia SX, et al: The social anxiety spectrum. Psychiatr Clin North Am 25(4):757–774, 2002

Schopp RG, Sturgis BJ: Sexual predators and legal mental illness for civil commitment. Behav Sci Law 13:437–458, 1995

Schützwohl M, Maercker A: Effects of varying diagnostic criteria for posttraumatic stress disorder are endorsing the concept of partial PTSD. J Trauma Stress 12:155–165, 1999

Shuman DW: The *Diagnostic and Statistical Manual of Mental Disorders* in the courts. Bull Am Acad Psychiatry Law 17:25–32, 1989

Shuman DW: Retrospective assessment of mental states and the law, in Retrospective Assessment of Mental States in Litgation: Predicting the Past. Edited by Simon RI, Shuman DW. Washington, DC, American Psychiatric Publishing, 2002, pp 21–46

Shuman DW: The tyranny of diagnostic labels: unmasking "forensic" diagnosis Int J Law Psychiatry (in press)

Simon RI: Toward the development of guidelines in the forensic psychiatric examination of posttraumatic stress disorder claimants, in Posttraumatic Stress Disorder in Litigation: Guidelines for Forensic Assessment, 2nd Edition. Edited by Simon RI. Washington, DC, American Psychiatric Publishing, 2002, pp 41–90

Stein MB, Walker JR, Hazen AL, et al: Full and partial posttraumatic stress disorder: findings from a community survey. Am J Psychiatry 154:1114–1119, 1997

United States v Brawner, 471 F.2d 969, 1011 (D.C. Cir. 1972) (Bazelon J, conc. and diss.)

United States v Torniero, 570 F.Supp. 721 (D.C. Conn. 1983)

Warshaw MG, Fierman E, Pratt L, et al: Quality of life and dissociation in anxiety disorder patients with histories of trauma or PTSD. Am J Psychiatry 150:1512–1516, 1993

Weiss DS, Marmar CR, Schlenger WE, et al: The prevalence of lifetime and partial post-traumatic stress disorder in Vietnam theater veterans. J Trauma Stress 5:365–376, 1992

## Suggested Readings

Gold LH: Psychiatric diagnoses and the retrospective assessment of mental states, in Retrospective Assessment of Mental States in Litigation: Predicting the Past. Edited by Simon RI, Shuman DW. Washington, DC, American Psychiatric Publishing, 2002, pp 335–367

Phillips KA, First MB, Pincus HA (eds): Advancing DSM: Psychiatric Dilemmas in Psychiatric Diagnosis. Washington, DC, American Psychiatric Publishing, 2003

Slovenko R: Psychiatry in Law—Law in Psychiatry. New York, Brunner-Routledge, 2002

CHAPTER 7

# The Forensic Examination and Report

Robert M. Wettstein, M.D.

## Introduction

The forensic evaluation is unlike a mental health evaluation for clinical or treatment purposes in several respects (Heilbrun 2001). The sharply contrasting role of the forensic evaluator has significant implications for the conduct of the forensic interview and evaluation. Clinical evaluators serve the health care needs of the individual patient and share mutual goals of beneficence and nonmaleficence. They typically rely on the patient's self-report in their decision making, and in most cases involving nondemented adult patients, they need not obtain information from family or other collateral data sources.

Forensic evaluators, however, are retained by third parties (e.g., attorney, court, or agency) whose goals are not clinical but legal or financial. Those third parties may have goals adverse to the evaluee's legal or financial interests, such as prosecution, incarceration, and loss of child custody. Forensic evaluators adopt an objective and skeptical approach to the evaluee's self-report and presentation and seek input from collateral sources of information as well as testing. They reach their opinions with a reasonable degree of clinical certainty and are not allowed to engage in speculation, which is permitted in a clinical evaluation.

Forensic mental health evaluations involve several phases: preparation for the case, data collection, data analysis, and forensic report writing (Heilbrun 2001).

## Clinical Vignettes

### Vignette 1

A psychiatrist in a general office practice had been treating a 30-year-old female nurse for anxiety and depressive symptoms who had difficulty functioning at work. Six months ago, on her way to work, the public bus on which the patient was riding was involved in a head-on collision with an oncoming truck. She was emotionally shaken but not physically injured and continued her trip to work at an urban public health clinic. Later that evening, while at work, she was sexually assaulted by a male patient at the clinic. As a teenager, she had been sexually abused for 3 years by an uncle.

The patient informed the psychiatrist that she filed a civil lawsuit against the public transportation agency and a workers' compensation claim against her employer, seeking monetary damages and expenses for the psychiatric treatment in both suits. She reported that her attorney wants the psychiatrist to assist her in this litigation, and she asked the psychiatrist to contact her attorney. The psychiatrist had no experience or training in forensic psychiatry, though some of his patients had been involved in civil litigation in the past.

### Vignette 2

A psychiatrist in general practice received a telephone call from his golfing partner, an attorney, who was representing a young man charged criminally with the homicide of his wife. The psychiatrist maintained a busy office psychiatric practice and had no experience evaluating criminal defendants charged with major crimes. He agreed to conduct the evaluation as a favor to his friend. He felt confident that he could properly evaluate the defendant and assist in lowering the defendant's criminal charges and sentence at the attorney's request, based on what his friend told him about the defendant.

### Vignette 3

The county public defender's office contacted a forensic psychiatrist to conduct a pretrial evaluation of a defendant accused of performing oral and anal intercourse, which occurred in a particularly sadistic manner, on a 5-year-old boy. The forensic psychiatrist had some experience with violent and sexual offenders but had not previously encountered such violent sexual activity perpetrated against a young child. The psychiatrist had two sons of preschool age and experienced intense feelings of revulsion and anger as the defense attorney introduced the case to him. The psychiatrist discussed his feelings about the defendant and the alleged crime with his wife, who encouraged him to accept the referral because it would be good for the psychiatrist's practice and income.

## Preparation for the Case

The forensic evaluator should address several issues before beginning work on the case (Table 7–1).

### Identify Forensic Issue and Clarify Expert Role

Once the forensic evaluator has been contacted by an attorney, court, or agency, the evaluator, like any consultant, must specifically identify the referral question. Some referral sources are not initially clear about the forensic issue; others may not know how a forensic mental health expert could assist them if they have not previously retained such experts. The evaluator should determine what role is being solicited. Three possible roles are forensic evaluator and court witness for the litigants or the court itself, court mediator between the litigants, and nonwitness consultant to the retaining party.

These differing forensic roles entail correspondingly distinct clinical and ethical responsibilities and obligations. Expert evaluators who conduct interviews of the litigant and render expert forensic opinions in the case do so while striving for objectivity (American Academy of Psychiatry and the Law [AAPL] 1995). In contrast, a mental health consultant to the retaining attorney who does not interview the litigant or testify in the case may serve as part of the legal "team" and thus advocate for that party's legal interests. That expert's role may include assisting in jury selection, testing mock trials, preparing witnesses to testify, or assisting with the preparation of cross-examination of the opposing experts (Strier 1999). Individuals should serve only one role in a given forensic case.

**TABLE 7–1.** Preparation of the case

- Identify the referral issue.
- Clarify role with the retaining party.
- Decide whether to accept the case.
- Accept referrals only within expertise.
- Establish fee and expense agreement.
- Other tasks
  - Know the relevant legal and forensic literature.
  - Inform retaining party of anticipated course of evaluation.
  - Obtain relevant documents.
  - Schedule interviews and testing.

## Decide Whether to Accept the Case

The evaluator should consider several issues before deciding to accept the forensic referral. The evaluator should have the expertise and training to work on the case; for example, a psychiatrist without child psychiatry training or supervised experience is unlikely to be able to appropriately perform a child custody evaluation involving young children. A general psychiatrist without forensic training and experience, as in vignettes 1 and 2, may not be able to competently perform the forensic evaluation, at least without considerable supervision from an experienced forensic expert. In such situations, the general psychiatrist is advised to refer the matter to an appropriate forensic expert or to at least collaborate with such a colleague.

Some states have enacted statutes setting minimum requirements for mental health professionals to conduct competency-to-stand-trial and criminal responsibility evaluations (Farkas et al. 1997). In these states, there may be training and experience requirements, as well as an examination and certification process that must be followed. These requirements were established as a result of concerns about the quality of existing pretrial evaluations.

The evaluator should not be so biased regarding the psychiatric or forensic issues on the case that an objective and fair evaluation cannot be performed. In vignette 3, the forensic psychiatrist was aware of intense negative feelings toward the defendant and the alleged crime and may have had difficulty putting those feelings aside. Similarly, previous contact or work with the retaining or opposing attorney should be considered as a potential source of conflict and as a barrier to objectivity in conducting the evaluation. The evaluator should be alert to such influences and able to decide to refuse the case if these barriers are substantial (Simon and Wettstein 1997). This is illustrated by vignette 2, in which the psychiatrist felt pressured to accept a referral as a favor to his attorney friend, though he was likely not to have the requisite training and experience to conduct the evaluation. That psychiatrist also may have had difficulty performing an objective evaluation if there was a perception of pressure or coercion to reach an opinion favorable to his friend.

A previous personal or professional relationship with the evaluee is similarly grounds for recusing oneself from the forensic evaluation (Strasburger et al. 1997). A treating psychiatrist may know her patient well and, therefore, be approached by the patient's attorney for participation in the litigation as a forensic expert. That psychiatrist, however, is well advised to refer the patient to another psychiatrist to perform the forensic evaluation. This may preserve the treatment relationship with the patient as well as ensure that a competent forensic evaluation is performed, which is perhaps beyond the therapist's experience. Treating psychiatrists do not typically bring the necessary skepticism, objectivity, and evaluation approach to their patients to be able to conduct a comprehensive and impartial forensic evaluation. In addition, attempting to perform a forensic evaluation of a current patient risks jeopardizing that treatment relationship, especially if the clinician is unable to support the patient's legal case.

### Establish Fee and Expense Agreement

The evaluator should secure agreement with the retaining attorney, court, or agency with regard to the evaluator's fees and expenses to conduct the evaluation. Such agreements are optimally secured in written form, whether with a formal contract provided by the evaluator or retaining party or in summary form through correspondence. Evaluators may be limited in their hourly or total fees by policy of the court or insurance carrier, and such resource limitations should be discussed in advance with regard to whether a proper evaluation can nevertheless be conducted. It is unethical for evaluators to contract with the retaining party (i.e., attorney, court, expert witness agency) on a contingency basis.

Expenses for consultants to conduct specialized medical or psychological testing may add considerably to the evaluator's fees and should be disclosed to the retaining party to the extent foreseeable. Fees for court testimony, waiting time, and travel time should also be formalized in advance. Court testimony is notoriously difficult to schedule in advance, and testifying psychiatrists who maintain a significant clinical practice will frequently suffer disruptions to their patient care activities. Some evaluators set higher fees for courtroom testimony as opposed to the forensic evaluation itself; such an increment, however, needs to be appropriately justified.

## Data Collection

### General Issues

The forensic evaluation must be a comprehensive review of the relevant clinical and legal information regarding the evaluee and the legal issue in question. It is typically essential for the forensic evaluator to obtain information from a variety of sources rather than solely from the evaluee (Heilbrun et al. 1994). Relevant records should be obtained, preferably before the interview with the evaluee (Table 7–2). Clinical records are typically obtained from retaining or opposing counsel.

**TABLE 7–2. Collateral document sources**

- Previous psychiatric evaluations and treatment
- Previous psychological testing
- Medical hospital and office records
- Academic records
- Occupational evaluations and employment documents
- Social Security disability records
- Military records
- Discovery regarding the legal case
- Diaries and journals written by the evaluee

Sometimes clinical records, or summaries of records, obtained from counsel are incomplete. Attorneys have been known to selectively provide information to their own expert witnesses, either inadvertently or with the intent of manipulating the evaluator (Gutheil and Simon 1999). In some cases, it will be important to obtain copies of an entire hospital or clinic chart rather than just a discharge summary. Evaluators may then need to obtain written consent from the evaluee for the complete record and request those records from the original source, such as a hospital or clinic. Retaining counsel should be aware that the evaluator is attempting to independently obtain such records and may later request a copy of them for their files once they reach the evaluator. Attorneys will ordinarily be the source of legal documents such as the litigation complaint or criminal affidavits, interrogatories, discovery depositions, hearing transcripts, and investigation and police reports.

It is usually necessary for the forensic interview to occupy far more time than a clinical evaluation, including the use of multiple forensic interviews with the evaluee (Simon and Wettstein 1997). Substantial contact with the evaluee often permits a more accurate assessment of an evaluee whose mental status could change over time because of a mood or other mental disorder. In rare cases, a face-to-face interview with an evaluee will not be possible, such as when the legal discovery deadline has passed, the court will not grant access to the litigant, or the litigant is deceased. Collateral interviews may nevertheless be possible, in addition to review of records. Any forensic opinions offered by the evaluator without a personal interview of the litigant must be explicitly qualified by that limitation.

The evaluator must attend to the conditions of the evaluation. Lengthy interviews can be stressful to the evaluee as well as the evaluator, and opportunities for bathroom use or other interruptions should be available. Daylong interviews may be necessary if there is great distance between the evaluator and evaluee. The presence of third-party witnesses or taping equipment potentially increases the adversarial nature of the evaluation process, distracts the evaluation, and distorts its results, but such procedures are sometimes compelled by applicable law (AAPL 1999). The presence of witnesses or taping can help to ensure a complete and accurate record and to challenge any misrepresentations by the evaluator (Simon 1996). The presence of interested observers potentially distorts standardized testing procedures such as neuropsychological testing (McSweeny et al. 1998). Nevertheless, some forensic evaluators routinely videotape their evaluations and make the tape available for use at trial. Opposing experts may then have an opportunity to review the tape or transcripts of the interviews and to identify distortions, errors, and omissions in the interviews.

Some forensic evaluation facilities employ a multidisciplinary staff to collect relevant information. Thus, a psychiatrist will obtain psychiatric data, a psychologist will perform psychological testing, a social worker will obtain family and social history, and an internist will perform medical and laboratory testing. Evaluators in solo practice usually obtain most information, albeit with the use of consultants or medical specialists as needed for additional testing (e.g., magnetic resonance imaging scan of the head, electroencephalogram, thyroid function tests, psychological testing, and neuropsychological testing). Team evaluations permit a greater number of forensic evaluations, but they create problems such as scheduling coordination, need for meetings to discuss and evaluate data, uncertainty regarding responsibility for the work product, and potential for inconsistency in the court testimony of the team (Bow et al. 2002).

Evaluators are responsible for initially informing the evaluee regarding the nature, purpose, and nonconfidentiality of the evaluation process. This notification procedure is distinguishable from the informed consent process conducted in a typical clinical evaluation or treatment session, as the forensic evaluation is usually a third-party evaluation, may be court ordered, and is undertaken ordinarily as a nonconfidential evaluation. Some evaluators request evaluees to acknowledge in writing that they received this notice, but evaluees in court-ordered evaluations ordinarily do not need to provide a release of information to the evaluator.

Forensic interviews are readily distinguished from clinical interviews with regard to general approach, technique, content areas, and skepticism of the evaluator. Though clinical interviews focus on such here-and-now issues as coping strategies used by the patient, ego strengths and weakness, and defense mechanisms, forensic interviews are directed to the assessment of cognitive or volitional capacities of the evaluee in the past, present, or future (Scheiber 2003). Forensic evaluations are focused around the particular forensic mental health issue in the case. Assessment of psychiatric symptoms and disorders is an essential component of both types of evaluation. Forensic evaluators maintain a skeptical attitude about self-reported data and are wary of the influence of others on the evaluee (Williams et al. 1999).

## Forensic Practice Guidelines

As in clinical psychiatry, practice guidelines for forensic evaluations can be useful to evaluators, especially because they have been developed by colleagues who are experts in the given area. These guidelines are typically considered aspirational rather than mandatory. Guidelines include clinical, forensic, legal, and ethical issues relevant to that particular forensic evaluation. Existing forensic practice guidelines include those for evaluations of child custody (American Academy of Child and Adolescent Psychiatry 1997b; American Psychological Association 1994), conduct disorder (American Academy of Child and Adolescent Psychiatry 1997a), juvenile sex offenders (American Academy of Child and Adolescent Psychiatry 1999), and criminal responsibility (AAPL 2002). Research data on forensic evaluators' adherence to professional guidelines have been published (Bow et al. 2002).

## Forensic Instruments

Forensic evaluators often use a nonstandardized, unstructured interview format, covering all relevant content areas. Open-ended rather than "yes–no" or leading questions are appropriate for exploring the forensic content in the interview, such as the defendant's account of the crime and mental status at that time. Standard psychological tests, including intelligence, projective, personality, and neuropsychological instruments, are variably used in forensic evaluations, depending on the forensic mental health issue in the case (Nicholson and Norwood 2000). However, traditional psychological testing measures do not specifically relate to forensic purposes such as competence to stand trial or criminal responsibility (Skeem and Golding 1998).

Evaluators may also choose to conduct structured interviews using forensic instruments. Indeed, there is a trend toward growing use of forensic assessment instruments when conducting forensic evaluations (Nicholson and Norwood 2000). Many such instruments, scales, and standardized psychiatric interview schedules have been published and may be useful to the evaluator, depending on the forensic or legal issues in the case (Grisso 2002; Rogers 2001). Several instruments relate to the risk assessment of violence or sexual violence (Rapid Risk Assessment for Sex Offense Recidivism [RRASOR; Hanson and Thornton 2000], Violence Risk Appraisal Guide [Barbaree et al. 2001; Loza et al. 2002]). Other instruments include evaluation of malingering (Structured Interview of Reported Symptoms [Rogers 1992]), psychopathy assessment (Psychopathy Checklist—Revised [PCL-R; Hare 1980]), assessment of criminal responsibility (Rogers Criminal Responsibility Assessment Scales [Rogers and Shuman 2000]), assessment of criminal competency (Georgia Court Competency Test [Ustad et al. 1996], MacArthur Competence Assessment Tool—Criminal Adjudication [Otto et al. 1998], Fitness Interview Test [Roesch et al. 1998]), and assessment of civil competency (MacArthur Competence Assessment Tool for Treatment [Grisso and Appelbaum 1998]). Some instruments rely on self-report data from the evaluee, but others (e.g., PCL-R) require that the evaluator incorporate third-party data as part of the assessment.

The instruments can be useful in conducting interviews, in obtaining relevant information, and in decision making regarding the forensic opinions in the case. Some instruments are useful as screening tests rather than as definitive measures of a forensic issue. The use of cutoff scores for the forensic instruments is discouraged, given that they may not correspond well with legal standards (Rogers et al. 2001). Forensic evaluators should be aware, however, that the reliability and validity of these instruments are often the subject of debate in the scientific literature (see Chapter 22: "Understanding Prediction Instruments," this volume). Moreover, these instruments, like psychological testing generally, may or may not satisfy legal criteria for admissible evidence under the law (Boccaccini and Brodsky 1999). Forensic evaluators should be familiar with the development, utility, administration, scoring, and limitations of the instruments before their use. In addition, familiarity with the research literature on forensic instruments is essential to their proper use.

## Issues in Using Self-Report Data

Several concerns arise regarding the accuracy of information obtained from evaluees. In clinical evaluations, self-report data are typically the basis for diagnostic and treatment decisions. Self-report tests are commonly used for screening for alcohol problems in primary care medicine (Allen et al. 1995). Traditional psychological tests such as the Minnesota Multiphasic Personality Inventory (MMPI) are self-report testing instruments. Research, however, has demonstrated that the accuracy of such data in medical and mental health settings is questionable. There is low agreement between patients and informants in the assessment of personality disorders (Riso et al. 1994) and adult attention-deficit/hyperactivity disorder (Zucker et al. 2002). In addiction psychiatry, patient self-report of illicit drug use can be highly inaccurate depending on the patient population (i.e., arrestees vs. patients in treatment), the context in which the data are collected, the type of drug, the method of survey, and the recency of use (Harrison and Hughes 1997; McNagny and Parker 1992; Weiss et al. 1998). In assessing major life stressors, there is a poor rate of agreement between subjects and informants as to whether a particular life event has occurred (Schless and Mendels 1978). Even the self-report of one's stature has been shown not to be accurate, at least for men (Giles and Hutchinson 1991).

Evaluees in forensic evaluations often have a reason or motivation to distort their history or presentation to the forensic evaluator based on their interest in the outcome of the litigation. Accused sexual offenders commonly deny, minimize, or distort previous sexual offenses in a self-serving manner consciously or unconsciously, and denial is a significant clinical issue in their assessment and management (Lanyon 2001). Head injury claimants in litigation retrospectively inflate their preinjury scholastic functioning to a greater degree than nonlitigating controls (Greiffenstein et al. 2002). Beyond this, memory for past events is generally reconstructive and often inaccurate; it is not complete and accurate like a videotape (Haber and Haber 2000; Hyman and Loftus 1998). An evaluee's memory for relevant events such as the presenting crime may be distorted as a result of intoxication, emotional arousal, psychosis, mood disturbance, or personality disorder (Porter et al. 2001; Stone 1992). The presence of clinical depression can affect neuropsychological functioning and reduce recollection memory (MacQueen et al. 2002), as well as cause overreporting of functional impairment (Morgado et al. 1991).

In addition, forensic evaluations often occur long after the legal incident in question, and memories change over time. Attorneys have been known to explicitly or indirectly coach their clients regarding how to behave in a forensic evaluation. Repeated forensic evaluations can inadvertently contaminate later forensic interviews when evaluees have learned how to respond to an evaluator's psychiatric questioning. Defendants who are incarcerated can be influenced by family members or other inmates regarding how to present in the forensic evaluation. For these reasons, it is standard practice for forensic evaluators to corroborate relevant information through multiple data sources and to explicitly assess the evaluee's response style as honest, deceptive, distorting, or otherwise (Heilbrun 2001).

## Issues in Conducting Collateral Interviews

In treatment settings, collateral data sources are routinely obtained in the practice of geriatric and child psychiatry because of the cognitive limitations of elderly and young subjects. Problems regarding confidentiality, however, generally arise in collecting collateral data in other subjects. Thus, clinicians may not be accustomed to considering when and how to obtain collateral data. In contrast, forensic evaluators are obligated to consider how to obtain collateral data, either from third parties or from written documentation. Third-party information can be challenged in court as inadmissible hearsay, but this is unlikely to occur to any significant extent in practice (Heilbrun 2001; Melton et al. 1997).

The forensic evaluator's initial task is the selection or identification of appropriate collateral contacts. Ethics obligations when striving for objectivity dictate that the evaluator seek information from all sides of the case and not just bolster a preformed expert opinion by contacting one set of collaterals. Even the appearance of unfairness in selecting collateral sources can form the nidus of cross-examination at trial or deposition. Established rules or procedures for selecting and conducting collateral interviews do not exist. The evaluator is obligated to adhere to the applicable professional ethics guidelines when contacting collateral sources as well as during the direct evaluation of the evaluee.

Nominations of specific contacts can come from a variety of sources such as the retaining agency or attorney, the evaluee, family members, coworkers, or crime victims. It is advisable to consult with the retaining attorney or agency before contacting any collateral sources. It may be awkward for the evaluator to contact collateral sources on the opposing side of the case; a crime victim or the arresting police officer might refuse to consent to an interview with a defendant-retained evaluator, but contact with such sources can be enlightening. Some spouses of litigants may refuse to be interviewed by opposing-side evaluators, but court orders to interview them can be obtained if they are named plaintiffs in the litigation. Evaluators can bolster or demonstrate their independence and objectivity by pursuing those collateral sources who are reluctant to be interviewed or those who provide information contrary to the position of the retaining side of the litigation.

The initial contact with the collateral source can occur through several means. In some situations, the evaluee or evaluee's attorney can request that the collateral sources contact the evaluator. When the evaluator is retained by the opposing side of the legal case from the evaluee, the evaluator may need to solicit collateral sources through the attorney who has retained the evaluator. In general, evaluators do not have significant direct contact, if any, with the opposing side attorney because of legal or ethical considerations such as confidentiality, contractual obligations, attorney-client privilege, or attorney work product.

The number of collateral interviews will depend on the particular facts, circumstances, and complexity of the case itself. A crime scene involving multiple victims and witnesses will require multiple interviews with those individuals. An employment law case involving a personality-disordered worker may require multiple interviews with coworkers and supervisors. More interviews, rather than fewer, are required when there is disputed information about the evaluee's mental state or behavior at the event in question or when the evaluator is attempting to reconcile conflicting accounts of what happened. Collateral sources can provide discrepant information from each other and from the evaluee about such matters as the existence of child physical abuse in the family (Kraemer et al. 2003). Mood disorders and intoxication can fluctuate over time, so that collateral interviews with exposure to the evaluee over time may be needed in those cases. Memories fade for collateral sources as well as evaluees, so more informants may be needed if the legal events in question occurred years earlier.

Collateral interviews can be conducted in person or, perhaps more frequently, by telephone, depending on time and availability of the collateral source (Heilbrun et al. 2002). Many evaluators prefer in-person interviews to telephone contacts, given the usefulness of nonverbal input in the interview.

Collateral interviews typically require the consent of the collateral source or the court but not of the evaluee. The collateral source will typically not be under court or agency order to appear for the collateral interview, though that could occur. Some evaluees will instruct the evaluator not to contact third parties or conduct collateral interviews, but these instructions can often be disregarded after consulting with the retaining attorney or agency. Audio- or videotaping of the collateral interview may require the collateral's consent.

The evaluator should inform the collateral source about who retained the evaluator, as well as the nonconfidentiality of the interview. Some evaluators provide a written notice of nonconfidentiality; they may further request that the collateral source sign an acknowledgement of that notice. The evaluator should ordinarily not release written or verbal information about the evaluee to the collateral source, absent consent from the retaining party. Information obtained from the collateral interview should be shared with the retaining party or attorney but not otherwise disclosed.

Obtaining collateral interview data can sometimes create problems or conflict between the collateral source and the evaluee once the evaluee has discovered the content of the collateral interview. In a child custody case, for example, a teacher or neighbor who provides information critical of one parent might thereafter have a strained relationship with the evaluee. Similarly, an evaluee in employment litigation could have more conflict with coworkers once he learns of their negative evaluation of him. One approach to this dilemma is for the evaluator to list the collateral sources of information in the report but to summarize the content of the collateral interviews without specifying their source (Bow and Quinnell 2002).

The evaluator must assess the collateral source's credibility and motivation with regard to the evaluee. The evaluator should not be surprised to discover that collateral sources can provide as much distorted information as the evaluee, given the presence and biasing effect of the litigation itself. Information obtained from neutral parties has higher credibility and is therefore more valuable to the evaluator. Nonestranged spouses of criminal defendants and civil plaintiffs will often be supportive and biased in favor of the evaluee to a considerable degree. Similarly, crime victims may have difficulty being objective in their recall of the defendant's behavior. Arresting police officers, too, may conceal information indicating that a defendant was irrational, delusional, hallucinating, or severely intoxicated. Child custody cases are notably prone to biased information provided by the respective parties (Austin 2002).

The collateral source's objectivity can be compromised by influence or input from the evaluee's attorney or staff; attorneys have been known to coach family as well as evaluees before contact with the opposing side evaluator.

On occasion, a collateral source will provide incriminating rather than mitigating or exculpatory information about a defendant to the evaluator, even if the evaluator was retained by the same side as the evaluee and collateral source. That information may necessitate additional interviewing of the evaluee.

## Data Analysis

Forensic evaluations often require many complex determinations. Evaluators must initially be thoroughly informed about the relevant legal standard including case law, statute, regulation, and policy. Data analysis is framed by the relevant legal issue in the case; for example, psychiatric diagnosis, violence risk, criminal or civil competence, voluntariness of action, criminal responsibility, and causation.

Forensic evaluators ideally approach each evaluation in a neutral manner without preconceived expectations and biases that could distort data collection or data analysis. Evaluee and collateral credibility must be assessed. As noted above, dissimulation and malingering must be considered through careful record review, interviewing, testing, and cross-checking of data sources. Knowledge of the natural course of the mental disorder in question is essential to assessing secondary gain issues.

In criminal responsibility evaluations involving multiple crimes committed over a period of time, the evaluator must separately evaluate the defendant with regard to each alleged act. This is typically an issue in white-collar crimes such as embezzlement, but it also occurs in multiple or serial homicides or sexual assaults. In such cases, multiple forensic evaluations are essentially required.

Causation is an important issue in most forensic evaluations. Scientific reasoning (i.e., hypothesis generation and testing) must be used to assess the connection between a clinical condition and the relevant psycholegal functional ability (Heilbrun 2001). Causation determinations require that the evaluator distinguish the respective effects of premorbid emotional problems, comorbid mental and physical disorders, and psychosocial stressors (e.g., deaths, job termination, victimization). Separating the effects of a manic episode, cocaine intoxication, and narcissistic personality disorder, and determining which was the main or a contributing cause of the criminal offense may be problematic. In vignette 1, the evaluator must separate the effect of three potentially traumatic life events (i.e., two sexual victimizations and one motor vehicle accident) in reaching forensic opinions appropriate to the litigation in question. Extensive interviewing and collateral data are likely to be essential in such situations. Accepted, rather than idiosyncratic, theories of causation must be used (Chadwick and Krous 1997).

Conducting personality disorder assessments can be challenging in many forensic evaluations, though this is often an essential task in both civil and criminal forensic evaluations. Forensic evaluations are relatively limited in time and direct exposure to the evaluee. Comorbid psychiatric disorders such as an evaluee's mood disorder can confound the assessment of personality functioning and lead to a false diagnosis of a personality disorder (Fava et al. 2002). Psychological testing can similarly fail to distinguish between personality disorders and comorbid mental or physical disorders. Ideally, personality assessments should be conducted in the absence of significant comorbid conditions and over an extended time interval to ensure personality trait stability. Previous mental health evaluations and treatment records are likely to be useful in compensating for the forensic evaluator's otherwise limited exposure to the evaluee. Collateral interviews can compensate for some of the limitations of the psychiatric interviews with the evaluee, but they have their own deficiencies.

Given that maintaining objectivity and credibility are such essential tasks to the forensic evaluation, evaluators often perform several integrity checks to ensure that their work is of the highest quality. An evaluator's opinions and conclusions should be similar if not identical regardless of which side retains that evaluator, though of course different evaluators may reach different expert opinions in a given case. Evaluators should question themselves when formulating their expert opinions and conclusions to ensure that the presence of a retaining party has not significantly influenced their forensic work on the case. They should be alert to the phenomenon of "forensic identification," which occurs when the evaluator comes to identify or ally with the retaining party as the case proceeds over time (Zusman and Simon 1983). Evaluators may permissibly choose to emphasize those aspects of the expert's conclusions that are favorable to the retaining side, but the expert's opinions should not fundamentally be different based on the identity of the retaining party. Similarly, the outcome of the legal case should not concern the evaluator. The evaluator is not a party to the litigation, and he or she is not being compensated according to the case outcome. The evaluator who is particularly pleased or dissatisfied with the legal outcome of the case may have unwittingly become over-invested in the case and may have sacrificed objectivity.

Some evaluators routinely maintain a log of their previous cases and ultimate opinions to monitor any patterns or distortions over time. Experts should have a significant percentage of cases for which their conclusions are unfavorable to the retaining party. They should be wary when they have been repeatedly retained by a given party and reach identical conclusions over an extended period of time. Finally, experts should be self-aware enough to monitor for the presence of significant countertransference in their forensic work, whether to a particular defendant, crime, accident, or legal cause of action. The literature has documented the significant presence of child sexual abuse in mental health professionals (Little and Hamby 1996), and this history could potentially bias the evaluation process. Individual consultation with an experienced forensic colleague, or a brief course of individual psychotherapy, can be useful to forensic evaluators in emotionally stressful cases.

Peer review of the expert's evaluation and testimony is another vehicle to enhance the quality of one's forensic work (American Psychiatric Association 1992, 1997). Peer review is available on a voluntary and confidential basis for members of AAPL, but it also can be arranged independently and privately by the evaluator. Such a peer consultation process provides an invaluable means of checking on the soundness of the expert's work and can illuminate any actual or potential problems in the evaluator's approach to this or similar cases (Chadwick and Krous 1997). State peer review statutes may or may not protect the peer review from legal discovery in subsequent proceedings. Peer review typically occurs after the evaluator has completed the evaluation rather than during it. If they discussed the case with a colleague, evaluators could be questioned when testifying at deposition or trial on what effect such consultation had on them. In such situations, the evaluator must, of course, testify honestly about the consultation.

## Forensic Report Writing

After completing the forensic evaluation, the evaluator is usually asked to prepare a detailed, written report of the evaluation. The evaluator should not, however, prepare a written report unless specifically requested to do so. Some retaining attorneys or agencies initially request a verbal report and may not seek a written report from the evaluator if the evaluator's findings and opinions are unfavorable to the evaluee's legal case. The absence of an unfavorable written report from the evaluator could protect the retaining attorney or agency from having to disclose the unfavorable evaluation results and prevent their being disclosed to the opposing side. However, some retaining parties will solicit a written report from the evaluator even if it is unfavorable, and then use that report to persuade the litigant to change legal tactics or dismiss the case; other retaining attorneys will use an unfavorable report to protect themselves against anticipated charges of ineffective assistance of counsel.

Some retaining parties request a preliminary written report from the evaluator. Providing such a report before the completion of the evaluation is often problematic, because proper analysis of the data requires that all relevant data be obtained before the expert reaches any forensic opinions on the case. An evaluator who provides a preliminary opinion may have difficulty reconciling the preliminary opinion with subsequently obtained data.

Even if the retaining party requests a written report from the evaluator, the evaluator and retaining party should discuss the length and substance of that report before it is prepared. Some retaining parties seek a brief report simply stating the examiner's forensic opinions, though not providing details of the evaluee's social, medical, or psychiatric history. Limitations in funds available to the retaining party could also limit the length and complexity of the expert's report, as extensive reports typically take considerable time to prepare. Advance discussion of the evaluator's opinions also minimizes the likelihood that the retaining party will later seek to edit the evaluator's report.

When the evaluator has been retained by a court rather than by a party to the litigation, the evaluation report might be more extensive and inclusive than if the evaluator has been retained by a party, though ideally there should be little difference in this regard.

## The Report

In general, the written report of the forensic evaluation must be comprehensive, detailed, precise, clearly written, and well substantiated. The purpose of the report is to communicate the evaluator's conclusions and supporting data to the retaining party and, ultimately, to the trial court or jury. The evaluator should assume that every word of the report is meaningful and exposes the evaluator to testimony on direct or cross-examination. He or she is likely to regret report writing characterized by casual, rushed, careless, or exaggerated statements or opinions. The evaluator will need to defend the report in court but can use the report to assist in presenting court testimony.

The evaluator's report should be well organized, with appropriate subject headings and subheadings for data sources, relevant history, collateral data, test results, mental status examination, diagnosis, and expert opinions. The report should specify the data sources used, including the dates of available records reviewed and the dates and time spent conducting interviews with the evaluee and collaterals. The report should also indicate that the evaluee was appropriately warned about the nature, purpose, and nonconfidentiality of the evaluation and that the evaluee understood this. The evaluator should refer to the evaluee as a litigant, plaintiff, defendant, or by name but not as a "patient." In their reports, evaluators should ordinarily not refer to the opposing experts by name or make personal attacks on their credibility or expertise.

The report should be precisely written with minimal use of technical jargon or explanations of such when appropriate. Casual or informal language should be avoided, but it is often useful to provide direct quotations from the evaluee or others. The source of statements in the report (e.g., defendant, crime victim, witness, and police) should be clear to the reader. Though the report should be focused around the referral forensic issue, related or even extraneous information about the evaluee is often appropriately included in the report, though retaining attorneys may not initially comprehend the justification for doing so. The evaluator must use judgment in deciding what is essential and relevant to include in the report; evaluators can be questioned in court regarding why some information was included or not included in the report. Sample expert reports are included in Melton et al. 1997.

Potential problems or errors in forensic report writing are numerous (Table 7–3). In accordance with the evaluator's ethical responsibility to strive for objectivity, the evaluator needs to explore and consider all data sources rather than ignoring, or even neglecting to explore, the data that fail to support the expert's diagnoses and expert opinions. The evaluator must remain within his or her expertise, use accepted rather than idiosyncratic psychiatric theories, correctly interpret the professional literature, use the data extant in the case, and not fabricate information (Chadwick and Krous 1997). Limitations to the expert's opinion should be disclosed to the extent feasible. Evaluators should be open to changing their diagnosis and expert opinion upon the receipt of additional information. They should state that no conclusions can be reached with the presently available database if that is the situation.

**TABLE 7–3. Problems in forensic reports**

- Failing to clarify data sources
- Providing preliminary reports
- Failing to consider all data sources in reaching opinions
- Mixing data and expert opinions
- Exceeding the data in the case
- Suppressing disconfirming data
- Including speculation or demonstrating overconfidence
- Relying on unsubstantiated diagnosis and expert opinions
- Addressing the wrong forensic issue
- Using idiosyncratic psychiatric theories
- Failing to disclose limitations of expert's opinion
- Aggregating multiple causes of a psychiatric disorder and legal damages
- Failing to analyze mental status for each criminal charge
- Allowing attorney-requested changes in expert's opinion
- Submitting inaccurate curriculum vitae

Perhaps the most significant deficiency in forensic mental health expert reports is the failure to adequately substantiate the evaluator's forensic opinions in the case (Skeem and Golding 1998). The legal system is the ultimate consumer or client for forensic consultation. Expert opinions without foundation are of limited value to the legal system. Evaluators should be able to fully explain their forensic opinions and to ground them in the available data. Experts who speculate, and those who "go beyond the data," are not properly serving the system. Such reports will be difficult for the evaluator to defend in court. Expert opinions need to be reached with "reasonable medical certainty," in the absence of which the report or testimony will not be admissible in court (Rappeport 1985). There is sometimes a narrow window between overstating and understating one's expert opinion. When there are substantial clinical or legal data to support more than one forensic opinion, then an accepted approach is to defer the ultimate opinion issue to the judge or jury rather than forcing an opinion that ignores substantial other data.

Retaining attorneys sometimes make a request to edit the report before turning it over to the opposing side. The attorney may ask that the evaluator delete certain factual information, change emphasis, or even change the ultimate expert opinion. Any substantial changes made at the attorney's request should be avoided; altering the expert's opinion at the attorney's request is unethical. Typographical and factual errors, and failure to address the appropriate legal standard, can be rectified without difficulty. A supplemental report can be provided to remediate any deficiencies in the original report (Simon and Wettstein 1997). Cross-examiners at deposition or trial sometimes inquire about earlier drafts of the expert's report, and a court may order the disclosure of such if available.

Evaluators should distribute their report only to the retaining party unless directed otherwise by the retaining party or the court. Requests for a copy of the report by the evaluee or the evaluee's treating physicians should be referred to the retaining party, who is responsible for all information disclosure resulting from the evaluation.

Evaluators are typically required to submit a recent copy of their curriculum vitae along with their report. Such resumes should be dated, be recent, and accurately reflect professional activities. Memberships on professional association committees or boards or other activities should not be overstated. Submission of an erroneous or misrepresented resume can subject the evaluator to charges of unprofessional conduct by a state board of medicine or of perjury by a court. Similarly, evaluators should not misrepresent their credentials if they advertise for their forensic services, whether in print media or on a Web site.

## Documentation

Documentation for risk management is an important area of forensic practice, as it is for clinical work. Forensic clinicians are at significant exposure to negligence or other legal liability, and they risk complaints of unethical conduct as well (Jensen 1993). Formal complaints against psychiatrists for alleged breach of ethical standards of practice in the conduct of forensic evaluations have been brought to the American Psychiatric Association. Dissatisfied litigants in either the criminal or civil arena readily bring lawsuits against the forensic evaluator, with or without counsel (Slovenko 2001). State licensure board complaints from a parent about the opposing expert regularly occur following child custody litigation (Glassman 1998; Kirkland and Kirkland 2001). Forensic evaluators need to maintain relevant records to later defend themselves against charges of unlawful or unethical conduct, the latter of which may have no statute of limitations. Beyond risk management, handwritten notes taken during the course of a forensic evaluation are discoverable in the litigation, and opposing attorneys may request to review them before or during court testimony.

## Stress of Forensic Psychiatry

For many reasons, forensic mental health work is often stressful, though experience and competence likely reduce its stressfulness (Strasburger et al. 2003). Sources of stress in forensic work include the lack of control over one's schedule, evaluating the perpetrators of horrific acts, exposure to emotional and physical trauma of evaluees, dealing with coercion from retaining attorneys, collecting fees from the retaining party, being physically or legally threatened by litigants and their associates, and being confronted in court with cross-examiners who make personal and professional attacks on the examiner's ability, performance, and character. Strong countertransference reactions to litigants and their alleged behavior commonly occur (Sattar et al. 2002). Professional isolation by forensic psychiatrists can contribute to the distress of a psychiatrist who does significant forensic work. Vicarious traumatization of practitioners can also occur, as it does when working with any traumatized population (Hegaty 2002).

## Conclusion

Forensic consultation, evaluation, and testimony are qualitatively distinct from evaluations for treatment purposes. Unlike clinical evaluations, forensic evaluations sometimes attract much media attention and visibility. Accountability for and scrutiny of forensic work are higher than those for clinical work (Otto and Heilbrun 2002). Even though forensic experts are not the ultimate decision-makers in the litigation, they wield considerable power, and the litigants and associated family can be injured by evaluators who are dishonest, corrupted by financial remuneration, unqualified, or otherwise disreputable. Clinicians without significant forensic training, experience, and relevant skills tread on thin legal and ethical ground when they undertake forensic work. Forensic experts must maintain objectivity, honesty, integrity, and humility in their evaluations and court testimony. Forensic work often requires diligence, conscientiousness, and hard work in fact finding.

As in clinical work (Unutzer et al. 2001), forensic evaluators should strive for excellence and undertake quality improvement efforts to the extent possible (Dietz 1996). These efforts require honest self-examination of one's work, enhanced by peer review by one's colleagues.

## Key Points

- The forensic evaluator should identify the forensic issue and clarify the expert role in the case.
- Forensic evaluations must be comprehensive and detailed.
- Forensic evaluations should be conducted without conflicts of interest.
- The evaluator should strive for objectivity and neutrality.
- The evaluator should use accepted psychiatric literature, theories, and definitions.
- The evaluator should not exceed his or her role or expertise or draw conclusions beyond those supported by the existing case data.
- The evaluator should clearly articulate forensic opinions in the written report and fully explain reasoning.

## Practice Guidelines

1. Self-monitor case selection.
2. Remain within one's expertise.
3. Obtain comprehensive data from original sources.
4. Perform multiple interviews with evaluee.
5. Obtain corroborative data.
6. Reconcile conflicting data.
7. Offer same opinion regardless of retaining side.
8. Self-monitor pattern of forensic opinions.
9. Attend to countertransference.
10. Fully substantiate basis for forensic opinions.
11. Disclose limitations of forensic opinions.
12. Do not become competitive with opposing experts.
13. Undertake peer review.

## References

Allen JP, Maisto SA, Connors GJ: Self-report screening tests for alcohol problems in primary care. Arch Intern Med 155:1726–1730, 1995

American Academy of Child and Adolescent Psychiatry: Practice parameters for the assessment and treatment of children and adolescents with conduct disorder. J Am Acad Child Adolesc Psychiatry 36:122S–139S, 1997a

American Academy of Child and Adolescent Psychiatry: Practice parameters for child custody evaluation. J Am Acad Child Adolesc Psychiatry 36:57S–68S, 1997b

American Academy of Child and Adolescent Psychiatry: Practice parameters for the assessment and treatment of children and adolescents who are sexually abusive of others. J Am Acad Child Adolesc Psychiatry 38:55S–76S, 1999

American Academy of Psychiatry and the Law: Guidelines for the Practice of Forensic Psychiatry. Bloomfield, CT, American Academy of Psychiatry and the Law, 1995

American Academy of Psychiatry and the Law: Videotaping of forensic psychiatric evaluations. Bull Am Acad Psychiatry Law 27:345–358, 1999

American Academy of Psychiatry and the Law: Practice guideline: forensic psychiatric evaluation of defendants raising the insanity defense. J Am Acad Psychiatry Law 30:S3–S40, 2002

American Psychiatric Association, Council on Psychiatry and Law: Peer review of psychiatric expert testimony. Bull Am Acad Psychiatry Law 20:343–352, 1992

American Psychiatric Association, Task Force on Peer Review: American Psychiatric Association resource document on peer review of expert testimony. J Am Acad Psychiatry Law 25:359–373, 1997

American Psychological Association: Guidelines for child custody evaluations in divorce proceedings. Am Psychol 49:677–680, 1994

Austin WG: Guidelines for utilizing collateral sources of information in child custody evaluations. Family Court Review 40:177–184, 2002

Barbaree HE, Seto MC, Langton CM, et al: Evaluating the predictive accuracy of six risk assessment instruments for adult sex offenders. Criminal Justice and Behavior 28:490–521, 2001

Boccaccini MT, Brodsky SL: Diagnostic test usage by forensic psychologists in emotional injury cases. Professional Psychology: Research and Practice 30: 253–259, 1999

Bow JN, Quinnell FA: A critical review of child custody evaluation reports. Family Court Review 40:164–176, 2002

Bow JN, Quinnell FA, Zaroff M, et al: Assessment of sexual abuse allegations in child custody cases. Professional Psychology: Research and Practice 33: 566–575, 2002

Chadwick DL, Krous HF: Irresponsible testimony by medical experts in cases involving the physical abuse and neglect of children. Child Maltreat 2:313–321, 1997

Dietz PE: The quest for excellence in forensic psychiatry. Bull Am Acad Psychiatry Law 24:153–163, 1996

Farkas GM, DeLeon PH, Newman R: Sanity examiner certification: an evolving national agenda. Professional Psychology: Research and Practice 28:73–76, 1997

Fava M, Farabaugh AH, Sickinger AH, et al: Personality disorders and depression. Psychol Med 32:1049–1057, 2002

Giles E, Hutchinson DL: Stature- and age-related bias in self-reported stature. Journal of Forensic Sciences 36:765–780, 1991.

Glassman JB: Preventing and managing board complaints: the downside risk of custody evaluation. Professional Psychology: Research and Practice 29:121–124, 1998

Greiffenstein MF, Baker WJ, Johnson-Greene D: Actual versus self-reported scholastic achievement of litigating postconcussion and severe closed head injury claimants. Psychol Assess 14:202–208, 2002

Grisso T: Evaluating Competencies: Forensic Assessments and Instruments, 2nd Edition. New York, Plenum, 2002

Grisso T, Appelbaum PS: MacArthur Competence Assessment Tool for Treatment. Sarasota, FL, Professional Resource Press, 1998

Gutheil T, Simon RI: Attorneys' pressures on the expert witness: early warning signs of endangered honesty, objectivity, and fair compensation. J Am Acad Psychiatry Law 27:546–553, 1999

Haber RN, Haber L: Experiencing, remembering and reporting events. Psychology, Public Policy, and Law 6:1057–1097, 2000

Hanson RK, Thornton D: Improving risk assessments for sex offenders: a comparison of three actuarial scales. Law Hum Behav 24:119–136, 2000

Hare RD: A research scale for the assessment of psychopathy in criminal populations. Pers Individ Dif 1:111–119, 1980

Harrison L, Hughes A: The Validity of Self-Reported Drug Use: Improving the Accuracy of Survey Estimates (NIDA Research Monograph 167). Rockville, MD, National Institute on Drug Abuse, 1997

Hegaty A: Vicarious traumatization, in Principles and Practice of Child and Adolescent Forensic Psychiatry. Edited by Schetky DH, Benedek EP. Washington, DC, American Psychiatric Publishing, 2002, pp 59–66

Heilbrun K: Principles of Forensic Mental Health Assessment. New York, Kluwer/Plenum, 2001

Heilbrun K, Rosenfeld B, Warren J, et al: The use of third-party information in forensic assessments: a two-state comparison. Bull Am Acad Psychiatry Law 22:399–406, 1994

Heilbrun K, Warren J, Picarello K: Third party information in forensic assessment, in Handbook of Psychology, Vol 11: Forensic Psychology. Edited by Goldstein AM. Hoboken, NJ, Wiley, 2003, pp 69–86

Hyman IE, Loftus EF: Errors in autobiographical memory. Clin Psychol Rev 18: 933–947, 1998

Jensen EG: When "hired guns" backfire: the witness immunity doctrine and the negligent expert witness. University of Missouri-Kansas City Law Review 62:185–207, 1993

Kirkland K, Kirkland KL: Frequency of child custody evaluation complaints and related disciplinary action: a survey of the Association of State and Provincial Psychology Boards. Professional Psychology: Research and Practice 32:171–174, 2001

Kraemer HC, Measelle JR, Ablow JC, et al: A new approach to integrating data from multiple informants in psychiatric assessment and research: mixing and matching contexts and perspectives. Am J Psychiatry 160:1566–1577, 2003

Lanyon RI: Psychological assessment procedures in sex offending. Professional Psychology: Research and Practice 32:253–260, 2001

Little L, Hamby SL: The impact of a clinician's sexual abuse history, gender and theoretical orientation on treatment issues of childhood sexual abuse. Professional Psychology: Research and Practice 27:1–9, 1996

Loza W, Villeneuve DB, Loza-Fanous A: Predictive validity of the Violence Risk Appraisal Guide: a tool for assessing violent offender's recidivism. Int J Law Psychiatry 25:85–92, 2002

MacQueen GM, Galway TM, Hay J, et al: Recollection memory deficits in patients with major depressive disorder predicted by past depressions but not current mood state or treatment status. Psychol Med 32:251–258, 2002

McNagny SE, Parker RM: High prevalence of recent cocaine use and the unreliability of patient self-report in an inner-city walk-in clinic. JAMA 267: 1106–1108, 1992

McSweeny AJ, Becker BC, Naugle RI, et al: Ethical issues related to the presence of third party observers in clinical neuropsychological evaluations. Clin Neuropsychol 12:552–559, 1998

Melton G, Petrila J, Poythress NG, et al: Psychological Evaluations for the Courts, 2nd Edition. New York, Guilford, 1997

Morgado A, Smith M, Lecrubier Y, et al: Depressed subjects unwittingly overreport poor social adjustment which they reappraise when recovered. J Nerv Ment Dis 179:614–619, 1991

Nicholson RA, Norwood S: The quality of forensic psychological assessments, reports, and testimony: acknowledging the gap between promise and practice. Law Hum Behav 24:9–44, 2000

Otto RK, Heilbrun K: The practice of forensic psychology. Am Psychol 57:5–18, 2002

Otto RK, Poythress NG, Nicholson RA, et al: Psychometric properties of the MacArthur Competence Assssment Tool-Criminal Adjudication. Psychol Assess 10:435–443, 1998

Porter S, Birt AR, Yuille JC, et al: Memory for murder. Int J Law Psychiatry 24: 23–42, 2001

Rappeport, JR: Reasonable medical certainty. Bull Am Acad Psychiatry Law 13: 5–15, 1985

Riso LP, Klein DN, Anderson RL, et al: Concordance between patients and informants on the Personality Disorder Examination. Am J Psychiatry 151: 568–573, 1994

Roesch R, Zapf PA, Eaves D, et al: The Fitness Interview Test, Revised Edition. Burnaby, BC, Mental Health, Law and Policy Institute, 1998

Rogers R: Structured Interview of Reported Symptoms. Tampa, FL, Psychological Assessment Resources, 1992

Rogers R: Handbook of Diagnostic and Structured Inteviewing. New York, Guilford, 2001

Rogers R, Grandjean N, Tillbrook CE, et al: Recent interview-based measures of competency to stand trial: a critical review augmented with research data. Behav Sci Law 19:503–518, 2001

Rogers R, Shuman DW: Conducting Insanity Evaluations, 2nd Edition. New York, Guilford, 2000

Sattar SP, Pinals DA, Gutheil T: Countering countertransference: a forensic trainee's dilemma. J Am Acad Psychiatry Law 30:65–69, 2002

Scheiber SC: The psychiatric interview, psychiatric history, and mental status examination, in Textbook of Clinical Psychiatry, 4th Edition. Edited by Hales RE, Yudofsky SC. Washington, DC, American Psychiatric Publishing, 2003, pp 155–187

Schless AP, Mendels J: The value of interviewing family and friends in assessing life stressors. Arch Gen Psychiatry 35:565–567, 1978

Simon R: "Three's a crowd": the presence of third parties during the forensic psychiatric examination. J Psychiatry Law 24:3–25, 1996

Simon R, Wettstein RM: Toward the development of guidelines for the conduct of forensic psychiatric examinations. J Am Acad Psychiatry Law 25:17–30, 1997

Skeem JL, Golding SL: Community examiners' evaluations of competence to stand trial: common problems and suggestions for improvement. Professional Psychology: Research and Practice 29:357–367, 1998

Slovenko R: Holding the expert accountable. J Psychiatry Law 29:543–574, 2001

Stone JH: Memory disorder in offenders and victims. Criminal Behavior and Mental Health 2:342–356, 1992

Strasburger LH, Gutheil TG, Brodsky A: On wearing two hats: role conflict in serving as both psychotherapist and expert witness. Am J Psychiatry 154: 448–456, 1997

Strasburger LH, Miller PM, Commons ML, et al: Stress and the forensic psychiatrist: a pilot study. J Am Acad Psychiatry Law 31(1):18–26, 2003

Strier F: Whither trial consulting? Issues and projections. Law Hum Behav 23: 93–115, 1999

Unutzer J, Rubenstein L, Katon W, et al: Two-year effects of quality improvement programs on medication management for depression. Arch Gen Psychiatry 58:935–942, 2001

Ustad KL, Rogers R, Sewell KW, et al: Restoration of competency to stand trial: assessment with the Georgia Court Competency Test and the Competency Screening Test. Law Hum Behav 20:131–146, 1996

Weiss RD, Najavits LM, Greenfield SF, et al: Validity of substance use self-reports in dually diagnosed outpatients. Am J Psychiatry 155:127–128, 1998

Williams CW, Lees-Haley PR, Djanogly SE: Clinical scrutiny of litigants' self-reports. Professional Psychology: Research and Practice 30:361–367, 1999

Zucker M, Morris MK, Ingram SM, et al: Concordance of self and informant ratings of adults' current and childhood attention-deficit\hyperactivity disorder symptoms. Psychol Assess 14:379–389, 2002

Zusman J, Simon J: Differences in repeated psychiatric examinations of litigants to a lawsuit. Am J Psychiatry 140:1300–1304, 1983

## Suggested Readings

Ackerman MJ: Essentials of Forensic Psychological Assessment. New York, Wiley, 1999

Goldstein AM: Handbook of Psychology, Vol 11: Forensic Psychology. Hoboken, NJ, Wiley, 2003

Grisso T: Forensic Evaluation of Juveniles. Sarasota, FL, Professional Resource Press, 1998

Heilbrun K: Principles of Forensic Mental Health Assessment. New York, Kluwer/Plenum, 2001

Melton G, Petrila J, Poythress NG, et al: Psychological Evaluations for the Courts, 2nd Edition. New York, Guilford, 1997

Rogers R, Shuman DW: Conducting Insanity Evaluations, 2nd Edition. New York, Guilford, 2000

Rosner R (ed): Principles and Practice of Forensic Psychiatry, 2nd Edition. New York, Chapman & Hall, 2003

Schetky DH, Benedek EP (eds): Principles and Practice of Child and Adolescent Forensic Psychiatry. Washington, DC, American Psychiatric Publishing, 2002

Simon RI (ed): Posttraumatic Stress Disorder in Litigation, 2nd Edition. Washington, DC, American Psychiatric Publishing, 2003

Wettstein RM: Ethics and forensic psychiatry. Psychiatr Clin North Am 25:623–633, 2002

CHAPTER 8

# Working With Attorneys

Robert L. Sadoff, M.D.

## Introduction

The practice of forensic psychiatry can be rewarding in a number of ways. It can be intellectually and clinically challenging, it is free of the constraints imposed by managed care, and it can be a good source of income for the practicing psychiatrist. More and more psychiatrists are requesting forensic training in accredited training programs and are entering the field. Despite the increase in the number of board-certified forensic psychiatrists, the bulk of testimony in civil and criminal cases is still given by practicing general psychiatrists. Most general psychiatrists work either alone in their offices or in a hospital or a group clinic setting. These clinicians need to familiarize themselves with the laws in the jurisdictions in which they work and become familiar with the general principles of forensic practice.

Practicing psychiatrists rarely have contact with attorneys unless they have personal legal problems such as a contractual dispute, a domestic relations issue, or a malpractice problem. Psychiatrists may also come into contact with attorneys when the patients they are treating become involved in civil or criminal legal matters. A patient's attorney may ask or require that the treating psychiatrist give testimony about the facts of the treatment rendered. In such cases, psychiatrists are considered fact witnesses.

In contrast, the forensic psychiatrist is often asked to evaluate an individual to give an expert opinion. Such opinions may be solicited in regard to a retroactive or past issue such as insanity, a present issue such as competency, or a future issue such as prediction of violence or prediction of harm from a particular injury and the prognosis for recovery.

These general psychiatric issues need to be placed in the context of a legal situation.

Research, academic, and treating psychiatrists are often called by attorneys to testify about questions of diagnosis, questions of treatment or use of various medications, or questions of the effect of a medication or combination of medications on a litigant's mental state. Psychiatrists crossing from a treatment or research setting to a forensic arena confront many questions that need to be addressed if they hope to participate successfully in the legal system as expert witnesses: When should psychiatrists become involved in litigtation, and when should they decline an attorney's invitation? How do the ethical guidelines differ between a forensic arena and a treatment or research setting? What can practicing psychiatrists expect when working with attorneys in various types of cases? How should psychiatrists respond to demands placed on them by attorneys seeking cooperation for help in presenting their legal claims?

There are many more attorneys than there are psychiatrists. Most psychiatrists do not know most of the attorneys in their geographic area. Therefore, psychiatrists may not know the reputation of attorneys who ask to retain their services. In most cases, this is not a problem. Many attorneys have a great deal of experience in working with experts. In some cases, however, attorneys may have unrealistic or unreasonable expectations. In some situations psychiatrists may have difficulty in collecting their fees, and in others they may have to contend with the attorneys' demands to change their reports by changing their opinions or leaving out essential information that may be harmful to the client. This chapter reviews some of the problem areas that frequently arise when psychiatrists work with attorneys on criminal and civil cases and includes some of the issues relating to testimony, subpoenas, and court orders.

## The Initial Phone Call

### Clinical Vignette

Dr. S had been treating Ms. J for many years for depression. She had a history of childhood sexual abuse and domestic violence as an adult. Ms. J became involved in a dispute with her employer and brought a suit charging intentional infliction of emotional distress. Ms. J's attorney contacted Dr. S, requesting that he forward all Ms. J's treatment records and asking that he serve as an expert witness in the case.

Dr. S was concerned that becoming involved in Ms. J's litigation will adversely affect her treatment. He was also concerned that he may not be able to protect the confidentiality of certain aspects of her history that are not relevant to the current litigation but may be highly embarrassing should they become public. For these reasons, he was hesitant to become involved. However, Ms. J and her attorney stated that it was his obligation as Ms. J's treating physician to testify, and demanded that he do so.

Many issues that create problems in providing forensic services can be addressed during the initial phone call from the attorney. For example, Dr. S was faced with a common dilemma that arises when a treating clinician's patient becomes involved in litigation. Patients and their attorneys often expect that the treating psychiatrist will be the best expert witness. However, these two roles are often incompatible for both ethical and practical reasons (Strasberger et al. 1997).

Dr. S was not sure what his obligations were. He therefore consulted Dr. B, a colleague experienced in forensic psychiatry. Dr. B advised Dr. S that he should decline to participate as an expert witness and should recommend to his patient and her attorney that they retain a forensic psychiatrist to act as the expert. However, Dr. B also told Dr. S that his patient's attorney or the defendant's attorney could subpoena him as a fact witness. In that case, Dr. S would have no choice but to fulfill his social and legal obligation to testify to the facts as he knew them.

## Role Clarification: Fact Witness Versus Expert Witness

Sometimes attorneys will call treating psychiatrists to testify in behalf of their own patients. When psychiatrists receive such calls, they should immediately clarify whether they are being asked to participate as a fact witness or an expert witness. The differences between these two roles are significant and have implications that affect both the patient and the treating psychiatrist. General practicing psychiatrists are most likely to be called to testify about the treatment rendered to a victim of an accident, the participants in a marital or other civil dispute, or the "competency" of patients that are under their care. In such cases, they may be asked to give expert opinions as well. Although psychiatrists are required to give testimony concerning the facts of the case, they are not generally required to give expert witness opinions unless they have agreed to do so.

In some cases, the line between being a fact witness and an expert witness may be blurred. However, fact witnesses should refrain from giving expert opinions unless they are designated as expert witnesses. Exceptions to the general rule of avoiding occupying both treatment provider and expert witness roles may arise. In some cases, the circumstances may be such that the treating psychiatrist's expert opinions may be the most relevant and knowledgeable in a given case. Nevertheless, the conflicts of interest inherent in occupying both roles of treatment provider and forensic expert have been clearly demonstrated (see Chapter 2: "Introduction to the Legal System," this volume; see also Strasburger et al. 1997).

The bias toward advocacy for patients generally makes treating psychiatrists' testimony as experts inappropriate. Psychiatrists providing treatment are ethically bound to be advocates for their patients. This creates a bias that will be revealed under good cross-examination. The ethics in forensic psychiatry mandate that the expert witness be impartial and strive for objectivity. The treating psychiatrist cannot be objective or impartial because the therapist wants the best therapy or outcome for the patient. The psychiatrist may believe that if the patient goes to jail, the patient will likely become suicidal, or that if the patient loses in the civil suit, he or she will become depressed, despondent, or even suicidal.

The appearance of financial gain on the part of treating psychiatrists will also cast doubt on the credibility of their testimony. In a criminal trial, psychiatrists may testify to help keep their patients out of prison and, therefore, in treatment for which the psychiatrist receives payment. In civil cases in which the patient has an outstanding bill, it may appear that the psychiatrist is testifying on a contingency basis to collect outstanding treatment fees. That is a conflict of interest and is clearly unethical according to the American Medical Association. Even if the patient's account is paid in full, ongoing treatment if favorable testimony is rendered will certainly affect the psychiatrist's income. Thus, such testimony can be viewed as being slanted to help the patient win so that the psychiatrist gets paid or to maintain a financial arrangement that benefits the psychiatrist.

One practical implication of clarifying the role of forensic expert or fact witness does involve the issue of appropriate compensation for time spent on the case, which may include document review, preparation of a report, preparation of testimony, and provision of testimony. Expert witnesses may charge an expert witness fee for all these services consistent with their hourly rate for treatment. If the attorney does not wish to pay this fee, the psychiatrist can decline to participate. In contrast, the fact witness may be paid only a daily rate that ranges between $9 and $30 per day for the time taken to present the testimony. Fact witnesses who are still treating patients involved in the litigation may be able to arrange more reasonable compensation directly from patients. Some patients are aware that requiring their psychiatrists to spend hours or days providing fact testimony with minimal compensation may compromise ongoing treatment. Psychiatrists called as fact witnesses may also be able to limit through their own attorneys the amount of time they are forced to spend providing fact testimony. This may mitigate the financial loss. However, fact witnesses cannot refuse to participate if they are summoned or court ordered to testify despite the low rate of compensation.

## Expertise

When an attorney calls, psychiatrists should obtain enough information to determine whether they wish to become involved in the case. This should include the nature of the case and whether it is within the psychiatrist's level of expertise. If the issue hinges on the combination of various psychopharmacologic agents and the psychiatrist is not an expert on psychopharmacology, he or she should decline and refer to known experts in the field. If the issue involves developmental problems in a young female patient and the psychiatrist is not board-certified in child psychiatry, he or she ought to refer to a subspecialist in the field. If psychiatrists are unfamiliar with such terms as "competency," "insanity," "weakened intellect," "voluntariness," and "undue influence," they should refer to a forensic specialist.

## Fees

Psychiatrists should also determine and agree on fees at the time of initial contact. Psychiatrists traveling away from their offices can charge for one half-day for time in court or for a full day if that is required. If they have to fly away from home or drive farther and stay overnight, they should negotiate fees with the attorney to cover expenses as well as time involved. During the first phone call, psychiatrists should advise attorneys regarding their hourly fees and give an estimate as to the number of hours required to complete the task. This allows attorneys to formulate a bottom-line estimate to pass on to their clients: the plaintiff, the insurance company, and the supervisor in a defender organization or a prosecutor's office.

Psychiatrists engaging in forensic work are well advised to obtain a retainer fee when working for the defense in criminal cases or the plaintiff in civil cases. Attorneys should also be advised of these fees at the time of the initial contact. Many experienced forensic psychiatrists prepare a retainer agreement for execution by both attorney and psychiatrist. The attorney's client may also sign the retainer agreement. However, the agreement should specify that the attorney is responsible for payment of all fees, regardless of the outcome of the case.

Retainer fees received in anticipation of services rendered are ethical and appropriate (American Academy of Psychiatry and Law 1995). Similarly, the expert should obtain a fee before going to court to testify. If the psychiatrist is retained by the defense in a criminal matter, bills are unlikely to be paid if the defendant loses and goes to jail. Attorneys working for plaintiffs in civil cases often work on a contingency basis and may expect experts' fees to be paid out of the settlement. However, if the plaintiff loses in court and receives no monetary compensation, expert witnesses may not be paid. Thus, psychiatrists should obtain retainer fees equivalent to their ultimate expected total fees.

A retainer agreement creates a binding contract that can go a long way toward ensuring recourse in the event of nonpayment for services. Nevertheless, payment in advance in either the form of advance fees or retainer payments ensures that professional services are properly compensated. The expression "your check is my key to the courtroom door" summarizes the recommended stance psychiatrists should take in regard to obtaining fees.

Attorneys may on occasion cancel an advance check after testimony is given, claiming that they "did not like" the testimony. Such behavior represents an ethical violation of canceling a proper check, for which the attorney may face sanctions. However, it is not unethical for attorneys not to pay their expert witnesses. Bar associations typically do not care whether or not attorneys pay their bills. They are only concerned with whether or not the attorney violates any ethical sanctions. A properly executed and designed retainer agreement may provide psychiatrists with legal recourse in the event their fees are unpaid.

## Conflict of Interest

If clinicians determine that the matter is within their expertise, they should then consider whether any conflict of interest would limit their participation in the case. Conflicts of interest relative to assuming the roles of both treatment provider and expert witness have already been reviewed. Other types of conflict of interest may also arise. Any possibility of such a conflict should be discussed with the attorney at the outset so that the attorney may determine whether the psychiatrist would be an appropriate expert witness in this particular case. In a psychiatric malpractice case, for example, clinicians should be certain that they are not familiar with any of the parties involved or have any positive or negative biases regarding the psychiatrist being sued.

## Bias

### Clinical Vignette

An attorney representing a skinhead charged with the murders of his parents and his siblings called a prominent local forensic psychiatrist for an evaluation. The psychiatrist happened to be Jewish. The psychiatrist told the attorney that he would not take the case. He was certain that the skinhead client would not want a Jewish or ethnic psychiatrist representing him. In addition, the psychiatrist himself did not feel comfortable working to help someone who had such extreme negative feelings about him and his ethnic background. The attorney agreed that his client would not be comfortable with the psychiatrist and thanked him for pointing this out. The psychiatrist referred the attorney to another forensic expert.

One of the most important areas for the general psychiatrist to consider when working in the forensic arena is the issue of bias. Such issues should be clarified on initial contact by the attorney. If the psychiatrist's bias is such that it cannot be addressed, the psychiatrist should decline the case. Psychiatrists may have a positive bias toward a particular defendant or plaintiff for a number of reasons. They may identify with the examinee or feel that the examinee holds similar qualities to their own. Psychiatrists may also hold a negative bias toward certain defendants accused of committing heinous crimes that they find intolerable and inexcusable. Other types of bias, such as that discussed above regarding testifying for one's own patients, may arise. In a psychiatric malpractice case, psychiatrists should not accept a case involving either a friend or a competitor for obvious reasons of bias. Striving for objectivity and recognizing and accounting for one's bias when taking on a case is a hallmark of a competent and ethical forensic psychiatrist.

# Conflicts That May Arise Between Attorneys and Experts

## Obtaining Records

Psychiatrists providing forensic evaluations should review all relevant records. The database on which the psychiatrist gives an opinion in court should be as broad and as deep as possible. However, experts can only review the records that the retaining attorney provides. Although psychiatrists should request to review all relevant records, attorneys will sometimes select the records they wish their expert to review and withhold others, often in the interest of saving money. Psychiatrists may also need to examine or interview individuals other than the plaintiff in a civil case or a defendant in a criminal case. Again, such collateral interviews are typically arranged through the retaining attorney, who may fail to see the importance of such examinations or who may not wish to pay for the time spent on them. Failure to include relevant information or to interview appropriate individuals may decrease the credibility or effectiveness of the expert's testimony. The psychiatrist who feels that the attorney's editing of records or unwillingness to arrange a collateral interview compromises the forensic evaluation should point this out to the retaining attorney.

## Third Parties at Forensic Examinations

### Clinical Vignette

Dr. A was asked by the defense to conduct a forensic examination of Mr. L, a plaintiff in a malpractice case. Mr. J, Mr. L's attorney, requested to attend the examination. Dr. A agreed. Soon after the interview began, however, Mr. J began interjecting questions, admonishing Dr. A not to ask about certain matters, and advising his client, Mr. L, not to answer some of the questions. When Dr. A stated that he would stop the interview if Mr. J continued to interfere, Mr. J became angry and insisted that he be allowed to participate as he saw fit. Dr. A was very uncomfortable but was not sure how to proceed.

Dr. A decided to stop the interview if Mr. J did not leave. He was so uncomfortable that he knew he could not perform an adequate evaluation with Mr. J in the room. Mr. L left with his attorney. The court then ordered an examination without Mr. J present but allowed the examination to be recorded.

Attorneys may wish to be present during the psychiatric evaluation of their clients in criminal defense cases or in civil plaintiff cases. Some psychiatrists have insisted that they conduct the examination alone with the individual to have a "pure examination." They resent the intrusion of others in their private work of examining evaluees. However, in forensic cases, the courts may order that an attorney representing the defendant or the plaintiff be present to protect the interests and the rights of the client. The court may also order the specifics of the examination, including ordering that the attorney not interfere with the examination or ordering that the examination be videotaped.

Requests for the presence of any third party, including attorneys, should be carefully considered. In general, the presence of attorneys is not disruptive if they sit behind the examinee and are asked not to interrupt. For the most part, attorneys will not interfere if the questions asked are appropriate and not insulting or harmful. The attorney is there to protect the interest of the client and to take notes for later cross-examination to ensure that the psychiatrist adheres to the information obtained and does not deviate (Simon 1996).

## Report Preparation

Psychiatrists should discuss with retaining attorneys their preferences regarding a written report. Some cases will not require a written report. Others may require extensive reports. Some attorneys may request only very brief reports, requiring the other side to obtain relevant details during deposition. Regardless, the nature and costs associated with writing the report should be clarified with the attorney as soon as possible in the case so there is no surprise or shock when the attorney receives the bill. Attorneys may not pay for excessive time in report preparation unless the matter is discussed before the report is prepared.

Psychiatrists should send the prepared report to the retaining attorney only and not to anyone else. Attorneys can then decide to whom they wish to forward copies of the report. The evaluee, family members, or other parties to the litigation may request copies directly from expert psychiatrists. Such requests should be referred to the retaining attorney, who then assumes both the responsibility and liability of any consequences that come from disseminating the information.

## Requests for Changes in the Psychiatric Report

### Clinical Vignette

Dr. S conducted a forensic evaluation of a plaintiff in a civil suit. The plaintiff, Mr. M, alleged that he had developed posttraumatic stress disorder (PTSD) as a result of a motor vehicle accident. Dr. S said in her report for the attorney that although Mr. M did have PTSD, his disorder was causally related to a traumatic assault that had occurred earlier that year. She believed that his current symptoms were exacerbated but not caused by the motor vehicle accident.

Mr. M had not told his attorney, Ms. B, about the earlier trauma. When Ms. B originally consulted Dr. S about the case, Dr. S stated that she believed that proximate causation could be demonstrated. However, because Ms. B did not know about the earlier trauma, she could not tell Dr. S about it. It was not until the evaluation was completed that this information became available.

Ms. B called Dr. S. She was very upset with Dr. S's report because she could not use it to demonstrate proximate cause, which jeopardized winning a large settlement in a case Ms. B had considered "open and shut." Ms. B asked Dr. S to delete the information regarding the earlier trauma and to change her opinion to reflect that Mr. M's symptoms were causally related to the motor vehicle accident.

Dr. S felt that she could not ethically provide a report regarding the causation of PTSD that did not include information that the plaintiff suffered a prior trauma that had caused the symptoms in question. She advised Ms. B that she could not make the requested change.

Attorneys often request that psychiatrists make changes in their reports. Psychiatrists should carefully consider such requests. Changes that address and correct factual inaccuracies or that add information that was initially missed or overlooked are generally inconsequential and proper. However, attorneys may request changes because the psychiatrist's opinions do not conform to the needs of the attorney. Some attorneys feel that because they are paying psychiatrists' fees, psychiatrists should acquiesce to such requests. Changes that alter the expert's opinions are not appropriate or ethical.

Problematic requests for changes may also include leaving out essential or relevant data that is harmful to the examinee. Changes that remove essential data are also not appropriate. Certain facts may not be relevant, depending on the purpose of the report, and so could be deleted without altering the nature of the opinion. For example, in a criminal case, the jury does not need to know about prior criminal acts. If the report is to be admitted into evidence, the psychiatrist may leave out the information about previous criminal charges or convictions. However, in the sentencing phase of the trial, the information about prior criminal cases is relevant and must be included.

Psychiatrists providing expert services may want to advise attorneys before writing a report if they become aware that their opinions or reports may not help the attorney's case. The attorney may choose to not use that expert's opinion. However, as in the case above, the fact that an opinion may not be helpful may not become evident until the evaluation is complete. Once an opinion has been formed, psychiatrists providing expert services need to inform the attorney, who will determine whether a report is needed.

Lawyers may also make requests for changes in opinions when those opinions must be formulated without benefit of a personal examination of the evaluee. Such circumstances can arise in cases involving wills and testamentary capacity, suicides, or criminal matters when defendants refuse to cooperate with examinations. Attorneys often like to have a diagnosis for a variety of reasons (see Chapter 6: "Psychiatric Diagnosis in Litigation," this volume). Psychiatrists should be very cautious in giving a diagnostic impression without having examined the individual. They can indicate that the symptoms noted in the records are consistent with a particular diagnosis, but they should refrain from giving a declarative diagnosis, even when the lawyer may request such a definitive response.

Some attorneys request to review a preliminary draft before the final report is issued. If drafts are prepared, they should be kept and not discarded. Psychiatrists who choose to prepare a draft should be prepared on cross-examination to acknowledge this and to produce the preliminary drafts. Failure to provide the drafts can result in the presumption on the part of the cross-examining attorney and perhaps even the court or the jury that the psychiatrist was attempting to conceal changes made in original opinions to suit the retaining attorney. However, some forensic psychiatrists routinely discard all previous draft reports and indicate this is their usual practice in all cases.

## Legal Proceedings

### Subpoenas and Court Orders

Once a report has been turned in and the attorney distributes it to opposing counsel, a subpoena for the records of the examining psychiatrist may be issued. A subpoena is a demand for records placed by one side of a case. The subpoena is a legal document and should never be ignored. However, psychiatrists need not respond to subpoenas simply by giving the information requested. On receiving a subpoena, psychiatrists should contact their retaining attorneys. In the case of a straightforward forensic evaluation, the opposing side is generally entitled to the records and there is little difficulty in complying with the subpoena request.

In contrast, when the subpoena involves a patient's records, questions regarding confidentiality may have to be addressed legally before turning the records over. In these cases, psychiatrists should contact the patient's attorney. Sometimes that attorney will determine that the subpoena is either invalid or irrelevant and will offer to go to court to have the subpoena quashed. The attorney will then request the psychiatrist to hold records until the court determines the validity of the subpoena. The case records should contain documentation that reflects the phone calls to the attorney, the instructions given, and the withholding of the records pending court order. Such documentation will prevent later questions regarding the psychiatrist's "failure" to respond to the subpoena.

A court order is a command for the records, rather than merely a demand. The psychiatrist must respond to the court order and has total immunity for sending the records to the opposing attorney in the event the records prove harmful to anyone. Psychiatrists refusing a court order to produce records put themselves in jeopardy of contempt of court charges. Conflict regarding the release of records should not reach this point. Psychiatrists concerned about the effects of the release of patients' records even under court order can contact the judge and discuss how best to protect patients' interests, leaving implementation of such considerations, such as redaction of the records, to judicial discretion.

## Depositions

Following a subpoena for records or a court order to send treatment records or a forensic psychiatric report, the attorney for the opposing side may wish to depose the treating psychiatrist or the psychiatrist who prepared the report. A deposition is a court hearing held out of court. It is sworn testimony and is considered to be the equivalent of testifying in court, though there is no judge present. The deposition can usually be held in the retaining attorney's office, the opposing counsel's office, or the psychiatrist's office, with a court reporter and the attorneys present.

Psychiatrists should be aware that what they testify to in deposition may be raised at the subsequent trial. Thus, the psychiatrist should have a copy of the deposition transcript before ever going to court so the psychiatrist can review the testimony given to be certain that he or she is consistent in court when cross-examined. Deposition transcripts should be reviewed for errors of omission, spelling, or typos, but they may not be changed for content or meaning.

Psychiatrists should also be aware that they are likely the only party without counsel at the deposition. Treating psychiatrists should therefore carefully consider the option of bringing counsel to a deposition regarding a current or former patient. Experts generally do not require such representation. However, they should remain aware that the attorney representing the patient-litigant is not the attorney for the psychiatrist and cannot tell the clinician not to respond to questions. The psychiatrist may refuse to answer various personal questions if they are not relevant to the matter at hand. The attorney for the patient may object, and the objection would be left to the judge, who would later review the matter.

## Cross-Examination

Testifying in court can be an anxiety-provoking experience, even for experienced forensic psychiatrists. Psychiatrists should never go into court unprepared. They should prepare as completely and as comprehensively as possible by spending time before testifying in court with the retaining attorney. When adequately prepared, many psychiatrists are more comfortable with direct testimony, as it has been reviewed and rehearsed.

Psychiatrists may nevertheless become anxious about cross-examination, in which questions are less predictable. With experience comes confidence that the questions on cross-examination may be easier than those on direct, where one has to develop the case. On cross, one merely has to anticipate the main weakness of the testimony or of the case and anticipate what questions will be asked. Psychiatrists should not become defensive but should respond truthfully, even if the response is not favorable to the side that has called the clinician. Psychiatrists should then trust the retaining attorney to rehabilitate them on redirect examination if necessary.

Some experts are concerned about personal questions that are asked, such as the age of the expert, how much money they make, marital questions if there has been a divorce, or other personal issues that need not be addressed. Questions asked must be probative or relevant or they may be objected to and sustained. Lawyers are free to ask just about anything they want. If the opposing attorneys are listening and attentive, they can be relied on to object to inappropriate questions. The judge will often sustain irrelevant, incompetent, or immaterial questions.

Attorneys will often ask about the testifying psychiatrist's opinion about the opposing expert. It is always best to praise one's colleague if praise is due. However, in one instance in a hearing without a jury, I was asked whether I respected the psychiatrist on the other side who was giving opposing testimony. In most cases, I do respect my adversaries and so indicate in court. This was a question that should not have been asked. The retaining attorney objected, but the judge said, "No, I'd like to hear what Dr. Sadoff says about that." I thought for a moment and responded, "I respect his right to disagree with me." The judge recognized the effect of my statement and did not pursue it further.

Psychiatrists may also be concerned about incurring liability when testifying in court. Psychiatrists can incur liability if they give false testimony, which may amount to the criminal charge of perjury. They may also incur liability if they are negligent in obtaining sufficient information on which to base their opinions or if they formulate such opinions in an incompetent manner that is below the standard of care (Binder 2002). For the most part, psychiatrists have immunity in court when testifying. This immunity is based on the principle that individuals under oath are obliged to testify to the truth, even if the truth hurts someone. Such immunity is granted to experts because courts recognize that without it, obtaining honest testimony would be limited by concerns involving liability.

## Problematic Practical Issues

### Presenting Expert Credentials to the Court

#### Clinical Vignette

Dr. Z was an aspiring forensic psychiatrist. He participated in a weekend seminar lasting 2 hours, given by a prominent forensic psychiatrist, Dr. A. Afterward, in the interest of "buffing" his curriculum vitae (CV), he listed himself as Dr. A's student. Shortly thereafter, Dr. Z was retained in a forensic case. Opposing counsel's expert, an actual student of Dr. A's, identified Dr. Z's claim as inaccurate: one seminar does not a student make. When Dr. Z testified that he was a student of Dr. A's in court, opposing counsel was armed with the information that Dr. Z was embellishing his credentials. This attorney was easily able to discredit Dr. Z's claim. This resulted in casting doubt on the credibility of the rest of Dr. Z's qualifications, as well as on his testimony.

Courts require that the experts have a CV that must be turned over to the other side in preparation for cross-examination. This may provoke concern in psychiatrists who are just beginning their forensic practices. They are presenting themselves as experts, but their CVs may not reflect the breadth of experience a more established forensic psychiatrist might have. Nevertheless, psychiatrists must never embellish their credentials or give false information about their accomplishments or achievements. The reader is referred to the book by Dattilio and Sadoff (2002) for a complete discussion of appropriately presenting one's credentials in court.

### Scheduling

Scheduling in forensic psychiatry takes precedence over scheduling for treatment cases. Forensic psychiatrists must make themselves available when courts order hearings and trials. On occassion, the court will schedule the trial or the hearing in accord with the psychiatrist's schedule. However, treating psychiatrists may claim that they cannot go to court because they have to treat sick patients. Sometimes the testimony can be put on videotape in the event the psychiatrist will be out of town or is involved in a family or patient emergency. The videotape will then be shown in court instead of the psychiatrist giving live testimony, a practice referred to as a *de bene esse* deposition.

Psychiatrists depend on appropriate scheduling for their income. Nevertheless, no matter how carefully psychiatrists manage their schedules, they are subject to the changing needs of the legal system. They may open their schedule to testify on a Thursday morning, canceling several patients, and then receive a call on Wednesday evening indicating the court case has settled or a plea bargain has been reached and the psychiatrist will not be needed for court on Thursday morning. Sometimes the rescheduling is for tactical or strategic reasons to disrupt the flow or to cause inconvenience for the experts' schedules. If the case is settled or canceled at the last minute, the psychiatrist will likely not be able to schedule any fee-bearing cases for the following morning. Another reason psychiatrists should be certain to receive advance payment for testifying is to avoid incurring a financial loss in these not uncommon circumstances.

## Avoiding Perils in the Practice of Forensic Psychiatry

Certain cases present perils for forensic psychiatrists (Sadoff 1998). The general psychiatrist inexperienced in working in forensic psychiatry should be wary of becoming involved in cases that may cause legal, personal, or professional difficulties. For example, psychiatrists working outside an institutional setting or an official capacity may encounter difficulty in examining a police officer for a return to duty. Officers are often evaluated to determine whether they can safely carry a gun after either previously misusing the weapon in the line of duty or attempting suicide with their service revolver (see Chapter 18: "Forensic Psychiatry and Law Enforcement," this volume). An evaluation that concludes that an officer may safely return to duty may appear incredible if, in the future, the same officer under stress again becomes suicidal or reckless. Psychiatrists cannot predict behavior that may be a response to unforeseen factors. If, however, the psychiatrist concludes that the officer is not fit to carry a weapon, the officer may sue the examining psychiatrist. The grounds of such a suit would be for negligence in conducting the examination because the psychiatrist will be depriving the officer of making a living. Thus, psychiatrists working privately and not under the aegis of the city or of a police department may risk both reputation and liability in performing such evaluations.

Similarly, psychiatrists may have difficulty examining an individual seeking a sex change operation. Such examinations raise unique issues that need to be addressed by individuals with specific expertise in the field. The same caveats apply to evaluations of the threat or danger to a community posed by sex offenders (see Chapter 16: "Forensic Assessment of Sex Offenders," this volume).

Forensic psychiatrists who become involved in workplace lawsuits, such as sexual harassment, sexual discrimination, or other racial or gender harassment cases, may encounter difficulties when taking a history. The damages claimed can only be compensable if they were caused by harassment. Plaintiffs' experts tend to believe the plaintiff's account and assume that harassment occurred; defense experts will often say that the plaintiff has no psychiatric diagnosis, or if a diagnosis of anxiety or depression is present, that it is not causally related to the workplace experience. Psychiatrists do not know what happened in the workplace; they only know what the plaintiff and the retaining attorney tell them.

Psychiatrists should refrain from making such conclusory statements. Whether the harassment occurred is the ultimate legal question in such cases. Lawyers like psychiatrists to give such opinions in a direct manner. Nevertheless, such statements lack credibility and can suffer under good cross-examination. Psychiatrists writing reports in such cases can avoid this potential pitfall by making subjunctive rather than declarative statements. That is to say, if the plaintiff's statements are true, the individual was sexually harassed and, if so, as a result of that harassment, he or she has suffered emotional damage.

## Mentoring

Mentoring is a very prominent part of the education and practice of forensic psychiatry. Forensic psychiatrists, even those who face each other from opposite sides of a case, traditionally provide assistance to their colleagues. Experienced forensic clinicians find that any number of general psychiatrists who become involved in legal cases call for consultation. Similarly, forensic psychiatrists at times need to consult child psychiatrists or psychopharmacologists to more fully understand the cases in which they are involved. Psychiatrists should and do share this information freely and help each other in a mentoring manner.

## Conclusion

The practice of forensic psychiatry presents perils, pitfalls, and problems. However, these need not be overwhelming and are not unresolvable. The complexities associated with the practice of forensic psychiatry cannot be too strongly emphasized. Situations that warrant consultation arise frequently. Practicing treating psychiatrists who find themselves in need of forensic information or consultation should not hesitate to call a respected colleague who has experience in forensic psychiatry. Such consultation can help clarify the complex issues that arise in this subspecialty, such as problems in working with the attorney, fee arrangements, testifying in court, and ethical issues related to a case.

## Key Points

- The practice of forensic psychiatry may present a number of problems with which the general clinician is unfamiliar.
- Many of these problems involve interactions with attorneys and with the legal system.
- An understanding of the nature of these interactions can help psychiatrists avoid the problems that arise by addressing them at the outset, responding to them appropriately, or referring cases to colleagues.
- Psychiatrists should contact more experienced colleagues for consultation when indicated.

## Practice Guidelines

1. Clarify issues regarding expertise, conflict of interest, bias, and fees during the initial contact with the attorney to avoid problems in these areas later in the case.
2. Carefully consider attorneys' requests. Comply only with those that do not detrimentally affect the evaluation or compromise ethical or professional integrity.
3. Become familiar with the relevant elements of the legal process such as discovery, deposition, and courtroom testimony. Such familiarity will improve performance and decrease anxiety.
4. Be respectful of colleagues involved in the legal process.
5. Provide and seek mentoring freely. Learning from the experience of others and passing on learned wisdom results in personal and professional growth.

## References

American Academy of Psychiatry and the Law: Ethical Guidelines for the Practice of Forensic Psychiatry. Bloomfield, CT, American Academy of Psychiatry and the Law, 1995

Binder RL: Liability for the psychiatrist expert witness. Am J Psychiatry 159:1819–1825, 2002

Dattilio FM, Sadoff RL: Mental Health Experts: Roles and Qualifications for Court. Mechanicsburg, PA, Pennsylvania Bar Institute Press, 2002

Gutheil TG, Simon RI: Risk management principles in recovered memory cases: the importance of the clinical foundation. Psychiatr Serv 48:1403–1407, 1997

Sadoff RL: The practice of forensic psychiatry: perils, problems and pitfalls. J Am Acad Psychiatry Law 26:305–314, 1998

Simon RI: "Three's a crowd": the presence of third parties during the forensic psychiatric examination. J Psychiatry Law 24:3–25, 1996

Simon RI, Wettstein RM: Toward the development of guidelines for the content of forensic psychiatric examinations. J Am Acad Psychiatry Law 25:17–30, 1997

Strasburger LH, Gutheil TG, Brodsky A: On wearing two hats: role conflict in serving as both psychotherapist and expert witness. Am J Psychiatry 154: 448–456, 1997

## Suggested Readings

American Academy of Psychiatry and the Law: Ethical Guidelines for the Practice of Forensic Psychiatry. Bloomfield, CT, American Academy of Psychiatry and the Law, 1995

Dattilio FM, Sadoff RL: Mental Health Experts: Roles and Qualifications for Court. Mechanicsburg, PA, Pennsylvania Bar Institute Press, 2002

Sadoff RL: The practice of forensic psychiatry: perils, problems and pitfalls. J Am Acad Psychiatry Law 26:305–314, 1998

Simon RI: "Three's a crowd": the presence of third parties during the forensic psychiatric examination. J Psychiatry Law 24:3–25, 1996

Strasburger LH, Gutheil TG, Brodsky A: On wearing two hats: role conflict in serving as both psychotherapist and expert witness. Am J Psychiatry 154: 448–456, 1997

# PART II

# Civil Litigation

CHAPTER 9

# Psychiatric Malpractice and the Standard of Care

Donald J. Meyer, M.D.
Robert I. Simon, M.D.

## Introduction

The standard of care is a legal concept that has a pivotal role in all allegations of malpractice as well as in other sources of liability to which a practicing psychiatrist may be exposed. The law requires that a professional provide a standard of ordinary, average, prudent care. In cases of medical malpractice, the standard of care is the legal yardstick of the duty that physicians owe their patients. If a professional has met the applicable standard of care, legal malpractice has not occurred, even if the patient has suffered terrible harm.

The applicable standard of care of a physician is usually outside the experience of laypersons. Rule 702 of the Federal Rules of Evidence allows scientific, technical, or other specialized knowledge to be admitted if it will assist the trier of fact (i.e., the jury or, in the absence of a jury, the judge) to understand the evidence or determine a fact at issue. Thus, courts admit the testimony of experts to assist in the adjudication of allegations of malpractice. Psychiatrists who testify as experts should therefore be familiar with the legal conceptualization of psychiatric malpractice and what is meant by the standard of care.

## Malpractice Liability and the Standard of Care

Under the law, individuals owe no duty of care to another beyond ordinary prudence. Doctors owe a duty of care to their patients of ordinary prudence of a physician. Failure to perform that duty with a satisfactory level of expertise may constitute either intentional or unintentional negligence and form the basis of a medical malpractice suit.

Malpractice has four separate elements, each of which the plaintiff must demonstrate to the court by a preponderance of the evidence (more likely than not) in order to prevail. The plaintiff must prove that

1. The psychiatrist had a duty of care due the patient as a result of a psychiatrist-patient relationship.
2. The psychiatrist breached this duty by conduct that did not meet professional standards.
3. The patient was harmed.
4. The psychiatrist's breach of professional conduct was the direct cause of the harm to the patient.

These four elements are sometimes referred to as the four D's of malpractice assessment (Table 9–1).

Each of these legal elements must be met for a court to find a psychiatrist liable for the act of malpractice. For example, the law of malpractice requires the establishment of a doctor-patient relationship. Therefore, a solo practitioner covering the practice of a vacationing colleague could not be held negligent for the suicide of his colleague's patient if the patient chose not to contact the covering doctor. Being on call for a practice would not be sufficient to establish a doctor-patient relationship with a particular individual. In the absence of a doctor-patient relationship, the doctor owes that person no duty of care.

The law also recognizes there are risks to medical treatment. Therefore, damage or harm that results from proper care may be tragic, but it is not malpractice, because there was no departure from the duty of ordinary, prudent care. Alternatively, if a psychiatrist provided substandard treatment but the patient was not harmed, legally, there is no malpractice.

**TABLE 9–1.** The four D's of malpractice assessment

| | |
|---|---|
| **Duty** | A duty of care, derived from a doctor-patient relationship, must be present. |
| **Deviation** | A deviation from the standard of care must have occurred. |
| **Damage** | Damage to the patient must have occurred. |
| **Direct cause** | Damage occurred directly as a result of deviation from the standard of care. |

In addition, no malpractice can occur unless the damage is a direct, causal result of the substandard treatment. Medical and legal concepts of causation are quite different. Legally, causation involves the consideration of two factors: cause-in-fact and proximate cause. *Cause-in-fact* is expressed by the "but for" rule and asks the question, But for the psychiatrist's misconduct, would the patient have been injured? If there are several causes acting together that brought about an injury, courts ask whether the misconduct was a substantial contributing factor in causing the damage. *Proximate cause* is the last factor in a series of events, the "straw that broke the camel's back," rather than the first primary cause of damage (Simon 1992).

A patient who was summarily terminated by his psychiatrist alleges in a malpractice suit that the abandonment caused a heart attack. Unless the court finds that the emotional stress of the psychiatrist's abandonment was both a substantial contributing factor to and a proximate cause of the patient's heart attack, the physician misconduct would not meet the legal standard as a cause of that particular damage.

The incidence of malpractice suits against psychiatrists and other mental health professionals has risen steadily since the early 1970s. In 1975, the annual incidence of claims against psychiatrists was about 1 in 45, or approximately 2.25%. In the 1980s, a psychiatrist's chance of being sued in any single year was 1 in 25 (4%). Thus, the rate of occurrence nearly doubled. Through 1995, the odds increased to approximately 1 out of every 12 psychiatrists. In some states, psychiatrists were sued at the rate of 1 in 6 every year (Simon 2001). The incidence of claims against psychiatrists, however, still remains lower than that of claims against other medical specialists. Moreover, plaintiffs are only successful in 2–3 out of every 10 claims (Simon 2001). Nevertheless, the rising incidence of malpractice claims against psychiatrists is expected to continue. Allegations of negligence in suicide cases is one of the most frequent bases for malpractice claims against psychiatrists.

## Malpractice and the Standard of Care

Malpractice cannot occur absent an individual doctor's departure from the relevant standard of care. The concept of a *standard of care* is not limited to professional liability. The *standard of care* is a legal concept, derived from English common law. Individuals must conduct themselves with the ordinary care and prudence of a layperson toward their fellow citizens. Individuals who disregard that ordinary care and prudence in their daily activities may have breached the standard of care of an ordinary citizen and may be guilty of negligence. For example, a person who operated a motor vehicle after having been informed the brakes were faulty could be liable for damages caused by an accident because of his violation of the standard of care applied to ordinary citizens.

As applied to professionals, the legal doctrine of the standard of care refers to the acceptable level of expertise of the professional group being considered. The law expects that professionals will conduct themselves with that degree of care, knowledge, and skill ordinarily possessed and exercised in similar situations by a member of the profession in the same field. This expectation forms the basis of the general definition of the standard of care. For example, in *Stepakoff v. Kantar* (1985), the standard of care applied by the court in a suicide case was that "the [defendant] psychiatrist owed a legal duty to treat the decedent in accordance with the standard of care and the skill of an average member of the medical profession practicing psychiatry."

The law of malpractice does not expect absolute certainty. Psychiatrists cannot guarantee a patient either the correct diagnosis and treatment or the desired treatment outcome. In addition, the legal system is not interested in punishing errors in judgment per se. Mistaken diagnostic and therapeutic assumptions and bad treatment outcomes may be made without the doctor incurring liability. Clinical judgments that later prove incorrect are not considered legally negligent when reasonable care was used and the reasoning documented. If the professional standard of care is breached, however, liability may arise.

## Standard of Care: Variations

Expert witnesses should always review the language of the specific statute or sentinel case that determines the legal definition of the standard of care in the jurisdiction in which they are about to testify. Jurisdictional differences will be reflected in the precise wording of the locally relevant legal standard. For example, the applicable law will have wording that defines whether the geographic region of average psychiatrists is the nation as a whole or the local jurisdiction in which the alleged malpractice occurred.

A national standard of care exists for most jurisdictions in the United States. The national standard of care is in keeping with the law's view that medical information and medical recommendations are widely disseminated across state and regional borders. Thus, an expert from California who testifies about the psychiatric standard of care in a general hospital in New York may base that opinion on experiences the expert has had in similar hospitals in California. In most jurisdictions that employ a national standard, the expert has leeway to consider locally available diagnostic and therapeutic resources. Such considerations in effect add a degree of geographic locality to national standards.

In some jurisdictions, the applicable standard of care is that of the local patterns of practice. Experts from a distant part of the country testifying in such jurisdictions can anticipate cross-examination regarding their knowledge of the local medical norms. Under these circumstances, attorneys often retain local practitioners as well as experts with specialized knowledge. This can assist attorneys in meeting the legal requirements of "the locality rule."

Jurisdictions may also vary in how they define the concept of "the skill and care ordinarily employed" by an average member of the profession. Tort law has traditionally relied on physicians' customary conduct to define the standard of reasonable care in medicine. Physicians have needed to conform their provision of care to the customary practice of their peers (Peters 2000). However, defendants in ordinary, nonprofessional negligence claims are required to have used reasonable care under the same circumstances. A number of states have now rejected the standard of medical custom based on the behavior of the group in favor of a standard based on a reasonably prudent physician (Peters 2000). This standard goes beyond a statistical "head count." These jurisdictions require that actual practice must bear a relationship to a reasonable, prudent standard of care. For example, courts have held that negligence cannot be excused because other physicians practice the same kind of negligence (Simon 2002).

## Foreseeability Versus Predictability and the Standard of Care

Cases involving suicidal or violent patients frequently raise the issue of the ability of psychiatrists to predict or "foresee" potentially disastrous consequences of their patients' illnesses. The law does not require an individual to "foresee events which are merely possible but only those that are reasonably foreseeable" (*Hairston v. Alexander Tank and Equipment Co.* 1984).

Legally, foreseeability is defined as the reasonable anticipation that harm or injury is likely to result from certain acts or omissions (Black 1999). A person who trips his friend as a joke is expected to foresee that harm could occur. A psychiatrist who assesses a patient to be at high risk for suicide is expected to foresee the significant risk of harm and take reasonable action within the standard of care of the profession to prevent this harm. However, experts should be careful not to confuse the foreseeability of an adverse outcome such as suicide with the predictability of such an outcome.

The term *foreseeable* in malpractice litigation is a legal term of art. As is often the case at the interface of law and psychiatry, this legal term does not translate neatly into a medical concept. Foreseeability is often confused with *prediction*. In contrast to foreseeability, prediction is an actuarial and scientific concept. Infrequent, so called low–base rate, events such as suicide and violence that occur within the context of frequent events such as feeling suicidal and feeling violent pose enormous barriers to mathematically and scientifically accurate prediction. No technology or tools currently exist that can accurately predict suicide in an individual case. Thus, although there is a standard of care for suicide risk assessment, there is no standard of care for the prediction of an individual suicide.

Consistent with this reasoning, a patient's demographic risk factors are relevant to the risk assessment process. However, courts generally do not regard listing individual demographic risk factors alone to be a sufficient clinical process of risk assessment to establish foreseeability. In *Williamson v. Liptzin* (2000), a patient sued his former psychiatrist for not having foreseen that the patient would commit violent murders 8 months after the termination of treatment. The appellate court held, "Evidence of 'risk factors' for potential violence, such as gun ownership, being under a certain age, or being of a certain gender, implicates a large portion of our population and is simply insufficient in and of itself to prove foreseeability." (*Williamson v. Liptzin* 2000, p. 1)

## The Standard of Care and Expert Testimony

A plaintiff who alleges psychiatric malpractice is required to establish both the applicable standard of care and the defendant psychiatrist's deviation from that standard. Usually this legal burden is met through the use of an expert witness. A jury or a judge needs no expert information to adjudicate claims of negligence if the alleged acts of commission or omission and their consequences are within the understanding of laypersons. However, a plaintiff's allegation of malpractice usually involves a series of facts, events, and customary practices that are beyond the experience of an ordinary person.

On rare occasions, the plaintiff alleging malpractice is relieved of the "burden of production" regarding proof of a departure from the standard of care. No expert testimony may be required if the facts of the case alone would allow for laypersons to discern a failure to conform to the applicable standard of care. For example, the plaintiff would not need an expert to prove there had been a departure from the standard of care if a doctor were to have significantly violated the hospital's own published policies regarding restraint or forced medication. Nevertheless, in such cases, an expert might still be used to testify to the damages or to the departure in conduct having directly caused the damages.

Expert witnesses in professional negligence cases should be prepared to demonstrate direct and current familiarity with the practices at issue based on their education, training, and experience. In general, medical expert witnesses must also be from the same discipline that typically practices the procedure or offers the treatment at issue. For example, in *Lundgren v. Eustermann* (1985), the Minnesota Supreme Court held that a licensed psychologist was not competent to give expert testimony about the standard of care in a medical malpractice case that challenged the use of chlorpromazine prescribed by the defendant physician.

Psychiatrists who do not see patients or who have little experience in treating certain types of patients should not offer testimony on elements of the standard of psychiatric care beyond their own expertise. As Principle V of the American Academy of Psychiatry and the Law's *Ethical Guidelines for the Practice of Forensic Psychiatry* (1995) states, "Expertise in the practice of forensic psychiatry is claimed only in areas of actual knowledge and skills, training and experience." A lack of relevant experience in the psychiatric practice at issue may result in disqualification as an expert. For example, in Massachusetts, a doctor who had never treated a person with the illness at issue (chlamydia) and "whose knowledge was based entirely of readings," was deemed unqualified as an expert (*Commonwealth v. Barresi 1999*, p. 909).

Thus, experts who testify about specific practices of psychiatric care should be able to prove the current basis of their expertise. The American Psychiatric Association (APA) "Resource Document for Peer Review of Expert Testimony" (American Psychiatric Association 1997) is a valuable guide to providing credible testimony. The appendices contain a checklist for both content and process of serving as an expert in addition to questions that deal with ethical issues. For the content of testimony, the checklist assesses whether the expert's testimony is within his or her area of expertise and whether the opinions are data based, scientifically accurate, and reasonable.

Expert witnesses offering testimony about the standard of care should consider the criteria of admissibility of their testimony at trial. The trial judge is responsible for the determination of the admissibility of expert testimony. Some jurisdictions retain the *Frye* rule of general acceptance (*Frye v. United States* 1923). In most jurisdictions, however, expert opinions about the standard of care should be formed with the expectation of meeting the standards and potential challenges expressed by United States Supreme Court decisions in *Daubert* (*Daubert v. Merrell Dow Phar-*

*maceuticals, Inc.* 1993), *Joiner* (*General Electric Co. v. Joiner* 1999) and *Kumho Tire* (*Kumho Tire Co., Ltd. v. Carmichael* 1999).

In lieu of the criteria of general acceptance from *Frye,* in *Daubert,* the Supreme Court provided trial judges with new criteria for the admissibility of expert evidence. Under *Daubert,* a trial judge's decision of the admissibility of testimony should be determined by the testimony's relevance to the case and by the reliability of the testimony. Judges can base their determination of the reliability of expert opinions on the general acceptance of the underlying foundations of the opinion within the relevant field; on whether the opinion is based on methods that are reliable, are testable, and have a known error rate; and on whether the methods have been published and peer reviewed.

The psychiatric diagnosis and treatment of the individual patient remains a clinical practice rather than a laboratory science. Aspects of the individual patient's treatment are beyond the reach of the scientific rigor described in *Daubert* that can be applied to a laboratory science. However, many of the foundations of psychiatric clinical practice have been subjected to the kind of scientific scrutiny described in *Daubert.* The diagnostic classification system of *Diagnostic and Statistical Manual of Mental Disorders,* 4th Edition, Text Revision (DSM-IV-TR; American Psychiatric Association 2000), many of the psychological tests used in forensic psychiatry, and many therapeutic interventions in psychiatry meet specific criteria noted in *Daubert.* They can be cited as sources of information in expert reports and testimony to assist the expert in meeting court admissibility criteria.

Although experience is admissible as one of several factors forming the basis of an expert opinion, experts should not base an opinion on the standard of care solely on their personal experience. As the court stated in *Joiner,* "Nothing in either Daubert or the Federal Rules of Evidence requires a district court to admit opinion evidence which is connected to existing data only by the ipse dixit of an expert" (*General Electric Co. v. Joiner* 1999, p. 520).

## Clinical Considerations in the Applicable Standard of Care

### Level of Expertise

The expert should consider what level of professional expertise the psychiatrist held out to the patient. The law differentiates between certain levels of training and experience in the consideration of professional liability. For example, specialists are held to a higher standard of care than nonspecialists, even in cases involving the same problem. A doctor with specialty training and certification in adolescent psychiatry is held to a higher standard of care than a general psychiatrist who treats the same teenager. In contrast, the law holds a trainee psychiatrist to the same professional standards as a psychiatrist who has finished training. Nonmedical therapists and primary care physicians who represent themselves as specialists in the treatment of emotional and mental illness may be held to the higher standard of the specialist. Similarly, a psychiatrist who undertakes the diagnosis and treatment of medical disorders will be held to the standard of care applicable to medical practitioners (King 1986).

## Schools of Treatment

From a legal perspective regarding malpractice, one school of treatment is not preferred per se over another. Psychiatry has a tradition of being hospitable to diverse and competing schools of thought. At present, there are more than 450 different schools of psychotherapy (Simon 2001). Psychiatrists may differ concerning the use of biologic, behavioral, and psychodynamic treatments for anxiety disorders. Honest disagreements among practitioners about the indications and effectiveness of psychotherapeutic modalities do not, of themselves, violate the standard of care. As one experienced expert opined, "If I think I could find a group of competently trained doctors who would have done the same thing in the same situation, then usually I think the standard of care was met" (Robert L. Sadoff, personal communication, May 2002).

Prescribed treatment or care, however, cannot be idiosyncratic. Courts have determined that a claimed treatment philosophy is considered legitimate if it is supported by a respectable minority of psychiatrists (Reisner and Slobogin 1990). This rule states that a psychiatrist is free to choose from any of the available schools of therapy—even ones that most psychiatrists would not use—if a respected minority of therapists would employ the same treatments under the same circumstances (Malcolm 1988). Unless egregious, even those forms of treatment that would not be employed by most psychiatrists may fall within the respected minority rule.

## Scientific Advances

Allegations of malpractice may involve the determination of the standard of care for novel or even experimental therapies. Innovation is important to developing new diagnostic and treatment methods in psychiatry (Simon 1993). Such developments in a professional field may change the standard of care. Psychiatrists have an ethical and professional duty to stay abreast of these therapeutic developments. *The Principles of Medical Ethics, With Annotations Especially Applicable to Psychiatry* (American Psychiatric Association 2001) states: "Psychiatrists are responsible for their own continuing education and should be mindful of the fact that theirs must be a lifetime of learning." The law has also imposed a duty on all physicians to stay abreast of changing concepts and new developments (Holder 1973). Specialists are held to have a clearer duty to be current with specialty advances than are general practitioners (Weintraub 1985).

The legal definition of the standard of care uses words such as "ordinary," "average," and "customary." Proving that a treatment is customary usually precludes liability if the treatment was not negligently performed. This concept would seem to discourage the development or use of innovative or novel treatments, which by definition are not customary. American psychiatry has welcomed credible treatments that hold promise for the alleviation of mental suffering. A professional vision that encourages innovation in research and treatment offers the best opportunities for progress.

The use of a treatment that is not customary is not necessarily an indication or evidence of professional negligence. For example, pharmaceutical companies must obtain approval from the Food and Drug Administration (FDA) for the prescription of their products. This approval is limited to indications for use of the product that have met the FDA's regulations for demonstrable efficacy. However, psychiatrists and other physicians commonly prescribe medications for non-FDA-approved indications. Standard-of-care issues that would apply to this practice include informed consent, the existence of scientific and clinical support for the non-FDA-approved treatment, and whether the treatment was based on thoughtful and prudent reasoning.

## Practice Guidelines

The expert witness formulating an opinion of the applicable standard of care for the individual case should consider a range of information including the medical literature, the unique circumstances of that case, and practice guidelines. Professional associations have developed and supported the use of clinical practice parameters and guidelines that may be introduced at trial as supporting or refuting evidence of the standard of care in a given case (Hirshfeld 1990). The American Medical Association is one professional organization that has supported the use of such guidelines. The APA, through its Task Force on Treatments of

Psychiatric Disorders, has published a number of official practice guidelines for the treatment of various psychiatric disorders (American Psychiatric Association 2002).

Practice guidelines generally have been established to define a spectrum of appropriate clinical care and are not intended to be followed rigidly. In a forensic setting, they are only one source for determining the standard of care and do not represent the standard itself. At the beginning of each APA practice guideline is a "Statement of Intent" that asserts, "This guideline is not intended to be construed or to serve as a standard of care. The ultimate judgment regarding a particular clinical procedure or treatment plan must be made by the psychiatrist in light of the clinical data presented by the patient and the diagnostic and treatment options available."

Not all the recommendations made in practice guidelines carry the same weight. Recommended interventions are generally based on the clinical or research evidence that supports their use, and the strength of such evidence may differ among the recommendations in any given practice guideline. The guidelines may indicate the degree of importance or relative certainty of each recommendation. They may also indicate which recommendations are evidence based.

Moreover, official practice guidelines are not static. They evolve and change according to new developments in practice and science, requiring frequent updating. Studies show that no more than 90% of practice guidelines are valid after 3.6 years. At 5.8 years, half of the guidelines are outdated (Shekelle 2001). This is another basis for disclaimers that emphasize that practice guidelines do not represent the proffered standard for clinical care, much less for a fact-specific case in litigation.

No official approved guideline in health care can substitute for sound clinical judgment in the diagnosis and treatment of individual patients, nor is any guideline alone probative of the standard of care of the profession. Courts recognize that these guidelines do not of themselves establish a legal standard of care. The court maintains full discretion in considering other evidence in establishing the appropriate standard of care. Indeed, the court may reach conclusions that are contrary to the practice parameter if it finds other evidence more persuasive (Hirshfeld 1991).

## Judicially Imposed Standard of Care

### Case and Statutory Law

The standard of care for certain issues may be defined by case law. In some cases, the courts have imposed their own version of professional practice standards even though those standards were not already customary professional practice. For example, in *Tarasoff v. Regents of the University of California* (1976), the court imposed a duty on psychiatrists and psychologists to protect endangered persons from foreseeably violent patients. In so doing it established a new element of the psychiatric standard of care in California. Many other jurisdictions have case law that follows the *Tarasoff* ruling. Other examples of judicially imposed standards of care of psychiatric practice include informed consent and confidentiality. In the landmark case *Canterbury v. Spence* (1972), the court imposed the "reasonable man" standard in informed consent litigation even though "professional custom" had been the prevailing standard up until that time.

An element of the standard of care may also be defined by statute. Some state legislatures have passed laws articulating a *Tarasoff* duty for mental health professionals practicing in that locality (e.g., Massachusetts General Law c.123, 36B). State laws mandating health care professionals to report child or elder abuse are additional examples of an element of the standard of care being defined by statute and not by the conduct of the average practitioner. Experts should consult attorneys to provide relevant case or statutory law on the particular clinical issue in question.

## Drug Manufacturers' Inserts and Other Sources of Information

The standard of care may also be informed by the drug manufacturers' instructions and by the medical literature. Again, courts have emphasized that a standard of care cannot be established by any one of these sources of information alone. In *Ramon v. Farr* (1989), for example, the court held that drug inserts do not by themselves set the standard of care. Rather, drug inserts are one factor to be considered.

## Regulatory Requirements

Governmental and nongovernmental regulatory agencies may specify requirements for health care delivery in different settings. Federal governmental efforts to control medical payments and monitor quality of care to recipients of federal health care programs inevitably affect standards of psychiatric practice by defining and funding "appropriate" care. These regulations may be considered relevant, but not solely definitive, in assessments of the legal standard of care.

Other nongovernmental sources of practice requirements, such as legislative mandates setting standards for peer review and record keeping, are becoming increasingly more common. Third-party payers such as private, state, and federal insurance programs are establishing requirements for covered treatments. Some managed care organizations have also created practice guidelines. These, too, may be considered in establishing standards of care in cases involving allegations of medical malpractice.

## Clinical Vignette

> Mr. S, a 37-year-old married man, was admitted to the psychiatric unit of a general hospital after telling his wife he intended to kill himself. The patient was depressed over financial reverses in his business. His marriage was unstable, and the couple had been discussing divorce. He had a history of recurrent depression but no previous suicidal ideation or hospitalization.
>
> The admitting psychiatrist made the diagnosis of major depression, recurrent. He recorded that Mr. S "currently denies suicidal ideation, intent, or plan." The nursing staff obtained a signed "no harm" contract from the patient. The patient was placed on 15-minute safety checks. The managed care organization authorized 5 days of hospitalization. The psychiatrist saw the patient individually each day for approximately 20 minutes. The treatment team provided daily group therapy. The psychiatrist started Mr. S on an antidepressant, a medication to which the patient had formerly had a positive response. The patient appeared improved on days 2 and 3 of his hospitalization. Mr. S consistently denied suicidal ideation, intent, or plan to the psychiatrist and the treatment team. He was taken off 15-minute safety checks on the third day of hospitalization.
>
> On day 4 of his hospitalization, Mr. S hung himself in his room with another patient's belt. Ms. S brought a wrongful death suit against the psychiatrist and the hospital, claiming negligent treatment and management of her husband. Both sides retained experts to provide testimony regarding the standard of care and whether the defendants deviated from that standard.

### Discussion

An inpatient suicide is a common precipitant of allegations of malpractice. Both defense and plaintiff's experts, Drs. B and W, were required to testify to the standard of care of the average psychiatrist. Both treated psychiatric inpatients. Both had to consider a variety of factors to provide well-informed and reasoned opinions regarding the standard of care and whether the defendants deviated from this standard. These factors included the multiple sources of medical information already reviewed as well as the individual circumstances of Mr. S's treatment. The experts' testimony in this case would have also been informed by the actual wording of the legal standard of care.

Two experts assessing the central issue of the standard of care can, and often do, come to different conclusions. No case at trial is wholly one-sided. Opposing experts routinely have access to different sources of information and to different levels of disclosure from corroborating witnesses. The plaintiff's expert, Dr. W, might give significant weight to the family's view that their worries about the decedent were not sufficiently included in the psychiatrist's clinical assessments. The defense expert, Dr. B, might view that same data as historical revisionism based on the family's need to defend against feelings of guilt and helplessness. Dr. B might emphasize the psychiatrist's regular, daily interviews with Mr. S, whereas Dr. W might credit the family's report that these visits were too short to adequately assess Mr. S's risk of suicide and to provide adequate treatment.

Although the plaintiff's attorney alleged multiple examples of negligent psychiatric practice, he focused on the absence of evidence that the defendant psychiatrist performed adequate suicide risk assessments of Mr. S. Both experts knew a standard of care for predicting suicide does not exist. However, a standard of care for assessment and management of patients who are foreseeably at significant risk for suicide does exist. The experts, and ultimately the court, would scrutinize the psychiatrist's assessment, treatment, and management of the patient to determine whether these standards of care were met and whether Mr. S's suicide had been reasonably foreseeable. They would also try to determine whether any deviations from these standards of care proximately caused Mr. S's suicide.

Dr. W, the plaintiff's expert, testified that Mr. S's care required ongoing suicide risk assessments to inform clinical treatment and management decisions. She further testified that the absence of systematic suicide risk assessments was below the standard of care. She noted that no suicide risk assessments were recorded by the psychiatrist or the treatment team in the daily treatment notes, other than the cryptic: "No SI, HI, CFS." Dr. W opined that merely recording that Mr. S did not have suicidal or homicidal ideation and had contracted for safety did not qualify as a suicide risk assessment. She acknowledged that a more extensive evaluation of suicide risk was recorded at the time of admission. However, she stated that adequate suicide risk assessment was not a single event that occurred at the time of admission but, rather, a process that needed to be repeated routinely during hospitalization. Dr. W referred to official practice guidelines that recommend systematic assessment of suicide risk factors to support her opinions. She testified that the absence of suicide risk assessment was the proximate causal factor in the patient's suicide.

Dr. W also identified other elements of Mr. S's treatment that she believed were below the standard of care. She stated that more rigorous assessment would have shown that the initial suicide risk factors, which had precipitated Mr. S's hospital admission, were all still present past the time when the 15-minute checks were discontinued. For example, the patient's marriage and financial status were still in jeopardy. Moreover, she opined, the fact that this patient had never before been suicidal was itself an indicator that this episode of illness was worse than his previous episodes. Finally, Dr. W testified that 3 days of antidepressant treatment was insufficient to have had a lasting and significant clinical effect on the patient's depression. Given the lack of change in Mr. S's risk factors and the short length of treatment time, she testified that Mr. S's appearing improved was a transitory change from having been admitted to the hospital and not a substantive improvement indicating a therapeutic response.

Dr. B, the defense expert, testified that Mr. S's suicide was not predictable (foreseeable) and that the treatment had met the applicable standard of care. According to both the hospital record and the treating psychiatrist's testimony, the patient was improving. Dr. B testified that the treating psychiatrist had been systematic in assessing the patient's potential for suicide. He agreed with the defendant psychiatrist's assessment that the patient's risk for suicide had been low to moderate.

Dr. B referred to medical literature that concluded that no suicide risk assessment method had been empirically tested for reliability and validity. He stated that research studies had not proven that suicide risk assessment can predict individual suicides or even serious suicide attempts.

Dr. B noted that the sworn deposition testimony of the treating psychiatrist indicated that she routinely assessed suicide risk, weighing both risk and protective factors, with all suicidal patients, including the decedent. The treating psychiatrist had also testified that it was not her practice to record the details of suicide assessments. Because Dr. B's retrospective assessment of the patient did not indicate that the patient had been forseeably at risk, Dr. B stated that even had the treating psychiatrist not performed these assessments, this omission could not be the proximate cause of Mr. S's suicide.

Ideally, he stated, all risk assessments should be reflected in a clinical record. However, in Dr. B's experience, busy inpatient psychiatrists often did not do so. He added that in the era of managed care, little time was allotted for the treatment of patients and even less for detailed documentation of risk assessments. He stated that physicians often used the same medical shorthand used by the defendant psychiatrist, although in actual practice, the assessments were more substantive. Dr. B opined that this problem in recordkeeping was, by itself, not a substantial departure from the standard of care and was not itself the proximate cause of the patient's suicide.

This vignette also demonstrates the importance of documentation in medical malpractice cases. The standard of care requires the documentation of important clinical assessments. The absence of documentation may or may not be the proximate cause of a suicide. In the case described, the testifying experts formed differing opinions about the gravity of the lapse of documentation. The final decision regarding the importance of this lapse in this case would be made by the trier of fact. Nevertheless, the relative lack of documentation may allow the court to focus narrowly on simpler aspects of the case while overlooking the numerous clinical complexities and ambiguities that exist with every patient.

## Conclusion

The standard of care is a legal concept that has a pivotal role in allegations of malpractice to which a practicing psychiatrist may be exposed. In the case of medical malpractice, the standard of care is the legal yardstick of the duty that physicians owe their patients. Psychiatrists who provide expert opinions in professional negligence cases are asked to testify to the applicable standard of care and to whether the defendant doctor conformed with or deviated from the standard. The law requires a standard of average or reasonably prudent care by a professional. Exceptional care is not required. Under the law, if a professional has met the standard of care, no malpractice has occurred, whether or not the plaintiff has been harmed.

Within the adversarial system, both plaintiff's and defendant's experts serve an educational function for the court, assisting "the trier of fact to understand the evidence or determine a fact in issue" (Fed. Rule Evid. 702). Psychiatrists should therefore be aware of the precise wording of the applicable legal standards, statutes, and sentinel case law in the jurisdiction in which they are testifying so that their testimony will conform with the locally relevant law. In determining the standard of care, expert witnesses should combine their training and experience with knowledge of the relevant scientific studies and consensus guidelines. These should then be applied to the specific facts at trial to offer the court an integrated opinion, broadly based on multiple, corroborative sources of information in the field.

## Key Points

- The standard of care is a legal, not a medical, concept.
- Psychiatric malpractice cannot be established without evidence of a duty of care, deviation from the standard of care, and damage to the patient as a direct result of that deviation.
- The standard of care is defined by statute or case law to which the relevant facts of a specific case can be applied. Expert testimony is generally required to establish the standard of care.
- Under the law, the standard of care requires average, ordinary, or prudent reasonable care in similar circumstances. It does not require exceptional care.
- Experts should not conclude that care is substandard simply because the expert practices differently or does not follow the practices of the majority of clinicians.
- A psychiatrist providing expert testimony regarding the standard of care should have training and experience with the relevant clinical issues in addition to an understanding of the applicable legal concepts.

## Practice Guidelines

1. Determine whether the relevant legal standard in regard to the standard of care is that of an average practitioner providing ordinary care, or that of a prudent, reasonable practitioner. The latter standard has been adopted by an increasing number of states.
2. Offer opinions only within your area of clinical expertise.
3. Base opinions on a careful review of the records, interviews, and examination of relevant person; knowledge of the relevant medical literature; and your training and experience.
4. Be cautious not to overreach a reasonable level of clinical certainty about the standard of care and foreseeability.
5. Remember that colleagues retained by the opposite side can and will come to different conclusions. Expert testimony on both sides of an adversarial process is intended to assist the trier of fact in understanding both sides of the legal arguments.

## References

American Academy of Psychiatry and the Law: Ethical Guidelines for the Practice of Forensic Psychiatry. Bloomfield, CT, American Academy of Psychiatry and Law, 1995

American Psychiatric Association: Resource Document on Peer Review of Expert Testimony. J Am Acad Psychiatry Law 25:359–373, 1997

American Psychiatric Association: Diagnostic and Statistical Manual of Mental Disorders, 4th Edition. Washington, DC, American Psychiatric Association, 1994

American Psychiatric Association: Diagnostic and Statistical Manual of Mental Disorders, 4th Edition, Text Revision. Washington, DC, American Psychiatric Association, 2000

American Psychiatric Association: The Principles of Medical Ethics With Annotations Especially Applicable to Psychiatry, Section 5, Annotation 1. Washington, DC, American Psychiatric Association, 2001

American Psychiatric Association: Practice Guidelines for the Treatment of Psychiatric Disorders. Compendium 2002. Washington, DC, American Psychiatric Association, 2002

Black HC: Black's Law Dictionary, 7th Edition. St Paul, MN, West Publishing, 1999

Canterbury v Spence, 150 U.S. App. D.C. 263, 464 F.2d 772 D.C. (1972)

Commonwealth v Barresi, 46 Mass.App.Ct. 907, 705 N.E.2nd 639 (1999)

Daubert v Merrell Dow Pharmaceuticals, Inc, 509 U.S. 579, 113 S. Ct. 2786 (1993)

Frye v United States, 54 App.D.C. 46, 47, 293 F. 1013, 1014 (1923)

General Electric Co v Joiner, 522 U.S. 136, 118 S. Ct. 512 (1999)

Hairston v Alexander Tank and Equipment Co, 310 N.C. 227, 233, 311 S.E.2d 559, 565 (1984)

Hirshfeld EB: Practice parameters and the malpractice liability of physicians. JAMA 263:1556–1562, 1990

Hirshfeld EB: Should practice parameters be the standard of care in malpractice litigation? JAMA 266:2886–2891, 1991

Holder AR: Failure to "keep up" as negligence. Best Law Med 116:107, 1973

King JH: The Law of Medical Malpractice, 2nd Edition. St Paul, MN, West Publishing, 1986, p 58

Kumho Tire Co, Ltd v Carmichael, 526 U.S. 137, 152, 119 S. Ct. 1167, 1176 (1999)

Lundgren v Eustermann, 356 N.W.2d 762 (Minn. Ct. App. 1984), rev'd., Lundgren v Eustermann, 370 N.W.2d 877 (Minn. 1985)

Malcolm JG: Treatment Choices and Informed Consent: Current Controversies in Psychiatric Malpractice Litigation. Springfield, IL, Charles C Thomas, 1988, pp 49–50

Peters PG: The quiet demise of deference to custom: malpractice law at the millennium. Washington & Lee Law Review 57:163, 2000

Ramon v Farr, 770 P.2d 131 (Utah 1989)

Reisner R, Slobogin C: Law and the Mental Health System, 2nd Edition. St Paul, MN, West Publishing, 1990, p 75

Shekelle PG, Ortiz E, Rhodes S, et al: Validity of the Agency for Healthcare Research and Quality Clinical Practice Guidelines. JAMA 286:1461–1467, 2001

Simon RI: Clinical Psychiatry and the Law, 2nd Edition. Washington, DC, American Psychiatric Press, 1992, pp 549–550

Simon RI: Innovative psychiatric therapies and legal uncertainty: a survival guide for clinicians. Psychiatric Annals 23:473–479, 1993

Simon RI: Psychiatry and Law for Clinicians, 3rd Edition. Washington, DC, American Psychiatric Publishing, 2001

Simon RI: Suicide risk assessment: what is the standard of care? J Am Acad Psychiatry Law 30:340–344, 2002

Stepakoff v Kantar, 393 Mass. 836, 473 N.E.2d 1131 (1985)
Tarasoff v Regents of the University of California, 13 Cal.3d 177, 118 Cal. Rptr. 129, 529 P.2d 553 (1974), reargued, 17 Cal.3d 425, 131 Cal. Rptr. 14, 551 P.2d 334 (1976)
Weintraub A: Physician's duty to stay abreast of current medical developments. Med Trial Technique Q 31:329–341, 1985
Williamson v Liptzin, 539 S.E.2d 313 (N.C. App. 2000)

## Suggested Readings

Dobbs DV: The Law of Torts. St Paul, MN, West Publishing, 2000
Melton GB: Psychological Evaluations for the Courts, 2nd Edition. New York, Guilford, 1997
Shuman DW: Psychiatric and Psychological Evidence, 2nd Edition. Colorado Springs, CO, Shepard's/McGraw-Hill, 1994

CHAPTER 10

# Civil Competency

Ralph Slovenko, J.D., Ph.D.

## Introduction

Webster's defines competency as "the quality or state of being functionally adequate or of having sufficient knowledge, judgment, skill, or strength (as for a particular day or in a particular respect)." In other words, competency depends on the activity or the task. In a dialogue in Richard Condon's *Prizzi's Honor,* a novel turned into a celebrated film, Charley (a Mafia hit man), wondering whether he can trust a woman he thinks he loves, asks, "Do I ice her? Do I marry her?" Replies girlfriend Maerose, "Just because she's a thief and a hitter don't mean she ain't a good woman in all other departments." Likewise, as a legal concept, competency refers to one's ability to perform an act or to make a decision in a certain situation. Its connotation is contextual, relating to the specific task to be accomplished or decision to be made. Therefore, incompetency in one area does not necessarily imply incompetency in another. Thus, in an Ontario case, an elderly man was found competent to marry though lacking in testamentary capacity (*In re* McElroy 1978).

In forensic or disciplinary proceedings, a witness qualified as an expert may be called on to address competency of a patient regarding medical care, competency of a witness, competency to make a will, competency to contract, competency of a minor to consent to treatment, professional competency, or impairment of an employee. Psychiatrists evaluate individuals to see whether they have an impairment related to a psychiatric problem that affects a function that is related to the competency issue at hand. The task of the psychiatrist is to make clear the relationship between a psychiatric symptom and a functional impairment related to issue-specific competence.

## Competency of a Patient Regarding Informed Consent for Medical Care

The doctrine of "informed consent" that has developed in regard to medical care calls for consideration of three elements: competency, disclosure (risks of a treatment and also alternative forms of treatment), and voluntariness. The three elements are interrelated. Competency involves the ability to understand relevant information and to appreciate the situation and consequences. In application, a patient's comprehension and decision are weighed against the value and risks of the treatment. A low test of competence is acceptable when the treatment has a high benefit-to-risk ratio, but a high test of competence is called for when the treatment poses a high risk or a questionable benefit-risk ratio.

When consent is given for a procedure or treatment but injury results because of an undisclosed risk, the basis of legal action in such a case is usually not battery but negligence. (An action based on negligence calls for expert testimony and is insurable.) In any event, where consent is lacking, it is of no moment that the treatment was skillfully performed. In *Zinermon v. Burch* (1990), the U.S. Supreme Court ruled that patient competency must be considered in regard to hospital admission as well as treatment.

> Darrell Burch was seen bruised and bloodied, wandering on a Florida highway without shoes. He was brought by a concerned citizen to a community mental health service. He was hallucinating, confused, and disoriented. He thought that he was entering heaven. He signed a form for voluntary admission and another form authorizing treatment. After 3 days of treatment with psychotropic medication, he was transferred to Florida State Hospital, where he again signed voluntary admission and treatment forms. As a voluntary patient, he was presumably free to leave at any time. He remained there for about 5 months. On discharge, he complained that he had been improperly admitted to both facilities and had thus been confined and treated against his will. He claimed that because he was not competent to sign any legal documents, he had a constitutional right to a judicial commitment before being admitted and treated and that because there had been no such hearing, he had been deprived of his liberty without due process of law.

The Supreme Court agreed. In a 5–4 ruling, the Court held that before being admitted and treated, Burch was entitled to a judicial hearing or at least some other hearing that would be a safeguard against arbitrary action by the state. The hearing would determine either that he was competent to consent to admission or that he met the statutory standard for involuntary commitment. The Court acknowledged that persons who are mentally ill and incapable of giving informed consent to admission would not necessarily meet the statutory standard for involuntary placement; namely, that they are likely to injure themselves or others or that their neglect or refusal to care for themselves threatens their well-being. The Court said:

> The involuntary placement process serves to guard against the confinement of a person who, though mentally ill, is harmless and can live safely outside an institution. Confinement of such a person not only violates Florida law, but also is unconstitutional.... Thus, it is at least possible that if Burch had had an involuntary placement, [he] would not have been confined at FSH. Moreover, even assuming that Burch would have met the statutory requirements for involuntary placement, he still could have been harmed by being deprived of other protections built into the involuntary placement procedure, such as the appointment of a guardian advocate to make treatment decisions, and periodic judicial review of placement.

Guardianship may not be used to circumvent commitment law, but a guardian may be appointed to decide on treatment. In or out of a hospital, the doctrine of *substituted judgment* is a method by which a decision about treatment can be made for an incompetent person. The goal of the doctrine is to make the decision that incompetent persons would make were they capable. In general, a guardian's decision as to what is in the person's best interests is granted only on a showing of clear and convincing evidence. Authorization for sterilization may be included in some jurisdictions under the broad equity powers of probate courts to act for incompetent persons (*In re* Guardianship of Hayes 1980).

Decisions concerning termination of life-support systems raise serious questions about competency. Can one ever be competent to make a decision about death? Ernest Becker wrote in his book *The Denial of Death* (1973) that "the idea of death, the fear of it, haunts the human animal like nothing else; it is a mainspring of human activity—activity designed largely to avoid the fatality of death, to overcome it by denying in some way that it is the final destiny of man" (p. ix). Becker's thesis is that under no condition can one make a rational decision about one's own death; rather, one is always in extremis, hence, non compos mentis on this matter.

In general, the courts have upheld the ability of a competent adult to refuse medical treatment, even if that care is deemed necessary to save or sustain life. The New York Court of Appeals upheld the termination of respiratory assistance to a patient who previously, while competent, had manifested a desire not to be placed on a respirator. The rule is more sparingly applied in the case of incompetent patients, however. In a companion case, the court refused to terminate treatment of a patient who had never been competent (Haber 1982).

In the ordinary course of medical practice, the physician discusses the illness and proposed treatment with the patient. The informed consent form is usually distributed by the nurse or administrator shortly before the procedure is to take place. Researchers have noted that these consent forms are written at a level too difficult for most people to understand (Mariner and McArdle 1985). Actually, the informed consent document is designed to provide evidence of consent, rather than to help a patient make a decision about treatment. In any event, the document as evidence may backfire under the theory that "if contracting parties write at all they must write it all because the law presumes they wrote it all if and when they write at all."

The obligation of physicians to disclose information has been expanded to include research or economic interests in connection with a proposed course of treatment. In *Moore v. Regents of the University of California* (1990), a landmark case, the California Supreme Court ruled that when a physician is seeking a patient's informed consent, the physician "must disclose personal interests unrelated to the patient's health, whether research or economic, that may affect the physician's professional judgment." In this case the physician obtained various body fluids and tissue samples for examination in connection with ongoing research. The court noted that the effect of such an economic or research interest on the exercise of clinical judgment represents information "that a reasonable patient would want to know in deciding whether to consent to a proposed course of treatment."

As a result of the failure of the medical profession to regulate itself successfully, the doctrine of informed consent has been expanded to include the risks of treatment by a particular physician (Miller 2000). In a relatively recent development, about which there is divided opinion, the doctrine of informed consent calls for information about the provider of health care. In *Hidding v. Williams* (1991), the Louisiana Court of Appeals ruled that a physician's failure to disclose his chronic alcohol abuse vitiated the patient's consent to surgery. There was a poor outcome but no evidence that the physician was under the influence of alcohol at the time of the surgery, that his hands trembled, or that the care fell below acceptable standards. Nonetheless, the court said, "Because this condition creates a material risk associated with the surgeon's ability to perform, which if disclosed would have obliged the patient to have elected another course of treatment, the fact-finder's conclusion that nondisclosure is a violation of the informed consent doctrine is entirely correct." It is a risk about which the patient should have been informed.

In contrast, the Arizona Court of Appeals declined to allow evidence of an anesthesiologist's alcoholism as a separate claim of negligence, absent a showing that he was intoxicated or impaired at the time of the surgery (*Ornelas v. Fry* 1986).

> The plaintiff argued that alcoholism necessarily diminishes a physician's capacity to render the proper standard of care and cited legislation regulating the medical profession wherein unprofessional conduct is defined to include habitual intemperance in the use of alcohol. The court recognized that an alcoholic doctor might present a danger to the public if allowed to continue to practice medicine but that it was a matter for the medical board to decide whether to revoke a license to practice. In a tort case, in contrast, the court said that the issue is whether the physician exercised the proper standard of care in treating a particular patient at a particular time.

Citing the decision of the Arizona Court of Appeals (*Ornelas v. Fry* 1986), the New Mexico Court of Appeals (*Reaves v. Bergsrud* 1999) ruled that a plaintiff in a medical malpractice action was not entitled to discovery of the defendant surgeon's mental health because she failed to produce evidence that his mental health had an effect on his performance and because disclosure would violate the psychotherapist-patient privilege.

> Sandra Reaves sued Dr. Richard Bergsrud, alleging he had been negligent in severing her median nerve during surgery to remove a benign mass in her hand. During discovery, Reaves learned that Dr. Bergsrud had bipolar disorder and that his medical license had been temporarily suspended a few years earlier when he inappropriately quit his psychiatric care and medication. Dr. Bergsrud refused to answer the plaintiff's interrogatories regarding his condition and treatment and raised the psychotherapist–patient privilege. The court ruled in favor of Dr. Bergsrud for the aforementioned reasons.

In a Wisconsin case (*Johnson by Adler v. Kokemoor* 1996), the plaintiff sued her physician for failure to inform her that he had very little experience in performing an operation on an aneurysm. As a result of the physician's inexperience, the plaintiff alleged she was rendered a quadriplegic.

> It was discovered that the physician had never performed surgery on a large basilar bifurcation aneurysm such as the plaintiff's. The physician argued that the trial court erred in admitting evidence about his own projected risk statistics, claiming that the doctrine of informed consent required that the risks generally involved with the procedure be communicated, but not those that might be associated with any particular physician.

The Wisconsin Supreme Court rejected the contention. The court stated that the duty to disclose information that is "material" to a patient's decision must be decided on a case-by-case basis. The court said that a bright-line rule that a physician must always give his qualifications to every patient would be impossible. In this particular case the court held that a reasonable person in the plaintiff's position would have considered such information material in making an intelligent and informed decision about the surgery.

Conversely, the Washington Court of Appeals has held that a surgeon's duty to obtain informed consent did not require him to disclose his lack of experience in performing a particular surgical procedure (*Whiteside v. Lukson* 1997).

> The plaintiff needed to have her gallbladder removed. The plaintiff's physician had never performed a gallbladder removal at the time he obtained the plaintiff's consent. The surgery was delayed, however, and during the delay, the physician performed a gallbladder removal on two patients. During the plaintiff's surgery, the physician misidentified and damaged her bile duct and, as a result, she suffered numerous complications after the surgery.

The Washington Court of Appeals stated that the duty to disclose material facts includes only those facts that relate to the proposed treatment. The court declined to follow the recent number of cases applying a broader construction of "material fact." Instead, applying the traditional approach, the court held that a physician's lack of experience in performing a surgical procedure is not a material fact for purposes of finding liability predicated on failure to secure an informed consent (LeBlang 1995; Petrila 2003; Slovenko 2002).

Another controversy arising under the informed consent doctrine is the need of health care providers to disclose that they are infected with the virus that causes AIDS. Is such a provider, in effect, to be excluded from health care?

> Spencer Waddell tested positive for HIV while employed as a dental hygienist for an Atlanta dentist, Eugene Witkin. The next year Witkin found out about Waddell's HIV status and removed him from his job treating patients. He was offered a clerical job paying half as much, but he refused and was fired. He sued, claiming discrimination under the Americans with Disabilities Act. He lost in the trial court, which found that the risk of HIV transmission, although negligible, was sufficient to justify his removal from a job in which he had contact with patients' mouths. The Eleventh Circuit Court of Appeals found that the exception applied to Waddell.

The Americans with Disabilities Act of 1990 (ADA; 42 U.S.C. §§ 12101–12213) states that an employer does not have to hire or retain an employee who poses a direct threat to others' health and safety. The Eleventh Circuit reasoned that AIDS is fatal and that Waddell could not avoid the possibility of some risk to patients perhaps through an accidental bite while he was cleaning teeth (*Waddell v. Valley Forge Dental Associates* 2002). In general, however, people infected with HIV are covered by the ADA. Most frequently, patients who believe they have been infected with AIDS bring an action alleging negligent infliction of mental distress rather than lack of informed consent (*Russaw v. Martin* 1996).

Reacting to negative publicity about physicians who have been disciplined elsewhere coming to Florida, the state enacted legislation, effective July 1, 1999, that requires the Florida Department of Health to compile a "practitioner profile" for all physicians seeking an initial license to practice medicine in the state or renewal of an existing license (Florida Statutes Title 32, ch. 456.041). The profile is made available to the public through the World Wide Web and other commonly used means of distribution.

The National Practitioner Data Bank, popularly known as "docs in the box," collects information (as of 1990) on medical malpractice, but the information may only be seen by official regulatory bodies such as hospital peer review boards, state licensing boards, and professional societies. The data bank is not open to the public.

In 1999, the Institute of Medicine (IOM) released a study, "To Err Is Human," regarding medical errors (defined as the failure of a planned action to be completed as intended or the use of a wrong plan to achieve an aim). The IOM estimated that at least 44,000, and perhaps as many as 98,000, people die in hospitals each year as a result of preventable medical errors. To date, some 37 states have variably addressed the issue, with 14 of them having enacted specific medical error reporting statutes. They call for informing the patient.

## Competency of a Witness

As a general rule, in civil or criminal cases, every adult witness is presumed competent to testify unless it can be shown that they do not have personal knowledge of the matters about which they are to testify, that they do not have the ability to recall the subject matter, or that they do not understand the duty to testify truthfully (Fed. Rule Evid. 601). In general, the decision whether or not to hold a competency hearing is a matter entirely within the discretion of the trial judge. Witnesses may be found competent despite the fact that in another case they may have been found criminally insane or incompetent to stand trial. In these or other cases, a psychiatrist or psychologist may be called to testify whether the witness has sufficient memory, understands the oath, and has the ability to communicate. Among the considerations to be taken into account in deciding whether to order a psychiatric examination is protection of privacy. As one court explained, "It is unpleasant enough to have to testify in a public trial subject to cross-examination the result of which will be spread on the record in open court to disqualify you, or at least to spice up your cross-examination" (*United States v. Gutman* 1984).

The rule that allows an individual deemed insane to testify assumes that jurors are capable of evaluating a witness's testimony. The court in *Gutman* stated, "If a lunatic takes the stand and babbles gibberish, the jury will ignore it and the defendant will not be harmed." In this case, the witness had been hospitalized 13 months earlier and was described as "highly depressed" with "some psychiatric thought disorder in addition to the difficulty he has in organizing and being relevant." This witness for the state was again hospitalized some 2 months after testifying. The court listed several factors in its decision not to order an examination of the witness's ability to testify: protection of the witness's privacy interests, the potential for harassment of witnesses, the possibility that a mental exam will hamper law enforcement by deterring potential witnesses from coming forward, whether the witness is a key to the case, and whether there are substantial indications that the witness was suffering from a mental abnormality at the time of trial.

It has long been established that age alone is not determinative of testimonial competency. The issue of competency of a child witness to testify came before the U.S. Supreme Court in 1895 in the oft-cited case *Wheeler v. United States.* The question was whether the 5-year-old son of a murder victim could testify. The homicide took place on June 12, 1894; the case was tried on December 21 of that year. In reply to questions asked on his voir dire, the boy said that he knew the difference between the truth and a lie and that he was going to tell the truth. When asked what they would do with him in court if he told a lie, he replied that they would put him in jail. He also said that his mother had told him that morning to "tell no lie." When asked what the clerk had said to him when he was told to hold up his hand, he answered, "Don't you tell no story." The Supreme Court said:

> That the boy was not by reason of his youth, as a matter of law, absolutely disqualified as a witness, is clear. While no one would think of calling as a witness an infant only two or three years old, there is no precise age which determines the question of competency. This depends on

> the capacity and intelligence of the child, his appreciation of the difference between truth and falsehood, as well as of his duty to tell the former. . . . [T]he boy was intelligent, understood the difference between truth and falsehood, and the consequences of telling the latter, and also what was required by the oath which he had taken. At any rate, the contrary does not appear. Of course, care must be taken by the trial judge, especially where, as in this case, the question is one of life or death. On the other hand to exclude from the witness stand one who shows himself capable of understanding the difference between truth and falsehood, and who does not appear to have been simply taught to tell a story, would sometimes result in staying the hand of justice. (*Wheeler v. United States* 1895, pp. 524–525)

The common law presumed that a child under age 14 years was not competent. At present, there is no fixed age below which a witness is deemed incompetent, although children under age 10 or 14 years are routinely examined by the court. The question in each case is whether the witness understands the obligation to tell the truth and has sufficient intelligence to give evidence. In general, it is sufficient if the child knows it is wrong to lie and that lying will be punished.

The suggestibility level of a witness is an important factor in determining competence. Of particular concern is the nature of certain kinds of evidence. For instance, sex offense cases are particularly difficult when they involve children or individuals with a mental disability. Recently, considerable attention has been given to the subject of children as witnesses in sexual abuse cases. In some jurisdictions, legislation specifically addresses the question of competency of children in such cases. For example, a Colorado statute (Colorado Stat. § 13-19-106) provides the following:

> The following persons shall not be witnesses: . . . (b)(I) Children under ten years of age who appear incapable of receiving just impressions of the facts respecting which they are examined or of relating them truly. (II) This proscription does not apply to a child under ten years of age, in any civil or criminal proceeding for child abuse, sexual abuse, sexual assault, or incest, when the child did not know the difference between telling the truth and lying.

In some jurisdictions, sex offense cases require corroboration of the minor's allegations as a matter of law (Melton 1981).

The vast majority of the literature on suggestibility shows that young children (under age 7 years) are susceptible to an experimenter's suggestion and that resistance to suggestion increases with age (Yarmey 1984). Under the law of evidence, courts recognize that leading questions are undesirable. Exception is made in the case of children, yet it is the child witness who is most likely misled by a suggestive question. Children are especially suggestible and compliant with those adults whom they seek to please and protect. Thus, the child's suggestibility greatly depends on the examiner. On cross-examination, attorneys ask questions that confuse the child—they often confuse adults, too. Children tend to speak and think slowly, and the adult world gets impatient with them. An adult may try to elicit a story that makes sense from one point of view. Children may have only one word for an object; they may not know the meaning of words such as *penis, vagina,* and *anus.* They may not have the same sense of time and chronology as adults; for example, children confuse lunch and dinner.

Psychological research confirms the popular view that children are more subject to suggestion than adults. However, Elizabeth Loftus and Graham Davies (1984) observe,

> Perhaps age alone is the wrong focus for these studies. Whether children are more susceptible to suggestive information than adults probably depends on the interaction of age with other factors. If an event is understandable and interesting to both children and adults, and if their memory for it is still equally strong, age differences in suggestibility may not be found. But if the event is not encoded well to begin with, or if a delay weakens the child's memory relative to an adult's, then age differences may emerge. (p. 63)

To obtain accurate information from young children, the danger of suggestion must be taken into account as well as the fact that children have greater communication difficulties than adults and are often need of assistance in this regard.

By and large, judges and juries view the testimony of child witnesses with suspicion. More than 60% of juries believe children are unreliable. Children fidget, their voices drop, and they look down or away. This can be interpreted as their not telling the truth or being less effective. For security, a child may hug a doll while testifying, which may impugn credibility.

The competency of elderly witnesses has also been questioned. Research shows the elderly experience a decline in episodic memory (which affects specific events such as what happened at yesterday's meeting), but not in implicit memory (which affects the large variety of mental activities that occur spontaneously, such as driving a car) or semantic memory (the overall storage of information and experience people accumulate over a lifetime). The elderly also tend to suffer from source amnesia, when they know something but cannot remember when or where they learned it.

## Competency to Make a Will

A will or testament is a legal document describing a person's wishes regarding the disposition of property on death. At the time of the making of the will, testators must have "testamentary capacity," which means the capacity to understand and remember the nature and extent of their property, the persons who are the natural objects of their bounty, and the disposition that they desire to make of the property. A person making a will does not necessarily have to have the capability to make a contract or engage in business matters. Even a considerable degree of eccentricity will not incapacitate a person in making a will. A guardian may not make a will for a ward, but the fact that a guardian was appointed does not of itself invalidate a will for lack of testamentary capacity.

The testamentary capacity concept is used at times to undo a will when necessary to further society's interests in family maintenance, but, in general, a will is difficult to overturn. Usually, the only way a disappointed heir can contest a will is on the grounds of a lack of testamentary capacity or susceptibility of the testator because of a mental condition to undue influence or duress in making the will. Most frequently, these challenges focus on some sort of bodily disease or infirmity, alcohol or drug use, or cerebral arteriosclerosis. In establishing capacity, incapacity, or undue influence, psychiatric testimony is usually presented. A presumption of undue influence arises when the beneficiary actively participated in the preparation and execution of the will and unduly profited from it.

In a will contest called "the largest, costliest, ugliest, most spectacular in American history" (Margolick 1993), on one side was strong-willed Barbara (Basia) Piasecka Johnson, a farmer's daughter who had only $200 when she left Poland in 1967, and on the other side were her six grown stepchildren—the progeny of J. Seward Johnson, an heir to a fortune earned by Band-Aids. The grand prize: $402,824,971.59 that Johnson left behind when he died in 1983. Mrs. Johnson, his principal beneficiary, swore not to give the children "the dust off half a penny." They contested the will, calling Mrs. Johnson a "conniving little witch" who exercised undue influence. She had met Seward Johnson when his second wife hired her as a maid at their New Jersey mansion. Just 31 when in 1971 she wed Johnson, then age 73, she is portrayed as a passionate woman who revitalized him. Of his children, he reportedly said his oldest child, Mary Lea, was "not worth the time to talk about," and he dismissed his other three daughters as "whores." The 3-year struggle, which culminated in a 17-week trial, was finally settled, with $5.9 million going to each child, $7.3 million to Mrs. Johnson's attorney, and $10 million to the legal team representing the children.

Persons who are addicted to drugs or liquor do not lack testamentary capacity if they are lucid or sober when the will was made. One who contests the will must establish that the influence of the drugs or liquor negated the "calm judgment" that the law requires. That is, the burden of proof is on the contestant of the will to establish that the testator was not lucid at the time of the making of the will. It is a heavy and difficult burden. Proof of addiction alone, for example, is not sufficient to carry the burden. The contestant must affirmatively show that the testator was intoxicated—affecting his or her lucidity—at the time the will was made.

Proof that a testator suffered from an insane delusion when making the will may be enough to render it invalid. An insane delusion is defined as a belief in things that do not exist and that no rational mind would believe exist. The subject matter of the delusion must have no foundation in fact, be unable to be dispelled by reason, and be the product of mental disorder or the product or offspring of a delusion. Delusional religious beliefs, a common source of litigation, do not generally affect capacity unless the mind of the believer assumes a chronic delusional state that controls and dictates the conduct of the testamentary act. A belief in witchcraft is not necessarily conclusive on the issue of a testator's capacity (*Rice v. Henderson* 1954).

## Competency to Contract

Usually individuals are considered competent to contract if they understand the nature of the contract and its consequences. If the individual is incompetent at the time of entering the contract but has not been declared legally incompetent, the contract is usually considered voidable rather than void. That is, the impaired individual can affirm the contract or nullify it through court action. The interests of commerce dictate preserving the validity of contracts, but at the same time, society has a *parens patriae* (father of the people) interest in protecting the welfare of impaired individuals in the case of contracting for basic necessities—shelter, clothes, food, and medical services—and the policy of protecting the mentally incompetent is less critical than in other cases because there is usually a fair trade in these matters.

> X, who is diagnosed as manic-depressive (bipolar), buys several expensive fur coats in the course of few days when he is manic. When out of his manic state, he consults an attorney seeking to rescind the contracts.

The traditional test of competence examples cognitive capacity, rather than motivation. Accordingly, the courts usually deny rescission to persons entering into contracts while afflicted by psychoses of the manic-depressive type because this particular illness impairs judgment but not understanding (*Smalley v. Baker* 1968). However, in an oft-cited case invoking the volitional test of criminal responsibility, a New York court held that a party is entitled to rescission of a contract executed during the manic phase of a manic-depressive psychosis (*Faber v. Sweet Style Mfg. Corp.* 1963). Rarely is volition a consideration in the law on contracts.

An individual unable to handle personal affairs with some degree of prudence may be adjudicated incompetent. A guardian or conservator (usually a family member or attorney) is then appointed to handle the person's affairs. Generally speaking, a guardian deals with the ward's physical or mental infirmities, whereas a conservator deals with his or her financial interests. Because the percentage of the U.S. population 80 years or older has tripled since 1950, there are more cases of impaired capacity, notably those resulting from Alzheimer's disease. In January 1996, at the urging of the elderly, a comprehensive competency law went into effect in California: the Due Process in Competence Determinations Act. It requires clear and convincing evidence of inability to appreciate the consequences of one's acts before appointing a conservator.

The physician's report about the need for a guardian should provide a detailed description of the individual's physical or mental infirmities; an explanation of how and to what extent each infirmity interferes with the individual's ability to receive or evaluate information in making decisions; a listing of all medications the individual is receiving, the dosage of each, and a description of the effects each medication has on the individual's behavior; a prognosis for improvement in the individual's condition and a recommendation for the most appropriate rehabilitation plan; and finally, the signatures of all individuals who performed the evaluations on which the report is based. The court sometimes requires that the physician provide an opinion on whether or not a guardian is needed.

The physician's report about the need for a conservator should describe in detail the individual's current condition and how this affects the individual's ability to conduct his or her financial affairs.

Problems arise when the physician fails to report that the individual has executed a health care power of attorney or patient advocate designation form. If the court is aware that an individual has appointed a patient advocate, it will not grant a guardian any of the same powers that are held by the patient advocate. Without this knowledge, a court listening to family of the individual may appoint a guardian or conservator who takes an action contrary to the understanding of the individual already named to act as agent or advocate, generating disputes, legal proceedings, and delays in acting in the individual's best interest.

In some states, the determination of incompetency is a blanket incompetency ruling that deprives the individual of any contractual capacity, including (theoretically) even buying groceries. In other states, a determination of incompetency may be limited, for example, to the managing of business affairs. In the ordinary course of events, a merchant would find it awkward and time consuming to go to the courthouse to check on the legal status of every contracting party. People do not wear badges indicating competency; hence, one contracts at a risk.

For centuries, there have been calls to simplify language in commercial transactions as well as in the law in general. (Napoleon simplified the civil code to make it understandable.) However, the devotion to archaic language is rooted in a desire for well-settled meaning. Furthermore, the use of seemingly redundant terms stems from a prudent effort to cover every contingency. The informed consent form used by physicians and hospitals in medical care likewise tends to be boilerplate. In recent years, there has been a crescendo of voices calling for plain and readable language. Some legislatures have enacted "plain English" laws calling for simple language in contractual forms in sales, mortgages, and leases.

## Competency of a Minor to Consent to Treatment

In general, minors (typically under age 18 years) are not considered legally competent to act on their own. Consent, express or implied, of a parent or guardian is necessary to authorize treatment or services. Absent that consent, treatment regardless of the outcome constitutes a battery (if there is physical contact) or possibly negligence. To this general rule, however, there are a number of exceptions: parens patriae, emergencies, emancipated minors, mature minors, and certain types of care. No longer does a parent have absolute legal control over a minor.

As parens patriae, the state may protect the best interests of a minor in the face of parental refusal to consent to treatment deemed necessary to preserve the life or health of the minor. Under this authority, for example, the state can compel vaccination or fluoridation. In addition, the state may override parental consent. Even with parental consent, sterilization or transplantation involving a minor is a procedure fraught with legal hazards, so court authorization is required or at least warranted. When a parent refuses on religious or other grounds to provide medical treatment for a child, courts are likely to grant an application to overrule the parent if the treatment is life threatening, but not if it will only improve the child's comfort or appearance (*In re* Green 1972). In the case of mental health hospitalization, the responsibility for the care and treatment of the patient becomes invested in the hospital or court, so a parent has no right of access to the minor's records (*In re* J.C.G. 1976).

In an emergency a physician may proceed with treatment without awaiting parental consent. Consent is implied from the emergency, defined as "a situation wherein, in competent medical judgment, the proposed surgical or medical treatment or procedures are immediately or imminently necessary and any delay occasioned by an attempt to obtain a consent would reasonably jeopardize the life, health or limb of the person affected, or would reasonably result in disfigurement or impairment of faculties" (Missouri Statutes Title 28, §431.063). When the question arises, the courts give a broad interpretation to emergency. Thus, the treatment of a fracture was deemed an emergency, though it was not lifesaving but done to stop pain and suffering (*Greenspan v. Slate* 1953). The Michigan Supreme Court (*Luka v. Lowrie* 1912) had this to say about implied consent in emergency situations:

> The fact that surgeons are called upon daily, in all our large cities, to operate instantly in emergency cases in order that life may be preserved, should be considered. Many small children are injured upon the streets in larger cities. To hold that a surgeon must wait until perhaps he may be able to secure the consent of the parents before giving to the injured one the benefit of his skill and learning, to the end that life may be preserved, would, we believe, result in the loss of many lives which might otherwise be saved. It is not to be presumed that competent surgeons will want only to operate, not that they will fail to obtain the consent of parents to operations where such consent may be reasonably obtained in view of the exigency. Their work, however, is highly humane and very largely charitable in character, and no rule should be announced which would tend in the slightest degree to deprive sufferers of the benefit of their services.

An emancipated minor—a minor who is legally free from the care, custody, and control of his or her parents—may give a legally valid consent. By dint of certain legislation, pregnancy amounts to emancipation. Alabama's statute, for example, provides: "Any minor who is married, or having been married is divorced, or has borne a child may give effective consent to any legally authorized medical, dental, health or mental health services for himself, his child or for herself or her child" (Alabama Code, Title 22 § 104[16]).

Under the mature minor doctrine, minors are permitted to consent to medical treatment if they are sufficiently mature to understand the nature of the procedure, its consequences, and the alternatives to that treatment. However, maturity is a matter of dispute, as it is a behavioral test. One pediatrician suggested that any child who could get to the doctor's Greenwich Village office by subway from the Bronx was, in her eyes, an adult.

The mature minor doctrine is applied in cases where the minor is at least 15 years of age, the treatment is for the benefit of the minor, and the procedure is something less than major or serious in nature. There is apparently only one case (*Bonner v. Moran* 1941) in which liability has been imposed on a doctor for treating a minor without parental consent. However, the operation in this case, a transplant operation, was not for the benefit of the minor, a 15-year-old, but rather for the benefit of a cousin (consent was given by an aunt). Yet the case has been cited or relied on in discussions of the need for parental consent in every situation.

In recent years, usually to help deal with problems that have high social costs, such as venereal disease, HIV, drug or alcohol abuse, contraception, and pregnancy, ad hoc exceptions (characterized as "general medical emancipation" statutes) have been made to parents' authority to consent. Underlying psychodynamics may be identical among individuals showing different symptoms or behavior, but it is only the named symptom or behavior that opens the door to care or treatment without parental consent. Some states set a minimum age for consent in these treatments or procedures. A number of state statutes authorize minors to receive mental health treatment without parental consent. For example, an Illinois statute provides: "Any minor fourteen years of age or older may request and receive counseling services or psychotherapy on an outpatient basis. The consent of the parent, guardian, or person in loco parentis shall not be necessary to authorize outpatient counseling or psychotherapy" (Illinois Statutes, ch. 91 1/2, § 3–5016 [a]).

The majority of states have enacted statutes permitting minors to consent without parental notice or consultation to receive treatment for venereal disease and drug or alcohol abuse and to receive counseling about contraception. In *Carey v. Population Services International* (1977), the Supreme Court upheld the right of minors to obtain contraceptives without parental consent. In the wake of that decision, the Sixth Circuit Court of Appeals in *Doe v. Irwin* (1980) ruled that contraceptives may be provided to minors also without the knowledge of their parents. A number of state statutes specifically provide that records concerning the treatment of a minor for venereal disease or the performance of an abortion shall not be released or in any manner be made available to the parent (New York Public Health Law ch. 763). However, in the event the minor is using a family insurance plan to pay for service, the parents may learn about it when they receive a benefit report from the insurer.

The U.S. Supreme Court in 1976, in *Planned Parenthood of Central Missouri v. Danforth,* ruled that a parent may not veto a minor's decision to have an abortion, but the Court went on to say, "We emphasize that our holding . . . does not suggest every minor, regardless of age or maturity, may give effective consent for termination of her pregnancy." This language might imply that immature or incompetent minors are required to obtain parental consent to abortion, even in the first trimester, just as they must for any other procedure. That issue came to the Supreme Court in 1979 in *Bellotti v. Baird*. In that case, the Court said that every minor has the right to go directly to a court without consulting her parents. Justice Powell said, "A pregnant minor is entitled in such a proceeding to show either: (1) that she is mature enough, well enough informed to make her abortion decision, in consultation with her physician, independently of her parents' wishes; or (2) that even if she is not able to make this decision independently, the desired abortion would be in her best interests."

As a matter of practice, the procedure set out by the Court in *Bellotti* has been and continues to be ignored. Abortion clinics around the country are carrying out abortions on minors just as they are on adults. No path is beaten to the courthouse door for a determination of maturity or best interests. Should there be complications, however, the minor will usually find that a hospital will not admit her without parental consent. Emergency care in a clearly lifesaving situation may be available, but even then the hospital (while administering such care) will as a matter of practice attempt to contact a parent or guardian.

What actually is the hazard in treating a minor without parental consent? In general, physicians and other therapists appear to be overly fearful in the care and treatment of minors, leading quite often to tragic results. Although the law defines an emergency broadly, many physicians and hospitals define it narrowly. One publicized case (Ramos 1981) involved a minor who split his lip and was spurting blood, but the doctor in the ER refused to suture it without parental consent. In actual fact, there has not been a reported case in any state since the aforementioned 1941 transplant case in which a physician or health facility has been held liable for treating a minor over age 15 without parental consent (Pilpel 1972).

Parental consent is no insulation against liability in the case of faulty treatment. Consent protects from a charge of battery but not from negligence or malpractice. In a case in which the treatment measures up to acceptable standards of care but there is no parental consent or applicable exception, the parents may claim that their expenses for the support and maintenance of their child were increased by an unfavorable result of the treatment, but that is not likely.

## Professional Competency

Competency is the essential requirement to enter or continue in a profession. Malpractice (professional negligence) may be an indication of incompetency in general, but not necessarily. Professionals held in highest esteem by colleagues may on occasion depart from standard of care and be sued and held liable in a malpractice action. Negligence as established in litigation is not equated with incompetency to practice. When egregious, however, malpractice may be cause for disciplinary action.

Every professional organization or licensing board must face up to the incompetency of its members. Institutional peer review is designed to restrict the practice of physicians to those procedures they are competent to perform. Hospitals have a duty to formulate, adopt, and enforce adequate rules and policies to ensure quality care for patients. Physicians are expected to report incompetent colleagues to the licensing authorities, who, in turn, are supposed to discipline or expel them from the profession, but that rarely happens. Marilyn Rosenthal, a sociologist at the University of Michigan who has collected data on what happened in more than 200 specific cases, found that it was a matter of months, or even years, before colleagues took action against an incompetent physician, however dangerous or incompetent his or her conduct may be (Rosenthal 1995).

Professionals, in particular, have an obligation to keep abreast of new developments in their field. Of medicine it is often said that half of what is taught in medical school will be outmoded in 10 years. Yet what is done to adequately keep up with new developments? Clinical practice lags research, and use of new interventions is haphazard. It is estimated that 25% of patients are disillusioned with traditional medicine and have turned to alternative medicine.

The various professions have different mechanisms for dealing with complaints. Expulsion or discipline of a member may be based on professional incompetence, misconduct, or emotional instability. The problem of incompetent professionals is not an aberration—they abound, appearing as the illustrious professional who has slowly gone senile or the long-respected professional with a drinking habit. The degree of proof necessary to justify loss of membership or suspension varies from state to state and from profession to profession. In some states, professional misconduct must be shown by a preponderance of the evidence, in others, by clear and convincing evidence. Seldom does a malpractice suit trigger a hearing by a disciplinary board. Seldom too, is mental or emotional instability a sufficient ground for disciplinary action. In general, acts or omissions that would themselves be grounds for discipline bring to light mental or emotional problems. Often, the issue of mental instability is raised in mitigation of the wrongful conduct.

In many cases, it can be difficult to determine whether incompetence lies with the person, with others, or with the system (Lapetina and

Armstrong 2002). Thus, for example, errors in filling a prescription can be reduced when a computer printout rather than handwriting is used. For patients, regardless of underlying medical conditions, the death rate in an approved ambulatory surgery center is much less than that of surgery performed in doctors' offices and clinics (Andrews 2002). Concern about medical errors committed by residents has spurred a push to reduce the number of hours and consecutive days that they may work (Mukherjee 2002).

In a first-of-its-kind ruling, the U.S. Seventh Circuit Court of Appeals in 2001 ruled that a professional society may discipline a member on account of testimony presented at trial that is deemed not up to standard. In *Austin v. American Association of Neurological Surgeons,* the court said: "Although [the expert witness] did not treat the malpractice plaintiff for whom he testified, his testimony at her trial was a type of medical service, and if the quality of his testimony reflected the quality of his medical judgment, he is probably a poor physician. His discipline by the Association therefore served an important public policy exemplified by the federal Health Care Quality Improvement Act."

> Dr. Donald Austin, a neurosurgeon who is often an expert witness in malpractice cases, testified on behalf of a woman whose recurrent laryngeal nerve was damaged during the course of an anterior cervical fusion performed by another neurosurgeon. According to Austin's testimony, which the trial judge ruled admissible, such an injury is always the consequence of the surgeon's negligence. Moreover, he maintained that the majority of neurosurgeons would agree with him. In contrast, expert witnesses for the defendant, a neurosurgeon who had performed 700 anterior cervical fusions without a similar injury, testified that the patient's injury was an unavoidable consequence of the surgery and not the result of negligence. The jury concurred, rejecting the patient's malpractice claim. Thereafter, the defendant filed an ethics complaint against Austin with the American Association of Neurological Surgeons (AANS), alleging that he had no factual basis for his testimony. The AANS suspended him from the association for 6 months.

The Seventh Circuit upheld the action by the AANS. The decision was rendered by a three-judge panel, including Judge Richard Posner, one of the country's leading jurists and the author of the opinion. In the opinion, Judge Posner explained at length why it is decidedly in the public interest for a professional organization to be able to sanction members who have provided irresponsible testimony. "It is no answer that judges can be trusted to keep out such testimony," Posner wrote. "Judges are not experts in any field except law. Much escapes us, especially in a highly technical field such as neurosurgery." Therefore, jurists need help from professional associations in evaluating the quality of expert testimony. "[T]he community at large had an interest in Austin's not being able to use his membership [in AANS] to dazzle judges and juries and deflect the close and skeptical scrutiny that shoddy testimony deserves." Finally, he said, "the judge's ruling that expert testimony is admissible should not be taken as conclusive evidence that it is responsible testimony" and so should not preclude an ethics proceeding by a professional organization (Appelbaum 2002, p. 389; Slovenko 2001, pp. 565–566). Actually, several years before the litigation, Dr. Austin had retired half-time from practice and had become, in the words of the vernacular, "a professional expert" (on behalf of plaintiffs).

In another case in which an ethics violation not involving competency of care was a basis for disciplinary action, the Mississippi Supreme Court upheld the withdrawal of a license on account of a breach of confidentiality (*Mississippi State Board of Psychological Examiners v. Hosford* 1987).

## Americans With Disabilities Act

In disputes involving employee disability, medical opinions are routinely offered on competency or disability as well as impairment, but although the terms "competency" or "disability" are often used interchangeably with "impairment," there needs to be an understanding that competency or disability involves more than a consideration of health status. Impairment is an alteration of an individual's capacity to meet personal, social, or occupational demands. Abraham Lincoln, the man regarded by most historians as the greatest president in U.S. history, suffered severe episodes of depression. To be able to render an opinion on competency or disability calls for knowledge about the particular act or work activity that is involved.

The courts, however, have generally not limited the testimony of experts to impairment but have allowed them to testify on virtually all issues under the ADA including disability status, ability to perform essential functions, and direct threat. For example, in *Fjellestad v. Pizza Hut of Am., Inc.* (1999), an expert testified to the number of jobs the plaintiff could not do in the geographic area in question. In *McKay v. Toyota Mfr. U.S.A.* (1997), experts testified on the plaintiff's physical limitations and how it affected her ability to work. In *EEOC v. Prevo's Family Markets. Inc.* (1998), experts testified on HIV status and whether the plaintiff posed a "direct threat" in his food handling position and on the need for physical examination to determine it.

A principal goal of the ADA is to increase employment opportunities for people who were kept out of the job market on the basis of disability—

other disability legislation (such as workers' compensation) provides compensation, not employment opportunities. It is the most important legislation that has been enacted in the United States to assist persons who are disabled (see Chapter 14: "The Workplace," this volume). When a disability meets the criteria for coverage under the legislation, an employer has an obligation to provide a "reasonable accommodation."

For those entitled to a "reasonable accommodation," the question is, What is a "reasonable accommodation"? The requirement of a "reasonable accommodation" is easier to implement when it comes to providing a wheelchair-accessible restroom than when it comes to accommodating an employee who develops an emotional hypersensitivity to workplace stress and supervisory criticism. For a psychiatric disability, flexibility in scheduling is the most frequently accepted form of accommodation; granting leave requests and changing supervisors are used far less often. Woody Allen's observation that "half of life is just showing up" is also true for employment. One who is depressed may have special difficulty showing up for work. Six percent of all complaints received by the Equal Employment Opportunity Commission (EEOC) are filed by people with depression (Stefan 2000). Although the courts will not require an employer to pay an employee for time the employee does not work, the ADA contemplates scheduling adjustments as an accommodation in appropriate cases.

The psychiatrist's recommendations in regard to accommodation for the severely mentally disabled are often unrealistic for an employer and tend to stigmatize the employee—things such as secluded work space, extreme quiet, and not working with others. Stress may be so inherent in an occupation that removal of the stress is not a reasonable accommodation that can be made. The functional assessment of the employee's disability must evaluate whether it is corrected or correctable through medication or other measures that mitigate the severity of the impairment's functional consequences.

An employer is not obliged to provide an accommodation when it would be an undue hardship. In determining undue hardship, the nature and cost of the accommodation, the number of persons employed, and the overall financial resources of the facility are considered. Furthermore, an accommodation may be considered an undue hardship if by nature it would be disruptive or would fundamentally alter the nature or operation of the business.

An employer also may refuse to employ or provide accommodation for individuals who pose a "direct threat" to themselves or other employees' health or safety. An expert or credible source must determine that the individual's condition poses significant risk of substantial and imminent harm that cannot be eliminated or reduced by reasonable accommodation. In *Reed v. LePage Bakeries, Inc.* (2001), the First Circuit held that insubordination was not protected by the ADA whatever the mental disability.

> During a meeting with human resources personnel, the employee refused to discuss her work restrictions and work assignment and instead insisted on discussing a shift change. After screaming obscenities at the human resources director, the employee was terminated for misconduct. After her verbal confrontation with the human resources director, the employee disclosed her diagnosis of mental illness (bipolar disorder) and asked for an accommodation, particularly permission to walk away from stressful confrontations. She sued, alleging that the employer failed to accommodate her disability. The district court granted the employer's motion for summary judgment, and the First Circuit affirmed, saying that "the ADA is not a license for insubordination at the workplace."

Upon the adoption of the ADA, there was debate whether it should cover mentally disabled as well as physically disabled individuals. Be that as it may, employees alleging any disability, but especially a mental disability, have little chance of prevailing in their claims against the employer. Surveys reveal that employers have won nearly 96% of discrimination cases filed in courts and 73% of cases filed as administrative complaints with the EEOC. Of 70 cases in which the disability was attributed to mental illness, the employee won only once (Allbright 2002). Nonetheless, it is maintained that this does not mean that the law has no effect—companies may settle those cases that have merit or be deterred from violating the law in the first place—but the system is far from predictable (Eviatar 2002).

## Conclusion

In law, competency depends on the context and is defined in relation to a particular act: writing a will, entering into a contract, or giving consent to treatment. Incompetency may result from the symptoms of an illness and may respond to treatment. Thus, impairment that results in incompetence may be permanent or may resolve on resolution or treatment of the illness. In forensic practice, the role of the psychiatrist in questions of competency is to identify the impairment or state that creates impairment in judgment related to a specific issue or capacity.

## Key Points

- Competency is an issue-specfic legal determination.
- All individuals are considered competent unless legally determined otherwise.

- The role of the psychiatrist in questions of competency is to identify the psychiatric impairment or state that creates an impairment in judgment related to a specific issue or capacity.
- The most common civil competency issues in which psychiatrists may be asked to provide opinions are competency to give informed consent to medical care, testamentary competency, and competency of witnesses.

## Practice Guidelines

1. Identify the specific capacity or capacities related to the competency issues in question.
2. Identify the impairment, if any, related to these capacities. If impairment is present, identify the specific psychiatric symptoms and related condition creating the impairment.
3. Offer an opinion regarding the severity and duration of the impairment, as well as whether the impairment is likely to be temporary, permanent, or amenable to treatment.

## References

Alabama Code, Title 22 § 104(16)
Allbright AL: 2001 employment decisions under the ADA Title I—survey update. Ment Phys Disabil Law Rep 26:395–398, 2002
Americans with Disabilities Act of 1990, 42 U.S.C. §§ 12101–12213
Andrews TW: The inherent risks of office surgery. Wall Street Journal, September 10, 2002, p 13
Appelbaum PS: Policing expert testimony: the role of professional organizations. Psychiatr Serv 53:389–390, 2002
Austin v Am Association of Neurological Surgeons, 253 F.3d 967 (7th Cir. 2001)
Becker E: The Denial of Death. New York, Free Press, 1973
Bellotti v Baird, 428 U.S. 132 (1979)
Bonner v Moran, 75 U.S. App. D.C. 156, 126 F.2d 121 (1941)
Carey v Population Services International, 431 U.S. 678 (1977)
Doe v Irwin, 615 F.2d 1162 (6th Cir. 1980)
EEOC v Prevo's Family Markets, Inc, 8 A.D. Cases 401 (1998)
Eviatar D: Is litigation a blight, or built in? New York Times, November 23, 2002, pp 21, 23
Faber v Sweet Style Mfg Corp, 40 Misc.2d 212, 242 N.Y.S.2d 763 (1963)
Federal Rules of Evidence, 88 Stat. 1926 (1975)
Fjellestad v Pizza Hut of Am., Inc, 188 F.3d 944 (8th Cir. 1999)
Florida Statutes Title 32, ch. 456.041
Greenspan v Slate, 12 N.J. 426, 97 A.2d 390 (1953)
Haber HG: In re Storar: euthanasia for incompetent patients, a proposed model. Pace Law Review 3:351–374, 1982
Hidding v Williams, 578 So.2d 1192 (La. App. 1991)

Illinois Statutes, ch. 91 1/2, § 3-5016 (a)
In re Green, 448 Pa. 338, 292 A.2d 387 (1972)
In re Guardianship of Hayes, 93 Wn.2d 228, 608 P.2d 635 (1980)
In re J.C.G., 144 N.J. Super. 579, 366 A.2d 733 (1976)
In re McElroy, 22 O.R.2d 381 (1978)
Johnson by Adler v Kokemoor, 545 N.W.2d 495 (Wis. 1996)
Lapetina EM, Armstrong EM: Preventing errors in the outpatient setting: a tale of three states. Human Affairs 21:26–39, 2002
LeBlang TR: Informed consent and disclosure in the physician-patient relationship: expanding obligations for physicians in the United States. Med Law 14:429–444, 1995
Loftus E, Davies GM: Distortions in the memory of children. Journal of Social Issues 40:51, 1984
Luka v Lowrie, 171 Mich. 122, 136 N.W. 1106 (1912)
Margolick D: Undue Influence: The Epic Battle for the Johnson and Johnson Fortune. New York, William Morrow, 1993
Mariner WK, McArdle PA: Consent forms, readability, and comprehension: the need for new assessment tools. Law Med Health Care 13:58–74, 1985
McKay v Toyota Mfr. U.S.A., 110 F.3d 369 (6th Cir. 1997)
Melton GB: Children's competency to testify. Law Hum Behav 5:73–85, 1981
Miller FH: Health care information technology and provider accountability: a symbiotic relationship, in Law and Medicine, Vol 3. Edited by Freeman M, Lewis ADE. New York, Oxford University Press, 2000, pp 27–45
Mississippi State Board of Psychological Examiners v Hosford, 508 So.2d 1049 (Miss. 1987)
Missouri Statutes, Title 28, §431.063
Moore v Regents of the University of California, 271 Cal. Rptr. 146 (Cal. 1990)
Mukherjee S: Resident aliens. New Republic, November 25, 2002, pp 14–18
New York Public Health Law, ch. 763
Ornelas v Fry, 151 Ariz. 324, 727 P.2d 819 (1986)
Petrila J: The emerging debate over the shape of informed consent: can the doctrine bear the weight? Behavioral Sciences and Law 21:121–133, 2003
Pilpel H: Minor's right to medical care. Albany Law Review 36:462–487, 1972
Planned Parenthood of Central Missouri v Danforth, 428 U.S. 52 (1976)
Ramos S: Insuring medical aid if parents are away. New York Times, January 22, 1981, p. 15
Reaves v Bergsrud, 982 P.2d 497 (N.M. App. 1999)
Reed v LePage Bakeries, Inc, 244 F.3d 254 (1st Cir. 2001)
Rice v Henderson, 140 W.Va. 284, 83 S.E.2d 762 (1954)
Rosenthal M: The Incompetent Doctor: Behind Closed Doors. Philadelphia, PA, Open University Press, 1995
Russaw v Martin, 472 S.E.2d 508 (Ga. App. 1996)
Slovenko R: Holding the expert accountable. J Psychiatry Law 29:543–574, 2001
Slovenko R: Psychiatry in Law—Law in Psychiatry. New York, Brunner/Routledge, 2002
Smalley v Baker, 262 Cal. App. 2d 824, 69 Cal. Rptr. 521 (1968)
Stefan S: Delusions of rights: Americans with psychiatric disabilities, employment discrimination and the Americans with Disabilities Act. Alabama Law Review 52:271–319, 2000

United States v Gutman, 725 F.2d 417 (7th Cir. 1984)
Waddell v Valley Forge Dental Associates, 276 F.3d 1275 (11th Cir. 2002), cert. denied, 535 U.S. 1096, 122 S. Ct. 2293, 152 L. Ed. 2d 1051 (2002)
Wheeler v United States, 159 U.S. 523 (1895)
Whiteside v Lukson, 947 P.2d 1263 (Wash. App. 1997)
Yarmey AD: Age as a factor in eyewitness memory, in Eyewitness Testimony: Psychological Perspectives. Edited by Wells GL, Loftus EF. New York, Cambridge University Press, 1984, pp 142–170
Zinermon v Burch, 494 U.S. 113 (1990)

## Suggested Readings

Berg JW, Appelbaum PS, Lidz CW, et al: Informed Consent: Legal Theory and Clinical Practice, 2nd Edition. New York, Oxford University Press, 2001
Bonnie RJ, Monahan J (eds): Mental Disorder, Work Disability, and the Law. Chicago, IL, University of Chicago Press, 1997
Ceci SH, Bruck, J: Jeopardy in the Courtroom: A Scientific Analysis of Children's Testimony. Washington, DC, American Psychological Association, 1995
Gawande A: Complications: A Surgeon's Notes on an Imperfect Science. New York, Henry Holt, 2002
Slovenko R: Psychiatry in Law—Law in Psychiatry. New York, Brunner/Routledge, 2002

CHAPTER 11

# Forensic Assessment in Personal Injury Litigation

Joan B. Gerbasi, M.D., J.D.

## Introduction

Forensic psychiatrists are frequently called on to evaluate plaintiffs in personal injury litigation. This litigation includes general tort law involving accidents and other injuries, the law of toxic torts, claims of sexual harassment, worker's compensation, and claims for infliction of emotional distress, either intentional or negligent. In general, plaintiffs claim that the defendant's act or omission resulted in a psychiatric condition that is disabling in some way or that caused significant distress, for which they should be compensated. Psychiatrists also become involved in cases in which plaintiffs claim physical injuries that cannot be fully accounted for on the basis of the medical findings.

Personal injury evaluations are some of the most difficult in forensic psychiatry. The evaluation involves not only an assessment of the claimant's current clinical and functional condition but also retrospective and prospective assessments of the claimant's condition. Opinions about the cause of the claimant's symptoms and the extent of impairment relative to the claimant's functioning before the trauma or event at issue are required. As has been noted elsewhere, retrospective assessments present with a myriad of problems (Simon and Shuman 2002).

These problems are intensified in the context of personal injury litigation, where claimants have an incentive to portray themselves as very healthy preaccident and significantly impaired postaccident. The issue of causation frequently involves the claimant's predisposition to mental disorder or the possibility that the claimant either had a preexisting mental disorder or some prodromal symptoms of a mental disorder. Finally, these evaluations require opinions about prognosis, which are complicated by evaluations of the claimant's present treatment and willingness to engage in further treatment.

Whenever evaluations occur in the context of litigation, ascertaining the truth of the claimant's situation becomes further complicated by the evaluator's stance in the case. As observed by Davidson (1965, p. 65):

> In a sense, the opposing doctors are examining different patients. The plaintiff-selected physician starts off with a good rapport. He is the helping doctor. The claimant trusts him—but sees the defense physician as the enemy. The first physician gets the picture of a sincere, trusting, and friendly soul. The defense examiner sees a surly and suspicious one. These differences obviously affect the examination technique, as well as the credibility of the history and subjective symptoms.

In addition, all personal injury evaluations should include an investigation of the possibility of malingering. This is true even for evaluators retained by plaintiff's counsel. Plaintiffs and their counsel will be better served if they hear of the vulnerabilities of the case from their own expert, rather than from the opposing side. Care should be taken to treat the claimant respectfully. Being challenging or confrontational will limit the evaluator's effectiveness. The evaluator should strive to maintain a neutral stance during the evaluation. When claimants sense that their veracity is being questioned, they are likely to feel threatened and respond by portraying themselves as "sicker" than they otherwise would.

This chapter focuses on the salient issues involved in conducting evaluations for personal injury litigation. These evaluations typically require that the following issues be addressed: complete psychiatric evaluation, psychiatric diagnosis, causation, evaluation of malingering, extent of impairment or disability, adequacy of current treatment, and prognosis. Practice recommendations are presented. These recommendations are aimed at helping evaluators perform and document thorough, reasoned personal injury evaluations.

## The Psychiatric Evaluation

Personal injury evaluations should include a thorough psychiatric evaluation of the claimant. This includes a detailed and complete history of the current psychiatric symptoms, as well as all of the other components of a complete psychiatric evaluation in a nonforensic setting. Inquiries must be made into social and developmental history, educational history, legal history, employment history, military history, substance abuse history, relationship and sexual history, medical history, and prior psychiatric history.

Although much of the information gathered in this inquiry will not bear directly on the questions posed to the expert, it is crucial in forming the relevant opinions in a personal injury evaluation. As will be discussed in greater detail below, the evaluator will be asked to render an opinion about the causal relationship, if any, between the traumatic event or injury and the claimant's symptoms or diagnosis. To form this opinion, the evaluator must have knowledge of other possible causes of the claimant's disorder. In addition, opinions about impairment are integral components of all personal injury evaluations. Impairment opinions cannot be formed without a detailed understanding of the claimant's past and current functioning.

In gathering the history, clinicians should be sure to keep in mind that claimants may tend to portray their preinjury functioning in an overly positive light. Lees-Haley and colleagues (1996) compared 34 litigants' and 80 nonlitigants' self-report of previous and current cognitive and emotional functioning. The primary finding was that litigants reported preinjury functioning superior to that of controls. This underscores the importance of collateral information, treatment records, and detailed questioning about life activities. This sort of information can often provide valuable objective evidence about the claimant's actual level of functioning.

The following clinical vignette demonstrates the importance of obtaining a complete history.

> Mr. B, a 55-year-old man, was driving with his 30-year-old son on a freeway when they were suddenly sideswiped and pushed off the road. Mr. B lost control of his car and drove into a tree at high speed. He suffered whiplash, multiple head and face lacerations, and a broken clavicle. His son was killed. After the accident, Mr. B recovered from his physical injuries but developed a severe depression. He is plagued by visions of his son dying in his arms and ruminates about his guilt over his son's death. He believes that if he had not lost control of the car, his son would have survived. At the time of the accident he was driving his son, who had AIDS, to a doctor's appointment. Mr. B worked as an accountant for 30 years, but he has been unable to return to work since the accident. He spends his time sitting alone at home, crying about his son. He is suing the other driver and seeking compensation for medical and psychiatric impairment.
>
> Mr. B has a previous history of four episodes of depression. He recovered from each with a combination of antidepressants and psychotherapy. He did not require hospitalization and was able to continue

working. His doctors recommended that he remain on medication indefinitely, but he did not follow this advice. He reported that he was resistant to being "dependent" on medicine. Mr. B was last in therapy 1 year before the accident. The major focus of the therapy was Mr. B's relationship with his son and his fears for his son's health. Mr. B's son had active symptoms of an opportunistic infection at the time of the accident, had a high HIV viral load, and had a very short life expectancy.

If an evaluator did not gather the social and psychiatric histories, the causation opinion would seem straightforward. However, with this history, the opinion becomes more complicated. Although the car accident may have caused Mr. B's depression, it may have merely exacerbated Mr. B's symptoms, or Mr. B might have developed the depression even if the accident had not occurred. Mr. B is grieving the loss of his son, who was in the end stages of AIDS at the time of the accident and had a short life expectancy. A detailed examination of Mr. B's current symptoms and any symptoms he had before the accident will be essential in sorting this out. Finally, Mr. B had a history of recurrent depression, and long-term medication was recommended. One could argue that medication could have prevented or lessened the severity of the current episode. Although the significance of Mr. B's medication refusal will be for the trier of fact to determine, clinicians should include this information in the evaluation.

With respect to collateral information, evaluators should review the following documents to the extent relevant to the particular examination at issue:

- Police reports and witness statements regarding the accident or injury
- Employment records, including performance evaluations, both pre- and postinjury
- Medical records, including medical records related to the alleged injury
- Ambulance records and emergency room records with respect to the accident
- All prior psychiatric records, including inpatient and outpatient
- Psychiatric records with respect to current treatment
- Depositions of plaintiff and other parties to the litigation

## The Psychiatric Diagnosis

The laws governing the various types of personal injury claims vary (see Chapter 12: "Personal Injury and the Legal Process," this volume). In general, however, a plaintiff can recover for all loss suffered as a result of the defendant's acts or omissions. Tort law does not require the presence of a specific DSM-IV (and its text revision, DSM-IV-TR; American Psychiatric Association 2000) disorder for the plaintiff to prevail. All the plaintiff needs to prove is some type of psychological condition that causes impairment. Impairment is broader than disability and merely requires "any loss or abnormality of psychological, physiological, or anatomical structure or function" (Stedman's 2003). Symptoms that result in impairment are compensable, even if they do not satisfy criteria for a specific DSM-IV diagnosis. In practice, however, the vast majority of cases involve the allegation of the presence of a disorder that is recognized in DSM-IV. In addition, some states (e.g., California) do require a DSM-IV diagnosis before the plaintiff can recover emotional damages in a personal injury suit (Melton et al. 1997, p. 375).

Many psychiatric disorders are based, in large part, on subjective symptoms and self-report. The problems inherent with this type of data gathering are exacerbated by the presence of litigation. Lees-Haley and Brown (1993) compared claimants with a control group with respect to self-report of neuropsychological symptoms. The claimants' litigation did not involve head injury, and no claims of neuropsychological impairment were being made. More than 50% of the claimants reported symptoms associated with neuropsychological impairment. In addition, a lower, but still significant, percentage of the controls also endorsed many symptoms.

In a related study, Lees-Haley and Dunn (1994) recruited college students and asked them which symptoms they thought an individual would experience if they were suffering from depression, anxiety, posttraumatic stress disorder (PTSD), or mild brain injury. They found that 96.9% of subjects were able to endorse criteria sufficient for a diagnosis of major depression, 96.9% were able to endorse criteria sufficient for a diagnosis of generalized anxiety disorder, and 86.0% were able to endorse diagnostic criteria for PTSD. With respect to mild brain injury, 63.3% of the subjects were able to endorse 5 of 10 symptoms associated with this condition.

Diagnosis can be further complicated by the concept known as "compensation neurosis." Although not a DSM-IV diagnosis, this concept has become important in personal injury litigation. In 1867, Hodges observed,

> It may be said, with emphasis, however, that in all cases . . . in which a claim for indemnity is made, no remedy equals an adjustment for damages. Until this result has been reached therapeutic measures are of little or no services. The curative effect of a pecuniary settlement shows itself more and more conspicuously with every case in which the facts are made known. So long as this issue is undetermined recovery must not be looked for. (Bellamy 1997, p. 96)

This phenomenon was formally termed "compensation neurosis" by Rigler after he observed that there was an increase in disability claims following railway accidents after compensation laws were enacted in Germany (Trimble 1981).

The essence of the syndrome is that, when involved in litigation, claimants report more symptoms than they would in the absence of litigation and that the resolution of the litigation results in a resolution of the symptoms. In 1961, Miller described five major characteristics of the patient with compensation neurosis (Miller 1961; see Bellamy 1997, p. 97):

- Failure to improve with treatment until the compensation issue is settled
- Accident occurring in circumstances in which there is potential payment of compensation
- Inverse relationship to the severity of the injury (compensation neurosis is uncommon in cases of severe injury)
- Low socioeconomic status
- Complete recovery after settling of the compensation issues

The concept of compensation neurosis has been criticized. First, some studies have found that accident victims who are seeking compensation do not endorse more symptoms than their counterparts who are not involved in litigation. Parker (1977) compared the psychiatric symptoms of accident victims reported in Spain and Australia. Spain has no compensation laws, but Australia does. Despite the seeming "advantage" of reporting symptoms in Australia, the two groups did not differ significantly. Likewise, Mendelson (1987) found that litigants with chronic low back pain did not describe their pain experience significantly differently than a control group of nonlitigants.

Moreover, recent work has demonstrated that many claimants do not recover after the settlement, as the compensation neurosis theory postulates (Mendelson 1981, 1984; Sprehe 1984). For example, Mendelson (1981) conducted psychiatric evaluations of 101 patients who had been involved in automobile or industrial accidents. He found that 67% of the patients had failed to return to work nearly 16 months after their compensation claims had been resolved.

However, as has been pointed out by Bellamy (1997), Halleck (1997), and others, the failure to improve after resolution of the litigation can be explained by another hypothesis. After adopting the posture of illness behavior in the context of litigation, claimants cannot recover afterward because they may fear this may be admission of fraud or that if they recover, benefits may be withdrawn or their claim may be reexamined. In addition, other benefits of ongoing impairment, including possible solicitude of others and freedom from responsibility, continue independent of any compensation issue (Blinder 1979). Claimants may be more or less conscious of this behavior and its related motivations.

One final consideration bears mentioning. Lanyon and Almer (2002) compared a group of compensable personal injury victims who chose to litigate with a group who chose not to pursue litigation. The results indicated that the choice to litigate reflected personality-related, rather than situational, factors. The litigants were found, by Minnesota Multiphasic Personality Inventory (MMPI) assessment, to be more dramatic and histrionic than their nonlitigating counterparts. This study raises the possibility that the symptoms reflected during litigation may not be caused by the litigation per se but rather are the result of ongoing personality traits and styles.

Given that self-report may not be a reliable indicator of true symptomatology, evaluators should be certain to gather collateral information, conduct detailed and comprehensive psychiatric examinations, and screen for malingering in every evaluation.

Plaintiffs can allege that an accident or other traumatic event caused any of the commonly recognized psychiatric illnesses, including the mood, anxiety, and psychotic disorders. As noted above, they also can allege impairment from symptoms that do not satisfy criteria for any of the DSM-IV diagnoses. However, several diagnoses are frequently alleged in personal injury litigation. These include PTSD, conversion disorder, and postconcussion syndromes and other sequelae of head trauma.

## Posttraumatic Stress Disorder

PTSD is defined by the development of characteristic symptoms following exposure to a traumatic stressor (American Psychiatric Association 2000, pp. 463–469; see Table 11–1). Unlike in other psychiatric disorders, the criteria for PTSD establish a causal link between the traumatic event and the potentially compensable symptoms. This is obviously advantageous in personal injury litigation because tort law requires that the plaintiff prove that the trauma was the proximate cause of the psychological impairment.

DSM-IV contains a specific definition of a "traumatic stressor." It requires that a person directly experience, witness, or be confronted with an event that involved actual or threatened death or serious injury or another threat to the personal integrity of self or others (criterion A1). In addition, the person must react to the event with intense fear, helplessness, or horror (criterion A2). Many injuries claimed by plaintiffs

**TABLE 11–1. DSM-IV-TR diagnostic criteria for posttraumatic stress disorder**

A. The person has been exposed to a traumatic event in which both of the following were present:
   (1) the person experienced, witnessed, or was confronted with an event or events that involved actual or threatened death or serious injury, or a threat to the physical integrity of self or others
   (2) the person's response involved intense fear, helplessness, or horror. **Note:** In children, this may be expressed instead by disorganized or agitated behavior

B. The traumatic event is persistently reexperienced in one (or more) of the following ways:
   (1) recurrent and intrusive distressing recollections of the event, including images, thoughts, or perceptions. **Note:** In young children, repetitive play may occur in which themes or aspects of the trauma are expressed.
   (2) recurrent distressing dreams of the event. **Note:** In children, there may be frightening dreams without recognizable content.
   (3) acting or feeling as if the traumatic event were recurring (includes a sense of reliving the experience, illusions, hallucinations, and dissociative flashback episodes, including those that occur on awakening or when intoxicated). **Note:** In young children, trauma-specific reenactment may occur.
   (4) intense psychological distress at exposure to internal or external cues that symbolize or resemble an aspect of the traumatic event
   (5) physiological reactivity on exposure to internal or external cues that symbolize or resemble an aspect of the traumatic event

C. Persistent avoidance of stimuli associated with the trauma and numbing of general responsiveness (not present before the trauma), as indicated by three (or more) of the following:
   (1) efforts to avoid thoughts, feelings, or conversations associated with the trauma
   (2) efforts to avoid activities, places, or people that arouse recollections of the trauma
   (3) inability to recall an important aspect of the trauma
   (4) markedly diminished interest or participation in significant activities
   (5) feeling of detachment or estrangement from others
   (6) restricted range of affect (e.g., unable to have loving feelings)
   (7) sense of a foreshortened future (e.g., does not expect to have a career, marriage, children, or a normal life span)

D. Persistent symptoms of increased arousal (not present before the trauma), as indicated by two (or more) of the following:
   (1) difficulty falling or staying asleep
   (2) irritability or outbursts of anger
   (3) difficulty concentrating
   (4) hypervigilance
   (5) exaggerated startle response

**TABLE 11–1.** DSM-IV-TR diagnostic criteria for posttraumatic stress disorder *(continued)*

E. Duration of the disturbance (symptoms in Criteria B, C, and D) is more than 1 month.

F. The disturbance causes clinically significant distress or impairment in social, occupational, or other important areas of functioning.

*Source.* Reprinted from American Psychiatric Association: *Diagnostic and Statistical Manual of Mental Disorders,* 4th Edition, Text Revision. Washington, DC, American Psychiatric Association, 2000. Copyright 2000, American Psychiatric Association. Used with permission.

will not meet these strict criteria. Although this will not make their symptoms noncompensable, it will eliminate the possibility of a formal diagnosis of PTSD (Simon 2002, pp. 56–65).

Consider the following case vignette:

> Mr. P is a 24-year-old professional race car driver. During the course of his career, he has been involved in several serious accidents but has always escaped without serious injury. One day, while driving with his infant son, Mr. P was rear-ended at a stop light. The other driver was using his cell phone and did not notice the red light. The speed at impact was 10 miles per hour. Immediately after the accident, Mr. P calmly exited the car, called an ambulance for his son and dealt with the other driver's insurance information. He recalls, "I wasn't particularly scared. I was involved in much more serious accidents on the track. I mean huge crashes with cars on fire and everything. I've even been trapped in a burning car more than once." There is no evidence that Mr. P dissociated during or after the accident. He had full recall for all details of the time period surrounding and including the accident. Mr. P was not injured in the accident. Unfortunately, his son, who was only 2 months old, sustained significant head injury during the accident.
>
> After a brief hospitalization, Mr. P's son began to have developmental difficulties. Eight months after the accident, Mr. P began to experience symptoms of PTSD: He had intrusive thoughts of the accident and nightmares, found himself "always on the alert" and unable to function calmly on the racetrack, was constantly fatigued, had difficulty initiating and sustaining sleep, withdrew from family and friends and formerly pleasurable activities, and reported feeling "resigned" to the fact that he would never live to see his son grow up. He described being "shattered" by the thought that he could not protect his son. He stated that he would lie in bed at night thinking, "How can it be—I'm a strong guy, a professional driver, and I couldn't stop this from happening. Now my son has all these problems—it's all my fault."

At first blush this appears to be a clear case of PTSD. However, notice that Mr. P did not react to the trauma with the requisite "fear, helplessness, or horror," as required by criterion A2 of DSM-IV. Although he has the required symptoms and the trauma itself could meet the definition of a trauma under criterion A1, a formal diagnosis of PTSD is not warranted. Other diagnoses, such as major depressive disorder, adjustment disorder, and anxiety disorder not otherwise specified, should be considered. Not reaching a formal diagnosis of PTSD does not deprive the claimant of his ability to be compensated for his injuries. The evaluator can still opine that the accident caused the disorder and, if accepted by the trier of fact, compensation would be allowed.

PTSD has been studied extensively in recent years. Blanchard et al. (1995) compared victims of motor vehicle accidents to a nonaccident control population and found that nearly 35% of the motor vehicle accidents group met diagnostic criteria for PTSD and approximately 28% demonstrated subsyndromal PTSD. These motor vehicle accident victims with PTSD also demonstrated a high comorbidity with major depression. Research has also shown that several factors make a person particularly vulnerable to developing PTSD after a trauma. These include being female, having a history of childhood trauma (including sexual trauma), parental poverty, having a behavior disorder in childhood or adolescence, parental separation or divorce before age 10 years, introversion, poor self-confidence in adolescence, prior psychiatric disorder, history of psychiatric illness among first-degree relatives, life stress before and after the trauma, and high neuroticism (Davidson 1993). In addition, dissociation at the time of the trauma is strongly associated with subsequent development of PTSD (Shalev et al. 1996; Ursano et al. 1999).

With the exception of the trauma itself, all of the symptoms of PTSD are subjective and are often not observable by the examiner. For example, the individual will report intrusive thoughts, recurrent nightmares and hyperarousal, and avoidant behaviors that the examiner will not necessarily be able to independently verify. When this fact is coupled with the presence of litigation, PTSD becomes ripe for malingerers. Although pure malingering is rare in PTSD, exaggeration of symptoms is quite common (Trimble 1981). For these reasons, an evaluation of PTSD requires a meticulous interview regarding history, symptoms, and treatment efforts. In addition, corroboration of the claimant report will be extraordinarily helpful. This should include police reports and witness statements about the event and treatment records (medical and psychiatric). If possible, relatives or associates of the claimant should be interviewed. Their observations about the claimant's behavior and functioning can be a valuable source of information.

Evaluators should insist on a detailed description of the claimant's symptoms. Claimants who are malingering may be able to report the basic symptoms but may not be able to report them convincingly when asked to describe them in the context of their lives. Evidence of irritability, difficulty concentrating, and exaggerated startle response on mental status examination would support the presence of a diagnosis of PTSD and not malingering. Of course, the absence of these signs would not rule out PTSD as an appropriate diagnosis (see Chapter 19: "Malingering").

Furthermore, with respect to symptoms of PTSD, evaluators should not give any clues to the claimant during the evaluation. Although many claimants will be familiar with the required symptoms, the evaluator should not supply the information to the claimant. If presented with a list of symptoms that will qualify for the diagnosis, many claimants are likely to endorse criteria that will justify the diagnosis, whether or not the claimant otherwise has a genuine diagnosis of PTSD. Furthermore, the evaluator should take care not to communicate any bias to claimants. If claimants view the evaluator as skeptical of their claims, they may feel a need to justify impairment by reporting more extreme symptoms (Resnick 1997).

Evaluators should familiarize themselves with recent research and literature on PTSD to be in a position to assess the credibility of the claimed symptoms (see e.g., Green and Kaltman 2002; Resnick 2002; Zatzick et al. 2002). For example, research has shown that genuine nightmares in PTSD show variations on the theme of the trauma (Garfield 1987). The malingerer may claim that the dreams always reenact the event in exactly the same way. Also, civilian adults with PTSD have different dream patterns with respect to the trauma than do veterans. In civilian adults, the nightmares fade rapidly within a few weeks of the trauma. These nightmares begin with a vivid, almost literal, reenactment of the trauma, and over time, the event becomes woven into the rest of the person's dream life. Considerable body movement almost always accompanies posttraumatic nightmares. This does not occur in non-trauma-related nightmares (van der Kolk et al. 1984). Veterans' nightmares are somewhat different. After the fading of the initial post-traumatic nightmares, the veteran may, even after a prolonged period of time, begin to wake up terrified and report that he dreamed of the event exactly as it happened. This dream may be repeated identically for many years (van der Kolk et al. 1984).

When evaluating the claimant's report of concentration difficulties or insomnia, the evaluator should explore a detailed history of living patterns before and after the traumatic event. This examination may reveal that certain symptoms were present before the trauma or that baseline activity before the trauma does not differ significantly from activity after the trauma. In addition, the evaluator should be certain to take a detailed trauma history, including history of physical abuse, naturally occurring disasters, and automobile accidents. Prior PTSD predisposes to reoccurrence of symptoms after further stressors. The prior trauma, rather than the alleged trauma that is the subject of the litigation, may be causing the present symptoms.

Some controversy exists regarding the use of subterfuge during a forensic evaluation. Some evaluators find this inherently unethical, whereas others promote its use as essential and relevant (Resnick 2002). Support for using misleading tactics is found in the insurance company practice of using surveillance to gather information of possible malingering (Resnick 2002). In an evaluation, the evaluator may choose to include symptoms unrelated to PTSD in the inquiry about specific symptoms. For example, after inquiring about dreams, a question about grandiosity or mania might be asked. Claimants who are malingering may endorse these symptoms.

Resnick has written extensively on malingering, including malingered PTSD (see e.g., Resnick 1997, 1998, 2002; Resnick and Harris 2002). He has devised a clinical decision model for establishing malingered PTSD. The model requires first a clear motivation for malingering (e.g., compensation). The second stage of the model requires the presence of at least two associated characteristics from the following list:

- Irregular employment or job dissatisfaction
- Prior claims for injuries
- Markedly discrepant capacity for work and recreation
- No nightmares or, if nightmares, exact repetitions of the civilian trauma
- Antisocial personality traits
- Evasiveness or contradictions
- Noncooperation in the evaluation

The final stage of the model requires confirmation of malingering, either by claimant admission or through unambiguous psychometric evidence or strong corroborative evidence of malingering (Resnick 1997).

With respect to psychometric tests, the MMPI-2 and the Illness Behavior Questionnaire (Clayer et al. 1984) may be helpful (Resnick 2002). The most specific diagnostic test for PTSD is psychophysiological measurement. This test measures physiological reactivity on exposure to cues that symbolize an aspect of the traumatic event, which is one of the diagnostic criteria for PTSD. After exposing the claimant to imagery of the trauma, heart rate, skin conductance, and tension in a muscle of the face are measured. This method has been found to be effective by several researchers (Orr and Pitman 1993; Pitman and Orr 2002; Pitman et al. 1994).

**TABLE 11–2.** DSM-IV-TR diagnostic criteria for conversion disorder

A. One or more symptoms or deficits affecting voluntary motor or sensory function that suggest a neurological or other general medical condition.
B. Psychological factors are judged to be associated with the symptom or deficit because the initiation or exacerbation of the symptom or deficit is preceded by conflicts or other stressors.
C. The symptom or deficit is not intentionally produced or feigned (as in factitious disorder or malingering).
D. The symptom or deficit cannot, after appropriate investigation, be fully explained by a general medical condition, or by the direct effects of a substance, or as a culturally sanctioned behavior or experience.
E. The symptom or deficit causes clinically significant distress or impairment in social, occupational, or other important areas of functioning or warrants medical evaluation.
F. The symptom or deficit is not limited to pain or sexual dysfunction, does not occur exclusively during the course of somatization disorder, and is not better accounted for by another mental disorder.

*Source.* Reprinted from American Psychiatric Association: *Diagnostic and Statistical Manual of Mental Disorders,* 4th Edition, Text Revision. Washington, DC, American Psychiatric Association, 2000. Copyright 2000, American Psychiatric Association. Used with permission.

Evaluators should recognize that, although physiological testing can verify a claimant's report of increased arousal and response to the trauma, the test results alone cannot satisfy diagnostic criteria for PTSD. In addition, published court opinions allowing psychophysiologic test results into evidence are not extant (Pitman and Orr 2002). Pittman and Orr (2002) have been involved in two cases in which the evidence was allowed, but no published opinion was issued.

## Conversion Disorder

DSM-IV-TR defines conversion disorder as the presence of symptoms or deficits affecting voluntary motor or sensory function that suggest a neurological or other general medical condition but whose origin is psychological and not a disease or physiological process. This judgment is based on the observation that the initiation or exacerbation of the symptoms or deficit is preceded by conflicts or other stresses (American Psychiatric Association 2000, pp. 492–498). In addition, to make this diagnosis, DSM-IV-TR requires that malingering be ruled out (Table 11–2).

First, the evaluator must rule out medical or neurological causes of the alleged symptoms. These workups are usually conducted in advance of the claimant being sent for psychiatric evaluation. If they were not, however, the evaluator should recommend that this workup be completed. Without an extensive medical evaluation, a diagnosis of conversion disorder will be impossible in the vast majority of cases. A history of other unexplained somatic or dissociative symptoms makes it more likely that a current apparent conversion symptom is not the result of a general medical condition. This is especially true when criteria for somatization disorder have been met in the past (American Psychiatric Association 2000, p. 493).

Once a physiological cause of the evaluee's symptoms is ruled out, the evaluator must then determine that the evaluee is not malingering. Differentiating between conversion disorder and malingering can be very difficult but is an essential part of the evaluation (see Chapter 19: "Malingering," this volume). Conversion disorder differs from malingering in that conversion disorder involves the unconscious production of symptoms for reasons unappreciated by the patient. Malingering, in contrast, involves the intentional production of false or grossly exaggerated symptoms. In addition, the symptoms are produced or exaggerated for the express purpose of achieving a goal; for example, avoiding military service or work, obtaining financial compensation, or evading criminal prosecution (American Psychiatric Association 2000, p. 739).

Observations about the behavior of patients who malinger in comparison to patients who have genuine conversion disorder and are producing their symptoms unconsciously provide valuable clues for evaluators. Patients with conversion disorder are unaware that they are producing their own symptoms and are, therefore, usually eager to find a medical explanation for their symptoms and will seek out treatment (Trimble 1981). An individual who is malingering, however, will often decline to cooperate with diagnostic or therapeutic procedures (Resnick 1997).

In addition, a person malingering is more likely than one with conversion disorder to refuse to work, even when the employment could be handled in spite of some impairment (Resnick 1997).

Furthermore, in response to an inquiry about the incident that produced the symptoms, a malingerer is likely to remember every detail, whereas the patient with conversion disorder is more likely to give an account that has gaps or inaccuracies (Huddleston 1932, cited in Resnick 1997).

A malingerer also often presents with very specific complaints and symptoms, whereas a person with conversion disorder may complain of vague and generalized symptoms (Chaney et al. 1984).

Finally, malingerers often present as suspicious, uncooperative, resentful, aloof, secretive, and unfriendly. Individuals with conversion disorder present themselves quite differently and are more likely to be cooperative, clinging, and dependent (Engel 1970, cited in Resnick 1997).

## Postconcussion Syndrome and Other Sequelae of Head Injuries

Approximately 1,500,000 traumatic brain injuries (TBIs) occur in the United States each year (Centers for Disease Control and Prevention 1999). These injuries can range in severity from mild, involving a brief change in mental status, to severe, with an extended period of loss of consciousness, prolonged amnesia after the injury, or a penetrating skull injury. 50,000 people die from TBIs each year, and an additional 80,000 to 90,000 experience the onset of long-term disability (Centers for Disease Control and Prevention 1999). TBI may cause many symptoms and functional deficits, including problems with cognition (concentration, memory, judgment, and mood), motor movement (strength, coordination, and balance), sensory abilities (tactile sensation, vision, hearing), and emotion (instability and impulsivity) (Thurman et al. 1999).

Studies of individuals who sustained minor head trauma and who were not involved in litigation indicate that a significant number of these individuals report memory impairment, concentration difficulties, fatigue, and increased irritability (Wrightston and Gronwall 1981). In addition, postconcussive syndrome is commonly reported following minor head injury. Postconcussive syndrome symptoms include dizziness, headaches, anxiety, emotional lability, blurry vision, concentration difficulties, and memory problems (Binder 1986).

Evaluating TBIs and their sequelae presents multiple layers of difficulties. The injury itself is usually not accompanied by hard evidence, such as findings on cervical spine X-rays or head magnetic resonance images. Assessing the severity of the injury is crucial. Evaluators should obtain evidence of the accident, including any associated police and ambulance reports, as well as full medical records. Individuals commonly report that they "lost consciousness" during an accident, when this was not the case. This can happen even in cases where the individual is clearly not malingering, perhaps as a result of incorrect knowledge about medical terminology.

All evaluations of psychiatric symptoms allegedly caused by head injury should include a screening examination for malingering. Evaluating the veracity of reports of vague psychiatric symptoms such as concentration problems, sleep difficulties, or irritability is problematic. Evaluators often find it helpful to have the claimant describe in detail a typical day and have this information verified by a relative or friend. If the examination reveals no impairment in social functioning or deteriorating of relationships, for example, irritability becomes suspect. In addition, a person who claims severe difficulty with concentration, but who spends his free time watching movies and reading newspapers and magazines, may be exaggerating his symptoms.

One common claim after head injury is ongoing memory deficits. Resnick (1997) suggests several clues that evaluators can explore in this regard. First, head injury is known to impair declarative memory (memory for events, things, places, etc.) but not procedural memory (memory that involves often conducted motor activities such as riding a bicycle or driving a car). Therefore, if a claimant reports forgetting how to do something that involves procedural memory, such as tying a shoe, the memory deficits may not be real. Second, if someone reports that they have difficulty with new learning but also has a full recollection for the incident that allegedly caused the injury, the report is suspect. This is because only extreme severely head injuries lead to impairment in new learning. These patients would be obviously impaired and would also typically not recall the alleged incident. A third clue to malingering is poor recollection when an examinee is informed that the questions are "memory testing" but a better performance for the other aspects of the evaluation. Fourth, if a claimant states that he or she doesn't know the answers to very easy questions (e.g., that a car has wheels) or misses easy autobiographical answers, the claimed memory deficits are suspect. Finally, in general, it is easier to recognize items or information than recall them. Therefore, if a claimant demonstrates recognition that is worse than recall, the reported memory deficit is suspect.

In addition, although complete neuropsychological evaluation is often necessary in claims involving cognitive deficits, psychiatrists may find the Ray Fifteen Item Test a useful tool (Resnick and Harris 2002). The test presents the material listed below:

| | | |
|---|---|---|
| A | B | C |
| 1 | 2 | 3 |
| a | b | c |
| ■ | ● | ▲ |
| I | I I | I I I |

The evaluee is told that he or she will be given a test that involves remembering 15 items. The evaluator implies that the test is difficult. Notice, however, that the test really only involves remembering three or four ideas to remember the majority of the material. The evaluee is given 10 seconds to study the items and then asked to reproduce what they remember of the material. In the absence of severe cognitive deficits, recalling fewer than three of the five character sets is suspect. Of course, if someone is claiming severe cognitive deficits, this test will not be helpful in ruling out malingering. In addition, this test should be employed as a screening tool only, because it has limited sensitivity and specificity (Cercy et al. 1997, p. 91). If the results of this screening are suspicious for malingering, a full neuropsychological evaluation should be pursued.

## Malingering

In all personal injury evaluations, evaluators must consider the possibility of malingering before arriving at a psychiatric diagnosis. *Malingering* is defined in DSM-IV-TR as the "intentional production of false or grossly exaggerated physical or psychological symptoms, motivated by external incentives, such as . . . financial compensation" (American Psychiatric Association 2000, p. 739). In addition to the clues and screening methods described above, some general principles should be kept in mind.

First, all diagnoses must be supported by objective evidence to the greatest extent possible. This evidence is collected through a thorough interview, exhaustive review of symptoms, review of treatment records, and other collateral documents and interviews with family and associates.

In conducting the interview, clinicians will find that first eliciting the evaluee's symptoms in response to an open-ended inquiry is helpful. After plaintiffs have reported all of their symptoms, the evaluator should then ask about the specific symptoms listed in DSM-IV-TR. Plaintiffs may be tempted to overendorse symptoms in this context, which may be a sign of malingering or exaggeration. Clinicians may also find it helpful to preface the list of symptoms with a statement such as, "I'm going to ask you about a variety of symptoms of mental disorders. No one has all of these symptoms, so don't be overwhelmed by the list." This may result in a more honest endorsement.

The hallmark of malingering is symptom inconsistency (Resnick 1999). This inconsistency can manifest in many different forms. There may be inconsistency between the claimant's report and the evaluator's observations. For example, a claimant alleging severe depression may present with psychomotor retardation, poor eye contact, and a sad affect. If, however, the claimant displays a bright affect without any evidence of sadness during the course of a several-hour interview, the diagnosis of depression is suspect.

In addition, there may be inconsistency between the claimant's report and his or her actual level of functioning. For example, a claimant may report extreme difficulties with concentration and memory but also be an active, vocal, and articulate member of the local city planning commission.

There also may be internal inconsistency in the claimant's report. For example, a claimant may report that he or she cannot remember the date or follow the news but have no difficulty maintaining concentration during an extended interview, recalling historical and recent information, and score perfectly on the Mini-Mental Status Examination.

Finally, there may be inconsistency between the claimant's report of symptoms and how genuine symptoms manifest themselves. For example, a claimant may report continuous auditory hallucinations and no strategies to decrease them. True hallucinations are usually not continuous, and patients often have developed ways to decrease their intensity (e.g., watching television, working) (Resnick 1999).

Evaluators should familiarize themselves with the literature on malingering the various types of psychiatric disorders. There is a growing body of literature in this area (see, e.g., Resnick 1998, 1999, 2002; Resnick and Harris 2002; Rogers 1997). Before conducting an evaluation, the evaluator should ask the hiring attorney about the claimant's allegations and should review psychiatric and medical treatment records and other collateral documents. This will provide guidance about which specific literature should be reviewed in advance of the interview. Finally, in any case where malingering is suspected on the basis of the clinical interview, psychological testing should be considered (see Chapter 19: "Malingering," this volume).

## Causation

Personal injury evaluations include an opinion about the causation of the disorder. In forming this type of opinion, evaluators should keep in mind that causation in medicine is fundamentally different from causation in the law. Clinical causation is often thought of as multifactorial. A number of different factors, including environmental, biological, and psychological factors, contribute to the eventual formation of psychiatric symptoms. Within clinical psychiatry, identification of any specific event as the "cause" of the symptoms is usually unnecessary and often impossible.

In contrast, the law requires that the claimant prove that the incident or trauma at issue caused the symptoms, either de novo or by precipitating, aggravating, or hastening the condition (Danner and Sagall 1977). Legal causation includes two findings. First, it must be determined that the defendant's acts or omissions are the cause in fact of the injuries (the "but-for" test). The but-for test requires a finding that, had the defendant's actions not occurred, the injury would not have happened. Although seemingly simple, this test implies causation forward into eternity. As noted by Keeton et al. (1984), citing *North v. Johnson* (1984):

> In a philosophical sense, the consequences of an act go forward to eternity, and the causes of an event go back to the dawn of human events, and beyond. But any attempt to impose responsibility upon such a basis would result in infinite liability for all wrongful acts, and would "set society on edge and fill the courts with endless litigation."

Because of these concerns, proximate cause—the second component of causation—developed. Proximate cause represents a policy determination that a defendant, even one who has behaved negligently, should not automatically be liable for all consequences of his act (Emanuel Law Outlines 1994, p. 139). Proximate cause is a complicated legal concept that has defied clear rules (Keeton et al. 1984). Most simply, proximate cause can be equated with foreseeability: if the consequences of a defendant's actions are unforeseeable, no causation will be found.

The fundamental difference between legal and medical causation is aptly illustrated by Danner and Sagall (1977, p. 305):

> [T]he proverb "the straw that broke the camel's back" may help to illustrate the differences in emphasis between the [differing views of causation.] . . . [T]o the physician, the proverb emphasizes the obvious predisposition to "breakdown" because of overload already present, and therefore suggests that the cause of the camel's collapse was the prior strain on his back, not the added straw. The attorney, on the other hand, seeks to gain legal recognition of the straw as the cause of the collapse, because his client stands to benefit from such recognition and from assignment of responsibility for the placing of the straw to a particular party.

Evaluators in personal injury litigation must recognize that they are being asked to render opinions based on the legal, and not medical, definitions of causation. Failure to do this will result in ineffective and misleading testimony and reports. If an evaluator is unable to render an opinion about legal causation, within a reasonable degree of medical certainty, they should convey this information to the hiring attorney.

The legal concept of the "eggshell skull" can be helpful in the causation analysis. In tort law, there is a general rule that a defendant "takes his plaintiff as he finds him." This is also known as the "eggshell skull" rule. Under this rule, defendants are responsible for the product of their negligence, independent of the vulnerability of the plaintiff. For example, if a defendant's acts would not cause the average person to be particularly traumatized, but the specific victim happens to be vulnerable to trauma by reason of prior sexual assault and PTSD, the fact that acute symptoms develop after the new injury cannot be excused by the previous history. The defendant cannot claim that the average claimant would not have been so affected and that he, therefore, should not be liable. Injured parties are taken as they are found, not as "normal" or average people, and are subject to whatever existing medical conditions and vulnerabilities were present at the time of the injury. This increased vulnerability does not excuse the defendant who inflicts the harm.

The eggshell skull principle can simplify the causation analysis. Psychiatric disorders and symptoms are often multifactorial, and predisposing factors, such as personality structure and other biopsychosocial factors, often coalesce around an inciting event such as an accident to produce the reported symptoms. Under the law, these predisposing factors do not lessen the defendant's liability; again, plaintiffs must be taken as they are found.

Hoffman and Spiegel (1989, p. 306) advocate a dual-pronged approach.

The psychiatrist should ask the question, But for the trauma, would the emotional disturbance for which compensation is sought have occurred? If the answer is, Probably not, then the claimant is entitled to be compensated. However, if it is demonstrated that there was a preaccident vulnerability in the plaintiff's mental constitution such that he or she would probably have developed a similar kind of emotional problem sooner or later, even in the accident had not occurred, then the plaintiff will fail in this aspect of his or her claim or may recover damages only to the extent that the trauma accelerated the condition.

The causation opinion involves comparing claimants' preincident functioning and symptoms to their presentation after the incident. The determination of whether the claimant had psychiatric symptoms before the trauma is crucial. Records should be made available of any treatment the claimant has received. In addition, the evaluator should collect a detailed history of the claimant's life circumstances for a period of time preceding the trauma. Especially relevant would be stressors that are known to be associated with the development of psychological symptoms, including loss of a spouse, loss of a job or change in employment, divorce, and death or birth of a child. If collateral information is available, it can be particularly important in this regard. Interviews of relatives or work associates, if possible, should be pursued.

Symptoms can be arranged along a timeline and their relationship to external events assessed. As discussed above, the possibility of malingering or symptom magnification must always be considered in the context of litigation. However, another process may be at work. Claimants may become more symptomatic during litigation because of the high level of stress involved in the adversarial process. Claimants are often, of necessity, challenged with respect to symptom validity and severity. Halleck (1997) has proposed that plaintiff behavior during litigation can be best explained by the concept of negative reinforcement (behavior produced as a way of avoiding painful stimuli). The easiest way for plaintiffs to refute allegations that their symptoms may be voluntary is to become more symptomatic and demonstrate that they are even sicker than anyone had previously thought.

Symptom exacerbation related to the fact of the litigation and not to the underlying event or trauma should be identified. Careful questioning about the course of the plaintiff's symptoms, activities, and functioning for a period of time spanning from before the incident up to and including the date of the evaluation is necessary. Evaluators should ask the claimant when the lawsuit was filed. This information will also be available from the hiring attorney.

Clinicians will often find it helpful to identify several key dates, including one before the injury, the date of maximum symptoms, a date before the initiation of the litigation, and the current date. Then the claimant can be asked about symptoms and function on each of those dates. This type of interviewing may help clarify whether symptoms have increased in response to litigation. In addition, simply asking the claimant whether the stress of the lawsuit has increased their symptoms can be a valuable source of information. Many claimants will readily acknowledge that the litigation has caused increased stress and that they expect to feel substantially better after it is settled.

Consider the following clinical vignette.

> Mrs. J is a 45 year-old married woman and mother of three young children who was involved in motor vehicle accident while taking her children to daycare. One of the children was hospitalized briefly for observation, but no one else in the car needed medical treatment. Mrs. J filed a claim against the driver of the other car, seeking damages for psy-

chological symptoms allegedly caused by the accident. She has no previous psychiatric history, either outpatient or inpatient. Mrs. J reported that almost immediately after the accident she developed severe depression and paralyzing anxiety. She stated she is afraid to drive and has panic attacks nearly every day.

Mrs. J has been married for 7 years. The marriage has been a difficult one, and 2 weeks before the accident her husband told her that he was in love with another woman and would be moving out of the family home. She found this news especially distressing because her own father left home under similar circumstances. Her mother was diagnosed with borderline personality disorder and depression and was hospitalized several times during Mrs. J's childhood. Mrs. J states that she fears she is like her mother and reports that, looking back, she has always been anxious and prone to bouts of depression. Mrs. J is in the early stages of menopause and reports that her anxiety had been increasing for several months before the accident. These symptoms improved somewhat when Mrs. J entered menopause. At the time she presented for evaluation, she had scheduled an appointment with her gynecologist to discuss hormone replacement therapy.

This vignette presents a complicated causation problem. Notice that a number of possibilities exist. They include that Mrs. J's symptoms are solely related to the accident, that her symptoms are solely related to the breakup of her marriage, that the combination of the stressors of her marital difficulties and the accident caused the symptoms, that Mrs. J has a history of untreated depression and anxiety and her symptoms have been aggravated by either the accident or the breakup or by a combination of both, that she has a history of untreated depression and anxiety and her current symptoms were precipitated by either the accident or the breakup, that Mrs. J has personality traits (Cluster B?) that make her vulnerable to stress and that have caused her to experience more symptoms in response to these stressors than the average person would, and that Mrs. J's symptoms are unrelated to any external stressor and are the effects of perimenopause.

In sorting out these possibilities, clinicians need to gather as much information as possible about Mrs. J's response to the marriage breakup. A detailed history of her functioning and symptoms during the 2-week period preceding the accident will be crucial. Note, though, that even if Mrs. J did not have symptoms before the accident, it does not necessarily mean that the marriage problems did not cause the depression and anxiety. Gathering a history of any previous accidents or other significant stressors and of Mrs. J's associated responses may be helpful. For example, if she has a history of multiple minor car accidents without any corresponding symptoms, it may make it more likely that her current symptoms are more significantly accounted for by her marriage difficulties. The evaluator may conclude that the two stressors combined to cause the current impairment. If this is the case, the expert should so opine and the trier of fact will sort out the apportionment issue.

In addition, Mrs. J presents with a possible history of depression and anxiety versus a personality style that includes some mood instability. She is also perimenopausal. These characteristics are examples of special vulnerabilities that would be included under the eggshell skull principle and that would not detract from her ability to recover. The evaluator should note the contribution of these characteristics to Mrs. J's presentation and leave it to the trier of fact to factor this into the compensation determination.

## Extent of Impairment

In rendering an opinion about the extent of impairment, evaluators should first become familiar with the requirements of the particular type of claim at issue. For example, workers' compensation claims require that evaluators use the American Medical Association (AMA) *Guides to the Evaluation of Permanent Impairment* (American Medical Association 2000) or other similar sources to evaluate impairment and related disability (see Chapter 13: "Disability," and Chapter 14: "The Workplace," this volume). The AMA *Guides* defines impairment as "a loss, loss of use, or derangement of any body part, organ system, or organ function" (p. 2). Disability is defined as "an alteration of an individual's capacity to meet personal, social, or occupational demands or statutory or regulatory requirements because of an impairment" (p. 8).

In tort law, the inquiry is broader, and any impairment that results from the injury is technically recoverable. Juries, however, are more likely to compensate only for those psychiatric symptoms that result in some functional impairment. In this respect, the AMA *Guides* can be a valuable reference because they stress linking the injury to functional impairment. In addition, if the AMA *Guides* are not used, the forensic examiner's testimony may be inadmissible as lacking in probative value (Simon 2002).

Evaluators should also rate the claimant on Axis V of DSM-IV-TR, the Global Assessment of Functioning (GAF) Scale. The GAF provides a rating of an individual's overall psychological functioning (including social, occupational, and school functioning) on a scale of 0–100 (American Psychiatric Association 2000, pp. 32–35). Although it has only modest reliability, the GAF is considered to be a reasonable measure of adaptive functioning (Simon 2002).

An assessment of impairment requires a detailed inquiry into the claimant's life before and after the event. Evaluators should ask claimants to describe their daily activities and to describe a typical day in detail. All activities of daily living should be covered, including dressing, preparing food and eating, using a watch and other common equipment, shopping, working, leisure activities, and the extent and quality of personal relationships. With respect to employment, the evaluator should ascertain the conditions of the employment and the particular requirements and demands of the claimant's position. Whenever the claimant describes a decline in functioning postevent, the claimant should be asked to quantify and describe the specific effects of this decline in detail. In addition, emotional symptoms should be reviewed in detail, and their effect on functioning should be assessed.

## Adequacy of Current Treatment

Evaluators are often asked to render an opinion about the claimant's treatment. The law places an affirmative duty on injured parties to limit their own damages, known as the "duty to mitigate." An example of this duty is the seat belt defense available in a number of states. Under this law, failure to wear a seat belt may deprive the plaintiff of recovery; if the defendant can show that the plaintiff would not have been injured had he or she worn a seat belt, the defendant may not be liable for the avoidable injuries (*Emanuel Law Outlines* 1994, p. 233). In civil litigation, plaintiffs have a duty to minimize their damages by obtaining appropriate treatment, even if the defendant did indeed cause the injury.

Evaluators should familiarize themselves with the accepted treatment for the mental disorder at issue. The APA's Practice Guidelines can be a valuable source of information in this regard. If it is the evaluator's opinion that the current treatment is inadequate, the opinion should include recommendations for adequate treatment, along with an estimated time when improvement could be expected, were the claimant to pursue the recommendations. For example, if a claimant has major depressive disorder and hasn't benefited from a 6-month trial of a selective serotonin reuptake inhibitor medication, a recommendation about alternative medication strategies would be appropriate.

## Prognosis

Finally, the evaluator is asked to render an opinion about the claimant's prognosis. This opinion is often twofold: one opinion based on the current treatment and another based on optimal treatment, if the current treatment is inadequate. Prognosis is extremely important in tort law because it will directly affect the amount of damages the claimant may receive. In tort law, the plaintiff's recovery is determined only once. The settlement and damage award is granted at the time of judgment and is final. Even if circumstances change, the damage award will not be reviewed in the future. The finality of the award makes the prognosis opinion crucial.

Again, as is true with many other aspects of the evaluation, the litigation context complicates this opinion. As mentioned previously, the very fact of the litigation creates an incentive for claimants to have impairments—appearing disabled will further the chances of securing compensation for injury. As stated by Blinder (1979, p. 88):

> Though not causative (in that secondary gain arises as an issue following injury), such secondary gain factors as financial compensation, the solicitude of others, freedom from responsibility and/or restitution for real or imagined past exploitation may greatly prolong convalescence and prevent recovery.

These individuals may have a poorer prognosis by virtue of the fact that they have pursued compensation. If evaluators believe that this "compensation neurosis" is relevant, they should so state and provide evidence for this belief. The determination of whether the claimant should be compensated for symptoms that are caused by the decision to pursue litigation will be made by the trier of fact.

Before preparing the prognosis opinion, evaluators should be familiar with the relevant psychiatric literature about the diagnosis at issue. In addition, studies have been conducted about prognosis following injury. For example, Mendelson (1985) found that older age, lower-back injury, and loss of libido are associated with a poorer prognosis after injury. Binder et al. (1991) studied 18 personal injury plaintiffs at varying times after the conclusion of the litigation. They found that plaintiffs who had more severe symptoms immediately following the injury had a poorer prognosis. They also found that a shorter time between injury and litigation settlement was associated with less current psychiatric impairment (see also Gardner 1991—correlation between early referral for psychiatric treatment and better rates of job return in workers' compensation cases).

Evaluators should consider the relevant literature and the specifics of the present case, including the progress the claimant has made to date and the adequacy of the current treatment in formulating opinions regarding prognosis. They should keep in mind that the goal of the tort system is to restore claimants to the place they would have occupied had the injury or accident not occurred. Despite the legal aphorism that the plaintiff should be made whole, this is not the goal of the law. Plaintiffs come to the table with psychiatric vulnerabilities and static personality traits that are not compensable. The goal of the compensation is to return the plaintiff to the previous, albeit imperfect, state. In determining prognosis, the evaluator must be careful to separate out treatment for the incremental increase in symptoms caused by the accident and full, complete treatment to render the plaintiff a normal, healthy individual.

## Conclusion

Forensic assessments in personal injury litigation present some of the most difficult issues in forensic psychiatry. In addition to requiring detailed assessments of both retrospective and prospective mental states, they include complicated evaluations of causation. Before conducting these evaluations, evaluators should heed one final word of caution: they should examine their own motives and strive for objectivity. Evaluators should take care not to be influenced by the retaining attorney. If the findings do not support the attorney's case, the expert will not be retained, which has implications for the expert's compensation and, potentially, for future case referrals. In addition, there is often a subtle need to "please" the retaining attorney. Evaluators may find themselves approaching the case looking for evidence that will support their side, rather than approaching the case objectively. Psychiatric evaluations are especially vulnerable because symptoms are subjective and, for the most part, not "provable" by hard evidence.

Alan Stone has questioned whether objectivity can ever be achieved in forensic evaluations. He attributes this to the nature of the adversarial process and suggests that experts are selected in a biased fashion to be partisan expert witnesses (Stone 1984). Goldstein (1986) shares this view and cautions that reports which contain information not supportive of the hiring attorney's side "will never see the light of day." There are many psychiatrists, however, who disagree and believe that objectivity can be obtained. As Hoffman (1986) states,

> Although the court and others may see me as biased, my goal is to be as thorough and objective as possible. I expect my written and oral testimony to be questioned and cross-examined in court. However, I would be embarrassed if my opinion were not supported by the facts, were biased by preconceived opinion, or were based on incomplete examinations. I do not suppress facts and opinions that weaken the argument of the lawyer who hired me.

The American Academy of Psychiatry and the Law (1995), in its ethics guidelines, recognizes the potential problem with bias and instructs forensic psychiatrists to "adhere to the principle of honesty and . . . strive for objectivity."

The recommendations outlined in this chapter can aid in achieving this principle. Insisting on and reviewing collateral information, looking for objective signs of illness and impairment, adhering to strict DSM-IV diagnostic criteria, and carefully assessing malingering all serve to strengthen the evaluator's conclusions. Although this makes the evaluator's opinions more helpful in court, it also helps ensure that the evaluation reflects accurately the plaintiff's diagnosis and impairment.

## Key Points

- Forensic personal injury evaluations are some of the most difficult in forensic psychiatry. They involve both retrospective and prospective assessments of the claimant's condition.
- The evaluation should include a complete psychiatric evaluation, including an evaluation of malingering. Opinions are typically required with respect to causation, the extent of impairment, adequacy of treatment, and prognosis.
- In conducting the evaluation and forming the required opinions, collateral information should be reviewed. This information may include police reports, medical records, psychiatric records, employment records, and depositions. Opinions should be based, to the extent possible, on objective or corroborated information, rather than on the plaintiff's subjective report.

## Practice Guidelines

1. Include a comprehensive psychiatric evaluation in all forensic personal injury evaluations. A complete evaluation is essential in reaching informed and reasoned opinions about causation and impairment. This should include a review of all relevant collateral documents.
2. Base diagnoses, to the extent possible, on objective, rather than subjective, data. This includes observations during the mental status examination and collateral data such as record review and interviews with family, friends, and associates.
3. Evaluate reported symptoms in light of the claimant's daily functioning.

4. Always consider the possibility that the claimant is malingering. Be familiar with hallmarks of this presentation, including symptom inconsistency, and consider formal psychological testing to support suspicions of malingering.
5. Use the legal rather than the medical model of causation, and address the causal relationship between the alleged symptoms and the alleged injury. Be certain to analyze symptoms in light of the alleged injury, the presence of unrelated stressors, and the claimant's past psychiatric history.
6. Assess the claimant's degree of functional impairment as a result of the psychiatric disorder or symptoms.
7. Evaluate the efficacy of current treatment. If inadequate, recommend specific changes.
8. Base opinions regarding prognosis on the psychiatric literature about prognosis for the specific disorder at issue as well as the specific facts of each case, including the effect of litigation. The reference point and goal of treatment should be preinjury functioning.

## References

American Academy of Psychiatry and the Law: Ethics Guidelines for the Practice of Forensic Psychiatry. Bloomfield, CT, American Academy of Psychiatry and the Law, 1995

American Medical Association: Guides to the Evaluation of Permanent Impairment, 5th Edition. Chicago, IL, American Medical Association, 2000

American Psychiatric Association: Diagnostic and Statistical Manual of Mental Disorders, 4th Edition, Text Revision. Washington, DC, American Psychiatric Association, 2000

Bellamy R: Compensation neurosis: financial reward for illness as nocebo. Clin Orthop March(336):94–106, 1997

Binder LM: Perissting symptoms after mild head injury: a review of the postconcussive syndrome. J Clin Exp Neuropsychol 8:323–346, 1986

Binder RL, Trimble MR, McNiel DE: The course of psychological symptoms after resolution of lawsuits. Am J Psychiatry 148:1073–1075, 1991

Blanchard ED, Hickling EJ, Taylor AE, et al: Psychiatric morbidity associated with motor vehicle accidents. J Nerv Ment Dis 183(8):495–504, 1995

Blinder M: The abuse of psychiatric disability determinations. Med Trial Tech Q 25(1):84–91, 1979

Centers for Disease Control and Prevention, National Center for Injury Prevention and Control: Traumatic Brain Injury in the United States—A Report to Congress. Atlanta, GA, Centers for Disease Control and Prevention, 1999

Cercy SP, Schretlen DJ, Brandt J: Simulated amnesia and pseudo-memory phenomena, in Clinical Assessment of Malingering and Deception, 2nd Edition. Edited by Rogers R. New York, Guilford, 1997, pp 85–107

Chaney HS, Cohn CK, Williams SG, et al: MMPI results: a comparison of trauma victims, psychogenic pain, and patients with organic disease. J Clin Psychol 40:1450–1454, 1984

Clayer Jr, Bookless C, Ross MW: Neurosis and conscious symptom exaggeration: its differentiation by the Illness Behavior Questionnaire. J Psychosom Res 28:237–241, 1984

Danner D, Sagall EL: Mediocolegal causation: a source of professional misunderstanding. Am J Law Med 3(3):303–308, 1977

Davidson H: Forensic Psychiatry, 2nd Edition. New York, Ronald Press, 1965, p 65

Davidson J: Issues in the diagnosis of posttraumatic stress disorder, in American Psychiatric Press Review of Psychiatry, Vol 12. Edited by Oldham JM, Riba MB, Tasman A. Washington, DC, American Psychiatric Press, 1993, pp 141–155

Emanuel Law Outlines: Torts. Larchmont, NY, Emanuel Publishing Corp, 1994

Engel GL: Conversion symptoms, in Signs and Symptoms; Applied Physiology and Clinical Interpretation, 5th Edition. Edited by MacBryde CM, Blacklow RS. Philadelphia, PA, JB Lippincott, 1970

Gardner J: Early referral and other factors affecting vocational rehabilitation outcome for the workers' compensation client. Rehabil Couns 34:197, 1991

Garfield P: Nightmares in the sexually abused female teenager. Psychiatric Journal of the University of Ottawa 12:93, 1987

Goldstein RL: Psychiatrists and personal injury litigation (letter). Am J Psychiatry 143(11):1487, 1986

Green BL, Kaltman SI: Recent research findings on the diagnosis of PTSD: prevalence, course, comorbidity, and risk, in Posttraumatic Stress Disorder in Litigation: Guidelines for Forensic Clinicians, 2nd Edition. Edited by Simon RI. Washington, DC, American Psychiatric Publishing, 2002, pp 19–40

Halleck SL: Perils of being a plaintiff—impressions of a forensic psychiatrist. Clin Orthop 336:72–78, 1997

Hoffman B: Reply to Dr. Goldstein's letter to the editor. Am J Psychiatry 143(11): 1488, 1986

Hoffman B, Spiegel H: Legal principles in the psychiatric assessment of personal injury in litigants. Am J Psychiatry 146(3):304–310, 1989

Huddleston, JH: Accidents, Neuroses and Compensation. Baltimore, MD, Williams & Wilkins, 1932

Keeton WP, Dobbs DB, Keeton RW, et al: Prosser and Keeton on the Law of Torts, 5th Edition. St Paul, MN, West Publishing, 1984

Lanyon RI, Almer ER: Characteristics of compensable disability patients who choose to litigate. J Am Acad Psychiatry Law 30(2):400–404, 2002

Lees-Haley PR, Brown RS: Neuropsychological complaint base rates of 170 personal injury claimants. Archives of Clinical Neuropsychology 145:632–635, 1993

Lees-Haley PR, Dunn JT: The ability of naïve subjects to report symptoms of mild brain injury, post-traumatic stress disorder, major depression, and generalized anxiety disorder. J Clin Psychol 50(2):252–256, 1994

Lees-Haley PR, Williams CW, English LT: Response bias in self-reported history of plaintiffs compared with nonlitigating patients. Psychol Rep 79(3):811–818, 1996

Melton BG, Petrila J, Poythress NG, et al: Psychological Evaluations for the Courts: A Handbook for Mental Health Professionals and Lawyers, 2nd Edition. New York, Guilford, 1997, pp 363–382

Mendelson G: Persistent work disability following settlement of compensation claims. Law Institute Journal 55:342–345, 1981

Mendelson G: Follow-up studies of personal injury litigants. Int J Law Psychiatry 7:179–188, 1984

Mendelson G: Compensation neurosis. Med J Aust 142:561–564, 1985

Mendelson G: Illness behavior, pain and personal injury litigation. Psychiatr Med 5(1):39–56, 1987

Miller MH: Accident neurosis. Br Med J 1:919–925, 992–998, 1961

North v Johnson, 58 Minn. 242 (1984)

Orr SP, Pitman RK: Psychophysiologic assessment of attempts to simulate post-traumatic stress disorder. Biol Psychiatry 22:127–129, 1993

Parker, N: Accident litigants with neurotic symptoms. Med J Aust 2:318–322, 1977

Pitman RK, Orr SP: Forensic laboratory testing for PTSD, in Posttraumatic Stress Disorder in Litigation: Guidelines for Forensic Clinicians, 2nd Edition. Edited by Simon RI. Washington, DC, American Psychiatric Publishing, 2002, pp 207–223

Pitman RK, Saunders LS, Orr SP: Psychophysiologic testing for post-traumatic stress order. Trial, April 1994, pp 22–26

Resnick PJ: Malingering of posttraumatic disorders, in Clinical Assessment of Malingering and Deception, 2nd Edition. Edited by Rogers R. New York, Guilford, 1997, pp 130–152

Resnick, PJ: Malingering of posttraumatic disorders. J Pract Psychiatr Behav Health 4:329–339, 1998

Resnick PJ: The detection of malingered psychosis. Psychiatr Clin North Am 22(1):159–172, 1999

Resnick PJ: Guidelines for evaluation of malingering in PTSD, in Posttraumatic Stress Disorder in Litigation: Guidelines for Forensic Clinicians, 2nd Edition. Edited by Simon RI. Washington, DC, American Psychiatric Publishing, 2002, pp 187–206

Resnick PJ, Harris MR: Retrospective assessment of malingering in insanity defense cases, in Retrospective Assessment of Mental States in Litigation. Edited by Simon RI, Shuman DW. Washington, DC, American Psychiatric Publishing, 2002, pp 101–134

Rogers R (ed): Clinical Assessment of Malingering and Deception, 2nd Edition. New York, Guilford, 1997

Shalev AY, Peri T, Caneti L, et al: Predictors of PTSD in injured trauma survivors: a prospective study. Am J Psychiatry 153:219–225, 1996

Simon RI: Forensic psychiatric assessment of PTSD claimants, in Posttraumatic Stress Disorder in Litigation: Guidelines for Forensic Clinicians, 2nd Edition. Edited by Simon RI. Washington, DC, American Psychiatric Publishing, 2002, pp 41–90

Simon RI, Shuman DW (eds): Retrospective Assessment of Mental States in Litigation: Predicting the Past. Washington, DC, American Psychiatric Publishing, 2002

Sprehe DJ: Workers' compensation: a psychiatric follow-up study. Int J Law Psychiatry 7:165–178, 1984

Stedman's: Online Medical Dictionary, 27th Edition. Philadelphia, PA, Lippincott Williams & Wilkins, 2003. Available at: http://www.stedmans.com.

Stone AA: The ethics of forensic psychiatry: a view from the ivory tower, in Law, Psychiatry, and Morality. Edited by Stone AA. Washington, DC, American Psychiatric Press, 1984, pp 57–76

Thurman D, Alverson C, Dunn K, et al: Traumatic brain injury in the United States: a public health perspective. J Head Trauma Rehabil 14(6):602–615, 1999

Trimble MR: Post-Traumatic Neurosis: From Railway Spine to the Whiplash. New York, Wiley, 1981

Ursano RJ, Fullerton CS, Epstein RS, et al: Peritraumatic dissociation and post-traumatic stress disorder following motor vehicle accidents. Am J Psychiatry 156:1808–1810, 1999

van der Kolk B, Blitz R, Burr W, et al: Nightmares and trauma: a comparison of nightmares after combat with lifelong nightmares in veterans. Am J Psychiatry 141(2):187–190, 1984

Wrightson P, Gronwall D: Time off work and symptoms after minor head injury. Injury 12:445–454, 1981

Zatzick DF, Kang SM, Muller HG, et al: Predicting posttraumatic distress in hospitalized trauma survivors with acute injuries. Am J Psychiatry 159:941–946, 2002

## Suggested Readings

Bellamy R: Compensation neurosis: financial reward for illness as nocebo. Clin Orthop March(336):94–106, 1997

Hoffman B: How to write a psychiatric report for litigation following a personal injury. Am J Psychiatry 143:164–169, 1986

Hoffman B, Spiegel H: Legal principles in the psychiatric assessment of personal injury in litigants. Am J Psychiatry 146(3):304–310, 1989

Melton BG, Petrila J, Poythress NG, et al: Psychological Evaluations for the Courts: A Handbook for Mental Health Professionals and Lawyers, 2nd Edition. New York, Guilford, 1997, pp 363–382

Resnick PJ: The detection of malingered psychosis. Psychiatr Clin North Am 22(1):159–172, 1999

Resnick PJ, Harris MR: Retrospective assessment of malingering in insanity defense cases, in Retrospective Assessment of Mental States in Litigation. Edited by Simon RI, Shuman DW. Washington, DC, American Psychiatric Publishing, 2002, pp 101–134

Rogers R (ed): Clinical Assessment of Malingering and Deception, 2nd Edition. New York, Guilford, 1997

Simon RI (ed): Posttraumatic Stress Disorder in Litigation: Guidelines for Forensic Clinicians, 2nd Edition. Edited by Simon RI. Washington, DC, American Psychiatric Publishing, 2002

CHAPTER 12

# Personal Injury and the Legal Process

Marvin Firestone, M.D., J.D.

## Introduction

Claims for personal injury arise in many contexts, including injuries on the job (see Chapter 13: "Disability," and Chapter 14: "The Workplace," this volume), injuries resulting from a defective product (product liability), and injuries caused by negligent or intentional tortious behaviors (e.g., toxic exposure, fire, gas inhalation, and vehicular collision). The type of psychological injuries for which the courts allow compensation in personal injury litigation has evolved over recent years. In the past, only plaintiffs who manifested mental symptoms secondary to a demonstrable physical injury were compensated. For example, if a person had spinal injury resulting in paraplegia and became depressed, he or she could be compensated not only for the paraplegia but for the depression as well. This was characterized as a "physical to mental" injury.

The courts then allowed plaintiffs to be compensated for injuries characterized as "mental to physical," that is, physical injuries for which psychological causal factors existed. An example of such an injury might be a heart attack secondary to acute stress. Most recently, an increasing number of courts have allowed compensation for "mental to mental" injuries; that is, psychological injuries secondary to stress. For example, posttraumatic stress disorder (PTSD) caused by a near-death experience may be compensable if it results from someone else's negligence.

Both plaintiff and defense attorneys often retain forensic psychiatrists to provide expert opinions and testimony in such cases. Such opinions both help determine the validity of the psychic injury and the extent of impairment and aid the attorney in developing legal strategies for prosecuting or defending such claims. Each case referred to the forensic psychiatrist will raise different questions that must be addressed by the expert's evaluation. The following vignettes provide examples of how claims of psychiatric harm can be triggered, aggravated, precipitated, or exacerbated by the events in question or can be a substantial causal factor in the development of a psychological injury. They also raise questions of misattribution of symptoms that may be unrelated to the events in question.

## Clinical Vignettes

### Vignette 1

T.G., a 50-year-old, married Caucasian woman, fell down some stairs at work. She was taken to the hospital emergency department, where she denied loss of consciousness but was noted to have a small hematoma on her scalp. She had a history of back pain, sciatica, and Hashimoto's thyroiditis before this acute injury. In addition, she had previously been in a car accident, in which she suffered a whiplash. She had taken an extended leave of absence from her work because of family problems and recurrent conflicts with her employer that also existed before her current injury. She did not return to work. She claimed that the fall caused memory problems and other cognitive dysfunction, PTSD, and major depression, for which she had been prescribed psychotropic medications. The forensic psychiatrist who evaluated T.G. had to address the distinction between her past impairments from illness and injury and her current injuries from her fall down the stairs. Was her depression causally related to her ongoing work or family conflicts or to the minor injuries she sustained during the fall?

### Vignette 2

J.S. was a 45-year-old, separated Caucasian woman whose car rolled over in a two-car collision. She was not sure whether she lost consciousness at the time of the injury. She developed symptoms of acute stress disorder a few months after the accident and persistent memory problems. She had a history of chronic fatigue syndrome, marital problems, and depression before the accident. Her husband left her shortly after the accident, allegedly because he was frustrated by her symptoms of depression and cognitive dysfunction. In this case the forensic psychiatrist must address a number of complex questions. Are J.S.'s cognitive deficits the result of a closed head injury or of depression? Had the accident aggravated the marital discord and depression? Was the breakup of her marriage related to the injuries from the accident or to the marital discord that existed before the accident?

## Vignette 3

E.N. was a 49-year-old intensive care nurse who was driving her minivan on an interstate highway when a big rig truck collided with her minivan, wedging her van between the truck and the center divide of the highway. She stated, "The truck came inside my minivan and dragged my minivan and then jackknifed in front of me. I struck the cab of the big rig head on. I was trapped in my minivan, and the engine was on fire with thick, black smoke." Because all doors were jammed shut, she was forced to escape through a smashed rear window of her van. Her physical injuries were considered minor, but she later experienced nightmares and flashbacks of smelling gasoline. She stated that she has given up all enjoyable activities outside work, but she continued to work at her nursing job without difficulty. E.N.'s history was consistent with PTSD, but the forensic psychiatrist may have the task of determining whether or not there is exaggeration of her PTSD symptoms, especially in light of her continuing to function well in her work as an intensive care nurse.

## Vignette 4

R.M., a 32-year-old pipe insulator, was working in a ditch and experienced a rotten-egg odor, later identified as hydrogen sulfide that was released from the insulation wrapping material. Within a few weeks, R.M. complained of symptoms of photophobia, fatigue, depression, and slowness of thought processes, which he attributed to the hydrogen sulfide exposure. He stopped working and entered a cognitive rehabilitation program. Toxicological studies revealed no chance of chronic toxic effects based on R.M.'s level of exposure. The referral to the forensic psychiatrist involved the determination of whether R.M. was manifesting a conversion disorder or a somatoform disorder or was malingering.

## Vignette 5

C.K., a 19-year-old man, was found unconscious by the side of the railroad tracks after having been struck by a train. Three different railroad companies ran trains over parallel tracks at about the time and place he was found. C.K. could not remember the events leading to the accident nor which train had struck him. His attorney sent him to a psychiatrist, who hypnotized C.K., after which C.K. identified the defendant railroad company by remembering the logo on the train that struck him. The attorney asked the psychiatrist to address the question of whether or not recovery of C.K.'s memory by hypnosis was valid or produced a "false" memory.

# Issues in Personal Injury Litigation

When evaluating any of these psychic injury cases, the forensic psychiatrist should keep in mind how such injuries will be perceived by the general public. Psychiatry and psychological injuries are often the objects of derision and bad jokes, and society is often unsympathetic to a plaintiff with these kinds of problems. Forensic psychiatrists assessing a plaintiff who has developed symptoms of mental disorder as a result of traumatic injury such as those in the vignettes above should take into consideration such societal bias and stigmatization. Such attitudes influence how a jury (and an attorney or judge) may view the psychiatrist or the plaintiff. Forensic psychiatrists should also have a good understanding of the necessary elements of legal proof and defenses to a claim of personal injury. Finally, they should have access to all relevant facts and circumstances to provide credible opinions that will be admissible in court.

The issues addressed in personal injury litigation usually relate to diagnosis, causation, the nature and extent of impairment, disability, and prognosis (see Chapter 11: "Forensic Assessment in Personal Injury Litigation," this volume). Psychiatrists may also be asked to evaluate how such impairment affects the plaintiff's personal functioning, relationships with family members, and need for and costs of future treatment. To be most effective in assessing these issues and presenting their opinions, forensic psychiatrists should understand basic tort law and procedure as they affect the assessment. Psychiatrists should also be aware of how their participation with attorneys and the court can best assist in the success of the prosecution or defense of a tort claim.

## The Law

Personal injury litigation is governed by principles of common law, discovery, and evidentiary rules, which are based primarily on *tort* theories. A *tort* is a civil wrong in which a defendant has breached a legal duty, causing injury to a plaintiff. To establish liability, the plaintiff must prove, first, that the defendant owed a legal duty to the plaintiff; second, that the defendant breached that duty; third, that the plaintiff suffered an injury; and fourth, that the defendant's breach of duty caused injury. The plaintiff is entitled to compensation not just for mental distress and pain, but for suffering, anxiety, depression, and fears. Pain connotes the physical; anxiety, depression, and fears connote the mental. Suffering is in-between the pain and emotional symptoms and is produced by both the pain and the emotional symptoms. The psychiatrist may also be asked to evaluate changes in the quality of the plaintiff's life, resulting from the mental disorder, in the past, present, and future. For example, psychological problems not uncommonly create or exacerbate some degree of impairment in everyday functioning, including disruption of family relationships or function at work.

Even the development of a somatoform disorder in which pains are considered psychosomatic in origin or are considered "imaginary" (in the sense that they are not the result of an organic ailment) may be compensable. In such cases, the plaintiff needs to demonstrate that the disorder was caused by the effect of the injury or by the aggravation of preexisting neurotic tendencies (*Bourne v. Washburn* 1971). The forensic psychiatrist should be able to effectively explain the dynamics of such mental disorders.

## Malingering

A common concern in personal injury litigation involves whether or not the plaintiff is malingering. If a plaintiff is exaggerating symptoms, is this malingering, a factitious illness, or a somatoform disorder? Consideration of the possibility of malingering begins even before the psychiatric examination (see Chapter 19: "Malingering," this volume). Such suspicions should arise when review of medical records and other discovery documents demonstrates inconsistency in the plaintiff's presentation of symptoms or inconsistent results of psychological testing, or when the physical manifestations or clinical course are inconsistent with the typical presentation or course of a known mental disorder. These issues should always be addressed when doing a forensic assessment (Resnick 1988).

Several tests have been developed that are directed toward assessment of malingering. If such tests have been administered, the forensic psychiatrist can incorporate them into his assessment. If the issue of malingering is raised and the person in question has not been formally evaluated with one of these instruments, the forensic psychiatrist may administer the tests or ask the retaining attorney whether the evaluee may be tested by a psychologist experienced in assessing this question, and then the results can be included as part of the forensic psychiatrist's overall assessment.

The psychiatrist must come to some conclusion, implicitly or explicitly, about whether or not the plaintiff is malingering. The ability to make such a determination, even when the criteria under DSM-IV (American Psychiatric Association 1994)—and its text revision, DSM-IV-TR (American Psychiatric Association 2000)—are fulfilled, has been widely debated and criticized (Arkes et al. 1990). Malingering lies on a continuum, ranging from exaggeration of symptoms to outright feigning (Millis 1992; Resnick 1988; Rogers 1988, 1990; Zielinski 1994). Although DSM-IV advises that malingering should be strongly suspected in medicolegal contexts, such suspicion should not be taken to mean evidence of malingering (Rogers 1990). Caution must be exercised to ensure that a person is not unjustly labeled. The diagnosis of malingering requires considerable clinical judgment because an erroneous diagnosis can have substantial negative consequences for all parties.

## Recovery of Memory by Hypnosis

Since the early 1990s, the effect of hypnosis on memory has received a lot of attention. In several civil and criminal cases, courts have addressed this question and have discussed the problems associated with testimony of witnesses based on hypnotically enhanced or recovered memory (e.g., *Kline v. Ford Motor Co.* 1975; *People v. Shirley* 1982; *State v. Hurd* 1981; *Wyller v. Fairchild Hiller Corp.* 1974). Hypnosis has been shown to increase the amount of information "recalled" by the individual who has been hypnotized (Shields and Knox 1986; Stager and Lundy 1985). However, substantial data exist to indicate that hypnotized individuals report both accurate and inaccurate or confabulated material (Orne et al. 1984; Smith 1983). Hypnotized individuals also have a greater confidence in information "remembered"—even the inaccurate information (McConkey and Kinoshita 1988; Nogrady et al. 1985). Furthermore, laboratory findings reveal a willingness by some hypnotized subjects to accept intentionally suggested alterations in their memories (Laurence and Perry 1983; McCann and Sheehan 1988; Spanos and McLean 1986). Some subjects will accept changes to their memory and incorporate those changes into their beliefs about the accuracy of their memory (Nogrady et al. 1985).

Because of the questions raised regarding reliability of hypnotically enhanced memory, testimony based on enhanced memory was precluded from admission by many courts in criminal matters. In contrast, courts have usually allowed such testimony in personal injury claims. In criminal cases, recent courts have allowed such evidence, but only if it meets certain conditions; for example, whether the hypnotist followed certain guidelines (e.g., California Evidence Code § 795). Regardless, opposing counsel would be likely to attack the credibility of a witness who had undergone hypnosis. Even the credibility of the expert witness who had used hypnosis to enhance memory would be subject to close scrutiny on cross-examination.

In 1979, Dr. Martin Orne proposed a number of safeguards to minimize potentially distorted memories by hypnotized witnesses, especially in criminal cases:

> (1) The hypnotist must be a psychiatrist or psychologist experienced in the use of hypnosis; (2) to avoid bias, the hypnotist must be independent

> of the prosecution or defense; (3) all information the police or defense give the hypnotist before the session must be recorded; (4) before the session the subject must describe in detail to the hypnotist the facts as he remembers them, and the hypnotist must avoid influencing that description; (5) all contacts between the hypnotist and the subject—i.e., the prehypnotic examination, the hypnotic session, and the posthypnotic interrogation—must be recorded, preferably on videotape; and (6) no person other than the hypnotist and the subject may be present during the session, or even during the prehypnotic examination and the posthypnotic interrogation. (Orne 1979)

Nevertheless, experts have recommended that therapists avoid such techniques as hypnosis and sodium amytal interviews to recover memories, as they may hopelessly confound the plaintiff's legal case (Simon 1996a).

## The Psychiatric Expert

According to evidentiary rules, an expert witness must have the education, training, skills, experience, or knowledge of the procedures or subject matter that is in dispute and may give opinions on the issues if they will assist the trier of fact (Federal Rules of Evidence). An expert witness is not necessary if the issue in dispute is common knowledge to the average person. Case law and statutes govern such questions, which may vary state by state (see Chapter 4: "The Expert Witness," this volume). Current law governing whether expert testimony based on a novel methodology has a valid scientific basis was recently clarified by the federal appellate courts and the U.S. Supreme Court (*Daubert v. Merrell Dow Pharmaceuticals, Inc.* 1993; *General Electric Co. v. Joiner* 1997; *Kumho Tire Co., Ltd. v. Carmichael* 1999). Such testimony may be challenged in a special hearing, at which time the judge will determine the admissibility of the expert's testimony. The judge must consider five questions if following the current line of federal court cases:

1. Whether the expert is proposing to testify about matters growing naturally and directly out of research conducted independent of the litigation, or expressly for purposes of testimony (*Daubert v. Merrell Dow Pharmaceuticals, Inc.* 1993)
2. Whether the expert has unjustifiably extrapolated from an accepted premise to an unfounded conclusion (*General Electric Co. v. Joiner* 1997)
3. Whether the expert has adequately accounted for obvious alternative explanations (*Ambrosini v. Labarraque* 1996; *Claar v. Burlington N.R.R.* 1994)

4. Whether the expert is being as careful as he would be in his regular professional work outside paid litigation consulting (*Kumho Tire Co., Ltd. v. Carmichael* 1999)
5. Whether the field of expertise claimed by the expert is known to reach reliable results for the type of opinion the expert would give (*Kumho Tire Co., Ltd. v. Carmichael* 1999)

On the basis of the U.S. Supreme Court cases of *Daubert v. Merrell Dow Pharmaceuticals, Inc.* (1993) and *Kumho Tire Co., Ltd. v. Carmichael* (1999), the theory and methodology underlying the testimony is further scrutinized before its admission, with the court addressing the following issues:

1. Whether the theory can be or has been tested (scientific methodology)
2. Whether the theory has been subjected to peer review and publication
3. The known or potential rate of error of the particular technique and the existence and maintenance of standards controlling the technique's operation
4. Consideration of general acceptance within the scientific community (*Daubert v. Merrell Dow Pharmaceuticals, Inc.* 1993)

The above factors addressed by the court are meant to be essentially a guide to judges, but judges have discretion in considering the nature of the case (*Kumho Tire Co., Ltd. v. Carmichael* 1999). Many state courts do not follow the federal line of cases but use the *Frye* test, which bases admissibility on whether the technique or theory has been generally accepted by the profession (*Frye v. United States* 1923).

## *Engagement by Attorney*

The forensic psychiatrist is initially contacted by an attorney, who will advise the psychiatrist of the nature of the case and elicit the psychiatrist's interest in participating in the case. The psychiatrist's experience in the matter in dispute is frequently discussed, as are fees and fee policies. A request is usually then made by the attorney for a copy of the psychiatrist's curriculum vitae. During these discussions, the psychiatrist may want to provide the attorney with an estimate of the time necessary for review of documents and for the completion of a competent assessment.

If the attorney wants to retain the psychiatrist, it is advisable to have a confirmatory letter from the attorney accepting the psychiatrist's fee arrangements, outlining the dates by which reports and testimony may be needed. Psychiatrists may prefer to send a letter to the attorney memorializing the financial and service arrangements so there will be no misunderstanding. Contingent fee arrangements for expert services are considered unethical (Reid 2002a).

Once the psychiatrist commits to providing services and is aware of the deadlines imposed by the court for reports or testimony, this should be acknowledged and memorialized in writing. Any conflicts with regard to deadlines should be discussed to seek possible alternatives. Agreement should also be sought on whether or not collateral interviews or depositions of key witnesses will be necessary to enhance the assessment. If collateral interviews may not be appropriate, questions might be suggested by the psychiatrist for the attorney to ask in depositions of such individuals.

At any time in the process of engagement or evaluation, it may become evident that the expert's opinions are adverse to the retaining party's position. This may become apparent immediately within the first few minutes of conversation with an attorney, or it may not become clear until documents are reviewed and the evaluee interviewed. If this situation arises, experts should communicate their opinions to the retaining attorney as soon as possible. This gives the attorney the opportunity to seek another expert or to settle the case before the parties have expended much time and money. If the evaluation by the forensic psychiatrist is supportive of the retaining attorney's position, then the psychiatrist may be involved as an expert witness in the matter until its conclusion.

## *Consultation With Attorney*

An attorney representing a plaintiff frequently seeks informal confidential consultation from an expert to determine whether or not a particular issue should be pursued on behalf of the client. A defense attorney likewise may seek informal consultation on whether there are any factual defenses to a plaintiff's claim of mental disorder. Attorneys may also seek advice regarding available current literature or seek an understanding of the pertinent neuropsychiatric issues. The attorney may provide certain literature obtained during the discovery procedures to seek the psychiatrist's opinions or to assist in educating the psychiatrist in the area under consideration. The attorney may be interested in an opinion about the opposing expert's or treating doctor's assessment or treatment. The attorney may also seek suggestions for appropriate consultants in other fields of expertise or for other psychiatrists who may be retained as treating or testifying experts in the matter.

Every effort should be made to prevent intrusion into the therapeutic relationship. If the psychiatrist is providing the plaintiff's treatment, an independent evaluation done by another forensic psychiatrist is desirable. This will help avoid the adverse effects inherent in providing both treatment and expert testimony. In all likelihood, the opposing attorney will be able to subpoena the treating psychiatrist for a deposition under oath if the psychotherapist-patient privilege has been waived. Certainly, the treating psychiatrist's records can be provided to the independent evaluator. Nevertheless, any testimony the treating psychiatrist gives under these circumstances should, if possible, be limited. The scope of such testimony should be confined to the facts and any bases for decisions made during therapy without rendering new opinions on the issues in dispute in the litigation.

Consultation of the forensic psychiatrist with attorneys before any decision to retain the expert to testify is confidential and protected from discovery by the opposing party under the attorney's work-product privilege. Once the attorney retains the psychiatrist to testify, further consultation is subject to discovery by the opposing party. In some jurisdictions, the decision to retain the expert may open the door to discovery of prior consultations between the expert and the attorney.

## *Information Provided by Retaining Attorney*

Information provided to the forensic psychiatrist will be the result of informal and formal discovery by the attorney. Products of informal discovery may include a literature search conducted by the attorney or records acquired through the client's permission, such as scholastic, military, medical, and psychiatric records. However, after the complaint is filed, served, and answered, formal discovery procedures are available to both parties. These include written interrogatories to be answered by the opposing party, requests for admission, requests for production of documents and things, depositions, and requests for independent psychiatric examination. A brief discussion of these formal discovery procedures will be helpful for the forensic psychiatrist to understand the limitations, as well as the uses, of the responses to such discovery.

**Interrogatories.** Interrogatories are written questions propounded to other parties involved in litigation to elicit the facts and circumstances relevant to the issues in dispute. The answers to interrogatories must be signed by the party under oath. In some jurisdictions, the number of written questions allowed is limited, and in others it is unlimited. The forensic psychiatrist may be consulted by the retaining attorney to assist in formulating relevant questions that may aid in this part of the discovery process.

**Requests for admission.** Requests for admission are factual statements made by one party to another party wherein the responding party must either admit or deny the factual statement. It may include facts about any relevant issue. In most jurisdictions, if the party does not admit or deny a request for admission within 30 days, the statement is admitted and may be relied on by the forensic psychiatrist as a basis for any expert opinion.

**Requests for production.** One party may request any relevant document or thing from the other party unless the document requested is privileged. Such requests usually include medical and psychiatric records when the plaintiff claims a psychiatric injury. Medical records, including psychiatric records, are important to understanding the diagnosis made by other physicians and the past and current care provided to the plaintiff. If psychological test reports are requested, the raw data on which these reports are based should also be requested.

**Depositions.** Depositions are oral questions posed by an attorney to any person who has relevant information about facts, circumstances, or opinions about the issues in dispute. The responses of the deponent are under oath and recorded by a court reporter. As a consequence, if collateral interviews of others would be helpful in doing the forensic psychiatric assessment and such other individuals are unwilling or unable to be interviewed by the psychiatrist, the psychiatrist may advise the attorney to take depositions of those individuals. The forensic psychiatrist can provide questions for the attorney to ask during the deposition that the psychiatrist would have asked if there were an opportunity to perform a collateral interview. In the alternative, the forensic psychiatrist may accompany the attorney to the deposition and provide questions in writing for the attorney to ask. The psychiatrist may also suggest necessary and helpful follow-up questions during the deposition. Such assistance to the attorney in the role of advisory witness is allowed in most jurisdictions.

**Independent psychiatric examination.** The defendant may request that the plaintiff be examined by the defendant's retained psychiatrist. The retaining attorney should provide all documents relevant to psychiatric issues for the psychiatrist's review before the expert examines the plaintiff. The attorney may have difficulty determining what is relevant to the psychiatrist's assessment. Therefore, the psychiatrist should request that all discovery material be provided. The psychiatrist then can determine which documents are relevant and which are not and review only those documents that are useful in evaluating the psychiatric issues under consideration.

The defendant will have only one opportunity for such an examination unless good cause exists (as determined by the court) for a second such independent examination. During this examination, it is not uncommon for the plaintiff to have his or her attorney or a family member present or to bring a tape recorder to the session (Simon 1996b). If such a condition is disruptive to the examination, it may be brought to the court's attention and the judge will rule on the issue. Results of the independent psychiatric examination and the forensic psychiatrist's opinions are documented in a report. This report is available to all parties in the litigation. The report of the examination is usually requested in advance of taking the forensic psychiatrist's deposition.

The psychiatrist should explain clearly to the evaluee at the outset of the clinical interview the purpose for the examination, the fact that no physician-patient relationship is being established to provide care, and to whom the report of the examination will be sent. The psychiatrist should elicit a complete and detailed history of the incident causing injury during the plaintiff's clinical interview. He should consider all contributing causes to the mental disorder claimed, including discussion of past medical and psychiatric history. All relevant medical records previously reviewed by the examiner may be discussed with the injured party during the interview. Any psychological testing previously performed may also be reviewed with the plaintiff, including the raw data, if pertinent.

### *Forensic Psychiatric Report*

The psychiatric expert usually provides an opinion letter or report to the retaining attorney following the clinical interview and mental status examination of the injured party and any collateral interviews relevant to the assessment. The retaining attorney then provides copies of this report to the opposing attorney. However, if the plaintiff's attorney requests the examination, he may not want a written report. Therefore, it behooves the psychiatrist to inquire at the outset if the plaintiff's attorney desires a written report (Reid 2002b).

Once all available facts of the claim are marshaled and there is an understanding of the factors that play a role in diagnosis, cause, extent of impairment, and prognosis, it becomes a matter of presenting the information clearly and credibly in a written report. The format of the forensic psychiatry report depends a great deal on the psychiatrist's writing style. Thus, the following discussion is based on this author's style. However, so long as the subjects are covered, they may be addressed in any reasonable manner (for an in-depth discussion, see Chapter 7: "The Forensic Examination and Report," this volume).

The report should contain a preamble describing the fact that the plaintiff was advised that the interview did not establish a physician-patient relationship, that the plaintiff understood the purpose of the examination, that the results of the examination and the examiner's opinions would be provided in writing, and that the examiner may testify about those opinions in a deposition or in court (i.e., there was no expectation of confidentiality by the plaintiff). Many attorneys appreciate the provision of a brief introduction and summary of the expert's opinions at the beginning of the report, and this can also be included in an introductory section.

The psychiatrist should then list the documents and any other references or sources of information that formed the database. A review or summary of the relevant data obtained from each of the documents in the database pertinent to the evaluation may be noted. A detailed history of the incident, including when, where, and how the injury occurred, as well as any background information such as preexisting illnesses that may have contributed to the severity of the psychiatric disorder, may be noted under separate headings. The psychiatrist should also note a complete history of the plaintiff's mental disorder, with documentation of the progression of symptoms; treatment received, including medications prescribed; responses; and side effects or complications of treatment. This should include descriptions of the symptoms the plaintiff manifested shortly after the injury; symptoms currently manifested; current and past treatment; the plaintiff's perception of the claimed mental disorder and care received; and how the illness (if any) is affecting work, family, and other aspects of the plaintiff's life.

The report should also document the results and interpretation of psychological testing administered and a complete Mental Status Examination noting pertinent signs and symptoms (or absence of signs and symptoms) relevant to the diagnosis claimed. Diagnostic assessment should follow DSM-IV multiaxial format (American Psychiatric Association 2000).

### *Discussion*

The discussion section is arguably the most important part of the forensic psychiatric report. It should address the parts of the database relevant to the opinions being rendered. The psychiatrist should note that all opinions are rendered with "reasonable medical certainty (probability)"

(Firestone 1984). The psychiatrist should discuss the criteria supporting any diagnosis under consideration, and the sources of information supporting or ruling out the diagnostic criteria should be clearly documented. The psychiatrist should also address recommended treatment, if any, and estimated costs of that treatment, as well as prognosis, bases for the opinions, and any other issues in dispute pertinent to the opinions. The effect of the mental disorder on quality of life, the effect of the mental disorder on other physical problems, and its anticipated effect on work and social and family relationships, as well as the effect of the mental disorder on the injured individual's well-being, should be discussed.

The attorney may not receive certain relevant documents before the psychiatrist's examination. If the psychiatrist is aware at the time of the preparation of the initial report that additional information will be obtained, he may note that his opinions may be subject to modification pending review of additional information. This statement helps maintain credibility if a change is necessary and reflects an openness to consider alternative opinions if the new facts so indicate. Documents received at a later date should be and usually are forwarded for the psychiatrist's review. An addendum regarding whether or not the additional information would change the psychiatrist's opinions and the reasons for such change, if any, may then also be requested. The retaining attorney may want to review a preliminary draft before submitting any final report of the psychiatrist's opinions. This helps ensure that the psychiatrist has addressed all important issues and may avoid the need for addendum reports.

### *Expert Witness Disclosures*

Disclosures of the expert witnesses and summaries of the experts' opinions are usually requested, either as a separate discovery procedure or in written interrogatories, as part of pretrial discovery. There may be a rule requiring simultaneous disclosure of experts or other order of disclosure, depending on jurisdiction and local court rules. Following such disclosures, depositions of the experts may then be taken. The psychiatrist should request the opportunity to review any such disclosures before they are submitted to other parties or the court. The forensic psychiatrist then has the opportunity to advise the retaining attorney of the need to modify the documents if they contain misleading or incorrect information.

### *Testimony at Deposition*

The discovery deposition provides the opposing party the opportunity to learn about the opinions that will be given by the expert witness at the trial and to explore all the bases for those opinions. The deposition also gives the opposing party the opportunity to assess the credibility of the expert witness and to assess how effective the witness will be in giving testimony at trial. The opposing attorney will attempt to confine the expert's opinion to the facts on which the opinion is based.

Expert witnesses should arrange to give deposition testimony in an environment in which they feel most comfortable. An opposing attorney, under the local court rules, may have the right to take experts' depositions in the attorney's or the court reporter's office or in a court conference room. However, if they prefer, experts may request that the deposition be taken in their own offices. Most opposing attorneys will accommodate the expert's request in hopes of acquiring future concessions.

The expert witness should meet with the retaining attorney in a predeposition conference. This important meeting will allow the psychiatrist to gain an understanding of the status of the litigation, how the testimony at deposition will be used, and whether the attorney is expecting to try the case or is using the testimony to attempt early settlement. If the case is not anticipated to go to trial, and the deposition testimony is primarily intended to assist in settlement, the attorney may want the expert to be elaborative in responding to questions without concerns about volunteering information. However, if the case is anticipated to go to trial, the attorney will usually ask that experts be succinct in their responses and not attempt to educate the opposition by volunteering information.

The expert should maintain an awareness of the implications of certain buzzwords, both in the written report and in testimony. For example, psychiatrists tend to use the word "feel" instead of the stronger "it is my psychiatric opinion that . . ." Psychiatrists are also prone to use the words "speculate" or "speculation." Such words are interpreted by most courts as meaning a "guess" and therefore will weaken any opinion intended to be admitted with "reasonable psychiatric probability." Similarly, the words "believe," "think," and "know" are frequently used interchangeably but may be interpreted differently by the court. "Believe" may be interpreted as something stated by a respected authority that the expert has read or heard. The word "think" may be interpreted to mean that the expert has seen other situations similar to the one under consideration in this litigation and that it is the expert's opinion that this situation is similar to the others. The court may interpret "know" as an indication that the expert has seen this exact situation on many occasions and thus is certain that his or her opinion is correct.

The use of inappropriate qualifying words in expert reports and testimony may adversely affect the outcome of the case even though all other aspects of the expert's evaluation and opinions are clear. For example, the words "possibility," "may," and "might" imply the lack of reasonable probability or certainty and will usually preclude the expert's opinion from being admitted. In contrast, the use of the words "likely," "more likely than not," and "probably" will usually allow the opinion to be admitted.

During deposition testimony, the expert must answer attorneys' questions even when there is an objection raised, unless the objection is that the information is subject to an evidentiary privilege. The percipient expert witness (e.g., the treating psychiatrist) may be obligated to raise privilege objections when a question invades the psychotherapist-patient privilege and the patient has not waived the privilege. If the patient's attorney is present, he may advise the expert witness before the deposition that the privilege has been waived or may state this during the deposition. Otherwise, any objections made by the attorney should not preclude answering the questions posed. Remember that the attorney does not represent the psychiatrist, but one of the litigating parties.

Experts should be aware that there is no need to rush to answer questions. They should always think carefully about both the questions asked by the opposing attorney and the answers to those questions. If the retaining attorney has advised keeping answers as succinct as possible, experts should take the time to think about the questions. They should then think about how to answer the questions, think about the answers, and only then answer the questions as succinctly as possible. When necessary, the expert may qualify the answer. At times, the expert cannot answer a question because of the manner in which the opposing attorney has phrased it. If this happens, the expert should not rephrase the question for the deposing attorney, but should merely express on the record that the question cannot be answered as phrased. The attorney may ask why it could not be answered and then rephrase the question.

At the end of the deposition, experts are usually asked whether they want to review the transcript to correct it or want to waive the review. Experts should always review the transcript of their deposition testimony. Court reporters sometimes make errors that may alter the meaning of an answer given. The expert may have misunderstood the question at the time it was posed. Reviewing the transcript provides the expert the opportunity to correct such errors and ensure that testimony is as accurate as possible. The party responsible for payment for the time involved in the expert's review and correction of the transcript should be clarified either before the deposition or on the record during the deposition.

Depositions may also be used to preserve testimony when the expert is unavailable to testify at the time of trial. The deposition testimony is considered as though it is testimony given at trial. One significant difference, however, is that the judge is not present to rule on objections. Such objections are preserved for ruling before or at the time of trial. Frequently, such depositions are taken by videotape and the testimony shown on a video monitor in the courtroom after any objectionable questions and answers sustained by the court have been edited out. Discovery depositions may also be taken by video, but this is not as common as in depositions to preserve testimony.

## *Trial*

The vast majority of personal injury cases are settled before trial. However, experts should never assume that a case will settle and that courtroom testimony will not be needed. The greater the familiarity of experts with courtroom procedure, the more comfortable they will feel giving testimony at trial. For example, if the expert witness has not previously testified before that particular judge or in that particular courtroom, the expert may wish to visit the courtroom or attend the trial of another case in which the assigned judge is presiding. Increased familiarity with the physical setting or the style of the presiding judge may provide the expert with a greater level of comfort in the courtroom.

A trial has an organized series of procedures. Familiarity with the organization of courtroom procedures will also increase the expert witness' comfort level as well as allow greater awareness of how the testimony fits into the entire scheme of the trial. Many evidentiary matters are resolved before trial, including whether or not certain issues are precluded and whether or not the expert witness will be allowed to testify about certain matters. These decisions may influence the psychiatrist's presentation of opinions at trial. A pretrial conference with the attorney is mandatory to address such issues, as well as other issues that may affect trial testimony.

Jury selection, referred to as voir dire, occurs at the outset of the trial. During this critical procedure, the attorneys have their only opportunity to interact directly with the panel of potential jurors to determine their suitability for selection as jurors in the case. In the voir dire questioning, the attorneys will attempt to elicit the potential jurors' biases for one party or another. It is not uncommon for an attorney to retain psychiatric or psychological consultants to assist in jury selection. Such consultants may help evaluate the manner in which the potential jurors answer questions and the meanings of their nonverbal behaviors. These may be indicative of bias that will either aid or detract from a particular party's strategy in prosecuting or defending the case at trial (Wagner 1981).

The court frequently allows expert witnesses to testify when it is most convenient for them. The court is aware that the parties are paying significant fees for expert testimony. In addition, the court allows this convenience in consideration of the experts' professional obligations and their need to return to their offices or hospitals as soon as possible. In such cases, lay witnesses may be excused temporarily from the witness stand.

## *Testimony*

As in the case of deposition testimony, the expert witness should meet with the attorney before testifying at trial. This meeting should address which issues to emphasize in trial testimony, what the witness can anticipate to be asked on cross-examination, and how the witness' testimony fits into the entirety of the evidence being presented.

A witness' testimony begins with direct examination by the retaining attorney. The first questions on direct examination are usually intended to establish the witness' expertise to qualify him or her as an expert. The retaining attorney will present the witness' credentials and curriculum vitae. Following this presentation, the opposing attorney may request a voir dire of the witness' credentials. Questions may then be posed by the opposing attorney as to whether the witness should be precluded from expressing opinions in particular areas in which the witness may not have the requisite education, knowledge, experience, training, or skills.

Direct examination questions are open-ended, frequently beginning with "What . . . ," "When . . . ," "Why . . . ," "Where . . . ," "How . . . ," or "How much . . ." This allows expert witnesses to present testimony in their own style. The court, however, will not usually allow a narrative-type answer that is unresponsive to the question. As a consequence, although the witness may wax eloquent in answering, the answer must be responsive to the question. The judge will rule on any objections made by the attorneys. If the judge sustains an objection, the witness must cease answering the question. If the objection is overruled, the witness may proceed to answer.

If testifying in support of the plaintiff's claim, the expert should carefully explain on direct examination how the psychological injury has reduced the plaintiff's emotional and intellectual capacity to confront the challenges of a competitive world. The forensic psychiatrist, when giving expert testimony, must therefore analyze the status of the plaintiff as a whole person. This analysis becomes more complicated when the plaintiff has a preexisting psychiatric disorder. When the experts cannot distinguish a condition that existed before the injury from a condition experienced after, the defendant may be held responsible for the entire indivisible condition that the plaintiff now suffers (*Blayne v. Byers* 1967). If the plaintiff was more susceptible to injuries because of a prior psychological condition, the defendant remains liable for any injuries caused by the act or omission. This is the case even if the plaintiff's injuries are greater than those suffered by an individual without plaintiff's preexisting psychological condition. The defendant is responsible for "breaking the camel's back," even though the contribution may have been only "one straw." In such cases, the expert witness should attempt to help the jury understand how the current injury aggravated the preexisting condition or predisposition. The expert should discuss whether this preexisting condition was active or in remission and whether it was stable or degenerative.

Following the direct examination, the opposing attorney will cross-examine the expert on any issues about which the expert testified on direct examination. On cross-examination, the attorney will usually ask leading questions that are closed-ended, requiring a "yes" or "no" answer by the witness. The expert witness should answer in this manner and defer any necessary explanation of those answers until the sponsoring attorney's redirect examination questions. At this time, any issues raised by the opposing attorney on cross-examination may be clarified or explained. If the question cannot be answered with a "yes" or "no," the witness may ask the judge to allow an explanation.

The opposing attorney may take several approaches in attempting to neutralize the value of the expert's testimony. Attorneys are taught, as a general rule of cross-examination, to challenge the factual bases for the opinions of the expert and, if unable to do this effectively, to challenge the credibility of the expert. Thus, opposing attorneys may challenge the expert witness' credentials or expertise in an attempt to impeach the witness' credibility. They may challenge the manner in which the evaluation was done or the expert's experience. The witness should not take the cross-examining attorney's challenges personally and should be careful not to respond to them in an angry or argumentative manner.

Typically, the judge will excuse the expert witness after the attorneys for both parties have indicated they have no more questions. Once excused, the witness should leave the courtroom rather than stay to observe the rest of the trial. Otherwise, jurors may have the impression that the witness has an interest in the outcome of the trial and is not being objective.

### *Demeanor of the Expert Witness*

Expert testimony is intended to assist the trier of fact (the judge or jury) in determining the merits of the case. Expert psychiatric witnesses should convey credibility. They should appear objective, and although they should be an advocate for their opinions, they should not advocate for any particular party. The expert witness should concede points in favor of the opposition during direct and cross-examination that can be explained or clarified during redirect examination, if necessary. The witness should communicate effectively by avoiding the use of medical or psychiatric jargon and should explain concepts so that a layperson can understand them. Any medical or psychiatric terms used should be explained. The expert witness should attempt to develop rapport with the jurors by speaking directly to them when explaining concepts (Reid 2002c).

## Conclusion

The forensic psychiatrist's assessment may be a critical component in both the plaintiff's proof and the defendant's defense in personal injury litigation. However, whether retained by plaintiff or defense, forensic psychiatrists should maintain credibility and integrity. They should confine their opinions to observed or documented facts rather than engage in speculation. They should endeavor to clearly communicate the meaning and implications of any psychiatric opinions that bear on the injured party's claims.

The basis of the forensic psychiatrist's testimony is a thorough, objective, and competent evaluation of the plaintiff's history and mental status. This evaluation should be coupled with an awareness of the issues in dispute and an understanding of how the rendered opinions fit into the resolution of those issues. The services of the forensic psychiatrist adhering to these principles in personal injury litigation will continue to be a critical and important contribution to the legal process.

## Key Points

- The forensic psychiatrist's assessment is an important component of both the plaintiff's proof and the defendant's defense in personal injury litigation.
- The forensic psychiatrist should maintain credibility and integrity.
- The forensic psychiatrist should confine opinions to observed or documented facts rather than engage in speculation.

- The basis of the forensic psychiatrist's testimony is a thorough, objective, and competent evaluation of the plaintiff's history and mental status.
- The psychiatric evaluation should be done with an awareness of the issues in dispute and an understanding of how the rendered opinions fit into the litigation and resolution of the issues in dispute.
- The forensic psychiatrist should endeavor to clearly communicate the meaning and implications of any psychiatric opinions that bear on the injured party's claims.

## Practice Guidelines

1. Have a clear agreement, preferably in writing, with the retaining attorney at the outset, addressing services and fee policies.
2. Determine the issues in dispute relevant to the psychiatric injury under consideration.
3. Discuss diagnosis, causation, and other pertinent issues based on a thorough review of provided documents and psychiatric examination of the injured person.
4. Understand the legal process and how best to effectively and credibly contribute to the process.
5. Understand forensic report writing, addressing the issues about which the retaining attorney is concerned.
6. Be objective in conveying opinions and bases for opinions.
7. Maintain credibility in report writing and testimony.
8. Do not provide opinions in the forensic report or during testimony that are beyond your expertise.
9. Insist on predeposition and pretrial conferences with the attorney.
10. Be yourself, be humble, and do not be argumentative when testifying.
11. Do not advocate for either party, but do advocate for your opinions.
12. Be truthful and concede points, even if unhelpful to the party that retained you.

## References

Ambrosini v Labarraque, 101 F.3d 129 (D.C. Cir. 1996)
American Psychiatric Association: Diagnostic and Statistical Manual of Mental Disorders, 4th Edition. Washington, DC, American Psychiatric Association, 1994
American Psychiatric Association: Diagnostic and Statistical Manual of Mental Disorders, 4th Edition, Text Revision. Washington, DC, American Psychiatric Association, 2000

Arkes HR, Faust D, Guilmette TJ: Response to Schmidt's (1988) comments on Faust, Hart, Guilmette, and Arkes (1988). Professional Psychology: Research and Practice 21:3–4, 1990

Blayne v Byers, 429 P.2d 397, 405–406 (Idaho 1967)

Bourne v Washburn, 441 F.2d 1022, 1026 (D.C. Cir. 1971)

California Evidence Code § 795: Testimony of hypnosis subject; admissibility; conditions

Claar v Burlington N.R.R., 29 F.3d 499 (9th Cir. 1994)

Daubert v Merrell Dow Pharmaceuticals, Inc, 113 S. Ct. 2786 (1993)

Federal Rules of Evidence § 700 et seq and similar state rules of evidence

Frye v United States, 293 Fed. 1013 (D.C. Cir. 1923)

Firestone MH: With reasonable medical certainty (probability). Legal Aspects Med Pract 12(6):1–4, 1984

General Electric Co v Joiner, 552 U.S. 136 (1997)

Kline v Ford Motor Co, 523 F.2d 1067 (9th Cir. 1975)

Kumho Tire Co, Ltd v Carmichael, 119 S. Ct. 1167 (1999)

Laurence JR, Perry C: Hypnotically created memory among highly hypnotizable subjects. Science 222:523–524, 1983

McCann T, Sheehan PW: Hypnotically induced pseudo-memories—sampling their conditions among hypnotizable subjects. J Pers Soc Psychol 54:339–346, 1988

McConkey KM, Kinoshita S: The influence of hypnosis on memory after one day and one week. J Abnorm Psychol 97:48–53, 1988

Millis SR: The recognition memory test in the detection of malingered and exaggerated memory deficits. Clin Neuropsychol 6:406–414, 1992

Nogrady H, McConkey KM, Perry C: Enhancing visual memory: trying hypnosis, trying imagination, and trying again. J Abnorm Psychol 94:195–204, 1985

Orne MT: The use and misuse of hypnosis in court. Int J Clin Exp Hypnosis 27: 311–341, 1979

Orne MT, Soskis DA, Dinges DF, et al: Hypnotically induced testimony, in Eyewitness Testimony: Psychological Perspectives. Edited by Wells GL, Loftus FF. New York, Cambridge University Press, 1984, pp 171–213

People v Shirley, 31 Cal.3d 18, 181 Cal. Rptr. 243, 250 (1982)

Reid WH: Law and psychiatry: forensic work and nonforensic clinicians, Part I. Journal of Psychiatric Practice 8(2):119–122, 2002a

Reid WH: Law and psychiatry: forensic work and nonforensic clinicians, Part II: reports and depositions. Journal of Psychiatric Practice 8(3):181–185, 2002b

Reid WH: Law and Psychiatry: Forensic work and nonforensic clinicians, Part III: testifying in court. Journal of Psychiatric Practice 8(4):246–249, 2002c

Resnick PL: Malingering of post traumatic disorders, in Clinical Assessment of Malingering and Deception. Edited by Rogers R. New York, Guilford, 1988, pp 84–103

Rogers R: Current status of clinical methods, in Clinical Assessment of Malingering and Deception. Edited by Rogers R. New York, Guilford, 1988, pp 293–308

Rogers R: Models of feigned mental illness. Professional Psychology: Research and Practice 2:182–188, 1990

Shields IW, Knox VJ: Level of processing as a determinant of hypnotic hypermnesia. J Abnorm Psychol 95:358–364, 1986

Simon RI: Bad Men Do What Good Men Dream: A Forensic Psychiatrist Illuminates the Darker Side of Human Behavior. Washington, DC, American Psychiatric Press, 1996a

Simon RI: "Three's a crowd": the presence of third parties during the forensic psychiatric examination. J Am Acad Psychiatry Law 24:3–25, 1996b

Smith MD: Hypnotic memory enhancement of witnesses: does it work? Psychol Bull 94:387–407, 1983

Spanos NP, McLean J: Hypnotically created pseudo memories. Br J Exp Clin Hypnosis 3:155–159, 1986

Stager GL, Lundy RM: Hypnosis and the learning and recall of visually presented material. Int J Clin Exp Hypnosis 33:27–34, 1985

State v Hurd, 86 N.J. 525, 432 A.2d 86 (1981)

Wagner W: Art of Advocacy: Jury Selection. New York, Matthew-Bender, 1981

Wyller v Fairchild Hiller Corp, 503 F.2d 506 (9th Cir. 1974)

Zielinski JJ: Malingering and defensiveness in the neuropsychological assessment of mild traumatic brain injury. Clin Psychol Sci Pract 1:169–183, 1994

## Suggested Readings

American College of Legal Medicine: Legal Medicine, 6th Edition. London, Elsevier, 2003

Blinder M: Psychiatry in the Everyday Practice of Law. New York/San Francisco, Lawyers Co-operative/Bancroft-Whitney, 1982

Hall HV, Pritchard DA: Detecting Malingering and Deception. Delray Beach, FL, St Lucie Press, 1996

Halleck SL, Law in the Practice of Psychiatry: A Handbook for Clinicians. New York, Plenum, 1980

Heilburn K: Principles of Forensic Mental Health Assessment. New York, Kluwer/Plenum, 2001

Lees-Haley PR: Pseudoscientific Mumbo Jumbo. Encino, CA, Grandmother Hunter's Own, 1991

Richards EP, Rathburn KC: Law and the Physician. Boston, MA, Little, Brown, 1993

Rosner R (ed): Critical Issues in American Psychiatry and the Law. Springfield, IL, Charles C Thomas, 1982

Scheflin AW, Shapiro JL: Trance on Trial. New York, Guilford, 1989

Simon RI: Clinical Psychiatry and the Law. Washington, DC, American Psychiatric Press, 1987

Simon RI (ed): Posttraumatic Stress Disorder in Litigation: Guidelines for Forensic Assessment. Washington, DC, American Psychiatric Publishing, 2003

Slovenko R: Psychiatry in Law—Law in Psychiatry. New York, Brunner-Routledge, 2002

C H A P T E R 1 3

# Disability

Albert M. Drukteinis, M.D., J.D.

## Introduction

Determining disability is the most common task of forensic psychiatry performed by the practicing clinician. Routinely, clinicians are asked by patients to authorize brief or extended periods away from work because of mental symptoms. Clinicians are also typically the ones to offer initial opinions about a patient's permanent disability.

Such psychiatric disability claims are frequent and not likely to diminish. The National Institute of Mental Health Epidemiologic Catchment Area Program and the National Comorbidity Survey have estimated 1-year mental and addictive disorder prevalence rates approaching 30% and lifetime rates approaching 50% (Kessler et al. 1994; Regier et al. 1984). Psychiatric disturbances have become the largest single reason for disability awards by the Social Security Administration, accounting for 22% of all claims (Leo 2002). More than half of all disability recipients have a mental disorder (Kochlar and Scott 1995). Psychiatric disability claims are estimated to cost about $150 billion a year (Sederer and Clemens 2002).

In addition to Social Security disability claims, clinicians are often asked to provide opinions on short-term and long-term disability for private insurance, worker's compensation, personal injury claims, accommodations under the Americans with Disabilities Act, fitness for duty evaluations, and incapacity under the Family and Medical Leave Act. Therefore, clinicians can expect to confront disability issues as a routine part of their practice and should learn ways to provide objective opinions and to avoid common pitfalls in the process. In forensic psychiatry, the issue of objectivity is so crucial that the American Academy of Psychiatry and the Law, in its code of ethics, recommends that psychiatrists not serve as both treating clinician and forensic evaluator (see American Academy of Psychiatry and the Law 1995). Practically, however, disability issues are so frequent that it would be impossible for a clinician to recommend an independent forensic evaluation on the question of disability every time it came up.

The purpose of this chapter is to provide guidelines for the treating clinician, both to assess a patient's disability objectively and to understand the inherent limitations of serving in both roles. We begin with a case vignette that demonstrates some of the key points in disability determinations.

## Clinical Vignette

Mr. G is a 58-year-old practicing trial attorney who is claiming disability because of depression. Shortly before being referred for outpatient psychiatric treatment, Mr. G was admitted to the psychiatric unit of the local community hospital with severe suicidal ideation. He reported that he had been very depressed and had symptoms of decreased appetite and weight loss, sleep disturbance, difficulty concentrating, withdrawal from family and friends, anxiety, and anger outbursts. Mr. G was diagnosed as having recurrent, severe major depressive disorder, without psychotic features.

Mr. G had a previous history of depression while in law school, for which he received counseling and a brief course of antidepressant medication. He had no other psychiatric or psychological treatment in his life. He has used alcohol regularly, more in recent months in conjunction with marital problems. Two weeks before his admission to the psychiatric unit, his wife left him, claiming that his time away from home and inattentiveness to her because of his practice had made her life miserable. With their children grown and out of the house, she claimed that she could no longer live with him.

During his 6-day hospitalization, Mr. G was placed on an antidepressant medication and directed to Alcoholics Anonymous meetings. A joint counseling session with his wife revealed her lack of interest in maintaining the relationship. In therapy, Mr. G discussed being overwhelmed by his law practice, his inability to concentrate, his difficulty meeting a demanding schedule of depositions and trials, and his problem facing the daily stress of an adversarial process. He reported becoming panicked when anticipating a court appearance.

Mr. G's treatment team at the hospital recommended that he not return to the same work. They suggested that he apply for Social Security Disability Insurance benefits, as well as benefits under a personal disability insurance policy.

## Defining Disability

A mental disorder does not automatically equate to disability. As elementary as that sounds, misconception about this principle is the main source of errors in disability evaluations. The American Medical Association (AMA) *Guides to the Evaluation of Permanent Impairment,* Fifth Edition (American Medical Association 2001) makes a distinction between impairment and disability. Impairment is defined as "a loss, loss of use, or derangement of any body part, organ system, or organ function" (p. 2). Such alteration of an individual's health status is assessed by medical means. In contrast, disability is "an alteration of an individual's capacity to meet personal, social, or occupational demands, or statutory or regulatory requirements because of an impairment" (p. 8). Disability is said to be assessed by medical and nonmedical means. Therefore, a mental disorder may or may not result in an impairment, and an impairment may or may not result in a disability.

Despite their distinction, the terms impairment and disability are often used interchangeably. For example, once a medical opinion is offered about work impairment, more than a medical consideration has been made, as the nature of the work must be understood from the nonmedical facts that are available. In addition, although the final determination of disability is made by a fact-finder (e.g., the court, a governmental agency, an insurance company panel), medical opinions on disability are not necessarily inappropriate. Routinely, medical opinions are offered on disability, including both its degree and expected duration (Drukteinis 2002). Again, however, the determination of disability requires more than a medical consideration of symptoms and health status. How and why the capacity to meet an occupational demand has been altered must be identified.

The AMA *Guides* offers a breakdown of impairment that can be used in making an assessment of disability. The categories for evaluating psychiatric impairment in the AMA *Guides* are activities of daily living; social functioning; concentration, persistence, and pace; and deterioration or decompensation in complex or worklike settings.

The AMA *Guides* provides a number of examples of impairment in each category as well as a system of classification ranging from class I (no impairment) to class V (extreme impairment). The focus of the *Guides* is said to be on impairment, not disability or work disability. However, a class V impairment is considered to significantly impede useful functioning and can probably be inferred to result in disability. In addition, because opinions about impairment should take into account work circumstances, they go beyond a purely medical consideration of health and may be tantamount to an opinion on disability (Drukteinis 2002). Therefore, an opinion on either impairment or disability may be appropriate and may not be that distinguishable as long as it includes an awareness of the patient's medical (clinical) and nonmedical (nonclinical or factual) circumstances.

In some states, a further caveat in disability determinations is the need to apply a percentage rating of impairment, regardless of whether the impairment is physical or mental. The AMA *Guides* specifically does not provide percentage estimates of mental impairments, indicating that "there are no precise measures of impairment in mental disorders. The use of percentages implies a certainty that does not exist" (American Medical Association 2001, p. 361). To circumvent this, some evaluators rely on the percentage criteria in the section on "Emotional or Behavioral Impairments" of Chapter 13 of the *Guides,* "Central and Peripheral Nervous System" (American Medical Association 2001, p. 325), arguing that mental disorders are in fact neurologically based. Although such an approach may be useful in states that require percentage impairment ratings, it clearly contradicts the AMA *Guides* itself. In general, percentage ratings of impairment should not be used, but where they are unavoidable, there should be a realistic awareness that such use is artificial and lacks objectivity.

Disability determinations for the Social Security Administration (SSA) involve their own set of rules. The SSA, the largest supplier of disability benefits in the country, offers benefits through Social Security Disability Insurance, supported by funds obtained from an individual's prior work (Federal Insurance Contributions Act), and through Supplemental Security Income, supported by revenued funds of the U.S. Treasury to individuals who have limited or no prior work history. For SSA purposes, a disabling psychiatric condition is one that renders an individual unable to engage in work for substantial gain by reason of a mental or physical impairment that has lasted or is expected to last at least 12 months (Leo 2002; Social Security Administration 1986). Mental impairments are listed as eight categories of mental disorders with varying levels of severity. The determination of disability, however, is based increasingly on vocational considerations, that is, nonmedical factors, rather than on the nature and level of impairment. The clinician is not asked or expected to determine whether the patient is disabled; he or she is asked or expected only to report on the mental disorder as an impairment. The categories that the SSA uses to determine disability are similar to those outlined in the AMA *Guides* (Social Security Administration 1986):

- Marked restriction in activities of daily living
- Marked difficulties in maintaining social functioning
- Deficiencies of concentration, persistence, or pace, resulting in frequent failure to complete tasks in a timely fashion in work settings
- Repeated episodes of deterioration or decompensation in work or worklike settings that cause the individual to withdraw from the situation or to experience an exacerbation of signs and symptoms (which may include deterioration of adapted behaviors)

As indicated above, the SSA requires that an applicant be unable to engage in work for substantial gain for at least 12 months. This means that the individual cannot work at all or, if 55 years of age or older, is unable to perform past relevant work (Leo 2002).

In some instances, such as in workers' compensation, levels of disability are broken down further, according to their degree and likely duration (Metzner et al. 1994), into temporary partial disability, temporary total disability, permanent partial disability, and permanent total disability.

Depending on the type of mental disorder, a temporary disability may be understandable but a permanent one would not be expected. Similarly, a given mental disorder may cause an individual to be disabled from one type of work but not another or prevented from working full-time but not part-time (one of the most common opinions provided by clinicians is that the patient can only work part-time). Such opinions may be reasonable, but only if formed from a complete understanding of the specific nature of the individual's work duties.

Another system of classifying disability was developed by an advisory committee for workers' compensation in California. The results of the committee's efforts have often been used by private disability insurance companies (Enelow 1991). In this system, the degree of disability is determined by assessing the individual's ability to comprehend and follow instructions; perform simple and repetitive tasks; maintain a work pace appropriate to a given workload; perform complex or varied tasks; relate to other people beyond giving and receiving instructions; influence people; make generalizations, evaluations, or decisions without immediate supervision; and accept and carry out responsibility for direction, control, and planning.

Private disability insurance policies typically define disability narrowly as an inability to perform the job functions of the job the insured had when he or she incurred the disability. For example, a social worker who practices psychoanalytic psychotherapy might be disabled if he can no longer practice this type of therapy, even if he can do other social work. Similarly, a vascular surgeon might be disabled even if she can practice another area of medicine. In the case of Mr. G, he may have difficulty in attaining Social Security Disability Insurance benefits because he would have to be totally disabled from any past relevant work for a year. However, if he had private disability insurance, he might be eligible for benefits if he could no longer practice as a trial attorney. Whether Mr. G is in fact so impaired that he is partially or totally disabled requires a comprehensive and objective assessment. This will now be addressed.

## The Assessment

The various classification systems for impairment discussed in the previous section, and others that may be used throughout the United States, show considerable overlap but also offer unique parameters for evaluation. The most important point to recognize in performing assessments of disability is that these classification systems provide a means of reporting impairment but not actually assessing it. Even the Global Assessment of Functioning Scale, Axis V in DSM-IV (American Psychiatric Association 1994) and its text revision, DSM-IV-TR (American Psychiatric Association 2000), only provides a means of reporting impairment. For example, a Global Assessment of Functioning score in the range of 41 to 50 connotes serious symptoms or a serious impairment in social, occupational, or school-related functioning. Inability to keep a job would certainly score in the 41–50 range and might offer a way of quantifying the level of impairment, but the scale itself does not help in making the assessment of whether the person was in fact unable to keep the job as opposed to merely not keeping it (Drukteinis 2002).

In the case of Mr. G, he reported an inability to concentrate as he should to work as a trial attorney and difficulty meeting a demanding schedule of depositions and trials. These symptoms could certainly qualify for impairment under the AMA *Guides* in the category of concentration, persistence, and pace. But how do you know that Mr. G was in fact unable to concentrate as he said or had difficulty meeting a schedule of depositions and trials? Is it really possible to determine this by speaking to him in your office? How much do you know about his actual schedule and whether or not he was keeping up with it in spite of his symptoms?

It may be possible through a mental status examination to observe his sluggish thought processes and infer that he would have difficulty concentrating as a trial attorney, but would these inferences be objective? Even if he appeared to have difficulty concentrating at the time of the mental status examination, can this performance be generalized to say that Mr. G will have this impairment indefinitely?

When Mr. G says he cannot face the stress of an adversarial process, how do you determine whether this is true? Is the mere fact of his depression enough? Are you relying on your assumption that the adversarial process must be stressful? What facts support Mr. G's claim? If he tells you that he has turned back at the courthouse steps because he could not face going to trial, you can report this under the SSA category of impairment that lists decompensation in a worklike setting that causes the individual to withdraw, but do you know if in fact this occurred? Do you know whether Mr. G's symptoms were the actual reason for his behavior?

Most of the time, clinicians make an assessment of disability based on the diagnosis of a sufficiently severe mental disorder and their intuition about the credibility of the patient's self-reports. Although this method may have merit, it is not particularly objective and typically relies on very scanty information about vocational abilities. In addition, because of the subjective nature of mental disorders and the investment of the patient in gaining disability status, self-reports of impairment may not be reliable. Even when those reports are reliable, they can never address the totality of the circumstances and tend to be anecdotal. Without following individuals in their everyday lives and monitoring their activities, it is impossible to completely understand their actual functioning. In that sense, all assessments of disability are only an approximation. The approximation can be made more reliable, however, by probing categories of function in detail, seeking clear examples of impairment, obtaining reliable corroboration, understanding the nature of the patient's work, using confirming clinical tools, and eliminating alternative explanations for disability claims.

Because a mental disorder does not equate to disability, clinicians should take extra steps after making a diagnosis to address whether there is a disability. Conclusory statements of the patient, such as "I can't take the stress of work anymore" or "I can't seem to function," should not be accepted at face value. The circumstances, degree, frequency, and context of those conclusory statements must be ascertained. Using the categories of functioning outlined in the AMA *Guides* is a reasonable way to start. Questioning should dissect each category in some detail, seeking specific examples. If the patient is unable to give reliable examples of impairment, is evasive, or can only discuss impairment in vague generalities, then he or she has not sufficiently demonstrated an impairment or disability. In contrast, concrete examples of impaired function can be compelling and are less likely to be contrived.

Corroboration of a disability can be either internal (i.e., within the history of the person being evaluated and mental status observations) or external (i.e., from outside sources, such as reports of family, friends, employers, or other witness observations). A complete forensic psychiatry evaluation of disability would also seek corroboration from medical and psychiatric records, employment files, and tax returns, all of which could help chronicle a person's functioning. Because a clinician may not have access to all of this information, he or she should be aware that an opinion on disability may have only a limited basis. The reliability of all sources of information must also be taken into account. For example, family members may be as equally invested in a disability claim as the person asserting it and may distort the patient's mental symptoms in support of the claim. However, especially in adversarial situations, such as personal injury litigation or workers' compensation, an employer or other party may be biased against a claim of disability and provide misleading information to indicate that the claim is fabricated. The inherent bias of all informants as well as the consistency of reported information must be scrutinized.

One method of obtaining internal corroboration from the patient is to survey a typical day in the patient's life. Tracing the day, hour by hour, can sometimes reveal areas of preserved functioning that demonstrate the potential for work or rehabilitation. Questioning a person in detail about his or her typical day makes it more difficult for the person to rely on sweeping descriptions of impairment. The person's hobbies, recreation, and social interactions can be a rich source of information. A full schedule of personal activities can demonstrate a lack of credible impediment to work. The absence of any activity may reveal someone who is passively accepting an invalid role.

To understand whether a patient is able to work or not, there must be an adequate understanding of the nature of the patient's job. Often, assumptions about a patient's job are poorly founded or based on stereotypes. Patients may sometimes misrepresent their work duties or overemphasize those duties that are particularly strenuous. Speaking to the employer, with the patient's permission, may reveal a more balanced description of what the work entails. It may also lead to an awareness of possible accommodations for the patient's mental disorder or opportunities for modified work duties. A formal job description may also be helpful. In Mr. G's case, practicing as a trial attorney sounds stressful, but when did it actually become stressful for him and why? How many depositions and trials was he facing? What income did he generate? Was he part of a firm where there was collegial support? Is there a way to modify his work?

Clinical tools can also help confirm impairment so that an opinion is not based solely on a patient's self-report. A carefully performed mental status examination or a battery of psychological tests may reveal cognitive impairment, severity of clinical complaints, vulnerability to fragmentation under stress, exaggeration, and other useful impairment parameters. Clinical observation can also provide a wealth of information: A dramatic or histrionic presentation, or one that is inconsistent with the history of complaints, can raise doubt about the severity of the mental disorder. An angry, belligerent presentation can at times lead a clinician to conclude that the patient is very symptomatic, when it actually represents a defensive posture to avoid scrutiny. A patient's ease during the clinician's interview and in conversation, as well as more formal testing of mental processes, may suggest proper cognitive functioning despite claims to the contrary.

In Mr. G's case, he may present as sullen, withdrawn, and depressed, consistent with his diagnosis, but is this the presentation he maintains in his personal life or the one he maintains just when he meets with the clinician? Will psychological testing demonstrate symptom exaggeration or manipulative personality traits that could cast doubt on his self-reports?

Finally, to make an objective disability assessment, the clinician must consider alternative explanations for the patient's disability claim. The most common alternative explanation for claims that are poorly supported is that the individual is choosing not to work rather than being unable to work. Because of the subjective nature of mental disorders, this is not an easy distinction for the clinician or any other evaluator to make; there is no bright line separating these two scenarios. Rather, choosing not to work and being unable to work because of impairment lie on opposite sides of a continuum in which both scenarios may be operative, with the task of the evaluator being to assess which is the more substantial factor. The best tool in this process is an accurate and reliable longitudinal history tracing the evolution of the claimed impairment in relationship to the individual's working life. For example, did Mr. G first become depressed and then unable to work? If so, was there a time when he was able to work through the depression? Why did the treatment he was receiving at that time fail to sustain him? Are there reasons why Mr. G would no longer want to pursue his trial practice irrespective of the depression? Did he make plans to leave his profession because of personal preference before the depression became more severe? Does his age suggest an interest in early retirement?

## Confounding Factors

Among the confounding factors facing the clinician in performing disability assessments, the thorniest is the potential damaging effect on the therapeutic alliance. Can a clinician give an objective opinion on disability when the patient is convinced that disability exists and is expecting a favorable opinion? For example, if you have been treating Mr. G for a period of time and your opinion on disability is now unfavorable, will he continue in therapy with you? Will he regress because he has lost his trust in you or suffered a financial setback?

Because of the therapeutic alliance, most clinicians are prone to give their patients the benefit of the doubt. A variety of clinician attitudes and countertransference dynamics may also enter into the decision-making process (Mischoulen 2002). Among these are judgments about the patient's character and work ethic, feelings of envy or disgust, hostility, identification with the patient, and rescue fantasies. A clinician should attempt to recognize these potential biases in assessing disability and minimize their effect.

If an opinion on disability is favorable to the patient, then at least in the short run the therapeutic alliance may be strengthened and legitimate financial security for the patient achieved. If the opinion on disability is unfavorable, then communicating this to the patient can be part of the therapeutic process (Mischoulen 2002). The clinician should address the underlying psychological issues leading to the patient's misperception of disability, taking care to do so in a nonjudgmental way, recognizing that the patient may genuinely perceive that he or she is disabled. It should be noted that an opinion in favor of disability may be considered by some patients to be unfavorable, as they may not want to consider themselves disabled and will insist on continuing to work even when a mental disorder is creating a significant impairment.

An alternative method of dealing with an unfavorable opinion is to limit your reporting to the diagnosis and claimed symptomatology, foregoing any conclusions about work impairment or disability. This allows the administrative fact-finder to make the determination. This is not unlike what the SSA expects anyway. However, it often falls short of what is sought by the inquiring party and may leave the patient stranded without the clinician's support.

In addition to the clinician's therapeutic alliance issues, malingering, symptom exaggeration, and secondary gain are other potential confounding factors in a disability claim and should be considered in the assessment. Malingering, as defined by DSM-IV-TR, is the intentional production of false or grossly exaggerated symptoms for an external incentive, such as disability payments (American Psychiatric Association 2000). The actual incidence of outright malingering is probably small. More importantly, to be reasonably certain that someone is malingering almost requires an admission of faking or an observation of flagrant contradiction to claims of impairment (Hurst 1940). Neither occurs often, and making the diagnosis of malingering inevitably has a pejorative effect. However, symptom exaggeration and magnification are common and may be unintentional, substantially unintentional, or at least partially unintentional. As with the difference between choosing not to work and being unable to work, symptom exaggeration and malingering are on opposite sides of the same continuum. Without evidence to the contrary, it is far better to explain to patients that their symptoms are inconsistent or without adequate objective basis rather than call them, in effect, liars.

Because disability benefits influence the reporting and perhaps the experiencing of symptoms (Lloyd and Tsuang 1985; Perl and Kahn 1983), the potential for secondary gain should always be considered. Secondary gain refers to those perhaps unexpected environmental responses to being sick that assist in reinforcing symptoms. Examples include financial reimbursement, attention from the family, or avoidance of less-than-satisfactory work conditions.

With Mr. G, what was his level of income before becoming depressed and claiming work impairment? Will his disability benefits be substantially the same? Are there reasons why not practicing as a trial attorney would be desirable for him whether or not he is depressed? Is he looking for a new career or overly involved with some avocation?

One way to assess the potential for symptom exaggeration or secondary gain is to explore whether there have been any rehabilitation efforts by the patient, which might demonstrate the patient's motivation toward recovery. Another way is to investigate whether the decision about a disability claim, especially one of long-term disability, was made before a full treatment effect was known. For example, for Mr. G to have precipitously decided that he will never again practice as a trial attorney after only a few days of hospitalization indicates an inadequate opportunity to see the effects of longer treatment and a lack of consideration of his ability to return to work part-time or in a modified capacity. In addition, questions should be raised if Mr. G has not complied with prescribed medication, has missed appointments for treatment, or is only seeking infrequent follow-up treatment.

Distortions in a patient's actual condition can also unwittingly be caused by the clinician, who at times can induce or reinforce disability, stymieing the patient's recovery and reinforcing an invalid role. This can be as simple as overpathologizing someone's condition. It can also occur through prematurely supporting a disability claim or extending it to the point that the patient cannot recover the initiative or energy to reenter the workforce. In addition, medication side effects can create their own impairments and should be regularly reevaluated for their potential role in maintaining invalidism, although there is little justification for a primary work impairment to be a side effect of medication. These iatrogenic factors can lead to a chronic, mutually reinforcing concept of invalidism between patient and clinician. Over the course of such long-term treatment, the perpetual focus on illness and impairment becomes a self-fulfilling prophecy (Seligman 2002).

## Disability and Specific Mental Disorders

Although patients with even very severe mental disorders can often work in a limited capacity or in a sheltered setting, certain disorders clearly are more likely to result in work impairment. Psychotic conditions such as schizophrenia or severe bipolar disorders routinely lead to major impairment in social and occupational functioning. Similarly, certain chronic anxiety and depressive disorders that are unresponsive to treatment can be disabling, if not for all work, then perhaps for the type of work that the patient was formerly capable of doing. Posttraumatic stress disorder, which is the subject of much litigation involving disability claims, is known to produce chronic and long-lasting symptoms. It may be quite disabling for certain types of work, in particular if the trauma occurred in a similar work setting. However, there is little objective data to support chronic total disability from posttraumatic stress disorder (Drukteinis 2002).

Somatoform disorders present a unique conundrum in disability claims in that the impairment is purportedly the result of physical symptoms, but the underlying pathogenesis is substantially psychological. In some of these cases, such as chronic pain disorders, a peculiar disability issue has emerged. Although the disability is said to be caused by physical symptoms, and therefore not technically a mental health issue, a secondary psychological reaction is asserted as an independent impairment (Drukteinis 2000). Therefore, for example, patients may claim disability because of back pain, but the medical evidence shows that a sedentary work capacity is still possible. Then, with what amounts to circular logic, patients say that it is their depression caused by an inability to work that makes them totally disabled. This scenario is often seen in situations in which percentage ratings of permanent impairment are required as part of settlement negotiations.

Even more controversial are disability claims for addictive and personality disorders (Frisman and Rosenheck 2002). Should disability be granted for an individual's maladaptive behavior, or are these conditions mental disorders over which an individual has no control? Political, philosophical, public policy, and social science considerations have been involved in this controversy, with research results often contradictory. Practically, however, if a period of disability can be used to help with psychological growth and recovery even in these conditions, it may very well be justified. Permanent disability, however, should be more carefully examined.

In general, disability determinations should take into account the natural course of a mental disorder, the expected effects of adequate treatment, and a realistic prognosis. Work, by and large, is healthy and restorative for most people, even those with mental disorders, and should be encouraged. Disability, in contrast, can have an eroding effect on the individual. As a consequence, opinions about disability should be judiciously considered and sparingly made. It may be that Mr. G cannot practice as a trial attorney any longer because his age and increased vulnerability to depression make placing him in a high-stress work environment undesirable. However, Mr. G's years of practice as a trial attorney were a resource for not only financial reward but also replenishment of self-esteem. Where is he to find that now if he remains totally disabled? Can he find a new source for intellectual stimulation and challenge? Every type of work has its drawbacks, stresses, and negative aspects, but the net product of Mr. G's practice may have been more valuable to him than he realizes. From the standpoint of his own recovery from depression, it should not be casually taken away.

## Conclusion

Disability determination is particularly challenging for the clinician and an area of forensic psychiatry that probably cannot be avoided. Clinicians should refer to accepted categories of potential impairment in addition to reporting symptoms and making a diagnosis. Assessing whether an impairment exists according to these categories is difficult but can be accomplished by a careful and detailed survey coupled with consistent corroboration. Disability must be demonstrated, not just presumed. The therapeutic alliance with the patient and its accompanying bias are challenging but not insurmountable. If disability status can be seen as both a benefit and potential harm to the patient, then a more objective judgment will be easier to make and to communicate to the patient as part of the therapeutic process.

## Key Points

- A mental disorder does not automatically equate to a disability.
- Disability determinations must involve nonmedical and vocational considerations.

- Disability must be demonstrated, not presumed.
- All disability determinations are an approximation, as it is impossible to completely know a person's functioning.
- The therapeutic alliance and countertransference issues can create an inherent bias for the clinician when evaluating patients for disability.
- Disability benefits can be an important safety net for a patient with a mental disorder, but they can also have an eroding effect that is unhealthy.

## Practice Guidelines

1. In addition to diagnosing a mental disorder and assessing its severity, address the various categories of function that can result in disability.
2. Take into account the natural course of the mental disorder, the expected effect of adequate treatment, and a realistic prognosis, in every disability determination.
3. Ensure that the patient convincingly demonstrates impairment by asking him or her to provide specific examples rather than generalized assertions of incapacity.
4. Enhance disability determinations by probing categories of function in some detail, obtaining reliable corroboration, understanding the nature of the work, using confirming clinical tools, and eliminating alternative explanations for the disability claim.
5. Consider if and to what degree choosing not to work, rather than being unable to work, is motivating the disability claim.

## References


American Academy of Psychiatry and the Law: Ethical Guidelines for the Practice of Forensic Psychiatry. Bloomfield, CT, American Academy of Psychiatry and the Law, 1995

American Medical Association: Guides to the Evaluation of Permanent Impairment, 5th Edition. Edited by Cocchiarella L, Landersson GBJ. Chicago, IL, American Medical Association, 2001

American Psychiatric Association: Diagnostic and Statistical Manual of Mental Disorders, 4th Edition. Washington, DC, American Psychiatric Association, 1994

American Psychiatric Association: Diagnostic and Statistical Manual of Mental Disorders, 4th Edition, Text Revision. Washington, DC, American Psychiatric Association, 2000

Drukteinis AM: Overlapping somatoform syndromes in personal injury litigation. American Journal of Forensic Psychiatry 21(4):37–66, 2000

Drukteinis AM: Disability determination in PTSD litigation, in Posttraumatic Stress Disorder in Litigation: Guidelines for Forensic Assessment, 2nd Edition. Edited by Simon RI. Washington, DC, American Psychiatric Publishing, 2002, pp 67–190

Enelow AJ: Psychiatric disorders and work function. Psychiatric Annals 21:27–35, 1991

Frisman LK, Rosenheck R: The impact of disability payments on persons with addictive disorders. Psychiatric Annals 32(5):303–307, 2002

Hurst AF: Medical Diseases of War. London, Arnold, 1940

Kessler RC, McGonagle KA, Zhao S, et al: Lifetime and 12-month prevalence of DSM-III-R psychiatric disorders in the United States: results from the National Comorbidity Survey. Arch Gen Psychiatry 51:8–19, 1994

Kochlar S, Scott CG: Disability patterns among SSI recipients. Social Security Bulletin 58(1):3–14, 1995

Leo RJ: Social Security disability and the mentally ill: changes in the adjudication process and treating source information requirements. Psychiatric Annals 32(5):284–292, 2002

Lloyd DW, Tsuang MT: Disability and welfare—who wants it? J Clin Psychiatry 46:273–275, 1985

Metzner JL, Struthers DR, Fogel MA: Psychiatric disability determination and personal injury litigation, in Principles and Practice of Forensic Psychiatry. Edited by Rosner R. London, Arnold, 1994, pp 232–241

Mischoulen D: Potential pitfalls to the therapeutic relationship arising from disability claims. Psychiatric Annals 32(5):299–307, 2002

Perl J, Kahn M: The effects of compensation on psychiatric disability. Soc Sci Med 17:439–443, 1983

Regier DA, Meyers JK, Kramer M, et al: The NIMH Epidemiologic Catchment Area Program: historical context, major objectives, and study population characteristics. Arch Gen Psychiatry 41:934–941, 1984

Sederer LI, Clemens, NA: The business case for high-quality mental health care. Psychiatr Serv 53(2):143–145, 2002

Seligman MEP: Authentic Happiness. New York, Free Press, 2002

Social Security Administration: Disability Evaluation Under Social Security (SSA Publ No 64-039). Washington, DC, U.S. Government Printing Office, 1986

## Suggested Readings

American Medical Association: Guides to the Evaluation of Permanent Impairment, 5th Edition. Edited by Cocchiarella L, Landersson GBJ. Chicago, IL, American Medical Association, 2001

Bonnie RJ, Monahan J (eds): Mental Disorder, Work Disability, and the Law. Chicago, IL, University of Chicago Press, 1997

Liberman RP (ed): Handbook of Psychiatric Rehabilitation. New York, Macmillan, 1992

CHAPTER 14

# The Workplace

Liza H. Gold, M.D.

## Introduction

Over the past years, labor and employment litigation has increased dramatically. The fact that 22% of the United States Supreme Court's decisions in the 2001–2002 term dealt with the relations between employers and employees reflects the upsurge in this area of law. The increase in employment litigation is related to a variety of factors. Recent changes in the law have allowed for jury trials and large damage awards. In addition, people are often less hesitant to bring a suit or claim against an employer than against another individual. A large company or corporation is easily perceived and portrayed as an impersonal entity that should bear responsibility for injustice or harm incurred in the workplace. People also often hold the belief that unlike individual defendants, these businesses can afford to pay large awards without incurring significant financial distress.

Employment litigation covers a wide array of complex legal, statutory, and administrative arenas. Claims against employers can be made under federal statutes such as the Americans with Disabilities Act of 1990 (ADA), the antidiscrimination laws embodied in the Civil Rights Act of 1964, or parallel state statutes. These claims can be brought through the Equal Employment Opportunity Commission, public or private disability insurance, and workers' compensation boards. Employment-related claims can also be brought under civil law, through torts such as premises liability, negligence, wrongful termination, and negligent or intentional infliction of emotional distress. Many employment-related claims are filed jointly. These suits can result in large awards, huge legal fees, administrative and court costs, and lost work time for many employees.

Forensic psychiatrists and psychologists are called on with increasing frequency to offer expert opinions regarding medicolegal issues in employment-related claims. Mental and emotional injuries constitute the bulk of exposure in much federal and civil litigation related to employment claims (Lindemann and Kadue 1992; McDonald and Kulick 2001). Virtually every federal employment discrimination lawsuit contains an allegation that the plaintiff suffered mental and emotional distress at the hands of the defendant employer (McDonald and Kulick 2001). Eligibility for public and private insurance benefits or workers' compensation benefits may hinge on a claim of psychiatric illness or disability as certified by an independent psychiatric evaluation. Psychiatric testimony may form the crux of legal arguments regarding causation, damages, and eligibility for benefits, as well as other issues that may affect the outcome of a claim or litigation.

## Clinical Vignettes

### Vignette 1

Ms. S worked as an administrative assistant in a large company. She was in the process of divorcing her husband. He had been violent in the past, and she had a restraining order against him. Despite the order, he had been calling and threatening Ms. S at work. The calls became more frequent and more threatening, and Mr. S also began to call and threaten one of Ms. S's coworkers. Ms. S and the coworker advised the company's security officer of the calls and of Mr. S's history of violence. The security officer dismissed the problem as a domestic matter and told Ms. S to keep her personal problems out of the workplace. A few days later, Mr. S entered the office. He shot his wife and three other employees before shooting himself. Mr. S, Ms. S, and one coworker were killed. The two wounded employees, one of whom was the coworker who spoke with the security officer, brought suit against their employer for premises liability and negligent infliction of emotional distress. Both employees claimed to have developed posttraumatic stress disorder (PTSD) in addition to physical injuries as a result of the incident.

### Vignette 2

Ms. A was one of a few female officers on a small city police force. Shortly after her employment began, she became the butt of jokes and insults regarding women. She frequently found pictures of naked women with graphic commentary taped to her locker. Male coworkers often commented that police work was "man's work" and that Ms. A did not belong on the police force. Ms. A reported this behavior to her supervisor, who told her to ignore it. The behavior escalated and began to include grabbing and touching. She complained to her supervisor again.

This time he told that her she was making things difficult for everyone and that she would be doing herself a favor if she quit. Ms. A was very upset but refused to quit her job. Shortly thereafter, Ms. A was sexually assaulted by a coworker while both were working a night shift. She brought a suit for sexual harassment against her employer, the city government, and claimed that she suffered severe emotional injuries as a result of sexual harassment and workplace discrimination.

### Vignette 3

Dr. B was a physician who owned his own practice, employing himself and a few other physicians. Over the course of years, he had become increasingly dysfunctional as a result of alcohol dependence. Dr. B denied that he had a problem with alcohol and ascribed his decreasing ability to function as a physician to "burnout." He stopped providing routine clinical care to patients and worked primarily as the administrator of his practice. His caseload was taken over by his physician employees, but he continued to provide patient care occasionally, such as when another physician was unexpectedly unavailable. As a result of concerns regarding his increasingly poor clinical judgment, one of the physician employees reported Dr. B to the state's impaired physicians program. Dr. B agreed to enter treatment for alcohol dependence to avoid losing his license. He applied for disability payments as per his private disability insurance plan.

After 1 year, Dr. B let his license expire, stating he had no desire to return to providing clinical care. He also refused ongoing treatment and claimed 1 year of complete sobriety. However, he also claimed he was completely disabled because of cognitive impairments that he ascribed to the effects of years of alcohol abuse. Neuropsychological testing revealed no evidence of cognitive deficits. Dr. B's insurance company referred him for independent medical evaluation to determine whether he was still eligible for his private disability benefits. The company noted that at the time of his claim, Dr. B was functioning primarily as an administrative rather than a clinical physician.

## Employment-Related Evaluations

In employment-related claims of emotional injury or disability, experts may be asked to assess one or more of the following issues (Brodsky 1987a; Metzner et al. 1994):

1. Whether the employee has a psychiatric diagnosis, and if so, its duration, symptoms, and prognosis
2. The etiology or causation of the disorder and, specifically, its relationship to work
3. Whether the disorder has resulted in a work-related impairment

Psychiatrists asked to provide opinions in employment-related claims should begin such evaluations by identifying the legal issues relevant to the specific type of employment litigation. This will allow experts to focus on those aspects of the case that will be most helpful in making the required legal determinations. Detailed review of the legal aspects of all types of employment claims is beyond the scope of this discussion. Regardless of the type of legal claim, however, three issues tend to form the core of employment-related evaluations: diagnosis, causation, and disability. As each of these issues relate to specific types of claims, the legal standards involved will be discussed.

## Diagnosis

In all types of employment litigation, examiners should first establish whether an emotional injury or disorder exists. The legal standard that must be met regarding diagnosis varies depending on the type of litigation. For example, in harassment or discrimination claims brought under Title VII of the Civil Rights Act of 1964, emotional injury does not have to be established for alleged discriminatory or harassing behavior to be actionable (*Harris v. Forklift Systems, Inc.* 1993). Similarly, common-law causes of action do not require that emotional distress be diagnosable as a mental disorder to be compensable. In contrast, entitlement to Social Security Disability Insurance (SSDI) benefits generally depends on establishing a disability based on a recognized category of mental disorder as defined by *Diagnostic and Statistical Manual of Mental Disorders* (DSM) criteria (DSM-IV-TR; American Psychiatric Association 2000).

Even when not specifically required by statute, however, both lawyers and forensic evaluators often think they must have a diagnosis for credibility. It may be difficult to establish damages or entitlement to compensation without a formal DSM diagnosis. This is particularly important in claims of emotional harm of disability as a result of emotional injury or psychological disorder. Such claims, when unaccompanied by physical injury, have historically been viewed with suspicion by the legal system. Recovery or award of benefits in such cases has been particularly problematic (Metzner et al. 1994; Shuman 2002).

For example, under workers' compensation statutes, claims in which a worker seeks compensation for a mental injury caused by a mental stimulus remain controversial. Many jurisdictions now find such claims compensable. Nevertheless, recovery for "mental-mental" injuries is often limited in ways that recovery for physical injury is not, even if there is a mental component to the claim (Brodsky 1987b; Melton et al. 1997; Metzner et al. 1994).

The formal diagnosis of a psychiatric illness supports arguments that a severe injury that entitles a claimant to damages or benefits actually occurred. In tort claims, both liability and damages may hinge on the existence of a DSM diagnosis. In claims of infliction of emotional distress, the element of severe emotional distress is required to prevail. Such claims may allege that the injury was intentional or nonintentional. In nonintentional infliction of emotional distress cases, the standard of recovery may be the impact rule, the zone of danger rule, or the foreseeability test. Nevertheless, regardless of the type of claim or the relevant standard of recovery, the emotional distress suffered must be severe. It is difficult, if not impossible, to establish severe distress if the plaintiff does not meet the criteria for a formal DSM diagnosis. Even in a discrimination claim, where psychological injury and, therefore, a DSM diagnosis is not required for a plaintiff to prevail, the Equal Employment Opportunity Commission will compute compensatory damages on the basis of a consideration of the severity and duration of harm (Strubbe 1999). A formal diagnosis strengthens such damage claims.

The value of DSM diagnoses to the legal system may differ significantly from the value of diagnoses to clinicians "because of the imperfect fit between the questions of ultimate concern to the law and the information contained in a clinical diagnosis" (American Psychiatric Association 2000, p. xxxiii; see Chapter 6: "Psychiatric Diagnosis in Litigation," this volume). Experts should be aware of these differences and of the uses (and misuses) of DSM diagnoses in litigation (Gold 2002b). A DSM diagnosis may not be the dispositive factor in a legal determination. In addition, a diagnosis does not specify the nature of the association between a specific etiological factor, relevant functional capacity, and symptom.

Nevertheless, the use of an established diagnosis can serve as a point of reference that enhances the value and reliability of psychiatric testimony (Gold 2002b; Halleck 1992; Shuman 1989). In making a diagnosis, evaluators identify a range of precipitants or possible symptoms that, in turn, may define associated impairments. This can allow experts to draw reasonable connections, restrain ungrounded speculation, or refute unreasonable claims between symptoms associated with a diagnosis and arguments regarding causation, impairment, and damages or disability.

In addition, when a diagnosis is established, the subject of the evaluation can be assessed in relation to others of the same diagnostic category. The application of a diagnosis allows the examiner to use the cumulative experiences and research of the fields of psychiatry and psychology. The longitudinal course of certain disorders, for example, can provide essential information relevant to legal issues. The identification of a chronic, episodic, or progressively deteriorating course of mental illness associated with various diagnostic categories provides a framework for assessment of causation. It also allows reasonable discussion of the course of a particular individual's illness and the likelihood of symptoms creating past, present, or future functional impairments. Often it provides clues as to the possible duration of such impairments and the efficacy of possible treatments.

In making diagnostic assessments, examiners should be careful to distinguish psychiatric illnesses from nonpathological emotional reactions. Most individuals experience employment-related problems and conflicts as stressful, especially if they result in adverse financial or social consequences. Adverse employment events and the stress and distress that accompany them may precipitate or exacerbate illness in individuals with preexisting diagnoses or vulnerability to psychiatric disorders. Nevertheless, in and of themselves, intense and distressing feelings and complaints associated with them, such as anxiety, insomnia, tearfulness, or irritability, do not amount to diagnosable psychiatric disorders: "Though it may be stressful, unhappiness is not a psychiatric condition; neither is injustice....One may be miserably and justifiably unhappy about a work experience and not be psychiatrically injured" (Savodnik 1991, p. 188).

If examiners determine that psychological symptoms rise to the level of a mental disorder, diagnoses should be made according to DSM criteria. Psychiatrists should be certain to use standard methods of evaluation and differential diagnosis. They should also be prepared to support diagnostic conclusions with specific information gathered from both the psychiatric interview and record review. Idiosyncratic diagnoses based on "clinical experience" will not withstand cross-examination or examination for scientific reliability. Clinical experience is a crucial element in evaluating psychiatric illness and formulating diagnoses. However, clinical experience will vary from practitioner to practitioner and is subject to personal interpretation of its relevance and meaning. Thus, it is cannot form the basis of a scientific methodology of diagnostic classification.

## Causation

Not all employment claims or litigation requires a finding of causation to determine awards or eligibility. For example, an individual's entitlement to public or private disability insurance benefits does not require that the injury alleged to be the source of disability be causally related to employment. In contrast, the principles of tort law allow individuals who have been injured by others to receive monetary compensation only if there is sufficient causal connection between the agency's illegal actions and the complainant's injury. Whether conduct is intentional or negligent and leads to direct or indirect infliction of emotional distress, an award for emotional harm will not lead to liability unless the conduct "proximately" causes injury. In both workers' compensation and tort law, a defendant cannot be held liable unless causation can be demonstrated.

Workers' compensation is an administrative remedy that was designed as an alternative to filing other types of claims and, when used, is typically considered an exclusive remedy. It is a no-fault system designed to provide medical treatment and disability benefits for workers who have suffered a work-related injury or illness. However, the "no-fault" component of workers' compensation means only that a finding of fault is not required as a prerequisite to awarding benefits. All other aspects of a claim may be and often are disputed and litigated, including the issue of causation. To receive compensation, workers must demonstrate by a preponderance of evidence that they have suffered an injury or disability arising out of and in the course of employment. This requirement involves establishing the causal relationship between the employment and the injury.

The legal concept of causation and the medical concept of causation are not congruent. The concept of proximate cause is an elusive one, even within the law. The law seeks to determine whether one particular event precipitated, hastened, or aggravated the individual's current condition. The legal requirement for establishing proximate cause generally is not scientific certainty but, rather, "probability," "50.1%," "more likely than not," or "reasonable medical certainty" (Danner and Sagall 1977). The traditional legal method of determining whether one event is the proximate cause of another is to ask whether one could "reasonably foresee" that the former would lead to the latter (Shuman 2002; Simon 1992). Practically speaking, proximate cause has come to mean the "recent" cause, that is, "the straw that broke the camel's back" (Simon 1992, p. 550).

In contrast, all behavioral and medical sciences consider axiomatic the concept that many factors contribute to a negative psychological outcome or the development of a psychiatric or medical illness. Psychiatrists examine and weigh multiple causative elements in the development of a theory of the etiology of any disorder. Psychiatric determinations of causation typically conclude that although certain factors may be more significant, a mental disorder has been precipitated by the interaction of a number of these factors.

Despite the conflicts inherent in these two approaches, it is clear that external events can precipitate psychological injury or emotional harm that falls within both legal and psychiatric parameters of causation. PTSD and adjustment disorders by definition develop in response to an external event. Other factors can play a role in the vulnerability to the development of these disorders. However, the psychiatric community acknowledges that an external event is necessary to precipitate or cause them. Stressful life events also have a substantial causal relationship with the onset of episodes of major depression (Kendler et al. 1999; Shalev et al. 1998). Genetic risk is a well-described factor in the development of a depressive disorder. Those at highest genetic risk have a considerably weaker association between stressful events and a first episode than do those at low genetic risk. Nevertheless, both initial and recurrent episodes of depression can be precipitated by stressful experiences.

Many distressing and potentially psychologically damaging events can arise out of or during the course of employment. Witnessing or experiencing events such as motor vehicle accidents, industrial accidents, or violence can result in both physical and psychological injuries. Traumatic exposure in the workplace is not uncommon. From 1990 to 1999, the average incidence of nonfatal workplace injury was 7.3 per 100 full-time workers. Motor vehicle accidents are a leading cause of severe workplace-related injury (Occupational Safety and Health Administration 1999). Terrorist attacks in the workplace, such as those that occurred in the Oklahoma City bombing in 1995 and in the World Trade Center/Pentagon attacks in 2001, can also cause emotional injury that may be considered to arise out of employment (Galea et al. 2002; North et al. 1999; Schlenger et al. 2002). In each year from 1992 to 1996, more than two million people experienced violent victimizations while they were working or on duty. These included simple assault (73.6%), aggravated assault (19.7%), robbery (4.2%), rape (2.5%), and homicide (0.05%). Approximately 12% of the nonfatal violent workplace crimes resulted in an injury to the victim (U.S. Department of Justice 1998).

Homicide was the second leading cause of death in the workplace between 1992 and 1996, exceeded only by motor vehicle–related deaths. More than 1,000 murders occurred each year (U.S. Department of Justice 1998). Women are more likely to die as victims of violence than from any other type of work-related injury, as the case of Ms. S demonstrates. These incidents occur typically in the larger context of domestic violence or stalking.

However, despite the stereotype of a disgruntled employee "going postal," the vast majority of workplace homicides (85%) are committed by a perpetrator who has no legitimate relationship to the business or its employees. The individual involved is usually committing a crime in conjunction with the violence. Barely 4% of people murdered at work are killed by another employee. Nevertheless, when such incidents occur, the degree of injury may be extreme. It is fairly common that the intended victim escapes harm while others are killed or injured (Merchant and Lundell 2001; National Institute for Occupational Safety and Health 1996; Southerland et al. 1997).

Claims of emotional injury caused by employment-related events, particularly when accompanied by physical injury, may be quite straightforward. Violence and accidents are readily acknowledged to cause or precipitate psychiatric harm under certain circumstances. No one would be surprised if Ms. S's surviving coworker developed PTSD or some other disorder. In the case of Ms. A, whose harassment experiences included a sexual assault, the development of PTSD would also not be unexpected.

Even absent physical injury, psychological harm is a real, possible, and at times legally compensable outcome of a horrific experience. Most events that can result in the development of PTSD are listed in DSM-IV-TR as examples of traumatic stressors (American Psychiatric Association 2000). Traumatic experiences such as these have also been associated with the development of depression, panic disorder, generalized anxiety disorder, and substance abuse or dependence (Briere 1997; Green and Kaltman 2002; Yehuda and Wong 2001). These are also the emotional injuries typically associated with employment claims (Aviera and Boehm 1994).

Nevertheless, examiners should not be too quick to assume a post hoc, propter hoc relationship between an employment-related incident, however traumatic, and a psychiatric disorder. Assessments of causation in employment litigation should always include consideration of exposure to another stressor, either in the past or concurrent with present events, as the cause of a new disorder; the extent to which the current exposure caused a new disorder or exacerbated a preexisting disorder; whether a disorder would have occurred at all but for the event in question; the presence and course of a preexisting disorder, with and without exposure to the events in question; and whether the dynamics of the individual or the workplace are contributing to either the perception of causation or the attribution of preexisting problems to conflict in the workplace.

Psychiatric theory does not propose or conclude that the inevitable outcome of any event is the development of a mental disorder. When evaluations are made retrospectively, as is often the case in litigation, estimates of pathology are inflated (Melton et al. 1997) and diagnosis of psychiatric illness is common (Long 1994; Rosen 1995). In a study examining assessments of survivors of the sinking of a fishing ship who subsequently become involved in litigation, mental health professionals diagnosed 86% of those seen while pursuing personal injury claims with PTSD (Rosen 1995). This rate is well in excess of any previously reported in the literature for any type of trauma with the possible exception of rape. On independent medical examination by a psychologist retained by the defense, only five individuals were diagnosed with PTSD. This yielded an incidence of 25%, a figure more congruent with rates observed generally in individuals exposed to trauma.

Epidemiological studies indicate that only 15%–24% of adults exposed to a traumatic event develop PTSD (Breslau 2001; Kessler et al. 1995; Yehuda and Wong 2001). For individuals exposed to violent crimes, deaths, or accidents, the PTSD lifetime prevalence rate is 7%–12% (Breslau 2001). How an individual responds to any experience, no matter how traumatic, depends on a variety of factors. These include duration, complexity, content, qualities, and kinds and amounts of associated losses. The dimensions of threat to life, severe physical harm or injury, exposure to grotesque death and loss, or the injury of a loved one are correlated to the likelihood of developing PTSD. The existence of a directly proportional dose-response relationship between stressor magnitude and subsequent risk of developing PTSD is well established (Briere 1997; Green and Kaltman 2002). In addition, the availability of support from friends, family, professionals, and institutions as well as therapeutic interventions can mediate the effects of traumatic or adverse experiences.

The evaluation of causation in employment litigation can become even more complex. Psychiatric illness may be alleged to have developed as a result of events that are adverse, distressing, and maybe even illegal but are not typically considered to be traumatic stressors. Claims of psychiatric illness or injury resulting from nontraumatic stressors or that are common (Gold 2002a). Attorneys will argue that unfair treatment in the workplace is so stressful and psychologically harmful that it has caused psychiatric injury. Clinicians who assess individuals involved in employment-related conflict often mistake the stress and distress that follows exposure to any adverse event for psychiatric illness (Long 1994; Rosen 1995).

Such claims should be carefully assessed. Job loss, unfair or discriminatory treatment, and employment-related conflict, whether real or perceived, are without doubt stressful. Such events may be associated with psychological symptoms and psychiatric disorders. However, an evaluation of causation should always consider alternate causation and preexisting disorders. Failure to consider the contribution of earlier or concurrent unrelated traumatic events or stressors to the evaluee's illness, regardless of the alleged precipitant, may result in the false attribution of current symptoms to the employment events being litigated.

Alternative sources of an individual's psychological problems may include past or present exposure to traumatic experiences other than the events involved in the litigation. One survey found that 60.7% of men and 51.2% of adults responded positively to questions regarding traumatic exposure (Kessler et al. 1995). Violence by an intimate partner accounts for about 21% of the violent crime experienced by women, and lifetime prevalence of these experiences ranges from 21% to 34% (Warshaw 2001). Other concurrent problems that can result in new-onset disorders include substance abuse disorders, medical conditions, and psychosocial stressors such as marital problems. Areas of inquiry should include family and personal relationships, financial problems, illness, death or loss of significant others, other job-related stress, and any other possible sources of tension or stress.

The possibility of diagnosed or undiagnosed preexisting disorders should also be considered. Disorders such as depression, panic attacks, and generalized anxiety are common. Panic disorder occurs in 1%–2% of individuals over their lifetime. The lifetime risk of major depressive disorder varies from 10%–25% for women and from 5%–12% for men (American Psychiatric Association 2000). Many preexisting illnesses may be exacerbated by adverse events. If the individual has not been previously diagnosed or treated, or if an adequate history is not obtained, such exacerbations may appear to be new-onset disorders.

Evidence of preexisting disorders will not prevent individuals from prevailing in their claims. Tortfeasors must take their victims as they find them in accordance with the "eggshell skull" doctrine. The law recognizes that relatively little trauma may cause injury to someone who is vulnerable to harm. An individual with a history of prior illness or trauma may have a more profound reaction to stressful events or conflict than would another individual without such a history. However, the presence of another major life stressor or trauma, or a disorder predating the employment events in question, will make proof of a causal connection between the employment events and the mental injury more difficult.

In such cases, an accurate evaluation may require some apportionment of causation, whether in circumstances of true traumatic exposure in the workplace or in the event of an extreme reaction to a relatively minor workplace event. In tort claims, this may affect findings of liability and awards of damages. In workers' compensation claims, an employee may only be entitled to benefits if workplace events "aggravated" or "accelerated" the course or severity of the preexisting disorder. If the injury existed or worsened independent of work, the claimant is not entitled to compensation (American Medical Association 2000; Melton et al. 1997).

In some cases, individuals with little or no insight into preexisting problems may genuinely but erroneously consider the workplace to be the cause of their psychological problems. Such false attributions may lead examiners to incorrectly assess causation by overlooking the central etiological significance of the individual's prior, long-standing emotional difficulties. This type of situation tends to arise in the context of adverse employment events or interpersonal conflict in the workplace, as often occurs when employees have personality disorders. Paranoid, antisocial, borderline, histrionic, and narcissistic disorders are those most frequently encountered in employment litigation (Lipian 2001; Price 1994).

In addition, personality disorders are commonly associated with a number of Axis I disorders, such as mood and anxiety disorders. When compounded by adverse events, such as lack of promotion, reprimand for poor performance, or job termination, personality disorders and the cognitive distortions, emotional reactivity, and maladaptive coping associated with them often worsen. Such work-related stress can also precipitate or exacerbate associated Axis I disorders. In these cases, the personality disorder rather than the workplace may actually be the cause of both the conflict and the Axis I disorders.

In making a diagnosis of a preexisting personality disorder, experts should be careful to distinguish the personality traits that define these disorders from characteristics that emerge in response to specific situational stressors. Clinicians are generally warned against the error of making a diagnosis of a personality disorder in the context of a specific external event or stressor (American Psychiatric Association 2000). This is particularly true in the context of employment conflict and litigation. The accurate diagnosis of a personality disorder requires an evaluation of the individual's long-term patterns of functioning. Personality disorders should therefore be evaluated across a life span from early adulthood. Evidence of repetitive patterns and symptoms that would be indicative of a chronic, rather than an acute, condition should be identified. These patterns should be evident in multiple spheres of functioning. Much of the evaluation involves analysis of the individual's documented life history and clinical presentation in comparison with self-report and information gathered from third parties.

The identification of a history of alternative trauma exposure or preexisting psychiatric history, even a personality disorder, should not be used to discount the stressful and at times traumatic nature of many events that may occur in relation to employment. Individuals can experience new-onset disorders or exacerbations of previous disorders as a result of work-related stress or distress. Regardless of preexisting vulnerabilities, psychiatric illness can develop in individuals without obvious risk factors in the face of a high-magnitude or -intensity stressor. Previously well-functioning adults can experience a sharp deterioration in functioning after exposure to severe trauma (van der Kolk and McFarlane 1996). However, examiners should not assume that any stressful, distressful, or even traumatic workplace event is causally related to any psychiatric diagnosis. The key to the evaluation of causation in any type of employment litigation lies in a thorough assessment of the workplace events, the circumstances surrounding these events, and the individual's life history.

## Disability

Degree of impairment and disability are relevant and often critical legal issues in almost all types of employment litigation. Eligibility for public or private disability insurance on the basis of a mental disorder requires a demonstration of disability, regardless of diagnosis. In workers' compensation, the benefit schedule hinges on the degree of disability and, specifically, on how the specific impairment affects earning capability. The nature of an accommodation that an employer is reasonably expected to make for a disabled employee under the ADA depends on the disability and how it specifically affects a work-related function. In tort law, an individual's level of impairment is the aspect of any psychiatric disorder most closely associated with assessment of damages (McDonald and Kulick 2001).

As noted above, the presence of psychological symptoms or even a psychiatric diagnosis does not necessarily equate with functional impairment or disability. The condition of the claimant before and after the occurrence of the incident in question is significantly more relevant to the assessment of disability in employment-related claims than is any diagnosis alone. A given illness may be more typically associated with certain types of impairments (Gold 2002b; Halleck et al. 1992). However, loss of function may be greater or less than a given diagnosis might imply. An individual's performance may fall short of, or exceed, that usually associated with that diagnosis. The degree of functional impairment is not even necessarily directly proportional to the severity of the disorder. As DSM-IV-TR warns, more information in addition to diagnosis is needed to establish legal standards such as disability: "It is precisely because impairments, abilities and disabilities vary widely within each diagnostic category that assignment of a particular diagnosis does not imply a specific level of impairment or disability" (American Psychiatric Association 2000, p. xxxiii).

An assessment of work-related function or dysfunction requires the evaluation of the particular abilities required by the workplace. The unique skills of the individual and the requirements and flexibility of the workplace should also be considered. Assessments of functional impairment and disability should be structured to meet the requirements of the type of litigation involved. Certain types of employment litigation, such as discrimination and tort law, do not require any specific degree of impairment or disability. In these cases, examiners are free to assess any and all types of dysfunction in relation to damages. In contrast, workers' compensation requires that the injury must affect earning capacity and, therefore, specific work-related functions. Other types of claims may expand or narrow the definition of a disability. An individual might be disabled according to the criteria of a private disability insurance but might not be disabled according to the criteria set forth by the Social Security Administration (SSA) or for purposes of ADA protection. Thus, psychiatrists should first determine the relevant definition of disability at issue.

### *Disability Insurance Benefits: Private Insurance and SSDI*

Some insurance companies offer individual policies designed to provide a disabled worker financial benefits, often based on a significant percentage of the income of the policyholder. These policies are generally expensive and are typically purchased by self-employed professionals rather than by employees of large organizations due to the significant payroll deductions needed to cover the premium expense. The standard for disability varies among such policies. The better policies define disability with specific reference to the policyholder's regular occupation. The policy may even supply definitions of "regular occupation" to identify particular professional subspecialties. Other policies may define disability more generally as the inability to perform one's regular occupation on a full-time basis or in terms of significantly decreased earning capacity related to injury or sickness. Dr. B's insurance policy covered his "regular occupation," which at the time of his claim was administrative, rather than clinical, medicine. As a result, he was not considered disabled for the purposes of his private policy.

The SSDI program, administered by the SSA, is a public disability insurance program. It provides benefits for those disabled workers and their dependents who have contributed to the Social Security trust fund through the Federal Insurance Compensation Act tax on their earnings. To qualify for benefits, the individual must be unable "to engage in any substantial gainful activity by reason of any medically determinable physical or mental impairment which can be expected to result in death or which has lasted or can be expected to last for a continuous period of not less than 12 months" (42 U.S.C. § 423[d][1][A] [1991]). This disability typically must be based on a recognized or "listed" disorder to meet the definition of a medical impairment. The SSA has eight listed diagnostic categories of mental disorders that are defined by DSM criteria.

Under SSDI regulations, individuals will not be eligible for benefits unless the impairment is so severe that claimants are not only unable to do their previous work but cannot "engage in any other kind of substantial gainful work which exists in the national economy" (42 U.S.C. § 423[d][2][A] [1991]). In private disability insurance, individuals may have to demonstrate only that they are disabled in relation to their specific occupation. Moreover, where impairment or disability is not specifically required, assessment of damages may still be significantly affected by specific areas of dysfunction. Therefore, even in these cases, clinicians should still focus on the ways in which the individual is less functional as a result of the causally related injury.

## *Americans With Disabilities Act*

In most other types of employment claims, individuals are seeking compensation because they cannot work as a result of disability. In contrast, individuals invoking the protection of the ADA are attempting to remain in the workforce despite disability. The ADA requires employers to provide reasonable accommodation to enable a qualified individual with a disability to perform essential job functions unless such an accommodation imposes an undue hardship on the employer. The ultimate determination of whether a particular condition is covered under the ADA is a complex legal process that requires a multistep analysis. A variety of issues related to legal disability, substantial limitation or impairment, and reasonable accommodation as defined by the ADA are subject to legal dispute.

Employers may refer individuals for psychiatric evaluation in an attempt to determine the nature of their legal obligations under the ADA in regard to claims of disability resulting from mental disorder. By statutory definition, a covered disability is one that substantially limits one or more major life activities as a result of a physical or mental impairment. (Individuals may also qualify for protection if they have a record of such impairment or of being regarded as having such impairment.) A recent unanimous Supreme Court decision (*Toyota Motor Mfg., Ky., Inc. v. Williams* 2002) narrowed this definition even further. The claimed disability must have a substantial effect on a person's daily life, and not just a work-related function, to qualify for protection under the ADA. Thus, psychiatrists should provide a careful assessment of the individual's degree of impairment resulting from the mental disorder and how it affects all spheres of the individual's functioning.

## *Assessment of Disability*

Impairment and disability are not equivalent concepts. An individual who is impaired as the result of a mental illness may have no work-related disability or may have no disability relative to some occupations yet be quite disabled relative to others. The AMA *Guides to the Evaluation of Permanent Impairment* defines impairment as "a loss, loss of use, or derangement of any body part, organ system or organ function" (American Medical Association 2000, p. 2). Disability, whether partial or total, temporary or permanent, is defined as "an alteration of an individual's capacity to meet personal, social, or occupational demands or statutory or regulatory requirements because of an impairment" (American Medical Association 2000, p. 8).

Whether an impairment is substantial enough to create disability is a difficult and complex assessment. The relationship between impairment and disability depends on the abilities and functional limitations of the individual, the employment environment, and the demands of a particular job (Bonnie 1997). Nevertheless, rarely are people totally impaired, either physically or mentally (Simon 2002). The evaluation of disability requires an appreciation of the interrelationships between each worker's unique medical and psychological status and his or her physical and social environment. Some workers who suffer an injury or develop an impairment become and remain disabled. Others with comparable injuries either do not enter into a disability status or role or recover much earlier if they do become disabled. No single factor can explain this or differentiate between such individuals (Brodsky 1987a).

The evaluation of disability resulting from injury or impairment should include an assessment of the severity of symptoms and the effect of these symptoms in all spheres of the claimant's functioning. The relationship between the claimant's occupation and the nature and severity of his or her symptoms will be a major determinant in whether the individual is disabled. Examiners should carefully review the history of the mental disorder, the history of the individual's ability to function over time, his or her response to treatment or rehabilitation, and the influence of other work- and non-work-related factors. The evaluation of disability also requires consideration of the individual's skills, education, work history, adaptability, age, job requirements, response to treatment, and medical status, including other medical problems.

Factors less obvious than the symptoms of the illness in question can determine the extent of a disability and should also be considered. Assessments of disability should therefore include consideration of the interaction of personal, work-related, and non-work-related factors. These include burnout, family conflicts or other dynamics, poor remuneration or high-risk jobs, poor working conditions, personality or interpersonal conflicts on the job, and perceptions of inequitable treatment by management (Brodsky 1987a). Such factors may in fact be the deciding features in the development of a disability from an impairment.

Even with all this information, translating specific impairments directly and precisely into functional limitations is a complex process. Little is known about many crucial issues relating to work disabilities arising from mental disorders. In addition, such evaluations are subject to the influence of an examiner's beliefs about work ethic, choice, and responsibility (Pryor 1997). The use of the impairment label has been suggested to provide a self-fulfilling prediction. Nevertheless, examiners should remain sensitive to the historical tendency of physicians and others to minimize psychiatric impairment because of lack of recognition of the significant symptoms associated with some mental disorders.

Individuals who develop psychiatric illnesses, particularly resulting from employment-related events, may suffer a degree of functional impairment as a result of their psychological symptoms such that their ability to work is severely compromised. However, this is not necessarily the case. For example, individuals with anxiety disorders, including PTSD, have employment rates comparable to those of persons without anxiety-related symptoms (Pryor 1997). The strongest predictors of work outcomes for individuals with mental illness are previous employment history and the individual's work-adjustment skills (Pryor 1997).

Other problems in addition to the primary psychiatric disorder in question can result in work-related disabilities. Examiners should consider whether individuals have work-related impairments resulting from their psychiatric illness or another concurrent illness, such as substance abuse or depression. In addition, individuals involved in employment litigation or making disability claims often are not working. Secondary damaging effects typically arise when the beneficial personal, social, and financial aspects of work become unavailable. Often financial and marital difficulties ensue. Examiners should distinguish impairment related to psychiatric illness from the consequences of not working.

Examiners should be certain to compare the individual's functioning before and after the development of the claimed disability. Only this type of comparative evaluation will allow examiners to arrive at a reasonable determination of severity of impairment and disability. Plaintiffs tend to assert that all functional difficulties began after the employment events in question. Regardless of current functional status, such assertions should not be initially accepted as factual (Simon 2002).

Psychiatrists should not rely on interviews and mental status examinations alone to determine level of disability. As noted in the AMA *Guides,* "Current research finds little relationship between psychiatric signs and symptoms identified during a mental status examination and the ability to perform competitive work" (American Medical Association 2000, p. 361).

Extensive review of relevant documentation is an essential part of the evaluation of disability related to the events or illness in question. An individual's level of functioning may vary considerably over time. Thus, evidence of functioning over a sufficiently long period of time before the date of examination should be obtained. Relevant documents include treatment notes, hospital discharge summaries, work evaluations, and rehabilitation progress notes if they are available. Clinicians should describe the length and history of the impairment, points of exacerbation and remission, any history of hospitalization or outpatient treatment, and modalities of treatment used in the past.

Prognostic assessments may also inform certain aspects of the litigation, including award of damages or entitlement to benefits for treatment. In workers' compensation cases, prognosis is a key factor in the determination of the likely duration of the impairment caused by the injury (Melton et al. 1997). The prognosis of the individual's illness is closely related to the degree and duration of an impairment or disability. Determination of the future degree of disability should be based on the assessment of current impairment and comparative assessment of functioning before and after the events in question. The assessment of prognosis should be informed by a thorough clinical evaluation as well as the epidemiological data regarding the natural course of the disorder.

In formulating opinions regarding prognosis, examiners should evaluate the extent to which treatment will restore the person's capacity to work (American Medical Association 2000). There are many variations in the course of recovery from an acute psychiatric disorder, ranging from complete remission to the development of a chronic illness. The effects of treatment can be a major factor in the course of the disorder and, therefore, in the determination of prognosis. The assessment of permanent impairment or disability should not be attempted until the claimant has received a sufficient trial of appropriate treatment. An individual who is quite symptomatic and impaired but has not obtained treatment may be someone whose condition will improve with appropriate treatment and, thus, have a good prognosis. In addition, examiners should also consider the presence or severity of factors that significantly worsen prognosis. Comorbid psychiatric disorders, such as substance abuse or personality disorders, complicate recovery or remission. The individual's life history, the availability of personal and social support, and the status of other related medical or psychosocial problems may also play a role in prognostic assessment.

The relationship between prognosis, functional impairment, and long-term disability requires assessment of issues such as secondary gain, malingering, and lifestyle. It may be difficult to untangle the effects of characterological depression, poor motivation, personality conflicts, the secondary gain of unemployment, and a lack of opportunity. Perhaps the most significant factor in recovery from impairment is motivation. Regardless of occupation, even minimal impairment may lead to permanent disability when the claimant is not motivated to obtain appropriate treatment or to recover previous level of functioning. Lack of motivation may be hard to distinguish from mental impairment, such as depression or avoidance, and requires careful assessment. Such determinations can be particularly difficult in the context of litigation, where remaining symptomatic and impaired may result in a better legal and financial outcome.

Finally, the evaluation should also consider the role of litigation in the clinical presentation and assessment of functional impairment (Gold and Simon 2001). Involvement in the litigation process is an extremely stressful experience. Litigation is widely acknowledged to exacerbate psychological symptoms regardless of diagnosis (Strasburger 1999). Extended litigation can also be disruptive to work functioning and can prove emotionally draining and demoralizing. In addition, it can lead to an interruption of treatment or therapy. These factors may combine to result in the appearance of severe impairment and disability. After the litigation is resolved, the individual's functioning may improve significantly. Thus, those aspects of functional impairment related to the stress of litigation should be identified separately from those of the underlying psychiatric disorder.

Assessments of all impairments should be as specific and detailed as possible. Psychological testing can be an important adjunct in this process. It may provide additional useful data, particularly regarding cognitive impairments, such as attention, comprehension, or memory (Gold and Simon 2001). Assessment of functional impairment should also include use of one or more of the widely available scales designed for this purpose. No analysis has examined the ways in which such impairment-rating guidelines apply to the evaluation of mental impairments (Pryor 1997). Nevertheless, the use of such scales minimizes the influence of examiner's biases related to beliefs regarding the differences between "can't work" and "won't work."

DSM provides the Global Assessment of Functioning Scale and the newer Social and Occupational Functioning Assessment Scale (American Psychiatric Association 2000). The most structured guidelines for assessment of impairment and disability are those delineated by the SSA for required use in SSDI claims. Limitations on functioning caused by the impairment must meet at least one of the "Paragraph B" criteria to qualify as a disability for purposes of these determinations. The AMA *Guides* (American Medical Association 2000) also provides scales for rating mental impairment modeled explicitly on the SSA rules for determining disability. Even when not required for use in litigation or claims, psychiatrists should consider the routine use of one or more of these scales. In tort cases, for example, the scales in the AMA *Guides* can provide a point of reference because they stress linking the injury to the activities in which the claimant normally engages. They are also useful in private disability evaluations because they focus on work-related injury.

## Conclusion

Psychiatrists have become increasingly involved in employment litigation over past years as a result of the increase in the amount of employment related claims. Expert testimony may be critical component in legal arguments or administrative decisions regarding damages, disability, prognosis, causation, and eligibility for private or public insurance benefits. Employment evaluations begin with identification of the legal issues relevant to the specific type of claim or lawsuit. The three most common issues in such assessments relate to diagnosis, causation and disability. Psychiatrists providing such assessments should familiarize themselves with the facts and legal requirements of the specific case, and provide opinions based on a thorough review of documents and evaluation of the claimant.

## Key Points

- The three primary aspects of psychiatric evaluation in employment litigation are diagnosis, causation, and disability.
- Diagnostic assessments should be made according to DSM criteria.
- Assessments of causation should always consider preexisting illness, alternate causation, and prior history of trauma.
- Assessments of disability must specifically correlate impairments related to psychiatric illness with specific work-related functions.

## Practice Guidelines

1. Determine the legal issues relevant to the type of litigation and structure the evaluation accordingly.
2. Establish or refute a diagnosis based on DSM criteria.
3. Base opinions regarding causation on a thorough evaluation of the incident in question, as well as prior psychiatric and trauma history. Consider the possibility of preexisting disorder and past or present alternate trauma exposure.
4. Base opinions regarding disability on a comparison of the individual's level of function before and after the onset of the disorder. Assess the individual's longitudinal functioning, current impairments, occupational requirements, and multiple other factors.
5. Use standard methods of forensic and clinical assessment in determining diagnosis and causation and in evaluating the level of functional psychiatric impairment. Support opinions with documented evidence from review of records, testing when indicated, use of standardized scales when available, and personal evaluation of the claimant.

## References

American Medical Association: Guides to the Evaluation of Permanent Impairment, 5th Edition. Chicago, IL, American Medical Association, 2000

American Psychiatric Association: Diagnostic and Statistical Manual of Mental Disorders, 4th Edition, Text Revision. Washington, DC, American Psychiatric Association, 2000

Aviera AT, Boehm WP: Mental disorders commonly claimed in employment litigation, in Mental and Emotional Injuries in Employment Litigation. Edited by McDonald JJ, Kulick FB. Washington, DC, Bureau of National Affairs, 1994, pp 32–67

Bonnie RJ: Work disability and the fabric of mental health law: an introduction, in Mental Disorder, Work Disability and the Law. Edited by Bonnie RJ, Monahan J. Chicago, IL, University of Chicago Press, 1997, pp 1–12

Breslau N: Outcomes of posttraumatic stress disorder. J Clin Psychiatry 62 (suppl 17):55–59, 2001

Briere J: Psychological Assessment of Adult Posttraumatic States. Washington, DC, American Psychological Association, 1997

Brodsky CM: Factors influencing work-related disability, in Psychiatric Disability: Clinical, Legal, and Administrative Dimensions. Edited by Meyerson AT, Fine T. Washington, DC, American Psychiatric Press, 1987a, pp 49–65

Brodsky CM: The psychiatric evaluation in workers' compensation, in Psychiatric Disability: Clinical, Legal, and Administrative Dimensions. Edited by Meyerson AT, Fine T. Washington, DC, American Psychiatric Press, 1987b, pp 313–332

Danner D, Sagall EL. Medicolegal causation: a source of professional misunderstanding. Am J Law Med 3:303–308, 1977

Galea S, Ahem J, Resnick H, et al: Psychological sequelae of the September 11 terrorist attacks in NewYork City. N Engl J Med 346(13):982–987, 2002

Gold LH: Posttraumatic stress disorder in employment litigation, in Posttraumatic Stress Disorder in Litigation, 2nd Edition. Edited by Simon RI. Washington, DC, American Psychiatric Publishing, 2002a, pp 163–186

Gold LH: Psychiatric diagnoses and retrospective assessment of mental states, in Retrospective Assessment of Mental States in Litigation: Predicting the Past. Edited by Simon RI, Shuman DW. Washington, DC, American Psychiatric Publishing, 2002b, pp 335–368

Gold LH, Simon RI: Posttraumatic stress disorder in employment cases, in Mental and Emotional Injuries in Employment Litigation, 2nd Edition. Edited by McDonald JJ, Kulick FB. Washington, DC, Bureau of National Affairs, 2001, pp 502–573

Green BL, Kaltman SI: Recent research findings on the diagnosis of posttraumatic stress disorder: prevalence, course, comorbidity and risk, in Posttraumatic Stress Disorder in Litigation: Guidelines for Forensic Assessment, 2nd Edition. Edited by Simon RI. Washington, DC, American Psychiatric Publishing, 2002, pp 19–40

Halleck SL, Hoge SK, Miller RD, et al: The use of psychiatric diagnoses in the legal process: task force report of the American Psychiatric Association. Bull Am Acad Psychiatry Law 20:481–499, 1992

Harris v Forklift Systems Inc, 510 U.S. 17, 114 S. Ct. 367 (1993)

Kendler KS, Karkowski LM, Prescott, C: Causal relationship between stressful life events and the onset of major depression. Am J Psychiatry 156:837–841, 1999

Kessler RC, Sonnega A, Bromet E, et al: Posttraumatic stress disorder in the national comorbidity survey. Arch Gen Psychiatry 52:1048–1060, 1995

Lindemann B, Kadue DD: Sexual Harassment in Employment Law. Washington, DC, Bureau of National Affairs, 1992

Lipian MS: Personality disorders in employment litigation, in Mental and Emotional Injuries in Employment Litigation, 2nd Edition. Edited by McDonald JJ, Kulick FB. Washington, DC, Bureau of National Affairs, 2001, pp 212–261

Long BL: Psychiatric diagnoses in sexual harassment cases. Bull Am Acad Psychiatry Law 22:195–203, 1994

Melton GB, Petrila J, Poythress NG, et al (eds): Psychological Evaluation for the Courts: A Handbook for Mental Health Professionals and Lawyers, 2nd Edition. New York, Guilford, 1997

Merchant JA, Lundell JA: Workplace Violence: A Report to the Nation. Iowa City, University of Iowa Injury Prevention Research Center, 2001

Metzner JL, Struthers DR, Fogel JD: Psychiatric disability determinations and personal injury litigation, in Principles and Practice of Forensic Psychiatry. Edited by Rosner R. New York, Chapman & Hall, 1994, pp 232–241

McDonald JJ, Kulick FP. Preface: the rise of the psychological injury claim, in Mental and Emotional Injuries in Employment Litigation, 2nd Edition. Edited by McDonald JJ, Kulick FB. Washington, DC, Bureau of National Affairs, 2001, pp xxxvi–xlv

National Institute for Occupational Safety and Health: Violence in the Workplace: Risk Factors and Prevention Strategies (Current Intelligence Bulletin 57). Washington, DC, National Institute for Occupational Safety and Health, June 1996

North CS, Nixon SJ, Shariat S, et al: Psychiatric disorders among survivors of the Oklahoma City bombing. JAMA 282(8):755–762, 1999

Occupational Safety and Health Administration: Occupational injury and illness incidence rates per 100 full time workers 1973–98, 1999. Washington, DC, Occupational Safety and Health Administration. Available at: http://www.osha.gov/oshstats/bltable.html. Accessed December 3, 2001.

Price DR: Personality disorders and traits, in Mental and Emotional Injuries in Employment Litigation. Edited by McDonald JJ, Kulick FB. Washington, DC, Bureau of National Affairs, 1994, pp 93–140

Pryor ES: Mental disabilities and the disability fabric, in Mental Disorder, Work Disability and the Law. Edited by Bonnie RJ, Monahan J. Chicago, IL, University of Chicago Press, 1997, pp 153–198

Rosen GM: The Aleutian Enterprise sinking and posttraumatic stress disorder: misdiagnosis in clinical and forensic settings. Professional Psychology: Research and Practice 26:82–87, 1995

Savodnik I: The concept of stress in psychiatry. Western State University Law Review 19:175–189, 1991

Schlenger WE, Caddell JM, Ebert L, et al: Psychological reactions to terrorist attacks: findings from the National Study of Americans' Reactions to September 11. JAMA 2888(5):581–588, 2002

Shalev AY, Freedman MA, Peri T, et al: Prospective study of posttraumatic stress disorder and depression following trauma. Am J Psychiatry 155:630–637, 1998

Shuman DW: The *Diagnostic and Statistical Manual of Mental Disorders* in the courts. Bull Am Acad Psychiatry Law 17:25–32, 1989

Shuman DW: Persistent reexperiences in the law and psychiatry: current and future trends for the role of PTSD in litigation, in Posttraumatic Stress Disorder in Litigation: Guidelines for Forensic Assessment, 2nd Edition. Edited by Simon RI. Washington, DC, American Psychiatric Publishing, 2002, pp 1–18

Simon RI: Clinical Psychiatry and the Law, 2nd Edition. Washington, DC, American Psychiatric Press, 1992

Simon RI: Forensic psychiatric assessment of PTSD claimants. In Posttraumatic Stress Disorder in Litigation: Guidelines for Forensic Assessment, 2nd Edition. Edited by Simon RI. Washington, DC, American Psychiatric Publishing, 2002, pp 41–90

Southerland MD, Collins PA, Scarborough KE: Workplace Violence: A Continuum From Threat to Death. Cincinnati, OH, Anderson Publishing, 1997

Strasburger LH: The litigant-patient: mental health consequences of civil litigation. J Am Acad Psychiatry Law 27:203–212, 1999

Strubbe MR, Lindemann B, Kadue DD: Sexual Harassment in Employment Law: 1999 Cumulative Supplement. Washington, DC, Bureau of National Affairs, 1999

Toyota Motor Mfg., Ky., Inc. v Williams, Supreme Court No. 00–1089, 2002

U.S. Department of Justice: National Crime Victimization Survey: Workplace Violence, 1992–96 (NCJ 168634). Washington, DC, U.S. Department of Justice, 1998

van der Kolk BA, McFarlane AC: The black hole of trauma, in Traumatic Stress: The Effects of Overwhelming Experience on Mind, Body and Society. Edited by van der Kolk BA, McFarlane AC, Weisaeth L. New York, Guilford, 1996, pp 3–23

Warshaw C: Women and violence, in Psychological Aspects of Women's Health Care: The Interface between Psychiatry and Obstetrics and Gynecology, 2nd Edition. Edited by Stotland NL, Stewart DE. Washington, DC, American Psychiatric Press, 2001, pp 477–527

Yehuda R, Wong CM: Etiology and biology of posttraumatic stress disorder: implications for treatment. Psychiatr Clin North Am Annual of Drug Therapy 8:109–134, 2001

## Suggested Readings

American Medical Association: Guides to the Evaluation of Permanent Impairment, 5th Edition. Chicago, IL, American Medical Association, 2000

Bonnie RJ, Monahan J (eds): Mental Disorder, Work Disability, and the Law. Chicago, IL, University of Chicago Press, 1997

Gold LH: Sexual Harassment: Psychiatric Assessment in Employment Litigation. Washington, DC, American Psychiatric Publishing (in press)

Meyerson AT, Fine T (eds). Psychiatric Disability: Clinical, Legal and Administrative Dimensions. Washington, DC, American Psychiatric Press, 1987

Simon RI (ed): Posttraumatic Stress Disorder in Litigation, 2nd Edition. Washington, DC, American Psychiatric Publishing, 2002

# PART III

# Issues in Criminal Justice

CHAPTER 15

# Competency to Stand Trial and the Insanity Defense

Phillip J. Resnick, M.D.

Stephen Noffsinger, M.D.

## Introduction

Forensic psychiatrists are frequently asked to perform competency to stand trial and sanity evaluations. Many general mental health clinicians will be asked at some point in their career to perform a competency or sanity evaluation. In this chapter we present practical guidelines for performing these evaluations.

A defense attorney, judge, or prosecutor may raise the issue of a criminal defendant's competency to stand trial at any point during criminal proceedings. In practice, defense attorneys most often raise the issue. A defendant's competency may be questioned when a defendant is obviously mentally ill, has a prior history of mental illness, or is having difficulty interacting with the court or defense counsel. Once the trial begins, the court should question a defendant's competency to stand trial if the defendant behaves irrationally or exhibits an unusual demeanor at trial (*Drope v. Missouri* 1974).

A defense attorney may raise an insanity defense if there is a possibility that the defendant's mental illness was a factor in the offense. Suspicions may be based on a defendant's present or past mental illness or reports that the defendant behaved bizarrely during or after the offense. After an insanity plea is filed, the court will order a sanity evaluation by a mental health professional. The prosecution, as well as the defense, may request additional sanity evaluations.

We discuss the following case example in the context of both competency and sanity.

## Clinical Vignette

Mr. B was charged with felonious assault for the serious assault of his neighbor. Mr. B had chronic schizophrenia with delusions and auditory hallucinations. He had a property dispute with his neighbor that had recently resulted in a lawsuit. In the days before the offense Mr. B delusionally believed that his neighbor was transmitting lethal brain waves that would soon kill Mr. B. On the day of the offense Mr. B telephoned his neighbor, demanding that the neighbor stop projecting the lethal brain waves. On the day of the offense Mr. B also complained to the police that his neighbor had trespassed on his property. When Mr. B encountered his neighbor at the property line, Mr. B said, "I gave you the chance to stop the brain waves—now you are going to pay!" Mr. B struck the neighbor several times with a hammer, threw the hammer in a trash can, and fled. A passerby called the police, who apprehended Mr. B after a foot chase and struggle.

Mr. B refused to cooperate with his defense attorney, believing that his attorney emitted the same lethal brain waves. Mr. B's defense attorney requested that the court order competency to stand trial and sanity evaluations. On the basis of a competency evaluation performed by a mental health professional, Mr. B was adjudicated incompetent to stand trial because his delusions interfered with his working relationship with his defense attorney. He was committed to a psychiatric hospital for treatment designed to restore his competency to stand trial. After several months in the hospital, Mr. B was restored to competency, and then he raised an insanity defense.

## Competency to Stand Trial

Competency, generally, is the capacity to understand, rationally manipulate, and apply information to make a reasoned decision on a specific issue. There are many types of competency, each with its own legal standard. Competency to stand trial is one specific type of competency.

The symptoms of many mental disorders may affect competency. However, a person may exhibit symptoms of a major mental illness and remain competent, as long as the symptoms of the illness do not impair the specific areas of functioning required for competence. Competency is based on an individual's present functioning. Because the symptoms of mental illness may fluctuate over time, an individual's competency may also change over time. A person in the midst of a manic episode may be rendered incompetent in a specific area because of racing thoughts, delusions, distractibility, and poor judgment. Once the manic episode has resolved, competency may be reestablished.

The right to be competent to stand trial is guaranteed by the U.S. Constitution, including the Sixth (right to confront witnesses, right to counsel) and Fourteenth Amendments (right to substantive and procedural due process of law). The prohibition against trying an unfit defendant is "a by-product of the ban against trials in absentia; the mentally incompetent defendant, though physically present in the courtroom, is in reality afforded no opportunity to defend himself" (Foote 1960).

## History of Competency to Stand Trial

The origins of competency to stand trial can be traced to thirteenth-century trials before the king's court in England. Criminal defendants who failed to enter a plea of guilty or not guilty were given three warnings by the court and then either confined and starved (*prison forte et dure*) or gradually crushed under increasing weights (*peine forte et dure*) until they entered a plea or died (Grubin 1996). The phrase "to press someone for an answer" originates from this practice. Before engaging such methods, the king's court first needed to determine whether the defendant was intentionally withholding a plea (mute by malice) or whether, because of a mental defect, the defendant was unable to understand that a plea was required (mute by visitation of God). Those defendants found mute by visitation of God were spared the extreme methods just described, and a not guilty plea was entered for them.

## Modern Standards for Competency to Stand Trial

In 1960 the U.S. Supreme Court articulated the modern American standard for competency to stand trial (*Dusky v. United States* 1960). This standard depends on whether a criminal defendant "has sufficient ability to consult with his lawyer with a reasonable degree of rational understanding, and whether he has a rational as well as factual understanding of the proceedings against him." All states, borrowing from *Dusky*, adopted a similar test for competency. A defendant is incompetent to stand trial if, because of a present mental disorder, either of the following conditions is true:

1. The defendant is unable to understand the nature and objectives of the court proceedings.
2. The defendant is unable to assist in the defense.

A defect in either part of the test may result in a finding of incompetence to stand trial. Incompetence to stand trial must be proven by a preponderance of the evidence (*Cooper v. Oklahoma* 1996) by the defense.

The standard in federal court for competency to stand trial is similar to the states' standards. Incompetence is found when the defendant "is presently suffering from a mental disease or defect rendering him mentally incompetent to the extent that he is unable to understand the nature and consequences of the proceedings against him or to assist properly in his defense" (18 U.S.C., § 4241).

## Procedures for Performing a Competency to Stand Trial Evaluation

When a defendant's competency to stand trial is questioned, the court will order the defendant to be examined by a mental health professional. Defense attorneys have doubts about their client's competence in 8%–15% of felony cases (Hoge et al. 1992; Poythress et al. 1994). Competency to stand trial evaluations are among the most frequently requested types of forensic evaluations performed by mental health professionals. Annually, 25,000–50,000 criminal defendants are referred for competency to stand trial evaluations (Hoge et al. 1997; Skeem et al. 1998). Many courts have associated mental health clinics responsible for performing competency evaluations. Other courts refer these evaluations to private practitioners (Grisso 1996). Most competency to stand trial evaluations are done on an outpatient basis, although provisions are usually available for inpatient evaluations if the outpatient evaluation is inconclusive (Grisso et al. 1994).

The clinician performing the competency to stand trial examination should

1. Be familiar with the competency to stand trial standard in the jurisdiction.
2. Review the defendant's relevant medical records.
3. Review relevant collateral sources of information (jail medical records, interview of family members, etc.).
4. Conduct a personal interview of the defendant, consisting of
    - A standard psychiatric diagnostic interview and mental status examination. The defendant's orientation, memory, concentration, mood, and affect and the presence of delusions, hallucinations, and loose associations are especially relevant.
    - An inquiry into the specific areas of competency to stand trial.
5. Provide a written report with a well-reasoned opinion on the competency to stand trial issue, applying the facts of the case to the legal competency standard.

Most states have statutes prohibiting data obtained from a competency to stand trial evaluation from being used to prove a defendant's guilt. For example, if a defendant confesses guilt to a clinician during a competency evaluation, the confession would be inadmissible at trial in most jurisdictions.

## Elements of the Competency to Stand Trial Evaluation

A number of specific inquiries must be made when performing a competency to stand trial evaluation. Using the two-part legal standard for competency to stand trial, described above, the clinician should examine the following areas:

1. Nature and objectives of the court proceedings
    a. *Charges.* Does the defendant understand the nature of the criminal charges? Knowledge of the official name of the charge is useful, but it is more important that defendants understand the nature of the specific act that they are accused of committing. For example, it is insufficient that defendants know that they are charged with aggravated robbery; defendants should understand that they are charged with robbing a specific victim on a specific date.
    b. *Severity of charge.* Defendants should understand the severity of the charge (misdemeanor or felony) and the possible range of sentences they face if convicted.
    c. *Pleas.* Defendants should understand the various pleas available, including guilty, not guilty, no contest, and not guilty by reason of insanity (and guilty but mentally ill, in some jurisdictions).
    d. *Courtroom personnel roles.* Defendants should understand the roles of the defendant, defense attorney, judge, prosecutor, jury, witness, and victim.
    e. *Adversarial nature of trial.* Defendants must understand which court personnel are acting adversely to their interests, and they must demonstrate self-protective behavior. Defendants who, because of a mental disorder, seek to confess to the prosecutor while waiting for the trial to begin may well be incompetent to stand trial.
2. Ability to assist in defense (including the ability to do the following)
    a. *Work with defense attorney.* Defendants must be able to have logical and coherent discussions with their attorneys and be free of paranoid thinking about their attorneys. Defendants should also be able to communicate relevant information to their defense

counsels. Incoherent or mute defendants are likely to be incompetent (Bonnie et al. 1997).

b. *Appreciate their situation as criminal defendants.* Defendants should understand that they are charged with a crime and are facing prosecution (Bonnie et al. 1997). Defendants who delusionally believe that they are immune from criminal prosecution are likely to be found incompetent to stand trial.

c. *Understand plea bargaining.* About 85% of criminal defendants plea bargain, by agreeing to plead guilty in exchange for a reduced charge and/or sentence. Therefore, it is important that defendants understand the concept of plea bargaining and have the capacity to rationally make decisions about plea bargaining in their own case.

d. *Consider a mental illness defense.* Defendants must possess sufficient insight into their mental illness to consider pleading not guilty by reason of insanity, guilty but mentally ill, or seeking mitigation due to mental illness, if relevant. Defendants who are otherwise competent to stand trial but irrationally refuse a mental illness defense may have such a defense imposed on them by the court and still proceed to trial (*Frendak v. United States* 1979).

e. *Appraise evidence and estimate likely outcome of trial.* Defendants must be able to evaluate evidence, determine which evidence is helpful or harmful to their case, and estimate their chances of conviction. Defendants must also be able to apply this knowledge in deciding whether to enter a plea.

f. *Possess sufficient memory and concentration to understand the events at trial.* Defendants must be able to pay attention during trial and have sufficient memory to retain and apply the information during trial.

g. *Understand appropriate courtroom behavior.* Defendants must understand appropriate courtroom behavior and possess sufficient impulse control to exercise appropriate courtroom demeanor. It is important to differentiate between a defendant who (because of a mental disorder) is not capable of acting appropriately and a defendant who elects to act inappropriately to make a political statement.

h. *Give a rational, consistent, and coherent account of the offense.* Defendants must be able to give a consistent and organized account of the offense. Such an account may help to achieve alibi, acquittal, insanity, or mitigation. However, a defendant with permanent amnesia for the offense is not categorically incompetent to stand trial (*Wilson v. United States* 1968).

i. *Formulate a basic plan of defense.* Defendants should be able to work with their attorneys to develop a basic plan of defense, working toward the goal of acquittal or mitigation.
j. *Make reasonable defense decisions.* Using their knowledge of the information listed above, defendants must be able to rationally apply their knowledge to their defense and make reasonable, logic-driven decisions.
k. *Have freedom from self-defeating behavior.* Defendants must be motivated to seek the best possible outcome for their criminal trial. Defendants who consciously seek an unfavorable outcome, because of mental illness, may be incompetent to stand trial. For example, a depressed, suicidal defendant who is seeking capital punishment is likely to be found incompetent to stand trial.

Many instruments have been developed to assess competence to stand trial, including the Competency Screening Test (Lipsitt et al. 1971), Competency to Stand Trial Assessment Instrument (U.S. Department of Health 1973), Interdisciplinary Fitness Interview (Golding et al. 1984), and Georgia Court Competency Test (Nicholson et al. 1988). Many of these instruments are of limited utility because they only assess a defendant's factual understanding, not reasoning ability (Hoge et al. 1997). The MacArthur Competence Assessment Tool—Criminal Adjudication (Mac-CAT-CA) is a recently developed instrument to assess "adjudicative competence," which includes competence to enter a plea, stand trial, and participate in pretrial proceedings (Hoge et al. 1997). It is a standardized instrument that assesses both factual knowledge and decisional competence (Bonnie 1993). Canadian researchers have developed the Fitness Interview Test, specifically designed to address the Canadian competency to stand trial standard (Zapf et al. 2001).

## Outcome of Competency to Stand Trial Evaluation

Once raised as a legal issue, a defendant's competency to stand trial is usually addressed by the court in a competency hearing (*Pate v. Robinson* 1966). The competency issue is ultimately a legal question, to be adjudicated by a judge. Clinical opinions on the issue of competence are admitted into evidence at a competency hearing. Courts usually (up to 90% of the time) base the adjudication of competence on the clinical opinion of the court-appointed forensic mental health professional (Freckelton 1996; Reich and Tookey 1986).

The majority of defendants clinically examined for competency to stand trial are found to be competent. The presence of a mental disorder is insufficient to conclude that a criminal defendant is incompetent to stand trial. In one study, almost one-third of defendants referred for competency evaluations who were found competent to stand trial had a psychotic disorder (Roesch et al. 1981). Although a mental disorder is necessary to conclude that a defendant is incompetent to stand trial, incompetency also requires that the mental disorder impair the defendant's performance on the specific functional areas relevant to the competency standard.

On average, 30% of defendants evaluated for competence to stand trial are adjudicated incompetent (Nicholson and Kugler 1991), although there is a wide range (4%–77%) of incompetency rates in different jurisdictions (Cochrane et al. 2001). From 37% to 50% of geriatric defendants are found to be incompetent (Frierson et al. 2002; Heinik et al. 1994; Riley 1998). Males and females are equally likely to be found incompetent to stand trial (Riley 1998). Younger adults are more likely to be incompetent because of a psychotic or mood disorder or mental retardation, whereas older defendants are more likely to be incompetent because of dementia (Frierson et al. 2002). Preteens and young adolescents are frequently incompetent because of numerous deficiencies, including inability to disclose relevant data to defense counsel, susceptibility to outside influence, inability to appraise the quality of their legal representation, and difficulty making decisions about their defense (McKee 1998; Slovenko 2000). Common reasons for incompetence to stand trial are listed in Table 15–1.

Defendants adjudicated incompetent to stand trial are usually committed to a hospital for treatment to restore them to competency. Approximately 7,000 defendants are involuntarily committed to public hospitals annually for restoration to competence (Steadman and Hartstone 1983). Restoration to competence is accomplished by treating the defendant's underlying mental illness and providing education about the trial process (Noffsinger 2001). About 80%–90% of defendants found incompetent to stand trial will eventually be restored to competence. This rate varies, however, depending on the severity of the defendant's illness and the statutory time allowed for restoration to competency.

Defendants adjudicated incompetent to stand trial are still presumed competent to make treatment decisions. However, an incompetent defendant who refuses antipsychotic medications may be involuntarily treated if so ordered by the court. In *Washington v. Harper* (1990) and, later, *Riggins v. Nevada* (1992), the U.S. Supreme Court found that the government may forcibly administer antipsychotic medication to a prisoner or

**TABLE 15–1.** Common reasons for incompetence to stand trial

- Low intelligence or dementia that impairs the defendant's understanding of the trial process
- Depression and self-defeating behavior that limit the defendant's motivation for the best outcome at trial
- Mania that impairs the defendant's ability to act appropriately in the courtroom
- Paranoid delusions that impair the defendant's ability to work with defense counsel
- Disorganized thinking that impairs the defendant's concentration and attention
- Irrational decision making about the defense as the result of delusions, disorganized thinking, low intellect, or dementia
- Hallucinations that distract the defendant from attending to the trial

criminal defendant. Such treatment may be given despite the individual's liberty interest to avoid unwanted medication, as long as the proposed medication was medically appropriate and furthered a legitimate governmental interest.

The U.S. Supreme Court has not directly addressed the issue of involuntary medication to restore competency to stand trial, but the issue has been addressed *en point* on the appellate level. In *United States v. Weston* (2001), the U.S. Court of Appeals ruled that the government's interest to make a defendant competent to stand trial by involuntarily administering antipsychotic medication overrode his individual liberty interests. The court found that restoring competence to stand trial with involuntary medication did not violate a defendant's right to a fair trial as long as the medication was medically appropriate.

Some defendants, because of the nature of their mental disorder, will not be restored to competency to stand trial. Common reasons for unrestorability include treatment-resistant psychosis, dementia, and moderate to severe mental retardation. Defendants who are incompetent to stand trial may not be committed for restoration to competency unless there is a substantial likelihood that they can be restored (*Jackson v. Indiana* 1972). Therefore, a clinician who opines that a defendant is incompetent to stand trial should offer an opinion about whether the defendant is likely to be restored to competency. Charges are dismissed or held in abeyance for defendants adjudicated incompetent to stand trial and not restorable. Incompetent, unrestorable defendants may remain involuntarily hospitalized only if they are civilly committed.

## Not Guilty by Reason of Insanity

### Clinical Vignette *(continued)*

Mental health professionals who performed several insanity evaluations on Mr. B had varied opinions regarding his mental status at the time of the crime. All the clinicians agreed that Mr. B met the threshold of having a severe mental disease, based on his delusions at the time of the offense. There was mixed evidence regarding whether his mental disease impaired his knowledge of the wrongfulness of the offense. His rational motive (anger regarding the property dispute) for the offense supported his knowledge of wrongfulness, as did hiding the weapon, fleeing the scene, and struggling with police. However, Mr. B's paranoid delusions caused him to believe that he was acting in (delusional) self-defense, which supported the view that he did not know the wrongfulness of the offense. There also was mixed evidence regarding his ability to refrain from the offense. His efforts to try lesser means to resolve the dispute prior to the offense (telephoning the neighbor, complaining to police) suggested that he could not refrain because he exhausted legal efforts. However, Mr. B's anger, not mental illness, may have caused his inability to refrain from committing the offense.

Mr. B was ultimately adjudicated not guilty by reason of insanity at trial, and he was committed to a state psychiatric facility. Approximately 1% of defendants charged with a felony plead insanity (Callahan et al. 1987). Overall, 15%–25% of defendants who plead insanity are adjudicated legally insane. Juries are much less likely to render an insanity verdict than judges. Eighty percent of successful insanity verdicts are not contested by the prosecution (Rogers et al. 1984); however, when clinicians disagree on the issue of sanity, an insanity plea is frequently unsuccessful.

A defendant adjudicated not guilty by reason of insanity is technically acquitted of the offense; the court may not punish defendants who are acquitted (Noffsinger and Resnick 1999). Insanity acquittees usually remain under the jurisdiction of the trial court or a legislatively created panel to supervise insanity acquittees. The disposition of an insanity acquittee balances the acquittee's need for treatment with concern about public safety. In most jurisdictions a legal finding of not guilty by reason of insanity results in commitment to a psychiatric inpatient facility; however, a small number of insanity acquittees are directly placed on conditional release in the community.

### History of the Insanity Defense

Under early English common law, courts sought to determine whether a child or mentally ill person could differentiate right from wrong (in the global sense) when determining whether the accused should be held responsible for an illegal act. Various tests were devised to determine whether a child or mentally ill person had the capacity to tell right from wrong, including counting 12 pence or other tests of intellectual function. William Lombarde (1536–1601) expressed the sentiment common in the sixteenth century toward accused children and mentally ill persons when he said, "If a madman or natural fool, or a lunatic in the time of his lunacy, or a child that apparently hath no knowledge of good nor evil do kill a man, this is no felonious act...for they cannot be said to have any understanding will."

A number of British and American insanity standards are summarized in Table 15–2. The M'Naghten standard (*McNaughtan's case* 1843) was highly influential because it was the first insanity case considered by an appellate court. Another approach to insanity standards is the irresistible impulse test (*Regina v. Oxford* 1840; American Law Institute 1955), which was concerned with whether the defendant, because of mental illness, could refrain from committing the offense. The majority of American jurisdictions now use the M'Naghten insanity standard. A minority of states add some variation of the irresistible impulse test to the M'Naghten standard (Giorgi-Guarnieri et al. 2002).

**TABLE 15–2.** Summary of insanity standards

- **Wild Beast Test** (*Rex v. Arnold* 1724)
  A man must be totally deprived of his understanding and memory, so as not to know what he is doing, no more than an infant, a brute, or a wild beast.
- **Irresistible Impulse Test** (*Regina v. Oxford* 1840)
  If some controlling disease was, in truth, the acting power within him which he could not resist, then he will not be held responsible.
- ***M'Naghten* Rule** (*McNaughtan's case* 1843)
  A mental disease or defect at the time of the act which caused the defendant not to know the nature and quality or the wrongfulness of the act.
- ***Durham* Rule** (*Durham v. United States* 1954)
  The accused is not criminally responsible if his unlawful act is the product of a mental disease or defect.
- **Model Penal Code** (American Law Institute 1955)
  A person is not responsible for criminal conduct if at the time of such conduct, as a result of mental disease or defect, he lacks substantial capacity to appreciate the wrongfulness of his conduct (cognitive arm) or to conform his conduct to the requirements of the law (volitional arm).

## Procedure for Conducting a Sanity Evaluation

When an insanity defense evaluation is requested, the clinician should carry out the following steps:

1. Determine the exact legal insanity standard currently used in the jurisdiction. This standard can be obtained from the court, prosecutor, or defense attorney who referred the defendant for assessment.
2. Ascertain the facts of the case. This is done by reviewing the following sources of information (discussed separately below):
   - Defendant's medical and psychiatric records
   - Observations of the defendant made at the time of the offense, including witness, victim, and police reports of the defendant's behavior
   - Personal interview of the defendant, including the defendant's account of the offense
3. Apply the relevant legal standard to the facts of the case and formulate an expert opinion on the insanity issue.

### *Determining the Facts of the Case*

**Defendant's medical and psychiatric records.** The clinician should obtain the defendant's medical and psychiatric records prior to interviewing the defendant. It is important for the clinician to be aware if the defendant has prior psychiatric illnesses, substance use disorders, or antisocial personality traits. It is imperative that the clinician review the defendant's psychiatric records closest in time to the offense because they may contain critical information regarding the defendant's mental state before or after the time of the offense. Some defendants are psychiatrically hospitalized after committing their crime. The psychiatric record for this hospitalization often contains detailed information regarding the defendant's mental status close to the time of the offense, and it may possibly contain statements from the defendant regarding the offense. If the defendant does not sign a release for these records, a court order should be sought to obtain them.

**Observations of the defendant at the time of the offense.** Victims, witnesses, and police often make detailed statements after a defendant has been arrested. These statements are a rich source of information regarding the defendant's mental state at the time of the offense. These statements should be reviewed for indications that the defendant was (or was not) behaving bizarrely, intoxicated, hallucinating, or delusional at the time of the offense. If statements are not available, a personal interview with the victim(s) or witness(es) should be attempted.

**Personal interview of defendant.** The defendant should be interviewed as close to the time of the offense as possible. Early evaluation reduces the likelihood that the defendant will have been coached about the legal criteria for insanity. As time passes, defendants may change their account of the offense because of unconscious distortion or conscious attempts to malinger insanity. Prompt examination also enhances the clinician's credibility in court.

At the outset of the interview the defendant must be told about the purpose of the evaluation, the disposition of the insanity report, and the lack of confidentiality. Most jurisdictions exclude from evidence any incriminating statements made during an insanity evaluation to prove guilt. However, in a limited number of jurisdictions, statements made by a defendant during a forensic evaluation can be admitted as a confession to the offense.

A careful psychiatric history should be obtained from the defendant, including inquiry into the nature of hallucinations and delusions and history of past treatment efforts. The clinician should be alert to the possibility that the defendant may attempt to malinger psychosis to succeed with an insanity defense. The clinician should obtain from the defendant a detailed account of the offense. It is often helpful for the clinician to have the defendant give a step-by-step account of the defendant's actions beginning 1 day prior to the offense. This account should include detailed information on psychiatric symptoms, medication compliance, and use of intoxicants.

The clinician should let the defendant tell the story uninterrupted and should not suggest any psychiatric symptoms that a malingering defendant may falsely endorse. After the defendant has given a detailed narrative account of his or her actions, the clinician may fill in the details by asking more specific questions. If the defendant admits doing the offense, the clinician should elicit the defendant's motivation for committing the offense. The clinician may wish to confront the defendant with inconsistent collateral information to clarify the defendant's account (Resnick 1999).

### *Formulating an Opinion*

The clinician should state an opinion in the exact language of the insanity standard used in the jurisdiction and explain the underlying basis for the opinion. The importance of a logical rationale underlying the opinion cannot be overestimated. Jurors and judges determine the credibility of an expert based on the soundness of the reasoning for the opinion.

In forming an opinion on insanity, the clinician should do the following:

1. Assess evidence of mental illness now, in the past, and at the time of the offense.
2. Determine the onset of the symptoms of mental illness and look for evidence of impaired functioning within a few days of the offense.
3. Carefully explore the motive for the offense.
4. Consider a detailed understanding of the defendant's thinking and behavior before, during, and after the offense.
5. Consider the defendant's prior legal history and personality style.
6. Consider whether the defendant's inability to know the wrongfulness or refrain from the act was caused by mental illness or other factors, such as voluntary intoxication or rage. The clinician should assess the nexus of causation between the mental disease or defect and the impairment in knowledge of wrongfulness or ability to refrain from the act.

Virtually all insanity standards require the presence of a mental disease or defect at the time of the offense. The term "mental disease or defect" is a legal term of art and is not defined in terms of specific *Diagnostic and Statistical Manual* psychiatric diagnoses. However, most courts have held that diagnoses such as schizophrenia, major depressive disorder, and bipolar disorder qualify as mental diseases for the purpose of insanity. Some jurisdictions have also recognized posttraumatic stress disorder, dissociative identity disorder, and other dissociative disorders. A mental defect usually requires intellectual impairment in the range of at least mild mental retardation. Diagnoses such as personality disorders, paraphilias, and voluntary substance intoxication do not usually qualify as a mental disease for the purpose of insanity. *Diagnostic and Statistical Manual of Mental Disorders,* 4th Edition (DSM-IV; American Psychiatric Association 1994), and its text revision, DSM-IV-TR (American Psychiatric Association 2000), include a disclaimer that the presence of a diagnosis in the diagnostic manual does not imply that it meets legal criteria for a mental disease in an insanity defense.

Most insanity standards focus on the defendant's knowledge of wrongfulness of the offense at the time of the act. The clinician should specifically look at the following factors when evaluating knowledge of wrongfulness:

1. *The defendant's behavior at the time of the offense* gives clues about the defendant's knowledge of the wrongfulness of the offense. Hiding evidence, lying about the offense, waiting to be arrested, and fleeing from the police or the scene of the crime suggest that the defendant knew the behavior was wrong. In contrast, leaving evidence in plain view, acknowledging the offense, and making no effort to flee usually imply a lack of knowledge of wrongfulness.
2. *The defendant's statements during or after the offense* provide information about the defendant's knowledge of wrongfulness. Explicit statements made by the defendant that he or she did or did not know the act was wrong are clearly helpful.
3. *The presence of a rational alternative motive for the offense* is important in the evaluation of knowledge of wrongfulness. A rational motive, such as revenge, profit, or sexual gratification may be helpful when determining knowledge of wrongfulness.
4. *The presence of a psychotic moral justification* is another important consideration. Some defendants commit an offense with knowledge that the act is illegal but believe the act is morally justified because of their psychosis. For example, a defendant who delusionally believed her children were in excruciating permanent pain may believe that killing the children to relieve their suffering is a morally correct act, even though she knew the act was illegal.

The Model Penal Code insanity standard contains a modified version of the irresistible impulse test. In evaluating a defendant's ability to refrain (volitional test) from committing the offense, the clinician may consider the following points:

1. Evaluate the defendant's ability to refrain from committing the offense versus the defendant's ability to defer the offense. For example, a defendant may wait until the victim is alone but still feel compelled to commit the act because of a delusional fear.
2. Assess the defendant's ability to refrain from the specific offense as compared to carrying out some other legal course of action. For example, a command hallucination to clean up the environment may lead to kidnapping the director of the Environmental Protection Agency or a decision to personally pick up litter.
3. For those defendants who were unable to refrain from committing the offense, examine the cause of their inability to refrain. Was the defendant's inability to refrain from committing the offense due to mental illness or some other factor, such as voluntary intoxication or rage?

4. Determine the consequences the defendant faced for failing to commit the offense. The magnitude, likelihood, and imminence of consequences for failing to act should be examined. For example, the consequences for failing to obey a command hallucination may range from restless sleep to a belief that one's soul will spend eternity in hell.
5. Determine whether the defendant had any legal alternative course of action available other than committing the offense. For example, a defendant might have sought help from the police rather than killing a neighbor due to a delusional belief that the neighbor was sending laser beams, causing extreme pain to the defendant.

Table 15–3 contains a checklist of common errors to avoid in compentency and sanity evaluations.

## Conclusion

Forensic psychiatrists routinely perform competency and sanity evaluations. General psychiatrists who agree to perform a competency or sanity evaluation must keep in mind that their opinion will be highly influential with the court and will carry serious consequences for the defendant. The competency and sanity evaluation guidelines in this chapter will assist the general psychiatrist in performing these evaluations more effectively.

**TABLE 15–3. Common errors in competency and sanity evaluations**

- Equating psychosis with incompetence to stand trial
- Confusing competency to stand trial with insanity
- Equating psychosis at the time of the act with insanity
- Conclusory reports that fail to state the basis for the opinion
- Psychodynamic explanation for the offense given as an excuse, rather than focusing on the legal standard for sanity
- Failure to read relevant medical records
- Failure to interview the defendant
- Desire for "just" outcome, influencing the accuracy of the report
- Failure to address the correct competency or sanity standard in that particular jurisdiction
- Evaluating competency in the past rather than the present
- Evaluating sanity in the present rather than at the time of the crime

## Key Points

- Standards for competency to stand trial do not vary appreciably among jurisdictions.
- There are two elements to competency standards: 1) whether defendants are able to understand the legal proceedings and 2) whether defendants are able to assist in their defense.
- A court-appointed clinician's opinion on competency to stand trial will be highly influential in the court's decision.
- Insanity standards vary among jurisdictions. All insanity standards require a threshold of mental illness. Almost all jurisdictions allow for a finding of insanity if the defendants' mental illness impaired their knowledge of the wrongfulness of the offense. One-third of jurisdictions allow for a finding of insanity if the defendants' mental illness caused them to be unable to refrain from committing the offense, even if they knew their act was wrong.
- Contested insanity cases are rarely successful.

## Practice Guidelines

1. In assessing competency to stand trial, focus on the defendant's present mental functioning.
2. In evaluating sanity, focus on the defendant's mental state at the time of the offense.
3. Assess the impact of the defendant's mental illness on the areas of functioning addressed by the competency and sanity standards. A defendant may be seriously mentally ill but still be competent to stand trial or legally sane. The critical issue is the impact of the defendant's mental illness on the areas of functioning addressed by the competency and sanity standards.

## References

American Law Institute: Model Penal Code, § 401.1(1), 1955

American Psychiatric Association: Diagnostic and Statistical Manual of Mental Disorders, 4th Edition. Washington, DC, American Psychiatric Association, 1994

American Psychiatric Association: Diagnostic and Statistical Manual of Mental Disorders, 4th Edition, Text Revision. Washington, DC, American Psychiatric Association, 2000

Bonnie R: The competence of criminal defendants: beyond Dusky and Drope. University of Miami Law Review 47:539–601, 1993

Bonnie RJ, Hoge SK, Monahan J, et al: The MacArthur Adjudicative Competence Study: a comparison of criteria for assessing the competence of criminal defendants. J Am Acad Psychiatry Law 25(3):249–259, 1997

Callahan L, Meyer C, et al: Insanity defense reform in the United States—post Hinckley. Ment Phys Disabil Law Rep 11:54–59, 1987
Cochrane RE, Grisso T, Frederick RI: The relationship between criminal charges, diagnoses, and psycholegal opinions among federal pretrial defendants. Behavioral Sciences and the Law 19(4):565–582, 2001
Cooper v Oklahoma, 116 S. Ct. 1373 (1996)
Drope v Missouri, 420 U.S. 163 (1974)
Durham v United States, 94 U.S. App. D.C. 288 (1954)
Dusky v United States, 362 U.S. 402 (1960)
Foote C: A comment on pretrial commitment of criminal defendants. UPA Law Review 108:832, 1960
Freckelton I: Rationality and flexibility in assessment of fitness to stand trial. Int J Law Psychiatry 19:39–59, 1996
Frendak v United States, 408 A.2d 364 (1979)
Frierson RL, Shea SJ, Shea ME: Competence-to-stand-trial evaluations of geriatric defendants. J Am Acad Psychiatry Law 30(2):252–256, 2002
Giorgi-Guarnieri D, Janofsky J, Keram E, et al: AAPL practice guideline for forensic psychiatry evaluation of defendants raising the insanity defense. J Am Acad Psychiatry Law 30 (2, suppl):S3–S40, 2002
Golding SL, Roesch R, Schreiber J, et al: Assessment and conceptualization of competency to stand trial: preliminary data on the Interdisciplinary Fitness Interview. Law Hum Behav 9:321–334, 1984
Grisso T: Pretrial clinical evaluations in criminal cases—past trends and future directions. Criminal Justice and Behavior 23(1):90–106, 1996
Grisso T, Cocozza JJ, Steadman HJ, et al: The organization of pretrial forensic evaluation services: a national profile. Law and Hum Behavior 18:377–393, 1994
Grubin D: Fitness to Plead in England and Wales. East Sussex, UK, Psychology Press, 1996
Heinik J, Kimhi R, Hes JP, et al: Dementia and crime: a forensic psychiatry unit study in Israel. Int J Geriatr Psychiatry 9:491–494, 1994
Hoge SK, Bonnie RJ, Poythress N, et al: Attorney-client decision making in criminal cases: client competence and participation as perceived by their attorneys. Behav Sci Law 10:385–394, 1992
Hoge SK, Bonnie RJ, Poythress N, et al: The MacArthur Adjudicative Competence Study: development and validation of a research instrument. Law Hum Behav 21(2):141–179, 1997
Jackson v Indiana, 92 Supreme Court Reporter 1845 (1972)
Lipsitt PD, Lelos D, McGarry AL: Competency for trial: a screening instrument. Am J Psychiatry 128:105–109, 1971
McKee GR: Competency to stand trial in preadjudicatory juveniles and adults. J Am Acad Psychiatry Law 26(1):89–99, 1998
McNaughtan's case, 8 Eng. Rep. 718 (1843)
Nicholson R, Kugler K: Competent and incompetent criminal defendants: a quantitative review of comparative research. Psychol Bull 109:355–370, 1991
Nicholson RA, Briggs SR, Robertson H: Instruments for assessing competency to stand trial: how do they work? Professional Psychology 19:383–394, 1988
Noffsinger SG: Restoration to competency practice guidelines. International Journal of Offender Therapy and Comparative Criminology 45(3):356–362, 2001

Noffsinger SG, Resnick PJ: Insanity defense evaluations. Directions in Psychiatry 19:325–337, 1999

Pate v Robinson, 383 Supreme Court Reporter 375 (1966)

Poythress NG, Bonnie RJ, Hoge SK, et al: Client abilities to assist counsel and make decisions in criminal-cases: findings from three studies. Law Hum Behav 18(4):437–452, 1994

Regina v Oxford, 9 Car. and P. 525, 546 (1840)

Reich J, Tookey L: Disagreements between court and psychiatrist on competency to stand trial. J Clin Psychiatry 47:29–30, 1986

Resnick PJ: The detection of malingered psychosis. Psychiatr Clin North Am 22: 159–172, 1999

Rex v Arnold, 16 How. St. Tr. 695 (1724)

Riggins v Nevada, 504 U.S. 127; 112 S. Ct. 1810 (1992)

Riley SE: Competency to stand trial adjudication: A comparison of female and male defendants. J Am Acad Psychiatry Law 26(2):223–240, 1998

Roesch R, Eaves D, Sollner R, et al: Evaluating fitness to stand trial: a comparative analysis of fit and unfit defendants. Int J Law Psychiatry 4:145–157, 1981

Rogers JL, Bloom JD, Manson SM: Insanity defenses: contested or conceded? Am J Psychiatry 141:885–888, 1984

Skeem JL, Golding SL, et al: Logic and reliability of evaluations of competence to stand trial. Law Hum Behav 22(5):519–547, 1998

Slovenko R: The prosecution of Nathaniel Abraham—a minor. J Am Acad Psychiatry Law 28(1):89–101, 2000

Steadman H, Hartstone E: Defendants found incompetent to stand trial, in Mentally Disordered Offenders. Edited by Monahan J, Steadman H. New York, Plenum, 1983, pp 39–64

US Department of Health, E. A. W: Laboratory of Community Psychiatry: Competency to Stand Trial and Mental Illness. Rockville, MD, U.S. Dept of Health, Education and Welfare, 1973

United States v Weston, 347 U.S. App. D.C. 145; 255 F.3d 873; 2001 U.S. App. LEXIS 16851

Washington v Harper, 494 U.S. 210 (1990)

Wilson v United States, 391 F.2d, 460 (1968)

Zapf PA, Roesch R, Viljoen JL: Assessing fitness to stand trial: the utility of the Fitness Interview Test (revised edition). Can J Psychiatry 46(5):426–432, 2001

## Suggested Readings

Ciccone JR: Competence to stand trial: efforts to clarify the concept and improve clinical evaluations of criminal defendants. Current Opinion in Psychiatry 12(6):647–651, 1999

Giorgi-Guarnieri D, Janofsky J, Keram E, et al: AAPL practice guideline for forensic psychiatry evaluation of defendants raising the insanity defense. J Am Acad Psychiatry Law 30 (2, suppl):S3–S40, 2002

Simon RI, Shuman DW (eds): Retrospective Assessment of Mental States in Litigation: Predicting the Past. Washington, DC, American Psychiatric Publishing, 2002

CHAPTER 16

# Forensic Assessment of Sex Offenders

Howard Zonana, M.D.
J. Adrienne Roth, Ph.D.
Vladmir Coric, M.D.

## Introduction

The last 10–15 years has seen a resurgence of public attention to sex offenders: individuals convicted of rape, child molestation, and other illegal paraphilias. The incidence of sexual victimization has increased over the past decade. The impact of sexual assault is devastating to both the victim and society (Briere 1992; Freeman-Longo and Knopp 1992; Prentky and Burgess 1990; Snyder 2000; West 1991). Additional physical violence is often associated with such crimes (Greenfeld 1997; Riggs et al. 2000). Victims may suffer chronic mental health problems, physical injury, loss of work productivity, and difficulties with interpersonal relationships.

Sexual victimization is routinely prosecuted, but many crimes remain unreported. Society has struggled with the problems posed by the long-term management of sex offenders because any recidivism is not well tolerated by the public. On a given day in 1994, there were approximately 234,000 offenders convicted of rape or sexual assault under the care, custody, or control of corrections agencies. Nearly 60% of these sex offenders are under conditional supervision in the community (Greenfeld 1997). The large number of known, convicted but released, sex offenders in community settings has created public outrage and anxiety.

The problems involved in the evaluation and long-term management of sex offenders have brought psychiatry and the legal system together in one of the most controversial arenas encountered by forensic psychiatrists. Concerns regarding the possibility of repeat offenses create social policy and legal issues that have increasingly involved psychiatric opinions. Both society and the medical profession have been faced with the challenging task of providing reliable assessment and management plans in the hope of decreasing future sexual victimization.

One response to this challenge has resulted in laws that bring sexual offenders into direct contact with psychiatrists and the mental health system. Changes in the criminal sentencing guidelines resulted in mandatory, but finite, terms of imprisonment for sex offenders. These laws replaced the indeterminate "one day to life" sentences that were previously common. Convicted offenders are now released after serving their full sentences. The publicity associated with repeated heinous crimes committed by some of these released sex offenders resulted in pressure on legislative officials to pass new laws to protect the public.

Washington State passed the first sexual predator statute that permitted the civil commitment of certain sex offenders deemed to be sexual predators at the end of their criminal sentences (Wash. Rev. Code 71.09 [1992]). Generally, civil commitment is based on the principle of *parens patriae*—that is, that the state has an obligation to care for those who are severely mentally ill and are unable to care for themselves. Commitments under the sexual predator laws resulted in bringing individuals with nonpsychotic disorders, antisocial personality disorders, and paraphilias—individuals not in need of acute mental health treatment—into mental hospitals until they could be deemed "safe." Most mental health professionals thought these new "civil" commitments of sex offenders undermined the *parens patriae* principle of involuntary hospitalization and overemphasized the *police power* principle (Zonana et al. 2003). The Supreme Court, nevertheless, has upheld the constitutionality of this commitment schema (*Kansas v. Hendricks* 1997). At least 15 states have followed the Washington model with similar sexual predator commitment statutes.

Some states have enacted separate registration statutes such as the widely known "Megan's Law," the statute specifying registry of sexual offenders in New Jersey. In fact, since 1994, federal law has required states to implement a version of Megan's Law that meets certain minimum requirements as a condition of receiving certain federal law enforcement funds. The Jacob Wetterling Crimes Against Children and Sexually Violent Offender Registration Act of 1994 (42 U.S.C. § 14071) required that all those convicted of a criminal sex offense against a minor, and all persons convicted of a sexually violent offense, be included in states' registries (42 U.S.C. § 14071[a][1]). This statute also afforded the states considerable discretion in designing their registration and notification laws, including how and to what extent they will disclose the information contained in the registry. Many states post the pictures and addresses of convicted sex offenders on the Internet, a practice that has been challenged but permitted by the U.S. Supreme Court (*Connecticut Department of Public Safety et al. v. Doe* 2003; Logan 1999).

Psychiatrists have become increasingly involved in these controversial and unsettled legal concerns and policies. For example, some states, such as New Jersey, require evaluations to determine how to classify sex offenders and what degree of publicity should be associated with that particular offender (N.J. Stat. Ann. 2C: 7–12 et seq.). Even in states that have not enacted "sexual predator" statutes, the heightened awareness and intolerance of repetitive sexual crimes have led departments of mental health, such as in Connecticut, to reexamine all of their current civil patients with a focus on risk assessments for problematic sexual behaviors. Mental health departments have also been more willing to admit nonpsychotic sex offenders released from prison who are themselves fearful of recidivism.

Thus, a variety of circumstances may result in requests for psychiatrists to evaluate individuals who may have been charged with or convicted of sexual offenses or exhibiting inappropriate sexual behavior. The nature of the evaluation, the status of the information, and the focus of the report or note will differ depending on the circumstances. In this chapter we review some of the relevant issues in approaching assessments of sexual offenders.

## Ethical Issues

### Clinical Vignette

Mr. A, a 52-year-old man with a history of two rapes, had been incarcerated for 15 years. As the time for his mandatory release approached, the state sought to have him committed to a mental hospital under the state's sexually violent predator act, and the state requested a psychiatric evaluation. Mr. A refused to talk with the psychiatrist. How does this effect the evaluation?

In some cases, the record may be sufficiently clear to fulfill the statutory criteria for involuntary commitment under sexual predator laws. In some states, prosecutors ask for court orders to coerce inmates to participate in evaluations. No court orders force psychiatrists to participate in such evaluations if they feel that doing so is not ethical. Yet, the referral question may not be answerable if the evaluation cannot be sufficiently comprehensive.

Psychiatrists should determine what limitations, if any, will be placed on their evaluations. As in the case of Mr. A, these may include an inability to interview the evaluee. Other limitations may include number of interviews, length of time to complete the evaluation, limitations on other collateral procedures such as CAT scans, MRIs, neurological evaluations, and psychological testing. The American Academy of Psychiatry and the Law (AAPL) ethical guidelines (AAPL 1995) suggest that, at a minimum, forensic psychiatrists make these limitations clear in their testimony.

Questions regarding the ethics of participating in the complicated area of assessment of sexual offenders are common. For example, in states with sexual predator statutes, many inmates are advised by their attorneys not to agree to interviews with evaluators because information may be revealed that could profoundly affect the life of the offender. As in the case of Mr. A, questions then arise as to the ethics of evaluators offering opinions without having performed a personal interview.

Confidentiality is another important ethical issue raised by the evaluation of sexual offenders. The importance of explaining the limits to confidentiality is critical. Sexual offenders are often caught in a bind created by a need to meet their own conflicting legal interests. It is not uncommon for therapists to encourage or even require the inmate or probationer to reveal all past inappropriate sexual behaviors. Some laws do not protect any information related to sexual offenses that is revealed in treatment settings. In such cases, additional charges (e.g., for perjury or new sexual assaults) can be brought as a result of the information revealed during treatment. However, if offenders refuse to participate, prosecutors can use a sexual offender's lack of therapy as an indication for involuntary civil commitment at the end of the sentence, creating a bind for the offender. It may also affect placement within the department of correction. In *McKune v. Lile* (2002), the Supreme Court upheld the transfer of an inmate back to a maximum security facility for refusing to participate in such a treatment setting.

Psychiatrists providing forensic evaluations are bound by a variety of ethical guidelines that address issues such as confidentiality and conducting an evaluation without an interview. These guidelines have been promulgated by professional associations and legislatures (Weinstock et al. 1990). Guidelines relevant to the evaluation of sexual offenders include those developed by the American Psychiatric Association (APA)

(2001), the American Medical Association (AMA), AAPL (1995), and the Association for the Treatment of Sexual Abusers (ATSA) (1997). Comparable ethical obligations exist for psychologists (American Psychological Association 1992). In problematic cases, consultation from local or national ethics committees may be helpful.

Ethical guidelines also help psychiatrists formulate a practical approach to evaluation. These guidelines require that psychiatrists clarify issues related to agency, that is, for whom they are working or by whom they have been hired. This issue is critical in the assessment of sexual offenders and should be the first practical issue psychiatrists address when asked to provide opinions in these cases. This determination informs psychiatrists about the status of the information with respect to confidentiality and whether a professional physician-patient relationship is being established with all of the fiduciary obligations concomitant with that status.

Generally, in a forensic evaluation, the psychiatrist's obligations are to provide information to an attorney, agency, or court as part of some legal proceeding. Such evaluations do not create a formal physician-patient relationship. However, the degree of confidentiality may vary considerably. If the psychiatrist is retained by the defense, the psychiatrist's evaluation may be covered under attorney-client privilege. If the psychiatrist is retained by a prosecutor or judge, the report is usually made available to both sides. Regardless, psychiatrists are ethically obligated to disclose the limits of confidentiality to the evaluee before beginning the assessment.

Ethical concerns may also arise in the evaluation of victims of sexual offenses. Victim rights concerns have in some cases resulted in statutorily mandated opportunities for victims to participate in proceedings. Some victims will avail themselves of these opportunities. Because these interviews can also be traumatizing, evaluators should generally go through prosecutors or attorneys rather than contact victims directly. Certainly, no victim should be coerced to participate. Contacting victims should generally be done through the hiring attorney and not directly, as there also may be limitations placed on access to victims or collateral informants.

Procedural as well as ethical issues may need to be considered before embarking on an evaluation. Some circumstances may require a competent defendant to meet due process or ethical requirements; others do not. Generally, this needs to be clarified before beginning the evaluation. Circumstances that do not require a competent defendant may arise, for example, when a private attorney representing the offender asks for an evaluation that is protected under the attorney-client privilege or when a court orders a competency to stand trial evaluation. Under these circumstances, an evaluation may proceed with notification of the limits of confidentiality.

## Determining the Nature of the Evaluation

### Clinical Vignette

Mr. J, an 18-year-old sophomore at a local university, was arrested after a computer repair service found two pictures of child pornography on his computer. Possession of child pornography is a federal crime. Mr. J's attorney wanted to minimize any penalty under the federal sentencing guidelines. To this end, he negotiated with the prosecutor about the specific charges. Mr. J's attorney contacted a psychiatrist and asked whether a psychiatric evaluation might help his client and, if so, how.

The psychiatrist informed Mr. J's attorney that a comprehensive psychiatric examination might help the attorney negotiate a lesser plea or, in the event of a conviction, a shorter sentence for his client. The attorney was aware that the possession of child pornography is a federal crime. In the past, three pictures were needed for a conviction; now, even the possession of one picture is sufficient (18 U.S.C.S. § 2252A [2003]). Negotiations regarding the charges and sentencing are common. Issues such as the rest of the defendant's history being clean are likely to be influential in the negotiations. In his defense, a defendant may claim, for example, that the picture was not requested and came in a package of hundreds of other adult pornography images on the Internet. Yet other evidence may challenge such a defense, for example, if a folder labeled "child pornography" had been found on the computer.

Increasingly, defense attorneys look for comprehensive psychiatric evaluations to negotiate with prosecutors for lesser pleas or to use at sentencing as a justification for a downward departure from the federal sentencing guidelines. The attorney should be familiar with the specific guidelines that need to be addressed by the psychiatrist. Indeed, at the sentencing guideline phase, specific factors relevant to psychiatric issues must be found to justify a departure. An opinion that states that jail is not an appropriate disposition for the defendant is generally not useful; disposition is a legal, not a psychiatric, decision. Discussion of diagnostic conclusions and indicated treatment recommendations, whether or not the defendant is incarcerated, is generally more useful.

Psychiatrists should clarify the nature of the evaluation at the outset, initially by consultation with the referring agency or attorney and, subsequently, in written form. Forensic evaluations involving sexual offenders will be geared to the specific question being considered: for example, competency, criminal responsibility, or predator commitment criteria. These are typically statutorily defined, or they can be determined by case law from the particular state. The legal question to be answered sets the tone and focus of the interview. A competency to stand trial evaluation is less comprehensive because it focuses on the present mental state and ability to understand the proceedings and the ability to work with an attorney. A criminal responsibility or presentence evaluation will be much broader and complete. In pretrial settings, evaluations can be critical in the plea bargaining or sentencing phases of criminal proceedings.

Obtaining detailed histories in these situations is essential to developing relevant diagnostic information. Specific and longitudinal sexual histories may elicit patterns or proclivities that will make for a better understanding of the individual defendant. Questionnaires such as the Derogatis Sexual Functioning Inventory (DSFI; Derogatis 1978) and the Multiphasic Sex Inventory (Nichols & Molinder Assessments; http://www.nicholsandmolinder.com) sometimes allow for a more comprehensive survey of attitudes and cognitive distortions that can be followed up in the interviews. Additionally, defendants may endorse a dysfunctional behavior or perception in a written questionnaire that they would not acknowledge in a face-to-face interview.

## Civil Commitment of Sexual Predators and Psychiatric Assessment

In contrast to issues of competency or criminal responsibility, evaluations related to the relatively new sexual predator statutes raise issues unique to sex offenders. Psychiatrists are often less familiar with legal criteria associated with these statutes and how they affect psychiatric evaluations. In addition, because of their relatively recent enactments, much less extensive literature is available to guide professionals. Psychiatrists involved in such assessments should develop an understanding of the current state of these new laws before providing opinions in such litigation.

The *predator* criteria vary to some degree from state to state but generally involve four elements: 1) a *conviction* for 2) a sexually relevant offense (sexually violent or harmful sexual conduct) and 3) the presence of a *mental abnormality* that 4) predisposes an individual to commit future sexually dangerous acts. In many states, conviction of a violent sexual crime is broader than a literal conviction and may include those found incompetent to stand trial, insanity acquittees, and juveniles. The relevant sexual crimes are generally specified by statute section number. A nonsexual crime may also be found to be "sexually motivated" (e.g., kidnapping) and satisfy the criteria. In some states, a sexually violent crime may be defined to include exhibitionism, especially if a child is involved. Some states, such as California, may exclude incest.

Legislatures intentionally included the broadly conceived *mental abnormality* element in the definition of a sexual predator. Mental abnormality is defined in at least eight states as "a congenital or acquired condition affecting the emotional or volitional capacity that predisposes the person to commit sexually violent acts." The use of this term was designed to allow inclusion of personality disorders as well as disorders that might not be found in the *Diagnostic and Statistical Manual of Mental Disorders,* Fourth Edition (DSM-IV; American Psychiatric Association 1994), and its text revision, DSM-IV-TR (American Psychiatric Association 2000). For example, some courts have accepted a diagnosis of "paraphilic rapism" because it is described in the research literature (Abel and Rouleau 1990) and can be marginally categorized as paraphilia NOS in DSM-IV.

Nevertheless, the use of the term *mental abnormality* in sexual predator statutes has created controversy. For example, because antisocial personality disorder has been found to meet these criteria, it is difficult to distinguish "the mad from the bad." The U.S. Supreme Court has recently begun to acknowledge this problem. The Court has found that there must be proof of both psychiatric diagnosis and serious difficulty in controlling behavior to justify indefinite civil commitment following completion of a prison term (*Kansas v. Crane* 2002). How lower courts will interpret this decision is not yet clear.

Psychiatrists may be specifically asked to evaluate a sexual offender's predisposition and risk of future crimes, the fourth element of statutory commitment criteria. To meet all the criteria, the evaluee's mental condition must be related to a specified degree of risk for committing future sexually violent acts. Difficulties in evaluations arise when psychiatrists find that the relevant statutes use legal terms that are not well defined or not part of their professional vocabulary. For example, 12 of the statutes use "likely" to denote the degree of risk. Some state courts have defined this as "more likely than not." Wisconsin uses "substantial probability" and has defined it as "considerably more likely to occur than not to occur" (*In re* Kienitz 1998). In such cases, consultation may be helpful, and states may evolve guidelines for specific evaluations.

## Evaluation of Risk of Future Sexual Offense

### Risk Assessment Instruments

Difficulty and controversy are associated with this fourth element of the criteria for the involuntary commitment of sexual offenders as a result of the requirement that psychiatrists provide predictions of future behavior. This endeavor is inherently fraught with problems. As the sexual predator statutes rapidly multiplied during the past decade, the need for data that could withstand courtroom scrutiny became more pressing, and a variety of risk assessment instruments were devised. These instruments have great appeal as they have the patina of a scientific approach to the question (Campbell 2000). However, as in any new field of scientific inquiry, the research supporting the use of these instruments in forensic settings is often inconclusive. Psychiatrists providing evaluations of risk of future sexual offenses should be familiar with the available instruments, as well as their strengths, limitations, and appropriate use in evaluation.

#### *Methodological Problems*

Many of the studies related to these risk assessment instruments have significant methodological problems. The multiple confounding variables make devising an adequately controlled study a formidable challenge. Obtaining a truly randomized control group is extremely difficult given legal and ethical constraints and limited availability of resources and data. For example, how could treatment be offered to one group and not another matched group when it is legally or ethically mandated?

Confidentiality needs are a challenge to the researcher in obtaining appropriate data. And more often than not, data sets differ both in information available and in the format in which they are kept. Outcome variables also depend on the foundation variable. We cannot say, "If this person is aroused by adolescent males, he is likely to be a sex offender." However, we may be able to say, "If he is a sex offender and is aroused by adolescent males, he is more likely to offend." Reverse probability errors are not uncommon when depending only on clinical judgment (Poole and Lamb 1998).

In addition, the available studies demonstrate little consistency in terms of operationally defining variables. For example, the operational definition of *recidivism* is as varied as *arrest, charge, conviction*, and *violation of probation/parole/conditional release*. Even these terms mean different things in different statutory settings. Using *arrest* as an operational definition would lead to false positives in that not everyone who is arrested is guilty. However, using conviction leads to false negatives, as most cases are resolved by plea bargaining and one would not know what charges were dropped or changed. Revocation, too, is problematic, as probation could be revoked for behavior not associated with sexual misbehavior (e.g., missing appointments).

Further, these definitions do not account for

1. Individuals who have recommitted the offense and have not been caught.
2. Individuals who would have re-offended were it not for their probation being revoked.
3. The variation of responses to the sexual offending or risk behavior by officers, treatment providers, and courts.

Recidivism studies require a long-term longitudinal approach to optimize inclusion of all caught recidivists. Otherwise, the base rate for caught recidivists is too low to assess the efficacy of treatment or any other intervention (Hanson 1997; Rice and Harris 1997; Seto and Barbaree 1999). Moreover, within-treatment studies (i.e., those that measure change in factors that are thought to be related to risk for re-offense) can support erroneous beliefs, derail assessments, and lead to inappropriate treatment. For example, it would appear that all sex offenders would benefit from insight therapy and empathy training, and so it is often provided; yet Rice et al. (1992) showed that psychopaths offended all the more when provided with such treatment.

Lack of resources and the political will to support research has resulted in limited long-term experimental design. This has led to mandated program development without validation. States have been required in one form or another to provide assessment, and even treatment, of sex offenders without benefit of good research. Thus, forensic experts may feel forced to give opinions based on data for which there is too often insufficient useful research. Therefore, they must be clear about the value of their findings and support these findings accurately and with honesty.

## *Psychophysiological Assessment*

Psychophysiological tests have long been sought as an accurate measure of deviant sexual arousal. The most widely known of such tests is penile plethysmography (PPG), also known as "phallometry." This technique, developed over 40 years ago, measures degrees of penile tumescence when a male subject is exposed to specific audio and visual sexual stimuli.

PPG results are used to characterize patterns of deviant sexual arousal, develop treatment plans, and monitor the effectiveness of treatment (Barker and Howell 1992). Two types of PPG used today measure changes in either penile volume or circumference (Kuban et al. 1999).

The PPG has been extensively researched. It is thought to provide objective data regarding sexual preference, both normal and dysfunctional, and promote self-disclosure. However, the use of PPG has been criticized for a variety of reasons (Simon and Schouten 1993). The acceptance of the use of the PPG is qualified because of the invasiveness and practical problems administering it. It lacks standardized testing and scoring techniques, and the validity of the testing is subject to question. In addition, the use of this test raises moral, ethical, and legal issues regarding the use of pornographic stimuli, particularly those involving children. The extent to which individuals can "fake" the instrument, the true nature of the ideation, and the behavioral implications of penile tumescence are unclear (Hale and Strassberg 1990; Quinsey and Bergersen 1976). Finally, while the numbers of female sex offenders are very small relative to male offenders, the lack of utility of PPG with females needs to be noted.

Another psychophysiological test, the Abel Assessment for Sexual Interest (AASI), is based on visual reaction time (VRT), that is, the correlation of reported arousal and attractiveness ratings with the length of time a subject looks at a stimulus (Abel 2000; Abel et al. 1998a, 1998b). This commercially available product consists of both subjective and objective components designed to measure sexual interest by age and gender. The first portion consists of a questionnaire that gathers information regarding the client's sexual preferences and behaviors, legal history, and self-reported ability to control his or her sexual behaviors. The questionnaire also contains items to address feigning and cognitive distortions about interest in sex with children, and it correlates responses with a profile of known child molesters. The "objective" measure of the AASI is the visual reaction time measured while the subject is asked to rate his or her degree of sexual arousal to the visual stimuli (160 slides depicting clothed children, teens, and adults). Data obtained are sent to Abel Screening, Inc. A detailed report of the results is then provided to the testing site.

The AASI was designed to aid therapists in the evaluation and treatment of sex offenders. It has been a popular instrument because it is easy to administer, takes less time, and, as intended, is less intrusive than PPG. However, there seems to be some variability regarding the importance given to AASI results (Fischer and Smith 1999; Smith and Fischer 1999). In addition, questions regarding its reliability and validity have been raised, as have concerns regarding the lack of standardized research, particularly in relation to meeting *Daubert* criteria. The AASI has not been subjected to peer review scrutiny and publication to any significant extent, particularly regarding the Risk Prediction Score, and the methods of analysis of data have not been made public. Thus, several courts have refused to admit testimony regarding the test (Sachsenmaier and Peters 2002).

Polygraphy is used in a number of states as part of the treatment or parole requirements for sex offenders. Individuals accused and convicted of sexual offenses have little incentive to provide truthful information regarding their offenses or compliance with mandated treatment programs. The polygraph has increasingly been used to verify information provided by sex offenders regarding both details of offense, conduct, and past sexual history. Many treatment programs use the polygraph to monitor a convicted offender's compliance with treatment plans or terms of probation and to modify treatment plans.

Studies have demonstrated that polygraph testing can be an effective means of obtaining a comprehensive sexual offense history and increasing the number of disclosures made by offenders (Ahlmeyer et al. 2000; Emerick and Dutton 1993). Nevertheless, polygraph data are not admissible as evidence in regard to any specific alleged crime. Polygraph results are highly dependent on the examiner's expertise. In addition, polygraph testing has been criticized for its lack of standardization.

Psychophysiological tests may be useful in part of the overall assessment of sex offenders. However, they may be more effective in addressing sentencing or disposition issues with admitted offenders when treatment is an option (Sachsenmaier and Peters 2002). The use of psychophysiological tests to accurately predict recidivism for any given individual has not been demonstrated in controlled studies. A disordered pattern of sexual arousal measured by length of gaze or penile tumescence does not prove that the individual is an offender, nor can these parameters be employed as tests of propensity toward committing a specific sexual act. The PPG and VRT screenings are limited in their use in risk assessment because of lack of technique standardization, absence of a widely accepted stimuli set, and difficulty generalizing from the laboratory to real-world circumstances (American Psychiatric Association 1999). Similarly, polygraph data cannot prove guilt or provide reliable information about recidivist tendencies, and their significance is limited by methodological problems and lack of standardization.

Psychophysiological testing can therefore have a limited role in the forensic assessment of sex offenders. Such test results should only be used in conjunction with a thorough psychiatric and psychological evaluation, comprehensive sexual history, and clinical expertise. Psychiatrists should not use test results to determine the truth of allegations. Care should be taken to avoid overgeneralizing results and making improper clinical extrapolations regarding risk assessments and predictions of recidivism.

## *Use of Hypnosis in Clinical Evaluation*

### Clinical Vignette

The police hypnotized Ms. P, a rape victim, in an effort to identify the rapist. Before hypnosis Ms. P was uncertain about the perpetrator's identity but thought it might be a man in the lineup. The police informed her that the leading suspect had several prior convictions for rape. Following the hypnosis, Ms. P was convinced that the man was, in fact, the rapist. The prosecutor requested that a psychiatrist review the case to obtain an expert opinion that Ms. P's recollection had not been rendered unreliable by the hypnosis. This opinion could facilitate the admission of Ms. P's testimony.

A number of years ago many police officers took brief courses training them to perform hypnosis. Some of the leading police trainers believed that human memory was like a videotape that records and stores most perceptions, which can be retrieved under hypnosis. However, many officers did not possess the necessary skills to avoid suggestive if not coercive procedures during hypnosis. Guidelines began to be introduced requiring substantial training and other professional credentials, as well as controls for setting up and using tape-recorded interviews. The hypnotist's behavior could then be reviewed for overly suggestive or coercive behavior during the sessions.

Dr. Martin Orne, in *State v. Hurd* (1981), originally outlined six procedural requirements used by the courts to determine whether the hypnotically refreshed testimony could be admitted:

1. A psychologist or psychiatrist experienced in the use of hypnosis must conduct the session.
2. The hypnotist must be independent of the prosecution, the investigator, and the defense.
3. Any information given to the hypnotist prior to the session must be recorded.
4. Before inducing hypnosis, the hypnotist must obtain from the subject a detailed description of the facts as the subject remembers them.
5. All contacts between the hypnotist and the subject must be recorded.
6. Only the hypnotist and the subject may be present during the hypnotic session or any prehypnotic testing or posthypnotic interview.

Dr. Orne also observed that subjects feel more convinced of their identifications following hypnosis as a result of suggestive conditioning surrounding and during hypnosis. He described this phenomenon as "hardening of memory." Gradually, courts began to feel that hypnosis was undermining the credibility of testimony. Because confabulations could be a by-product, the risk of admitting such testimony was felt to be too great.

Hypnosis continues to be a controversial matter for the courts in the post-*Daubert* era, although suggestibility of testimony is an issue independent of hypnosis. Use of hypnosis has been sharply curtailed in most jurisdictions, except when defendants are involved or when all leads have fizzled and police are looking for new leads. Some police departments are still using hypnosis, as the cases previously described here illustrate. Hypnosis has yielded useful information in some cases, but it is generally useful only if other independent confirmatory evidence is found. In criminal cases, many states have totally excluded witnesses or victims from giving evidence if they have been hypnotized. In some jurisdictions they have been permitted to testify only about documented, relevant evidence they were able to recall before the hypnosis.

Some jurisdictions do not totally exclude witnesses who have been hypnotized but require the court to consider the totality of the circumstances before deciding whether to let the witness testify. The court in *State v. Fertig* (1996), for example, when faced with the proffered testimony of a previously hypnotized state's witness, declined to abandon *Hurd*. Nevertheless, as of 1996, 26 states considered hypnotically refreshed testimony inadmissible per se. However, the majority of courts allow witnesses other than the defendant to testify to statements made prior to hypnosis if well documented (see also Fleming 1990 and 1998 Supp.).

## Collateral Data

### Clinical Vignette

Mr. G, a 42-year-old man, was involved in a custody dispute. His ex-wife requested that his visitation with their 9-year-old daughter be stopped when the girl told her new psychologist that he had taken a shower with her. The incident had allegedly occurred 1 year before the girl reported it to the psychologist, although she had been in treatment continuously before that time with another therapist. The child's guardian *ad litem* requested a psychiatric evaluation of the father to determine the risk of danger to his daughter. Mr. G categorically denied the allegation. The guardian refused to allow the psychiatrist to communicate with the daughter, the ex-wife, or the therapist. Should the evaluation be undertaken?

The psychiatrist had to explain to the guardian *ad litem* that the limitation on his ability to collect collateral data prevented him from coming to any conclusion in this case given the father's denial of the incident. In the face of such denial, some evaluators might use PPG (see discussion in previous subsection) to determine whether Mr. G exhibited any clear arousal to children. Although such testing is not evidence or proof of the allegation, such "evidence" might be useful in attempts to negotiate a settlement of the custody dispute.

However, evaluation in this type of case requires collateral data. Contact with both therapists is essential. The evaluator has to be able to try to determine why that information came out when it did and under what circumstances, especially in light of the fact that it did not emerge in the earlier therapy. For example, it would be critical to learn if therapist suggestion played a role in the late disclosure. If there are too many unanswerable questions by the end of the restricted evaluation, then there may be no clear conclusions possible. The psychiatrist in this case might be well advised to decline the evaluation if access to this collateral data cannot be obtained.

Regardless of the type of sexual offense involved, psychiatrists should endeavor to obtain as much collateral data as possible. Family members' perspectives of the defendant's history, although potentially biased, may be helpful. Comprehensive record reviews are necessary to confirm histories and general reliability of the interview data. Such records will include past psychiatric treatment, criminal justice records including confessions, military records, general hospital summaries, and school records where appropriate. Collateral data should be actively sought, but permission should be obtained from the referring agency, as there might be legal constraints to making unauthorized contacts.

## Clinical Evaluation

### Clinical Vignette

Mr. B, a 47-year-old man, exposed himself to two 12-year-old girls 15 years ago. At that time, he was found not guilty by reason of insanity (NGRI) and has been hospitalized since then. Over the course of his hospitalization, Mr. B has had a long-standing delusional belief that people's subconscious minds communicate with him in the form of hallucinations. One chronic delusion involved the belief that his former girlfriend had been telling him to call her. As a result, he harassed her for many years, believing that she was still romantically interested in him.

Mr. B had no history of violence or physical assault and had responded well to medications. It became clear to him that his former girlfriend was no longer interested in him. He exposed himself once on the ward to a staff psychologist when his medications were being altered. The review board that determines whether Mr. B can be conditionally released requested a psychiatric assessment about the risk of recidivism he posed when he was to be transferred to a less restrictive setting.

The consulting psychiatrist noted Mr. B's history of repeated exposures, as well as the long history of harassing phone calls based on his delusional belief about his former girlfriend. Mr. B's lack of a violent history was not a significant issue because he only requested a transfer from a maximum- to a moderate-security facility. The psychiatrist reviewed his response to treatment, the lack of contact associated with the sexual offense, and the increased ability to relate to others in a functional and appropriate manner displayed over the years. The psychiatrist recommended that Mr. B be transferred to the less restrictive setting.

The review board decided to allow the transfer to a step-down, moderately secure facility but would not approve visits into the community. In many jurisdictions, insanity acquittees are often held longer in mental hospitals than they might have been had they pled guilty to the original offense and served a determined sentence in jail or prison. Review boards are often mandated to use public safety as their primary concern. Many NGRI acquittees have mental disorders that are chronic and require medication to maintain remissions. Because these individuals can never be "cured," and it is hard to guarantee compliance, they may be subjected to long terms of monitoring and only gradually gain privileges. Thus review boards will often maintain their commitment status for the maximum permissible period.

The case of Mr. B raises the issue of how to make an assessment of the risk of recidivism in sexual offenders. Heilbrun (1997) points to the need to differentiate between assessments used for prediction (inclusion/exclusion) purposes and those used for management (treatment/supervision) purposes. The latter tend to be more valuable in terms of what the forensic expert can offer and what the community needs, and they tend to be more responsive to the legal context (Dvoskin and Heilbrun 2001).

Both clinical and research instruments have focused on a dichotomous approach to addressing this critical issue: Will the offender recidivate, or will he not? A nondichotomous approach, which considers factors such as imminence, frequency, and severity, represents a far more complex examination but may be more responsive to treatment and disposition issues (Sjostedt and Grann 2001). For example, the question of whether a child molester poses future danger may be more usefully answered by a discussion of the time frame for which such an assessment would be reasonable, the entrenched nature of the problematic sexual behavior, the ability to incorporate and use treatment, the need for monitoring, and what sort of monitoring would be most effective.

In addition, a conceptual development of definitions and purpose needs to be considered in both clinical and forensic evaluations. Hart (1998) speaks of the necessity of identifying dangers (risky situations, states) to better reduce risk as opposed to merely making a passive prediction. What puts people at risk to re-offend? Under what conditions are they more likely to offend? Incarcerated or hospitalized pedophiles are not nearly the risk they would be in the community. Yet, some people may pose only minimal risk in the community if they have only supervised contact with children, are randomly tested for alcohol, remain involved in treatment, work in an adult-only environment, and are monitored for access to pornography or children via the computer.

Research and clinical experience have identified factors that play a role in recidivism of sexual offenses. Psychiatrists conducting these evaluations should assess such variables in detail through obtaining an extensive sexual, personal, and legal history. No single factor is determinative of future risk. However, certain constellations will be more significant than others and will lead the evaluator toward a conclusion regarding possible recidivism. This conclusion can then be presented in terms of risk assessment: which situations will increase the risk of recidivism, and which will decrease this risk? Therefore, experts should consider approaching evaluations of recidivism from a perspective other than the provision of a "yes" or "no" answer. A more useful question to answer would be, Under what circumstances is the offender more—or better yet, less—likely to offend?

Factors that contribute to the evaluation of future risk of violence and sexual recidivism fall into two general categories: those that are static and those that are dynamic (Table 16–1). Static factors include elements such as Psychopathy Checklist—Revised (PCL-R) score (Hare 1991, 1998); DSM diagnosis of personality disorder; failure on previous conditional release; history of alcohol abuse and male victim in index offense; contact sex offense; any stranger victim sexual offense; contact sexual offense against a relative; and number of prior sex offenses and sex offense convictions. Dynamic variables include intimacy deficits, tolerant sexual attitudes, treatment dropout and lack of cooperation with supervision, and psychological identification with children (Hanson and Harris 2001; Seidman et al. 1994; Wilson et al. 1999).

A method that borrows from the relapse prevention model has come to be known as the *anamnestic* approach. This involves a microanalysis of

**TABLE 16–1.** Factors in the evaluation of future risk of violence and sexual recidivism

| Static variables | Dynamic variables |
|---|---|
| PCL-R score | Intimacy deficits |
| Personality disorder | Tolerant sexual attitudes |
| Failure on prior conditional release | Chemical use |
| History of alcohol abuse | Proximity to target victims |
| Contact offense(s) | Psychological identification with children |
| Male victim in index offense | Deviant sexual arousal needs |
| Prior sex offenses and sex offense convictions | Treatment dropout and lack of cooperation with supervision |
| Stranger victim sexual offense | |
| Contact sex offense with relative | |

the person's history that examines the conditions, situations, thoughts, and behaviors that preceded the event. To the extent these variables are currently present, the risk is assessed as higher.

## Clinical Versus Actuarial Approaches

The question of whether a clinical or an actuarial approach to the determination of the risk of recidivism in sexual offenders is unresolved. Some experts believe actuarial methods are superior in making risk assessments (Grove et al. 2000). There is no shortage of studies in which expert evaluators failed to distinguish between low-risk and high-risk offenders. The predictive accuracy of the typical clinical judgment is only slightly above chance level (Hanson and Harris 2000). Actuarial instruments based on large numbers appear more reliable and accurate than clinical interviews. This is not surprising, because clinical acumen varies widely. A few experts have gone so far as to opine that interviews may hinder the assessment due to lack of clinical objectivity (Grove et al. 2000).

However, findings from studies that compare both actuarial and clinical approaches on the same populations, taken as a whole, are inconclusive (Litwack 2001). A review of the literature indicated that actuarial risk assessment tools, while apparently superior to solely clinical assessment, are not as effective as hoped. They are more effective in predicting imminent and nonsevere re-offending than long-term and serious offending. They are particularly poor at assessing risk with intrafamilial recidivists. Additionally, their variability was quite high when elaborated criteria (imminence, frequency, nature, and severity) were included (Sjostedt and Grann 2001). If such findings are replicated, it would appear that actuarial risk assessment tools are too unreliable to be useful for individualized prediction. Moreover, inasmuch as most of the actuarial variables are static, they cannot provide information about the effectiveness of treatment, rehabilitation, or even confinement.

Actuarial instruments used in forensic settings must also be evaluated in light of *Daubert* criteria and the Federal Rules of Evidence. (For a comprehensive explication and analyses of these issues, see Sachsenmaier and Peters 2002.) Finally, as with any type of testing, the inappropriate use of such tests can be misleading. For example, it is not unusual for an assessment to include several instruments whose items or scales either are related or measure the same variable. These scores are sometimes added or averaged and then said to have more validity than any single score. This invalid procedure is poor practice. It actually negates the results of all the testing. If one is measuring the role of various foods in the triggering of allergy, one would not include lactic acid in all of them. It adulterates the findings.

To avoid the blind man's problem in the parable, that of describing only one part of an elephant, psychiatrists should use as many different data types as possible to come to a comprehensive and well-reasoned conclusion. They must understand the context of the sexual offense, such as the base rates of occurrence and re-offense within which an individual falls. They must also consider the idiosyncratic situation and the high-risk variables for each evaluee. They should remain aware of research that results in the increased standardization in the administration, definition, and application of actuarial instruments, and therefore the availability of increasingly valid and reliable findings.

Purely actuarial approaches often have problems related to their utility; purely clinical approaches often have problems related their accuracy. Many forensic experts advocate a combined approach that uses a structured clinical assessment and a clinically adjusted actuarial approach. There is, indeed, a continuum of assessment methods between the purely actuarial and purely clinical. And perhaps the differences employed are more in degree than kind. Still, nothing has proven both accurate and efficient enough to allay fears of a "bad call." Errors in risk assessment are fraught with troubling consequences. They can result in contributing to depriving individuals of deserved freedom or releasing dangerous perpetrators back into society.

## Psychological Testing

A variety of psychological instruments are available and have been used to help determine future risk of sexual offense. These tests have both strengths and limitations. A full psychological battery of tests may be appropriate and helpful in answering relevant questions (e.g., differential diagnosis, intellectual functioning, impulse control, ego functioning) regarding disposition and management. However, such evaluations are neither intended nor validated for use as assessments of risk for sexual offending.

In contrast, specific tests for the assessment of risk have been devised. The Violence Risk Appraisal Guide (VRAG) was developed to classify perpetrators of violence and assess their risk of future violence by assessing multiple variables weighted on relative strength as predictors of violence. Although not specific to sexual-offending behavior, the VRAG has been effective in the prediction of sex-offending recidivism (Hanson and Harris 2000; Seto and Barbaree 1999). The authors of The Sex Offender Risk Appraisal Guide (SORAG) attempted to fine-tune the VRAG to predict the likelihood of sex offense by replacing some of the VRAG variables with variables found specifically useful in regard to sexual offenses (Quinsey et al. 1995, 1998). There has been a dearth of published research on the SORAG to date. Interestingly, the SORAG seems to have the same measure of success in predicting sex offense as the VRAG. One possibility for this is the measuring, in both, of psychopathy that may well be the best predictor of both risk of violence and sex offending.

Another tool and actuarial instrument, the Rapid Risk Assessment of Sex Offender Recidivism (RRASOR; http://www.sgc.gc.ca/az-index/sindex_e.asp) was based on the findings from 61 studies (Hanson and Bussière 1996). The RRASOR has been cross-validated and appears to be useful primarily as a screening device, to select individuals who are likely to benefit from more comprehensive and individualized assessment. Four items (prior sex offenses, offender age, male victims, extrafamilial victims) were found to be variables most often predictive of recidivism. It is an exceptionally short and easily applied test that requires minimal training. Given the simple procedures, it is not surprising that interrater reliability is high (Barbaree et al. 2001; Sjostedt and Langstrom 2001).

There has been significant empirical support for the validity of the RRASOR, particularly among forensic and correctional subjects and when recidivism is defined as conviction for a sex offense (Doren 2002). The obvious weakness of the RRASOR is that it does not directly consider deviant sexual preferences, which were among the strongest recidivism predictors in Hanson and Bussière's (1996) meta-analysis. It also does not consider the effects of monitoring and cooperation with treatment, which may have significant effect on risk of future behavior (Hanson and Harris 1997).

Structured Risk Assessment (SRA; http://www.sgc.gc.ca/az-index/sindex_e.asp) is a three-part test for the assessment of risk of sexual offense. Step 1, the Static-99, is the most researched and widely known of the three. First used in 1999, this instrument combines the four RRASOR items with some variables of a less-published test, the Structured Actuarial Clinical Judgment—Minimum (SACJ–Min) (Grubin 1998). The Static-99 has been exposed to published peer review, standardized scoring information, and a potential error rate. It also enjoys general acceptance. Studies have been done in multiple geographic areas with correctional and forensic subjects that support the validity of this instrument (Doren 2000).

Though the research indicates that the Static-99 is a better predictor than either the RRASOR or SACJ–Min alone, it does not appear to be a lot better (Hanson and Thornton 2000). Therefore, although appropriate as rough screens and pretreatment assessments, the Static-99 and the RRASOR should not be used as individualized predictors of sex-offending behavior, as a measure of progress, or for dispositional decisions.

Step 2 of the SRA, the Initial Deviance Assessment (IDA), and step 3, which is still under development, represent some of the newest research in the assessment of risk. The IDA and step 3 consider dynamic variables in the assessment of risk, such as the effects of intervention, treatment dropout, lack of cooperation with supervision, and progress in treatment (Hanson and Harris 2001; Seidman et al. 1994; Wilson 1999). The ability to assess and predict the effects of treatment would be particularly useful for those offenders who have psychopathic traits and highly deviant sexual arousal needs. Literature review indicates that these two variables are significant in the risk of sex offending. To date, no instrument has met sufficient empirical testing to address this major problem. Neither the IDA nor step 3 has the empirical support of the Static-99. In time, research and standardization procedures may lead to measures of reliability and validity that will further popularize these aspects of the SRA.

Other available tests include the Minnesota Sex Offender Screening Tool—Revised (MnSOST-R), developed for use by the Minnesota Department of Corrections to identify high-risk sex offenders who would be released from prison; the Sex Offender Needs Assessment Rating (SONAR; http://www.sgc.gc.ca/az-index/sindex_e.asp), developed to monitor the risk of a sex offender in community supervision (Hanson and Harris 2000, 2001; available at http://www.sgc.gc.ca/epub/corr/e20001a/e200001b/20001b.htm); and the Historical, Clinical, Risk Management-20 (HCR-20; Webster et al. 1997), a structured interview that focuses on violent behaviors rather than sex offenses. All of these hold some promise of developing into useful risk assessment instruments.

However, they suffer from a lack of research supporting their validity, which currently limits their usefulness in sex offender evaluations (Barbaree et al. 2001; Doren 2002; Doren and Roberts 1998; Fanning et al. 1999; Quakenbush 2000).

Forensic psychiatrists should be familiar with these instruments and use them only when appropriate. The power of actuarial findings is impressive. However, psychiatrists should also be mindful that the usefulness of such instruments is limited by their tendency to yield generic information with static variables. Static variables are of limited utility in addressing ongoing individualized risk, treatment, and disposition, and in assessing the effectiveness of treatment interventions. Finally, because they yield group norms, these assessment tools cannot adequately address the multiple issues unique to any individual forensic assessment.

## Conclusion

Given the current state of the art, psychiatrists who provide assessments of risk of recidivism in sexual offenders should acknowledge both the strength and limitations of their findings in their reports and testimony. Questions regarding optimal length, type, and setting of treatment; differentiation of the population; role of monitoring and evaluating; and the data and tools that are needed in doing these assessments remain unresolved. In each case, judgments must be made both on research data and the individual facts at hand.

Assessment of sexual offenders is a relatively new area of forensic evaluation. The psychiatric and legal implications of such assessments have not yet become clear and are fraught with problems. Experts who provide such opinions should be certain that they understand the questions they are being asked to address, the tools available to help address those questions, the strengths and limitations of those tools, and the uses that will be made of their opinions.

## Key Points

- Research and its application in the area of sex offender assessment and treatment are still in the early stages of development. Empirical and statistical evidence has been lagging behind practice.
- The importance of individualized relapse prevention and management factors has not been sufficiently addressed through research, and the forensic expert is left with a significant gap in providing comprehensive evaluations.

- Controversy over the relative value of actuarial and clinical assessments exists: the former tends to provide generic information, which has been supported via research; the latter is more individualized but yields less reliable and valid findings.
- Forensic experts are advised to use a combination of both approaches and to keep in mind the limitations and strengths of each in answering the referral question.

## Practice Guidelines

1. Identify the nature of the evaluation and limitation issues regarding the evaluation at the outset.
2. Attend to and clarify ethical issues regarding confidentiality and agency before beginning the evaluation.
3. Identify the static and dynamic variables that will contribute to the issue of risk rather than attempt to simply answer whether or not the offender will offend again.
4. Use appropriate psychological and psychophysiological instruments to gather relevant information. Testing should be administered by a qualified and experienced expert, and results should be considered in light of both strengths and limitations of the instruments used.
5. Given the variables, identify the circumstances that will increase or decrease risk of recidivism.
6. Use all available data from collateral sources, interviews, and testing to formulate well-reasoned opinions.

## References

Abel GG: The importance of meeting research standards: a reply to Fischer and Smith's articles on the Abel assessment for sexual interest. Sex Abuse 12(2): 155–161, 2000

Abel GG, Huffman J, Warberg B, et al: Visual reaction time and plethysmography as measures of sexual interest in child molesters. Sex Abuse 10:81–96, 1998a

Abel GG, Lawry SS, Karlstrom E, et al: Screening tests for pedophiles. Criminal Justice and Behavior 21:115–131, 1998b

Abel GG, Rouleau JL: The nature and extent of sexual assault, in Handbook of Sexual Assault: Issues, Theories, and Treatment of the Offender. Edited by Marshall WL, Laws DR, Barbaree HE. New York, Plenum, 1990, pp xvii, 9–21

Ahlmeyer S, Heil P, McKee B, et al: The impact of polygraphy on admissions of victims and offenses in adult sexual offenders. Sex Abuse 12(2):123–138, 2000

American Academy of Psychiatry and the Law: Ethical Guidelines for the Practice of Forensic Psychiatry. Bloomfield, CT, American Academy of Psychiatry and the Law, 1995

American Psychiatric Association: Diagnostic and Statistical Manual of Mental Disorders, 4th Edition. Washington, DC, American Psychiatric Association, 1994

American Psychiatric Association: Dangerous Sex Offenders: A Task Force Report of the American Psychiatric Association. Washington, DC, American Psychiatric Association, 1999

American Psychiatric Association: Diagnostic and Statistical Manual of Mental Disorders, 4th Edition, Text Revision. Washington, DC, American Psychiatric Association, 2000

American Psychiatric Association: The Principles of Medical Ethics, With Annotations Especially Applicable to Psychiatry. Washington, DC, American Psychiatric Association, 2001

American Psychological Association: Ethical Principles of Psychologists and Code of Conduct. Washington, DC, American Psychiatric Association, 1992

Association for the Treatment of Sexual Abusers: Ethical Standards and Principles for the Management of Sexual Abusers. Beaverton, OR, Association for the Treatment of Sexual Abusers, 1997

Barbaree HE, Seto MC, Langton C, et al: Evaluating the predictive accuracy of six risk assessment instruments for adult sex offenders. Criminal Justice and Behavior 28(4):490–521, 2001

Barker JG, Howell RJ: The plethysmograph: a review of recent literature. J Am Acad Psychiatry Law 20(1):13–25, 1992

Briere JN: Child Abuse Trauma: Theory and Treatment of the Lasting Effects. Newbury Park, CA, Sage, 1992

Campbell TW: Sexual predator evaluations and phrenology: considering issues of evidentiary reliability. Behav Sci Law 18:111–130, 2000

Connecticut Department of Public Safety et al v Doe, 123 S. Ct. 1160 (2003)

Derogatis LR: Derogatis Sexual Functioning Inventory. Baltimore, MD, Clinical Psychometrics Research, 1978

Doren DM: Being accurate about the accuracy of the commonly used risk assessment instruments. Paper presented at the 18th Annual Research and Treatment Conference of the Association for the Treatment of Sexual Abusers, Lake Buena Vista, FL, November 2000

Doren DM: Evaluating Sex Offenders. Thousand Oaks, CA, Sage, 2002

Doren DM, Roberts CF: The proper use and interpretation of actuarial instruments in assessing recidivism risk. Paper presented at the 17th Annual Research and Treatment Conference of the Association for the Treatment of Sexual Abusers, Vancouver, British Columbia, October 1998

Dvoskin JA, Heilbrun K: Risk assessment and release decision-making: toward resolving the great debate. J Am Acad Psychiatry Law 29:6–10, 2001

Emerick RL, Dutton WA: The effect of polygraphy on the self-report of adolescent sex offenders: implications for risk assessment. Annals of Sex Research 6:83–103, 1993

Fanning T, Zimmel T, Jaskulske D, et al: An assessment of recidivism in juvenile/young adult sex offenders. Unpublished manuscript, Ethan Allen School, Department of Corrections, Wales, WI, 1999

Fischer L, Smith G: Statistical adequacy of the Abel assessment for interest in paraphilias. Sex Abuse 11(3):195–205, 1999

Fleming TM: Annotation, admissibility of hypnotically refreshed or enhanced testimony, 77 A.L.R. 4th 927 (1990 and 1998 Supp.)

Freeman-Longo RE, Knopp FH: State of the art sex offender treatment: outcome and issues. Annals of Sex Research 5:141–160, 1992

Greenfeld LA: Sex Offenses and Offenders: An Analysis of Data on Rape and Sexual Assault (NCJ 163392). Washington, DC, U.S. Department of Justice, Bureau of Justice Statistics, 1997

Grove WM, Zald DH, Lebow BS, et al: Clinical versus mechanical prediction: a meta-analysis. Psychol Assess 12(1):19–30, 2000

Grubin D: Sex Offending Against Children: Understanding the Risk (Police Research Series Paper 99). London, Home Office Development and Statistics Division, Policing and Reducing Crime Unit, 1998

Hale VE, Strassberg DS: The role of anxiety on sexual arousal. Arch Sex Behav 19(6):569–581, 1990

Hanson RK: How to know what works with sexual offenders. Sex Abuse 9(2): 129–145, 1997

Hanson RK, Bussière MT: Predictors of Sexual Offender Recidivism: A Meta-analysis (User Report 96-04). Ottawa, Ontario, Department of the Solicitor General of Canada, 1996

Hanson RK, Harris AJR: Predicting sexual offender recidivism in the community: acute risk predictors. Presentation at the Keeping Risky Men Out of Trouble: Ongoing Research on Sex Offenders symposium at the annual convention of the Canadian Psychological Association, Toronto, June 1997

Hanson RK, Harris AJR: Where should we intervene? Dynamic predictors of sexual assault recidivism. Criminal Justice and Behavior 27:6–35, 2000

Hanson RK, Harris AJR: A structured approach to evaluating change amongst sexual offenders. Sexual Abuse: Journal of Research and Treatment 13(2): 105–122, 2001

Hanson RK, Thornton D: Improving risk assessments for sex offenders: a comparison of three actuarial scales. Law Hum Behav 24(1):119–136, 2000

Hare R: Manual for the Hare Psychopathy Checklist—Revised. Toronto, Ontario, Multi-Health Systems, 1991

Hare R: The role of psychopathy in assessing risk for violence: conceptual and methodological issues. Legal and Criminological Psychology 3:121–137, 1998

Hart SD: Psychopathy and risk for violence, in Psychopathy: Theory, Research and Implications. Edited by Cooke DJ, Forth AE, Hare RD. Dordrecht, the Netherlands, Kluwer, 1998, pp 355–373

Heilbron K: Prediction versus management models relevant to risk assessment: the importance of legal decision-making context. Law Hum Behav 21(4): 347–359, 1997

In re the Commitment of Peter Kienitz, 221 Wis.2d 275; 585 N.W.2d 609; 1998 Wisc. App. (July 30, 1998)

Kansas v Crane, 534 U.S. 407, 122 S. Ct. 867 (January 22, 2002)

Kansas v Hendricks, 521 U.S. 346, 138 L. Ed. 2d 501, 117 S. Ct. 2072 (1997)

Kuban M, Barbaree HE, Blanchard R: A comparison of volume and circumference phallometry: response magnitude and method agreement. Arch Sex Behav 28:345–359, 1999

Litwack TR: Actuarial versus clinical assessments of dangerousness. Psychology, Public Policy, and Law 7:409–443, 2001

Logan WA: Liberty interests in the preventive state: procedural due process and sex offender community notification laws. Journal of Criminal Law and Criminology 89:1167–1231, 1999

McKune v Lile, 536 U.S. 24 (2002)

Poole D, Lamb M: Investigative Interviews of Children: A Guide for Helping Professionals. Washington, DC, American Psychological Association, 1998, p 295

Prentky R, Burgess AW: Rehabilitation of child molesters: a cost-benefit analysis. Am J Orthopsychiatry 60(1):108–117, 1990

Quakenbush R: The assessment of sex offenders in Ireland and the Irish sex offender risk tool. Unpublished manuscript, Granada Institute, Dublin, Ireland, 2000

Quinsey VL, Bergersen SG: Instructional control of penile circumference. Behavior Therapy 7:489–493, 1976

Quinsey VL, Harris GT, Rice ME, et al: Violent Offenders: Appraising and Managing Risk. Washington, DC, American Psychological Association, 1998

Quinsey VL, Lalumiere ML, Rice ME, et al: Predicting sexual offenses, in Assessing Dangerousness: Violence by Sexual Offenders, Batterers and Child Abusers. Edited by Campbell JC. Thousand Oaks, CA, Sage, 1995, pp 114–137

Rice ME, Harris GT: Cross-validation and extension of the violence risk appraisal guide for child molesters and rapists. Law Hum Behav 21(2):231–241, 1997

Rice ME, Harris GT, Cornier CA: An evaluation of maximum security therapeutic community psychopaths and other mentally ill disorder offenders. Law Behavior 6(4):399–412, 1992

Riggs N, Houry D, Long G, et al: Analysis of 1,076 cases of sexual assault. Ann Emerg Med 35(4):358–362, 2000

Sachsenmaier SJ, Peters JM: Sex offender risk assessment methods and admissibility as scientific evidence, in Assessment and Management of Sex Offenders: What Prosecutors Need to Know. Edited by Peters JM. Washington, DC, U.S. Department of Justice, Child Exploitation and Obscenity Section, 2002

Seidman BT, Marshall WL, Hudson SM, et al: An examination of intimacy and loneliness in sex offenders. Journal of Interpersonal Violence 9:518–534, 1994

Seto MC, Barbaree HE: Psychopathy, treatment, behavior, and sex offender recidivism. Journal of Interpersonal Violence 14(12):1235–1248, 1999

Simon WT, Schouten PG: The plethysmograph reconsidered. J Am Acad Psychiatry Law 21(4):505–512, 1993

Sjostedt G, Grann M: Risk assessment: what is being predicted by actuarial prediction instruments? International Journal of Forensic Mental Health 1(2): 179–183, 2001

Sjostedt G, Langstrom N: Actuarial assessment of sex offender recidivism risk: a cross-validation of the RRASOR and Static-99 in Sweden. Law Hum Behav 24(3):271–296, 2001

Snyder H: Sexual Assault of Young Children as Reported to Law: Victim, Incident, and Offender Characteristics (NCJ 182990). Washington, DC, U.S. Department of Justice, Bureau of Justice Statistics, National Center for Juvenile Justice, 2000

State v Fertig, 143 N.J. 115 (1996)

State v Hurd, 86 N.J. 525 (1981)

Webster CD, Douglas KS, Eaves D, et al: HCR-20, Assessing Risk for Violence, Version 2. Burnaby, British Columbia, Mental Health, Law and Policy Institute, Simon Fraser University, 1997

Weinstock R, Leong GB, Silva JA: The role of traditional medical ethics in forensic psychiatry, in Ethical Practice in Psychiatry and the Law. Edited by Rosner R, Weinstock R. New York, Plenum, 1990, pp 31–51

West DJ: The effects of sex offenses, in Clinical Approaches to Sex Offenders and Their Victims. Edited by Hollins CR, Howells D. Toronto, Ontario, Wiley, 1991, pp 55–77

Wilson DB, Gallagher CA, Coggeshall MB, et al: A quantitative review of the effects of sex offender treatment on sexual reoffending. Corrections Management Quarterly 3:19–29, 1999

Zonana H, Bonnie R, Hoge S: In the wake of Hendricks: the treatment and restraint of sexually dangerous offenders viewed from the perspective of American psychiatry, in Protecting Society From Sexually Dangerous Offenders: Law, Justice, and Therapy. Edited by Winick BJ, LaFond JQ. Washington, DC, American Psychological Association, 2003, pp 131–145

## Suggested Readings

Marshall WL, Fernandez YM, Hudson SM, et al: Sourcebook of Treatment Programs for Sexual Offenders. New York, Plenum, 1998

Quinsey VL, Lalumiere ML: Assessment of Sexual Offenders Against Children, 2nd Edition. Newbury Park, CA, Sage, 2001

Winick BJ, LaFond JQ (eds): Protecting Society From Sexually Dangerous Offenders: Law, Justice, and Therapy. Washington, DC, American Psychological Association, 2003

C H A P T E R 1 7

# Psychiatry in Correctional Settings

Jeffrey L. Metzner, M.D.
Joel A. Dvoskin, Ph.D., A.B.P.P.

## Introduction

Local jails, which are usually administered by city or county officials, are facilities that hold inmates beyond arraignment, generally for 48 hours but less than a year. Prisons are state or federal correctional facilities in which persons convicted of major crimes or felonies serve sentences that are usually in excess of a year. Six states (Alaska, Connecticut, Delaware, Hawaii, Rhode Island, and Vermont) and the District of Columbia have combined jail and prison systems (Metzner 1997).[1]

There were 1,965,495 persons incarcerated in the nation's prisons and jails at midyear 2001. Prisoners in the custody of state and federal prisons and the District of Columbia accounted for two-thirds of the incarcerated population (1,334,225 inmates). Prisoners accounting for the other third were held in local jails (631,240). The total correctional population included 94,336 female prisoners, who accounted for 6.7% of all prisoners (Beck et al. 2002). A total of 3,932,751 adult men and women were on probation at year-end 2001, in addition to an adult parole population of 732,351 (Glaze 2002).

---

[1]Despite the clear legal status differences between pretrial detainees in jails and inmates in prisons, the term *inmate* will be used throughout this chapter to refer to both.

Recidivism rates are high, as demonstrated by a study of 272,111 state prisoners discharged from prisons in the United States during 1994, which revealed that 67.5% were rearrested for a new offense (almost exclusively a felony or a serious misdemeanor) within 3 years following their release (Langan and Levin 2002).

Psychiatric hospital populations have dwindled during the past five decades, and the locus of psychiatric treatment has increasingly shifted from long-stay state hospitals to acute general hospitals and community-based treatment. As a result, the frequency with which persons with the most serious psychiatric diagnoses interact with the criminal justice system has dramatically increased. It is not our intention to debate the wisdom of community-based treatment; for many consumers it has resulted in a richer and more fulfilling life, whereas for others it has resulted in frequent incarcerations. It is clear, however, that this change in the mental health treatment system has resulted in a "pooling" of some persons with diagnoses of serious mental illness in correctional settings.

Studies and clinical experience have consistently indicated that 8%–19% of prisoners have psychiatric disorders that result in significant functional impairments and that another 15%–20% of prisoners will require some form of psychiatric intervention during their incarceration (Dvoskin et al. 2003; Metzner 1993; Morrissey et al. 1993). Thus, even if the prevalence of mental illness within correctional populations has remained the same, the 71% increase in correctional populations between January 1990 and June 2001 (Beck et al. 2002) has resulted in at least a corresponding increase in the number of mentally ill prisoners.

Psychiatrists should become familiar with these settings and their particular stressors because persons with serious mental illnesses are increasingly being incarcerated in jails and prisons. Psychiatrists, along with other mental health professionals, are needed for their expertise in providing the appropriate mental health treatments to these persons. There are more than 5,000 jails in the United States, and only the larger ones have full-time psychiatrists or mental health staffing. Thus, while correctional psychiatry is an increasingly important and valued specialty, it remains true that the majority of psychiatric care, in local jails especially, will be provided on a part-time or contracted basis, often by general psychiatrists.

## Standards of Care in Correctional Mental Health Programs

Numerous sets of standards and guidelines for correctional mental health care programs have been promulgated by national organizations. The most widely recognized are those promulgated by the National Commission on Correctional Health Care (1999) (NCCHC) and by the American Psychiatric Association (2000). The American Psychiatric Association's published guidelines, which use the NCCHC standards as a foundation, recommend that the fundamental policy goal for correctional mental health care is to provide the same level of mental health services to each patient in the criminal justice system that *should* be available in the community.

By definition, of course, this standard is generally higher than that applied to people in the community; it is appropriate to ask why arrest, and perhaps commission of a crime, would entitle individuals to better mental health services than they would receive if they had obeyed the law and stayed out of trouble. The answer lies in both constitutional and common law. Because inmates are prevented from seeking their own food, clothing, shelter, and medical care by the very fact that they are locked up, those who incarcerate have legally been charged with providing these *necessities* of life to the people they incarcerate. This "necessaries doctrine" and subsequent constitutional law make it illegal for jails and prisons to be "deliberately indifferent" to the serious medical needs of prisoners. State and local governments, perhaps sadly, have no similar constitutional duty to meet the medical needs, however serious, of free citizens (Cohen 1998).

There is, however, a more positive public policy reason to provide a reasonably high "floor" of mental health services to prisoners. Steadman (H. Steadman, personal communication, November 2002) has spoken of the American jail as a "public health outpost," where those in need of services can be started on a course of physical or mental hygiene that will prevent future, expensive exacerbations of serious illness, including consequences such as crime. Correctional officials have a literally captive population that has demonstrated an inability to live safely and freely in the community, one that, under the stress of jail, may be more in need of psychiatric treatment and amenable to such treatment. This is not to suggest that jail or prison is the *preferred* method of entry into the mental health system, but, as is the case with illiteracy, jails and prisons have an opportunity to address some of the failures of other social and health systems in our society. To ignore this opportunity would be bad public policy.

## Forensic Evaluations in Correctional Settings

In addition to the essential treatment role that a psychiatrist provides in a correctional mental health system, a general psychiatrist will often have the opportunity to participate in various types of forensic evaluations within the correctional setting. In jails, forensic mental health evaluations involving pretrial detainees most commonly address issues related to competency to stand trial, diversion programs (related to sex offender treatment, substance abuse treatment, or mental health treatment), presentencing recommendations, and civil commitment. In the prison setting, forensic mental evaluations are most frequently requested to assess parole board issues (e.g., psychiatric suitability for parole, need for mental health treatment upon parole, risk assessments for violence), consultation for classification purposes (i.e., security-level questions), competency and dispositional issues relevant to disciplinary infraction proceedings, and the so-called *Hendricks* (*Kansas v. Hendricks* 1997) assessments related to evaluations of sex offenders for commitment following completion of their prison sentences. As correctional systems become increasingly aware of the legal and ethical obligations to inmates, formal assessments of competency to consent or refuse treatment will become increasingly important and common, and these will require forensic expertise.

The vast majority of correctional or forensic psychiatric evaluations have one thing in common: they require the psychiatrist to make an assessment of risk of interpersonal violence. Although a thorough review of violence risk assessment is beyond the scope of this chapter (but see Dvoskin and Heilbrun 2001), we recommend at the very least that psychiatrists familiarize themselves with the most important types of risk assessment: actuarial, anamnestic, and guided clinical assessment.

Actuarial prediction or assessment (see, e.g., Monahan et al. 2001; Quinsey et al. 1998) is a strictly statistical method of assessing risk that reports a person's risk of violence based on the violent behavior of groups with similar characteristics. Thus far, actuarial instruments have relied predominantly on static, historical variables and have been criticized as overgeneralizing from the populations on which they were normed (e.g., Canada) to populations with quite different base rates of violence. So far, actuarial instruments have not spoken to the severity or imminence of violence risk, but they have demonstrated an impressive ability to assess the likelihood of interpersonal violence.

Anamnestic assessment (Dvoskin 2002) uses the person's own history and patterns of behavior to predict the circumstances under which the person is likely to offend in the future and to guide clinical interventions aimed at reducing the likelihood of re-offending.

Finally, guided clinical assessment (e.g., Hart 1998) includes elements of both actuarial and anamnestic assessment. Guided clinical assessment typically involves a structured set of questions that are investigated, each based on a characteristic that has shown some empirical relationship to violent behavior, either among similar groups of people or in the person's own history.

As in all forensic assessments, the psychiatrist should inform the inmate, prior to beginning the assessment process, about the purpose of the evaluation and limits of confidentiality. Psychiatrists who provide treatment to inmates in various correctional settings should be aware of limitations related to confidentiality. Inmates should be informed about these limitations prior to beginning treatment (except in unusual circumstances—e.g., when the inmate is psychotic and unable to provide informed consent for treatment). These exceptions to confidentiality often vary from one state to another. For example, parole boards by statute often have access to an inmate's health care record, which will include mental health evaluations and treatment notes. The correctional staff is usually provided information by mental health staff that an inmate is on the mental health roster and is generally aware that an inmate is receiving psychotropic medications. Psychiatrists performing forensic evaluations of inmates should attempt to receive informed consent from the inmate, unless not required by law or regulations, to obtain relevant information, both oral and written, from past and current mental health providers.

The nature of the forensic issue to be addressed will certainly help to structure the interview so that relevant information will be obtained and assessed by the psychiatrist. In general, a standard psychiatric examination as described in standard textbooks (Nicholi 1999) should be performed. Depending on the specific referral question, the inmate's history relevant to substance abuse, mental health treatment, support systems, employment, plans if granted release, legal history, and adjustment to the correctional setting are often issues that need to be comprehensively assessed. See Chapter 6 ("The Forensic Examination and Report") for information relevant to writing the forensic report.

Dual-agency issues commonly arise in the correctional mental health setting. This potential problem becomes apparent when disclosing to the inmate one of the exceptions to confidentiality that may occur, such as when the inmate has been assessed to be a threat to staff or other inmates. This issue may also become prominent if the health care record is available to the parole board. There are circumstances in which the treating psychiatrist is asked to perform a forensic evaluation concerning a patient. Under some circumstances, this dual role is not inappropriate or avoidable, but generally speaking, dual-agency roles should be avoided.

## Clinical Vignette 1: Evaluation of an Inmate Suicide

Dr. J is a forensic psychiatrist who, in the past, consulted on a part-time basis to local jails. Dr. J received a call from a plaintiff's attorney concerning the death by suicide of Mr. S at the local jail two weeks following his incarceration. Dr. J was asked whether he would serve as an expert witness for the estate of the deceased, which had initiated a lawsuit against the sheriff and mental health director alleging negligence (in contrast to a Section 1983 constitutional rights violation claim). How should Dr. J proceed?

As in all forensic cases, Dr. J first needed to determine his level of relevant expertise, if any, in the issues being litigated. Dr. J had relevant experience in correctional psychiatry and agreed to review this case. He also checked his own records to ensure that he had not personally treated Mr. S, which might create a real or apparent conflict of interest.

Because of the increased risk of suicide among incarcerated jail inmates, especially among those with mental illness, correctional institutions are expected to have suicide prevention programs for identifying and responding to each suicidal inmate. To provide a competent forensic report, Dr. J will need to be familiar with the standard of care relevant to suicide prevention programs in a correctional facility. His opinion concerning this standard of care should not be idiosyncratic to Dr. J; rather, it should reflect and be grounded in statements by recognized experts, prior judicial decisions, published literature, empirical studies, and, perhaps most important, policy statements from relevant professional organizations.

The National Commission on Correctional Health Care (1999) and the American Psychiatric Association (2000) have provided very clear guidelines relevant to this issue. Both organizations require policies and procedures designed to identify newly arriving inmates who may require mental health evaluation and/or treatment. The APA guidelines describe three separate processes (receiving mental health screening, brief mental health assessment, and comprehensive mental health evaluation) that should be in place to identify inmates requiring psychiatric treatment. The NCCHC provides procedures for identifying inmates requiring psychiatric treatment via receiving screening, comprehensive health assessment, and mental health assessment procedures. All of these processes include assessments relevant to an inmate's potential for suicide and procedures to follow when actions are required as a result of positive findings.

The essential components (American Psychiatric Association 2000; National Commission on Correctional Health Care 1999) of an adequate suicide prevention program in jails include the following:

1. Training of all staff who have regular contact with inmates concerning recognition of danger signs and procedures to follow when an inmate may be suicidal
2. Procedures for identification, referral, and evaluation of all newly admitted inmates who may be suicidal, in addition to other inmates who may become suicidal at other times during their confinement
3. Policies and procedures to ensure adequate communication between the arresting/transporting officer and correctional staff, among the jail staff (including correctional, medical, and mental health personnel), and between facility staff and the suicidal inmate
4. Housing options that facilitate adequate monitoring of suicidal inmates by staff
5. Timely provision of mental health interventions to the suicidal inmate
6. Policies and procedures for reporting and notification of suicide attempts or completed suicides
7. Administrative reviews and critical incident debriefing in the event of a completed suicide

Awareness of these standards-of-care issues should result in Dr. J advising the plaintiff's attorney to request via the discovery process the following documents:

1. Policies and procedures relevant to the jail's mental health program, which will include a written description of the suicide prevention program
2. Training records, including the curriculum and the percentage of staff that have received this training, concerning the suicide prevention program
3. The complete health care record of Mr. S
4. A list containing the funded allocated mental health staff positions, which should include vacancies, at the jail during the period of time surrounding Mr. S's suicide
5. The number of suicide attempts and completed suicides during the past 2–5 years, which may help to identify systemic issues at the jail
6. A copy of the administrative review and investigations of Mr. S's suicide, including statements of all staff and inmate witnesses, autopsy and toxicology reports, external investigations, and the like

Dr. J will need to closely examine issues related to the screening procedures administered to Mr. S on admission (e.g., adequacy, timeliness, response to any positive findings), whether the officers with whom he interacted had received the relevant suicide prevention training, adequacy of the policies and procedures relevant to the suicide prevention program, and whether the jail successfully implemented these policies and procedures. As in other forensic evaluations, the initial review of this basic material will generate other questions and discovery requests to formulate an opinion relevant to liability issues.

After reviewing all of these materials, Dr. J may also want to obtain information from relevant witnesses, assuming that investigations have been completed. These may include other inmates, who either witnessed the event or knew the deceased, family members of the deceased, and various mental health, medical, and correctional staff. This information may be obtained in a variety of ways, such as interrogatories, deposition, and interviews. The specific method is usually determined by discovery procedures.

Ultimately, Dr. J will render an opinion concerning the presence or absence of negligence in regard to the death of Mr. S, if the suit is a simple tort claim of wrongful death or malpractice. In rendering this opinion, Dr. J must be careful to avoid the retrospective bias that may result from his knowledge that Mr. S is dead. Instead, Dr. J must try to judge whether the appropriate standard of care was met.

## Clinical Vignette 2: Adult Jail Diversion

> Dr. S consults with a local community mental health center (CMHC). Recently, the sheriff has entered into an intergovernmental agreement with the CMHC to provide a jail diversion program in an effort to reduce the unnecessary incarceration of persons with serious mental illness. The first candidate for this program is Mr. H. What are the relevant issues that Dr. S should address in his evaluation?

Jail diversion programs are organized interagency efforts to identify inmates with serious mental illnesses and establish mental health treatment programs that meet their needs in the least restrictive environment that does not appear to endanger the community. These programs negotiate with prosecutors, defense attorneys, courts, and community mental health providers to develop a comprehensive mental health disposition outside of the jail, either instead of prosecution or as a condition of reduction in charges, or at least to transfer defendants into treatment while awaiting trial. These dispositions usually occur when the charge is for a relatively minor crime (Hoff et al. 1999), although many diversion programs focus on felony defendants.

The first set of questions to be addressed by Dr. S will likely involve the criteria for inclusion into the program. Typically, there will be a requirement that the patient has a diagnosis of serious mental illness. Further, various types of offenses, especially crimes of violence, may disqualify the person for inclusion in the program. Dr. S will need to review recent psychiatric records, which will assist in the determination of Mr. H's diagnosis, and relevant legal documents to determine his current charges and criminal history.

Assuming that Mr. H meets the program's minimum criteria, the next set of questions will address his appropriateness for release and the conditions under which his release is least likely to result in harm to the community. Both of these questions are best answered by a competent risk assessment for violence. Dvoskin and Heilbrun (2001) have summarized the literature on violence risk assessment, including a description of actuarial, clinical, and anamnestic approaches to the task. Briefly, actuarial instruments, despite many limitations, appear to have value in determining the *likelihood* of violence, which is one important aspect of violence risk assessment. However, it is not the only axis, nor is it necessarily the most important. *Severity*, *imminence*, and *duration* of violence risk are all important determinants of Mr. H's appropriateness for diversion and must be considered by Dr. S.

To do so, Dr. S must conduct either a guided clinical evaluation (Hart 1998) or anamnestic (Dvoskin 2002) assessment of violence risk. Anamnestic assessment looks at the person in context and over time, examining and learning from his or her life story. In a sense, it is an ethnographic way of studying people. There should be few differences between this type of assessment and a good clinical evaluation. Both types of assessments should carefully review prior incidents of violence, including the clinical and situational aspects of Mr. H's life at the time of these incidents. This analysis will result in identification of risk-laden situations, clinical risk factors, skill deficits, and strengths or protective factors (which were likely in evidence at times that Mr. H did *not* commit any acts of violence).

This risk assessment will lead to a set of specific recommendations for services, supports, and monitoring that will address the situational and clinical risk factors identified in Dr. S's assessment. These recommendations must include recognition of the role of various social service and criminal justice agencies, in addition to mental health and psychiatric services in the community. Dr. S and the diversion program staff must take time to familiarize themselves with the practices and resources of local probation, parole, and police agencies and gain an awareness of various federal and state entitlement programs and how to access them.

Finally, no matter how well-crafted the diversion plan is, it must be accepted by prosecutors and judges. To this end, Dr. S or a program representative must have access to the courts and enjoy a high level of credibility in the eyes of judges and prosecutors. To accomplish this goal, diversion programs must avoid taking marginal cases early in the program's life. Early successes set the stage for later risk taking, but establishing the program as consistent with public safety is essential, so that the inevitable failure will be seen an exception to an otherwise safe and responsible process.

## Clinical Vignette 3: Juvenile Sex Offenders

> Dr. D, who is the clinical director of a sex-offender-specific treatment program for adolescent males, is asked by the juvenile court to evaluate a 14-year-old boy for treatment as part of a diversion program. What are the likely issues that will need to be addressed concerning confidentiality and double agency?

Dr. D will obviously need to have expertise in the evaluation and treatment of adolescent sex offenders to accept the appointment by the juvenile court. It is beyond the scope of this chapter to summarize issues relevant to the sex-offender-specific assessment required, which can be found elsewhere (Colorado Sex Offender Management Board 2002; Metzner and Becker 1999). However, this vignette does provide the opportunity to discuss issues of confidentiality and dual agency in the context of a mandated assessment or treatment ordered by a court.

In many states, such as Colorado, the standard of care relevant to mandated treatment concerning confidentiality is as follows:

> Juveniles who have committed sexual offenses must waive confidentiality for purposes of evaluation, treatment, supervision, and case management to obtain the privileges attached to community supervision. This waiver of confidentiality must be based on complete informed consent of the parent/legal guardian and voluntary assent of the juvenile. The juvenile's parent/guardian must be fully informed of alternative dispositions that may occur in the absence of consent/assent. (Colorado Sex Offender Management Board 2002)

Under such circumstances, the psychiatrist needs to be sure that both the juvenile and the parents or legal guardian fully understands the meaning of this waiver.

These same standards clearly state that "the highest priority of the standards and guidelines is community safety. Whenever the needs of juveniles who have committed sexual offenses conflict with community safety, community safety takes precedence" (Colorado Sex Offender Management Board 2002). In other words, the evaluating or treating psychiatrist is now in the potentially conflicting role of a double agent. However, this situation may be one of the exceptions to the general rule of avoiding dual agency.

This waiver of confidentiality and dual-agency role are often obstacles to establishing a therapeutic alliance with the juvenile offender. However, this difficulty can be decreased by including the juvenile, when possible, in the process that involves sharing of information with others. For example, this information sharing occurs during treatment planning and review meetings, which often include the juvenile's probation officer, social worker, residential treatment staff, and mental health clinicians. The adolescent should attend part of all such meetings (with few exceptions). Discussing issues relevant to the staffing with the adolescent, prior to the actual staffing, can be very helpful in establishing a therapeutic alliance. Including the parents or legal guardian in this process is also helpful. Providing the adolescent with a draft copy of reports sent to the court or probation officer prior to actually sending the reports is consistent with this straightforward approach.

## Clinical Vignette 4: Evaluation for Disciplinary Board

Inmate L was charged with disobeying a direct order from a correctional officer and destroying state property. During the investigation, Mr. L appeared to be agitated and demonstrated disorganized thinking. Dr. S received a referral from the disciplinary board hearing officer for a mental health evaluation of Mr. L prior to going forth with the disciplinary hearing. How should Dr. S proceed?

Dr. S needs to be familiar with the policies and procedures in the correctional institution relevant to such a mental health evaluation. Unfortunately, this area of correctional psychiatry is frequently very unclear, with little guidance being provided in the psychiatric literature (Krelstein 2002).

In general, these types of evaluations focus on the following three questions:

1. Are there any mental health factors that may cause the inmate to not be able to competently participate in the disciplinary hearing process?
2. If the inmate has a mental disorder, did the disorder contribute to the behavior(s) that led to the alleged disciplinary infraction?
3. If the inmate is found guilty of the offense, are there any mitigating mental health factors that should be considered by the hearing officer in determining the punishment?

It is also not unusual, although it is somewhat controversial, for some correctional systems to ask for consultation relevant to a responsibility (i.e., equivalent to a plea of not guilty by reason of insanity) examination. Many correctional mental health professionals are not trained to do such a forensic assessment, and most systems requesting the specific responsibility evaluations lack adequate standards and definitions for these examinations. It is beyond the scope of this vignette to further discuss issues relevant to responsibility examinations in the correctional setting. However, Dvoskin et al. (1995) have argued against formal evaluations of criminal responsibility in prison, preferring an informal process that will divert fewer clinical resources from treatment and allow the prison mental health professionals to maintain the trust of staff and inmates alike.

Dual-agency issues arise if the mental health assessment is provided by the inmate's treating clinician. In general, the treating clinician should be made aware of the alleged infraction because the inmate's actions leading to the alleged rule violation are often clinically significant. However, to minimize dual-agency issues, the actual consultation provided to the disciplinary board should be provided by a clinician who is not treating the inmate.

## Conclusion

Historically, jails and prisons were viewed as the least desirable settings in which to practice psychiatry. However, it has been our experience that correctional settings can be financially, intellectually, and clinically rewarding places to work. In many states, it is sadly true that the most mentally disabled citizens are likely to be found in jails and prisons, and these institutions often have more resources available for the treatment of these individuals than can be found in traditional mental health settings. Finally, medical schools are increasingly contracting out as service providers, creating exciting opportunities for advancing the field by serving the people who need us most.

## Key Points

- Forensic evaluations that are relevant to correctional psychiatric issues generally require either of the following:
    1. Knowledge of specific legal standards (e.g., Was the appropriate standard of care followed? Did the inmate have the capacity for a specific competency such as competency to stand trial or competency to refuse treatment?)

2. Familiarity with relevant treatment resources and their availability, because the forensic question being addressed is related to dispositional issues (e.g., Is diversion an option? What psychiatric conditions, if any, should be part of an inmate's parole requirements? Are there treatment settings available that will decrease a particular inmate's participation in dangerous activities if released?)

## Practice Guidelines

1. Be familiar with standards and guidelines for mental health services in correctional facilities promulgated by key national organizations such as the National Commission on Correctional Health Care and the American Psychiatric Association. Treatment of inmates should be consistent with these standards.
2. Stay current with accepted risk assessment procedures, which are generally important elements of forensic evaluations in a correctional setting and often relevant to treatment in jails and prisons.
3. Ensure that inmates are fully informed about the many exceptions to confidentiality in a correctional setting, and remain sensitive to treatment issues related to these potential breeches of confidentiality.
4. Avoid dual-agency roles whenever possible. Dual-agency conflicts, similar to issues related to confidentiality, can adversely affect the therapeutic alliance.
5. Be straightforward and respectful in interactions with inmates.

## References

American Psychiatric Association: Psychiatric Services in Jails and Prisons: A Task Force Report of the American Psychiatric Association, 2nd Edition. Washington, DC, American Psychiatric Association, 2000

Beck AJ, Karberg JC, Harrison PM: Prison and Jail Inmates at Midyear 2001 (NCJ 191702). Bureau of Justice Statistics Bulletin, April 2002, pp 1–16

Cohen F: The Mentally Disordered Inmate and the Law. Kingston, NJ, Civic Research Institute, 1998

Colorado Sex Offender Management Board: Standards and guidelines for the evaluation, assessment, treatment and supervision of juveniles who have committed sexual offenses. Available at: http://dcj.state.co.us/odvsom. Accessed October 13, 2002.

Dvoskin JA: Knowledge is not power—knowledge is obligation. J Am Acad Psychiatry Law 30(4):533–540, 2002

Dvoskin JA, Heilbrun K: Risk assessment and release decision-making: toward resolving the great debate. J Am Acad Psychiatry Law 29:6–10, 2001

Dvoskin JA, Petrila J, Stark-Riemer S: Case note: *Powell v Coughlin* and the application of the professional judgment rule to prison mental health. Ment Phys Disabil Law Rep 19(1):108–114, 1995

Dvoskin JA, Spiers EM, Metzner JL, et al: The structure of correctional mental health services, in Principles and Practice of Forensic Psychiatry, 2nd Edition. Edited by Rosner, R. London, Arnold, 2003, pp 489–504

Glaze LE: Probation and parole in the United States, 2001 (NCJ 195669). Bureau of Justice Statistics Bulletin, August 2002, pp 1–8

Hart SD: The role of psychopathy in assessing risk for violence: conceptual and methodological issues. Legal and Criminological Psychology 3:123–140, 1998

Hoff RA, Baranosky MV, Buchanan J, et al: The effects of a jail diversion program on incarceration: a retrospective cohort study. J Am Acad Psychiatry Law 27:377–386, 1999

Kansas v Hendricks, 117 S. Ct. 2072 (1997)

Krelstein MS: The role of mental health in the inmate disciplinary process: a national survey. J Am Acad Psychiatry Law 30(4):488–496, 2002

Langan PA, Levin DJ: Recidivism of prisoners released in 1994 (NCJ 193427). Bureau of Justice Statistics Bulletin, June 2002, pp 1–16

Metzner JL: Guidelines for psychiatric services in prisons. Criminal Behavior and Mental Health 3:252–267, 1993

Metzner JL: An introduction to correctional psychiatry, Part I. J Am Acad Psychiatry Law 25:375–381, 1997

Metzner JL, Becker J: Juvenile sex offenders, in Dangerous Sex Offenders: A Task Force Report of the American Psychiatric Association. Washington, DC, American Psychiatric Association, 1999, pp 81–101

Monahan J, Steadman H, Silver E, et al: Rethinking Risk Assessment: The MacArthur Study of Mental Disorder and Violence. New York, Oxford University Press, 2001

Morrissey JP, Swanson JW, Goldstrom I, et al: Overview of mental health services provided by state adult correctional facilities: United States, 1988 (DHHS Publ No SMA 93-1993). Washington, DC, Dept of Health and Human Services, 1993, pp 1–13

National Commission on Correctional Health Care: Correctional Mental Health Care: Standards and Guidelines for Delivering Services. Chicago, IL, National Commission on Correctional Health Care, 1999

Nicholi AM: History and mental status, in The Harvard Guide to Psychiatry. Edited by Nicholi AM. Cambridge, MA, Belknap Press, 1999, pp 26–39

Quinsey V, Harris G, Rice M, et al: Violent Offenders: Appraising and Managing Risk. Washington, DC, American Psychological Association, 1998

## Suggested Readings

American Psychiatric Association: Psychiatric Services in Jails and Prisons: A Task Force Report of the American Psychiatric Association, 2nd Edition. Washington, DC, American Psychiatric Association, 2000

Anno J: Prison Health Care: Guidelines for the Management of an Adequate Delivery System. Chicago, IL, National Commission on Correctional Health Care, 1991

Cohen F: The Mentally Disordered Inmate and the Law. Kingston, NJ, Civic Research Institute, 1998

Wettstein R (ed): Treatment of Offenders With Mental Disorders. New York, Guilford, 1998

CHAPTER 18

# Forensic Psychiatry and Law Enforcement

Debra A. Pinals, M.D.

Marilyn Price, M.D.

## Introduction

Recent interest has grown in the relationship of forensic psychiatry and law enforcement. This relationship has evolved along many fronts as psychiatrists are increasingly called on for consultation, training, or assessment. First, especially since deinstitutionalization, police are frequently first responders to community emergencies that involve persons with mental illness. Authors have referred to police as quasi-mental health professionals and have labeled them "streetcorner psychiatrists" (Teplin and Pruett 1992) and "frontline mental health workers" (Green 1997). Given this important social function, law enforcement agents have a heightened need to recognize manifestations of mental illness and appropriately triage individuals who come to their attention. As a result, psychiatrists may be asked to collaborate with police departments and provide mental health training for officers.

Additionally, encounters between police and persons with mental illness have increasingly received public scrutiny, especially when the encounter results in a lethal outcome (Appelbaum 2000). A review of these encounters at times points to excessive force on the part of the officer. At other times, however, an individual motivated by suicidal intent provokes the use of lethal force in what has become known as "suicide by cop." Psychiatrists become involved in these issues through a variety of circumstances, including postmortem reviews of suicide by cop in civil litigation, criminal forensic evaluations, and police investigations. Psychiatrists may also work with patients who have a history of attempting suicide by cop or may be at risk of engaging in this type of behavior. Attempts to reduce negative outcomes in police encounters have included calling on psychiatrists to assist police with crisis negotiation, at times involving hostage and/or barricade situations.

Finally, as psychiatrists have gained expertise in working more closely with police, there has been a parallel growth in understanding aspects of psychiatric disability specifically related to law enforcement officials. Police departments often seek evaluations of officer fitness for duty. Unique job stress, exposure to violence and death, and substance abuse are just some of the factors that contribute to the potential for psychological sequelae affecting occupational functioning. Given the tight social network among officers, peer relations are important to consider in police fitness for duty assessments. Suicide risk is also important to weigh, because this group has easy access to firearms. Psychiatrists conducting independent medical examinations of officer fitness for duty must carefully balance risks to the officer and to others in light of the social importance of bearing a firearm and the implications for its removal.

The areas just described represent focused arenas where psychiatry and law enforcement intersect. Many psychiatrists have developed specialized involvement with police along these lines. This chapter presents a more detailed review of each of these areas, in an effort to highlight some of the unique aspects of work with law enforcement and with cases that involve police encounters with persons in crisis.

## Mental Health Training for Law Enforcement

Police have long been called to help with crisis situations for persons with mental illness. Although community resources and crisis services have come a long way, Liberman noted in 1969 that the police would continue to serve a role in the care of the mentally ill as long as there were gaps in community treatment. The release of persons from state hospitals in the late 1960s and 1970s has been touted as a primary reason why police encounters with the mentally ill have risen over the years.

Studies have shown that arrests of homeless persons and those discharged from psychiatric facilities are quite common (Belcher 1988; Lamb and Lamb 1990). Most officers, ranging from 60% to 92% in some studies, report responding to one mental health crisis call each month (Borum et al. 1998; Gillig et al. 1990). Between 42% and 84% said they had responded to more than one such call in the same time period.

Police departments vary in their approach to training and managing crisis calls involving persons with mental illness. In a survey of police departments in 194 U.S. cities with a population of 100,000 or more, responses indicated that 7% of all police contacts involved persons believed to be mentally ill (Deane et al. 1999). In that same study, over half of the departments reported having no specialized system in place to handle the issues that arose from these contacts (Deane et al. 1999). Husted et al. (1995) found in their survey of California law enforcement agencies that police were called to a robbery as often as they were called to handle a mental health crisis (Husted et al. 1995). Yet, in that same study, most law enforcement officers reported they were given insufficient training to identify, manage, and appropriately refer the mentally ill offenders they encountered.

Several authors have described various organized strategies used by some police departments to manage citizens with mental illness who are in crisis (Borum 2000; Deane et al. 1999; Dupont and Cochran 2000). These strategies have been labeled based on the agency responsible (i.e., police-based or mental health–based) and the primary discipline of the responder (i.e., specially trained police officer or mental health professional). For example, a police-based specialized police response is used by a small number of police departments. In this strategy, a selected group of police officers within a particular department receives specialized training to act as liaisons to the mental health system and manage crisis intervention. These specially trained officers respond to mental health emergencies. In a second scheme—the police-based, specialized mental health response—mental health consultants work for police departments and are available for on-site and telephone consultations.

More commonly, a mental health–based, specialized mental health response has been used to handle mental health crises. This strategy involves the use of mental health crisis teams that function as mobile crisis units. Often these teams represent an arm of local community mental health centers or public agencies whose mission is to be available at all hours to provide evaluations, treatment, and triage decisions. Many of these crisis teams work hard to foster relationships with local police, who may still be called on to assist in emergencies. Lamb et al. (2002) cautioned that mental health professionals who are members of mobile crisis teams need to be mindful of their role and not try to act as police officers. The importance of working within one's expertise during a crisis further highlights the importance of collaboration between mental health professionals and police officers and calling on each as needed.

Mental health professionals should familiarize themselves with the type of mental health crisis response system that exists in their community. Especially in jurisdictions where there is no formal relationship between police and mental health, forging a relationship between a psychiatric department and a police department can go a long way toward assisting persons with mental illness who are in crisis (Lamb et al. 2002). For example, police mental health training could alert officers how to access mental health services and avoid unnecessary incarceration of certain individuals. Mental health professionals, through such collaborations, could capitalize on the expertise of the police. Police often desire these relationships, and at times they will seek out specialized mental health training. Meetings between mental health providers and police are a forum that can be used to develop target topics to cover in training and to develop approaches to mutual problem solving.

Increased knowledge of mental illness, verbal skills, and crisis intervention strategies related to encounters with persons with mental illness are at the forefront of desired goals of police officer training. Police may be motivated for such training because of concern for their potential for liability in the management of encounters with persons with mental illness.

Education alone, however, will not provide solutions to the challenges officers face in managing crises that involve persons with mental illness (Borum 2000; Dupont and Cochran 2000). For example, an earlier study examining the effect of a mental health educational program on police officers found that police showed greater knowledge related to working with emotionally disturbed persons following training, although their attitudes were not altered (Godschalx 1984). Studies examining overall efficacy of crisis intervention training for officers have also been reported to be equivocal (Borum 2000).

Nevertheless, many psychiatrists involved in police mental health training would argue that improvement of an officer's knowledge about mental illness is significant and possibly a first step in changing overall attitudes over time. Limited mental health training may not be afforded the emphasis needed to really change attitude and behavior, although further study would be helpful in assessing this.

Officers must be trained in a wide variety of topics, both as recruits and during in-service training, ranging from education about policies to use of service weapons. Police departments are thus faced with difficult choices to make in determining how many hours of specialized mental health education to provide for officers. Given the competing agendas, the psychiatrist planning mental health training needs to develop a list of educational priorities.

Negative attitudes toward persons with mental illness are likely a factor in how police work with them, so that education should, in part, be aimed to reduce the stigma associated with mental illness. Decreasing stigma may ultimately enhance communication skills of officers responding to a call involving an emotionally disturbed person. Training can be used to help the law enforcement community recognize basic psychopathology so that individuals may get help when needed.

Training should also help police understand that people are not just "crazy" and that numerous diagnoses can manifest themselves as emotional disturbance. Emphasizing the biological underpinnings of serious mental illness can serve to further diminish stigma. Such emphasis can also highlight the potential need of persons in crisis to receive medical attention to rule out any medical causes of acute symptomatic exacerbations. Factors contributing to behavioral emergency can be explained to include stressors, mental illness, substance use, and medical causes.

Topics of interest may also include suicide and violence risk reduction, assessment of a person for signs of a psychiatric disorder, assessment of a scene of an emotionally disturbed person, communication with a suicidal person, communication with people with psychotic symptoms, written communication regarding observations, and mental health law. Borum (2000) identified several additional areas worthy of focus in officer training, such as mediation skills, anger control, verbal skills to deescalate conflict, education aimed at helping to shift negative attitudes toward persons with mental illness, and training to counter popular misconceptions that could negatively effect perceptions or attributions during stressful encounters.

Officers trained in handling criminal behavior are taught to use their authority as a means of control. However, as Fyfe (2000) commented, it is critical for police to understand that the forceful approach used with rational offenders may, in fact, paradoxically lead to an escalation of behavior in irrational offenders. Patient, one-on-one communication, with minimal distraction from others at the scene, can make a difference in a highly charged situation. Yet, police are called to manage the heights of psychopathology, often after failed attempts to do so by others. Therefore, mental health professionals must recognize the extreme stress of such situations. Psychiatrists conducting training should be cautious and avoid going beyond their expertise. Issues such as the use of weapons are best left to police to decide on the basis of their own policies, training, and practices.

Husted et al. (1995) noted that cross-training between police and mental health professionals is also highly desirable and may help to create attitude changes through improved communication and interagency satisfaction. Cross-training identified as being useful includes in-service training to officers presented by mental health agency representatives and mental health personnel exposure to police activities related to crisis calls, such as through ride-alongs and briefings.

Numerous studies have examined how officers make decisions related to the management of persons with mental illness at the time of contact. Dispositional decisions often rely on "extrapsychiatric" variables at play in handling encounters with persons in crisis, rather than on symptom presentation alone (Teplin and Pruett 1992). Officer discretion, rather than legal regulation, is commonly the guiding force behind dispositional decisions. Green (1997) noted that police generally attempt to reserve arrest for more violent actions, yet they are faced with difficulties in involuntarily hospitalizing persons with mental illness who have engaged in some type of potentially criminal act.

Use of individual discretion can become problematic when officers exceed their authority through unwarranted arrest. Thus, officer mental health training should include time for case discussions and problem solving around the challenging decision making required in these encounters. Information about available mental health resources can also be of use. Given the inevitable intersection of mental health professionals and police, mental health training should allow a mutual sharing of experiences. In addition, establishing openings to direct communication with mental health professionals and developing collaborative specialized response mechanisms are examples of approaches that can ultimately assist in the management of persons with mental illness who are in crisis.

## Suicide by Cop

### Clinical Vignette

Mr. S was shot to death by police after a 1-hour confrontation. He had recently been released from a 1-month hospitalization, precipitated by an attempt to stab himself in the abdomen. Prior to his hospitalization, Mr. S had lost his job and his wife had left him. He was treated with an SSRI [selective serotonin reuptake inhibitor] and an atypical antipsychotic medication for his depression and preoccupation with wanting to die. Mr. S considered himself a failure for having unsuccessfully attempted suicide. He appeared to respond to medications and was discharged home, with a plan for a family member to reside with him.

Several days after discharge, Mr. S began shouting at his neighbors, saying they were part of a conspiracy, that there was no hope, and that he needed to find a way out. The neighbors noted that he was wielding a knife, and they became frightened and called the police.

The police arrived on scene and tried to calm Mr. S by speaking with him, but he continued to escalate, threatening to kill his neighbors and himself. He suddenly raised the knife he was carrying and showed it to the officers. The officers told him to drop the knife, but he did not. Instead he lunged forward as if to stab one of the officers. An officer fired his service weapon, hitting Mr. S in the chest. Mr. S died within moments.

When an individual engages in behavior intended to provoke police to use lethal force, the question may be raised as to whether the individual behaved in such a way because of suicidal ideation. There is little psychiatric literature regarding this phenomenon. Several terms have been proposed to describe it, including the most colloquial and the most commonly used term, *suicide by cop*. Other terms that have been used include "victim-precipitated homicide" (Wolfgang 1959), "law enforcement-forced-assisted suicide" (Hutson et al. 1998) and "law enforcement officer–assisted suicide"(Homant and Kennedy 2000).

Regardless of the label attached, this phenomenon has gained increasing attention in recent years. It has been defined as an incident in which a suicidal individual intentionally engages in life-threatening and criminal behavior with a lethal weapon or what appears to be a lethal weapon toward law enforcement officers or civilians to specifically provoke officers to shoot the individual in self-defense or to protect civilians (Hutson et al. 1998). The police involved may or may not be aware that they are being used to accomplish an individual's suicide. Other definitions have not specifically required the use of a weapon or object appearing as a weapon. For example, Stincelli (2003) offered the definition of suicide by cop as "a colloquial term used to describe a suicidal incident whereby the suicidal subject engages in a consciously, life-threatening behavior to the degree that it compels a police officer to respond with deadly force."

In an early, classic paper, Wolfgang (1957) identified 150 cases of victim-precipitated homicides over the course of a 5-year period in Philadelphia and spoke to the notion that a victim's behavior is often an important factor in criminal homicide. Although Wolfgang's study did not address victims who provoke police, his commentary highlighted the intense interpersonal dynamic that may be involved in some homicides. His subsequent paper went on to describe the dynamics involved when suicide is a motivating force in victim-precipitated homicide (Wolfgang 1959).

More recently, the literature has expanded in its examination of incidents involving police who are provoked into shooting a suicidal individual. Categorizing these cases as homicides (based on the intent of the police) or suicide (based on the intent of the victim) is complicated, and forensic pathologists do not always agree on the best approach to this dilemma (Wilson et al. 1998). Hutson et al. (1998) conducted one of the more carefully designed studies of suicide by cop in their review of all files of officer-involved shootings investigated by the Los Angeles County Sheriff's Department from 1987 to 1997. Of note, in the lethal shootings that met the authors' criteria for suicide by cop, all deaths were classified by the coroner as homicides.

Although the methodology has varied, studies have found that at least 10% of incidents of police using deadly force may be attributed to suicide by cop (Hutson et al. 1998; Kennedy et al. 1998). It has been suggested that the incidence of suicide by cop is on the rise, although this may be related, in part, to better reporting (Mohandie and Meloy 2000). Furthermore, the overall incidence examined in the literature does not speak to additional cases of attempted suicide by cop. This may be harder to study, as it can include nonfatal police shootings or situations in which lethal force does not end up being used at all. Thus, these incidents can look like routine police contacts rather than failed attempts at suicide by cop.

Several authors have identified general characteristics of persons who engage in suicide by cop and of the behavior itself by retrospective review of cases purported to be incidents of suicide by cop (Hutson et al. 1998; Mohandie and Meloy 2000; Wilson et al. 1998). In those analyses, suicide by cop was more commonly associated with males. Ages of suicidal persons across studies ranged from late teens to almost 60, although average ages tended to be in the 20s and 30s. Most of the suicidal individuals, although not all, had histories of psychiatric problems, most commonly including histories of suicidal ideation and depression.

Histories of substance abuse and prior arrests were also seen in the majority of the suicidal persons. Intoxication with alcohol at the time of the incidents was seen in approximately 40% of cases (Wilson et al. 1998). Use of drugs was less common but was noted in some cases. Use of firearms or facsimile firearms as the provoking weapon was most common, followed by knives and blunt objects. In one study, 10 of 15 victims verbally communicated suicidal threats during the incident, whereas 8 of 15 had communicated their suicidal intent in writing prior to the incident (Wilson et al. 1998). Interestingly, some of the subjects who had written of their suicidal intent did not verbally communicate it to officers, who may thus have been unaware that the victim was using them to assist in their suicide.

A typological construct of suicide by cop developed by Mohandie and Meloy (2000, pp. 384–385) divided the goals of the victim into instrumental and expressive subtypes. In the instrumental subtype, individuals engaged in suicide by cop behaviors in an attempt to 1) avoid consequences of criminal or shameful acts, 2) reconcile a failed relationship, 3) avoid exclusion clauses of life insurance policies, 4) resolve the spiritual sanction against suicide by allowing oneself to be killed, or 5) seek an effective and lethal means of accomplishing death. The expressive goal of engaging in suicide by cop was identified as effecting a means of communicating sentiments of 1) hopelessness, depression, desperation; 2) ultimate identification as victim; 3) need to save face by dying rather than surrendering; 4) intense power needs; 5) rage and revenge; or 6) need to draw attention to a personal issue. To achieve these goals, varying degrees of physical threat to police may be initiated.

Certain deaths are often difficult to identify as motivated by suicide (e.g., motor vehicle accidents). In an effort to categorize reports of police shootings, two police officers with master's degrees in criminal justice cataloged 240 news reports of police shootings into five categories with regard to the motivation of the person who was shot. The categories included 1) probable suicide, 2) possible suicide, 3) uncertain, 4) suicide improbable, and 5) no suicidal evidence (Kennedy et al. 1998). Of the incidents reviewed, 14 (5%) involved either homeless persons or persons with known mental illness.

Kennedy et al. (1998) also reported that between 16% and 47% of the cases reviewed were found to involve probable or possible suicidal motivation, although unclear and missing facts made the characterization of these incidents difficult and the methodology of reviewing news reports has limitations. Nevertheless, the authors commented on the need to maintain an awareness of the possibility that suicide may be a motivation in police shootings. They identified a goal of improving interpersonal communication skills for officers, who they note must make reasonable attempts to avoid having to use deadly force, regardless of the victim's determination to die.

In a review of 143 incidents of suicide by police gathered from newspaper reports, prosecution cases, and legal literature, Homant and Kennedy (2000) proposed dividing suicide by cop behavior into three categories: 1) direct confrontation, 2) disturbed intervention, and 3) criminal intervention. These categories were each further divided into subcategories. Direct confrontation involved situations in which the subject plans ahead of time to attack law enforcement officers in order to be killed by them. Subcategories reflected the manner in which subjects interacted with police, including sudden attacks on officers, controlled confrontation with demands that police kill the subject, and manipulated confrontation when the subject sets up a situation so that the police will come and investigate. When police arrive, the subject confronts police with a threat of deadly force. Examples of manipulated confrontation include traffic stops leading to high-speed chases and reporting crimes to the police so that they will go to the scene.

Disturbed intervention involved the majority of incidents reviewed by Homant and Kennedy (2000). In these situations, the subject was acting irrationally and either was overtly suicidal prior to police arrival or became suicidal on their arrival. These situations include police calls for suicide interventions (such as police calls to manage ambivalent suicide attempts and domestic calls to police to help manage a suicidal family member), calls of general domestic disturbances, and disorderly behaviors that result in police calls. In the disturbed intervention category, the disturbed behavior was not specifically designed to bring police to the scene, but behavior leading to suicide by cop came about after their arrival.

The third major category described by Homant and Kennedy (2000) is one that comes about through routine police work in criminal intervention. In these situations, people engaged in ordinary criminal activity are under the impression that they will avoid detection, so police involvement is unwelcome and unexpected. The subject, feeling there is no hope for escape, prefers to be killed by police. Suicide by cop behavior may ensue in an effort to avoid incarceration when a major crime is involved, or as a matter of principle when the crime is a minor one.

Suicide by cop following criminal intervention was found to occur in only a handful of cases, yet what was noteworthy was that the resistance to police escalated from a seemingly routine incident to a fatal outcome. The authors speculated that unconscious suicidal motivations may be at play in those incidents, even though the suicide by cop was not planned or articulated in advance. The term *unconscious* has different meanings for psychiatrists and law enforcement agents. From a psychiatric perspective, unconscious motivations are difficult to prove in cases involving litigation. Psychiatrists should thus be cautious about interpreting an individual's actions as unconsciously suicidal without strong collateral data supporting suicidality prior to the incident.

The case of Mr. S reflects an individual who communicated homicidal and suicidal threats, possibly with the goal of instrumentalizing an effective means of accomplishing death. He either manipulated a scenario to bring police to the scene or created a disturbance that caused the neighbors to call the police. Mr. S may have previously expressed the idea or plan to die at the hands of the police because his own direct attempt at suicide was unsuccessful. The neighbors, family members, witnesses, and other collateral sources should be questioned about this, if possible. A note at the scene, if present, might provide additional information.

Psychiatrists may be called to examine suicide by cop from a number of different perspectives, including post hoc review of an incident related to litigation involving police, questions for life insurance policies, and even medical malpractice where a decedent's cause of death is at issue. In addition, psychiatrists may conduct evaluations of suicide by cop survivors related to issues of criminal responsibility (Bresler et al. 2003) and ongoing suicide risk assessment.

Generally, in cases involving completed suicide by cop, a psychological autopsy is necessary to gather comprehensive information about the manner of death through a variety of collateral sources. These might include examining the coroner's report, contacting family members and friends of the decedent, contacting police, and reviewing police, criminal, and medical records as available. In conducting this review, psychiatrists should be cognizant of methodological limitations of the retrospective data (Hawton et al. 1998) that may be at issue in the litigation process.

Psychiatrists evaluating individuals who have had volatile encounters with police should be aware that suicide by cop may have been a motivating factor in their behavior. However, clinicians should consider the possibility that a patient or evaluee is malingering in accounts of suicide by cop. Individuals reporting attempted suicide by cop retrospectively may be trying to present a version of events to exonerate their actions. As with any forensic evaluation, collateral data and a comprehensive review of an individual's premorbid functioning are critical in an analysis of such incidents.

Legal cases have addressed specific questions that are important considerations in a psychiatric evaluation involving suicide by cop. In *Graham v. Connor* (1989), the U.S. Supreme Court held that claims alleging that officers used excessive force in the course of their work should be analyzed using an "objective reasonableness" standard. Such a standard would take into account the facts and circumstances confronting the officer at the time, rather than data learned retrospectively. In *Palmquist v. Selvik* (1997), the U.S. Court of Appeals for the Seventh Circuit held that failure to train officers to adequately handle calls involving emotionally disturbed individuals can be a basis of liability in certain situations. The court noted, however, that officers in the suicide by cop case in question had received some training and that the police department had not been deliberately indifferent to the need to train its officers in this area. Exposure to some training, no matter how limited, protected the police from liability in that case.

Suicide by cop involves a complex interplay between people in high-intensity encounters. It has become a relatively common term and is an increasingly recognized occurrence. Thus, police and psychiatrists should continue to learn about the phenomenon of suicide by cop as it gains more attention in the literature and in popular culture.

## Crisis Negotiations

### Clinical Vignette

Police responded to a call from Mr. and Mrs. H concerning a domestic dispute. The H's reported that the couple living in the apartment next door, Mr. and Mrs. J, had been fighting all night. The H's were concerned because they had overheard Mrs. J screaming, "Get away from me. Don't hurt me."

Mr. J had been drinking heavily since losing his job as a computer programmer in a recent company downsizing. The J's were experiencing serious financial problems and had received an eviction notice. The couple's marital problems had escalated. Mrs. J confided that she was thinking about asking for a trial separation. Earlier that day, Mr. J had asked Mr. H to recommend an attorney so that Mr. J could get his affairs in order. Mr. J was a Desert Storm veteran and had several guns in the home.

As police were interviewing the neighbors, Mr. J stepped onto his balcony, holding a gun to his wife's head. He threatened to kill his wife if the police officers did not leave immediately. Mr. J insisted that he had the situation in control, and this was none of their business.

Police called in a psychiatrist to act as a consultant to the crisis team while they negotiated with Mr. J. The psychiatrist monitored the progress of the negotiations and offered suggestions to the team. The recommendations were helpful in resolving the situation. Mrs. J was released unharmed, and Mr. J later surrendered to police.

The modern era of crisis negotiation began in the 1970s after a series of incidents highlighted the need for specific training and preparation in crisis/hostage negotiations. In 1970 an El Al flight was hijacked, and in 1971 the Attica prison uprising resulted in the deaths of 39 people, including 11 correctional officers. During the 1972 Munich Olympics, 13 Arabs, demanding the release of 200 Arab prisoners, killed Israeli athletes who had been taken hostage. In response to this growing threat, in 1972, New York City Police Department Commissioner Simon Eisendorfer requested that Frank Bolz, a police lieutenant, and Dr. Harry Schlossberg, a police psychologist, develop a verbal alternative to the use of force in resolving hostage situations. The techniques developed by Bolz and Schlossberg have been credited with creating the discipline of hostage negotiation (Hatcher et al. 1998; Louden 1998). In 1973, building on the experience of the NYPD, the FBI began to promote the principles of negotiation by instructing police officers around the country on negotiation skills and practices (Noesner 1999).

Although the field of crisis negation has evolved since the 1970s, the goal of crisis/hostage negotiation remains to provide nonviolent resolution options. Verbal strategies are used to secure the safe release of the hostages/victims and when possible the arrest of the perpetrator without violence. In barricade situations, the aim is the safe release of the subject. In most cases the initial approach is focused on de-escalating and defusing an incident by lowering emotions and reducing the tensions at the scene. Newer strategies incorporate techniques derived from the field of conflict management and mediation (Fisher and Ury 1991). There has been an effort to develop an understanding of terrorist incidents and to develop strategies to effect resolution (Gilmartin 1996; Raven et al. 1999; Wilson 2000)

## Classification of Crisis Incidents

The FBI characterizes critical events as either hostage or nonhostage situations and suggests tailoring strategies to effect resolution based on this classification (Noesner 1999). During true hostage situations, perpetrators take hostages to force their demands on a third party, usually law enforcement. The FBI's national database of crisis incidents notes that these traditional hostage situations account for only 7% of crisis negotiation incidents (FBI Hostage Barricade Study 2001). The perpetrators use their hostages as leverage. They usually make overt or implied threats to harm the hostages unless demands are met. There are clearly recognizable objectives and substantive demands such as money, a means for escape, and political or social change. It is in the interest of the hostage takers to keep the hostages alive, or they risk losing their leverage. The hostage takers are aware that if their hostages are harmed, police may consider a tactical intervention (Noesner 1999; Noesner and Webster 1997; Price and Kelly 2002).

An example of a classic hostage incident would be when a bank robber is unable to escape because police have arrived on the scene earlier than expected. The robber finds himself trapped inside the bank. He holds employees and customers hostage because he is hoping to negotiate with police for a car and safe passage. The hostages have no special meaning to the bank robber other than as bargaining chips. There has been no previous relationship. Law enforcement strategies include using delay tactics, making subjects work for every concession, and using highly visible containment. This approach serves to lower the perpetrators' expectations and promotes discussion about the benefits of surrender in contrast to the risk of further confrontation. Noesner (1999) suggests that the negotiator offer "safe surrender with dignity." The strategy is based on the premise that the hostage taker's desire to survive is greater than the need to have his demands satisfied.

In contrast, subjects in a nonhostage situation generally act in an emotional, irrational, purposeless, and often self-destructive manner. If the subject is holding anyone, the person or persons being held are not being used as bargaining chips. They are really victims at risk of being harmed, possibly in a suicide or homicide scenario. The perpetrator makes no substantive demands or has completely unrealistic ones. Goals are emotionally driven. A barricade is another example of a nonhostage situation that requires crisis intervention, and this situation accounts for 59% of crisis incidents. The barricaded subject is often threatening suicide. In the nonhostage situation the barricaded subject or the subject who is holding someone against his or her will may be expressing anger, frustration, and feelings of being wronged by others or by events (Noesner 1999).

The case example of Mr. and Mrs. J is an example of a nonhostage situation; the rejected husband holds his wife against her will. Emotionality is driving the situation. A different strategy is used to resolve such situations, as perpetrators have what they want, the victim. Noesner (1999) suggests maintaining low-profile containment, using patience and understanding, and giving without requesting something in return. He also recommends using active listening skills to lower emotion, defuse anger, and create rapport. The FBI Hostage Barricade Study (HOBAS) data note that 92% of all law enforcement incidents are emotionally driven, with the subjects having no clear goal (FBI Hostage Barricade Study 2001).

A hostage or barricade incident can be resolved in one of five possible ways: a negotiated surrender, SWAT team tactical assault and apprehension of the perpetrator, perpetrator killed, perpetrator suicide, and perpetrator escaped (Hatcher et al. 1998). Fortunately, negotiation strategies are highly successful. According to the HOBAS data, 87% of incidents involving victims are resolved through the negotiation process (FBI Hostage Barricade Study 2001). In 90% of cases there is no loss of life; 64% of incidents are resolved in 4 hours or less; and 91%, in 9 hours or less. Certain risk factors in the perpetrator are associated with a higher risk that the incident will not be resolved by negotiation alone. These include multiple stressors, lack of family supports, forcing confrontation with police, notification of others of intent, similar incidents and threats to injure victim in the past, and verbalization of intent to commit suicide (Fuselier 1991).

## Role of Psychiatrists

The guidelines of the National Council of Negotiation Associations advise that negotiation teams consider establishing a consultative relationship with a mental health professional. The mental health professional should "serve as a team advisor and not as a negotiator, participate in negotiation team training, respond to team call outs as requested, focus on behavioral assessment of the subject and assist in team debriefing after a critical incident" (National Council of Negotiation Associations 2001, p. 3).

Traditionally, psychiatrists have been less commonly involved in crisis negotiation consultation than other mental health professionals. Psychiatric professional guidelines for this type of work are not available. Psychiatrists who become involved would do well to limit their roles to functions within their area of expertise, acquire appropriate training and mentoring, consult with colleagues around issues that arise, and be mindful of potential pitfalls. Psychiatrists should also consider liability issues that could surface from their work in this arena and protect themselves accordingly.

As indicated by the guidelines issued by the National Council of Negotiation Associations in 2001, crisis/hostage/barricade management is a very specialized area within law enforcement requiring additional focused training. If an incident is not managed in an optimal manner, death or serious injury can result (Vecchi 2002). Lacking the training of a police officer, the mental health professional functions best as a consultant to the team, with clear delineation of responsibilities and expectations.

Some departments, such as the Los Angeles Police Department, have a behavioral science service. One of the many functions of the service is to consult with the crisis negotiation team. Other agencies have consulting relationships with outside providers. Mental health consultants are usually recruited for the crisis negotiation team because of past involvement with providing more traditional services. Credibility is gained over time and may lead to an invitation to consult with the hostage/crisis negotiation team (Hatcher et al. 1998). Only a few police departments offer pre- or postdoctoral training in police psychology to mental health professionals.

National guidelines recommend the use of a mental health consultant. However, few studies document whether hostage negotiation teams derive any benefit from the use of mental health professionals as consultants. Butler et al. (1993) surveyed 300 law enforcement agencies in the United States that used a negotiator in hostage incidents. They found that 39% of the agencies with a negotiator employed a mental health professional as a consultant to the negotiation team and that these teams did demonstrate some benefit from this combined approach. Crisis/hostage negotiation teams with a mental health professional had more hostage incidents ending by negotiated surrender and fewer hostage incidents ending with the use of a tactical team assault and the arrest of the perpetrator. When mental health professionals were used as consultants for the assessment of the perpetrator, fewer hostage incidents resulted in serious injury or death of the hostage. The use of a mental health professional did not result in better outcome in barricade incidents.

Hatcher et al. (1998) estimated that from 30% to 58% of agencies with a crisis/hostage negotiation team use a mental health professional to provide on-scene or off-scene consultation. Hatcher et al. reported that 88% of these mental health professionals are psychologists as opposed to psychiatrists, social workers, or others. In hostage and barricade situations, non–law enforcement personnel have functioned in one of four roles: consultant/adviser, integrated team player, primary negotiator, or primary controller (Butler et al. 1993; Hatcher et al. 1998).

The most common role assumed by a mental health professional is that of consultant or advisor (Hatcher et al. 1998). Despite the complexity of the task, Butler et al. (1993) estimated that 40%–56% of consultant advisers function without training or field practice in actual negotiation. Off-scene, mental health providers may help in the selection of members of the negotiation or tactical team. They may provide training, especially in understanding the manifestations of mental illness and teaching application of therapeutic communication (Slatkin 1996). Mental health providers can consult on the development of instruments to screen, interview, and debrief witnesses and hostages. An important function is to foster a collaborative atmosphere among the on-scene commander, the tactical team, and the negotiation team during practice call outs and during incidents (Bahn and Louden 1999; Vecchi 2002).

Hatcher et al. (1998) noted that 40% of the agencies surveyed had used a psychologist as an on-scene advisor during incidents. The on-scene mental health professional may be asked to profile the suspect and hostages and provide a risk assessment (Trompetter and Honig 1999). The mental health professional may evaluate the perpetrators to determine their motivation, agenda, and vulnerabilities. The vulnerability of each hostage and the importance and value of the hostage(s) to the perpetrator may be assessed (Hatcher et al. 1998).

The field of profiling is quite complex. Any mental health professional embarking on this work should have the requisite training. Additionally, risk assessments in these situations would likely be limited. At times, officers on the scene are looking for information describing symptomatic behavior (e.g., a description that someone with mania could be irritable and/or would not likely need much sleep through the night), which is information a psychiatrist could certainly provide. However, when requests are made for input that goes beyond psychiatrists' professional expertise, they need to explain the limits of what they can offer.

Monitoring dialogue and suggesting strategies can be of benefit in negotiations, especially when there are impasses (Rogan and Hammer 1995; Taylor 2002a). The mental health professional can provide insight into the dynamics of the interaction and suggest modifications. Taylor (2002b) found that the likelihood of negotiation success was reduced when the dialogue was rated as competitive. Another important function for the mental health professional is to monitor the negotiation team's stress level.

Negotiation teams frequently rely on mental health professionals to interface with relevant mental health providers and family members to collect data about the subject or hostages. Mental health professionals may provide advice about the use of a third-party intermediary (Romano 1998). Mental health professionals may also play a role in debriefing hostages as they are released and in interviewing witnesses (Feldman 1998).

Mental health professionals have assumed roles other than that of consultant in the negotiation process, such as primary negotiator, integrated team member, and primary controller (the person directing the operation) (Hatcher et al. 1998). One study estimated that 7% of law enforcement agencies used psychologists in the role of the primary negotiator (Butler et al. 1993).

The authors strongly advise that psychiatrists act only as consultants because of ethical and procedural concerns (Feldman 1998, 1999; Price and Kelly 2002). By assuming any other role, psychiatrists would be accepting direct responsibility for the operation. The National Council of Negotiation Associations also recommends limiting the psychiatrist's role to that of consultant (National Council of Negotiation Associations 2001).

Many objections have been raised to psychiatrists acting as primary negotiators. For example, Hatcher et al. (1998) noted that hostage takers may resent any inference that they are mentally ill. In addition, psychiatrists and police officers have very different perspectives, experience, and training related to violence and aggression. If suspects insisted that they would only come out if the negotiator were present, this would create a dilemma for the police on scene. The police would not wish to place a psychiatrist without police training or experience in potential danger, and yet the failure to do so could negatively affect the outcome. Furthermore, a psychiatrist would not be able to advise the subject about the specific process for surrender, which would demand knowledge of police procedure and safety issues. A controller role requires the assessment of options, which may include a tactical approach, an area clearly outside the expertise of a mental health professional.

Ethical concerns for psychiatrists acting as primary negotiators also militate against psychiatrists taking on this role. Primary negotiators may be asked to distract a hostage taker while the tactical team enters, possibly leading to the death of the suspect in the interest of saving hostages. Participation leading to the death of the hostage taker would be at variance with ethical obligations of physicians.

Ethical issues arise in relation to informed consent requirements when psychiatrists act as primary negotiators. Dietz has questioned whether the psychiatrist as a primary negotiator would be acting as a forensic evaluator and would be required to obtain informed consent from the subject (Burns et al. 2001). Full disclosure could interfere with the negotiation process. However, psychiatrists could possibly be viewed as forming a doctor-patient relationship with the subject by initiating direct contact in the absence of informed consent (Burns et al. 2001).

In contrast, the police officer faces different obligations to the subject, as defined by case law (Burns et al. 2001). An officer is not required to provide a warning about the limits of confidentiality (Price and Kelly 2002). The police negotiator may not even be required to give a *Miranda* warning so that statements made to negotiators during the crisis will be admissible in court (Higginbotham 1994). *Miranda* only applies if the suspect is in custody. Generally, because the perpetrator is not within the complete control of the police during a hostage incident, the perpetrator is not in custody. Thus, *Miranda* does not apply. According to *People v. Gantz* (1984), the nonviolent resolution of a hostage/crisis situation is not an interrogation. The U.S. Supreme Court has ruled that the *Miranda* rule does not apply when questions are reasonably prompted by concerns for public safety, including questions relating to the safety of persons who have been abducted by the suspect.

The U.S. Supreme Court has also ruled that emergencies relating to life and safety excuse the normal warrant requirement (Higginbotham 1994). In *Mincey v. Arizona* (1978) the Court concluded, "The need to protect or preserve life or avoid serious injury is justifiable for what would be otherwise illegal" (*Mincey v. Arizona* 1978, p. 393). When the negotiator agrees to a subject's demands that seem to have serious legal implications, the government is not bound to enforce them (Higginbotham 1994).

When litigation arises out of such cases, a formal accounting of the level of training of negotiators involved in significant events is commonly requested (Becker 1995; Pruessner 2001). The mental health professional acting as a primary negotiator does not have the requisite background and training in law enforcement to perform all the functions of the position. Limiting one's role to that of a consultant and working within one's expertise exposes the mental health professional to fewer ethical dilemmas and decreases liability. Thus, although the literature suggests that the use of mental health professionals as consultants to a hostage team may decrease the risk of hostage injury and death, consultants need to carefully delineate their role in advance.

## Fitness for Duty Evaluations of Law Enforcement Officers

### Clinical Vignette

Officer L had been with the New City police department since the age of 22. She started as a dispatcher and advanced to the rank of patrol officer. Officer L had been sexually abused as a youth. In addition, she had been involved in a relationship with a man who was physically abusive. She had sought counseling after the termination of this relationship. She was treated briefly with medication for anxiety and depression. These symptoms resolved completely long before she was assigned to patrol duty.

As a patrol officer, Officer L had primarily been involved in minor community incidents, until one day when she was called to the scene of a homicide. She was the first to arrive on scene. While there, she heard family members shouting and yelling and witnessed a woman lying in a pool of blood on the floor. The woman had obviously been beaten and shot. She had bruises all over her body, and her clothes were torn and bloody.

Within a month of this incident, Officer L began to develop nightmares of the incident. She became tremulous and hypervigilant at work. She avoided the neighborhood where the homicide took place, despite the fact that it was her beat. She became irritable, snapping at her coworkers, whom she felt had not handled the homicide scene according to policy. She felt very strongly that she could continue her work. She wanted to keep working to provide a good role model for her 13-year-old daughter. Her supervisor insisted that she be placed on light duty but noted that even then her concentration was so poor that she could not focus on her work. The supervisor requested an independent medical examination regarding disability and causation.

Law enforcement is commonly viewed as one of the most dangerous, stressful, and health-threatening occupations. Officers are at risk for physical injury, homicide, and accidents, as well as psychological injury (Violanti et al. 1996). Officers face psychological harm as a result of exposure to death, human misery, inconsistencies in the criminal justice system, and negative public image (Violanti and Paton 2000).

The effects of stress on an officer's physical and emotional health are well documented. Problems include an increased risk of alcohol or drug abuse, ischemic heart disease, marital problems, excessively aggressive conduct, premature retirement, disability, and possibly an elevated suicide risk (Boxer et al. 1995; Davey et al. 2000; Forastiere et al. 1994; Hem et al. 2001; Neylan et al. 2002; Richmond et al. 1998; Tuchsen et al. 1996), although recent data have raised some questions about this latter factor (Marzuk 2002).

Police are repeatedly exposed to critical incidents. This exposure predisposes them to the development of acute stress disorder and posttraumatic stress disorder (Carlier et al. 1997; Kopel and Friedman 1997; Rivard et al. 2002; Sims and Sims 1998; Stephens and Miller 1998). Given the stressful nature of law enforcement, performance can become impaired because of any combination of personal, biological, and work-related factors. These can include exposure to trauma, ineffective coping strategies, difficulties in interpersonal relationships, marital conflict, and health concerns. Impairment of performance can place the officer and others at risk.

A law enforcement officer could become involved in many areas of workplace litigation because of this occupational exposure. This section is limited to fitness for duty evaluations for law enforcement officers. (For a general approach to workplace litigation, see Chapter 14: "The Workplace.")

Departments have an interest in promoting the mental well-being of their officers. Departments have been held to have a legal duty to monitor the psychological fitness of officers and take reasonable precautions to avoid hiring and retaining officers who are psychologically disturbed (*Bonsignore v. City of New York* 1982). The courts have also held that administrators have the right to monitor the psychological health of officers by ordering fitness for duty evaluations (McNaught and Schofield 1998).

In *Conte v. Harcher* (1977), a police officer faced allegations of having used excessive force when taking a suspect into custody. The officer refused to undergo a fitness for duty exam as requested by the chief. The U.S. Supreme Court held that the chief had the authority to order the exam based on the need to protect the public interest and the efficiency of the department and to keep informed about officers' ability to perform their duties. In *Yin v. State of California* (1997), the U.S. Court of Appeals for the Ninth Circuit upheld the department's prerogative to order a fitness for duty evaluation as constitutional and not in violation of the Americans with Disabilities Act (ADA). The examination could be compelled to ensure the public safety and guarantee a stable, reliable, and productive workforce.

Law enforcement agencies often have policies that guide referral for fitness for duty evaluations. The model policy suggested by the California Peace Officers Association in 2001 provides for assessment of officers' ability to perform the essential function of their positions. Such assessments may be ordered when an officer's conduct, behavior, or circumstances indicate to a reasonable person that continued service by the employee may be problematic in certain ways. These include presenting a threat to public safety, the safety of other employees, and the safety of the particular employee and potentially interfering with the agency's ability to deliver effective police services (Hyams 2001).

Even when indicators of possible impairment are present, the supervisor always has discretion in ordering a fitness for duty evaluation. Most law enforcement agencies recognize the need for programs to deal with the stress inherent in police work. The fitness for duty evaluation should not serve as a replacement for a comprehensive policy for providing mental health interventions for at-risk officers and a venue for confidential referral. The supervisor may well suggest that the officer seek treatment on a voluntary basis rather that proceeding with a formal fitness for duty evaluation.

Many departments use an external Employee Assistance Program (EAP), an in-house treatment program or contract with outside providers to provide a variety of mental health services. These programs usually allow for self-referral and referral by peer counselors (Finn and Esselman-Tomz 1998). They provide for voluntary referral of an officer by a supervisor or an agency chief executive if there is suspicion of psychological problems contributing to poor or erratic work performance.

Some departments have special provisions for officers exposed to a critical incident including a requirement to see a mental health professional. A critical incident is any event that has a stressful impact that proves sufficient to overwhelm the usually effective coping skills of an individual (Kureczka 1996). Critical incidents may include line-of-duty shootings; death, suicide, or serious injury of coworkers; homicides; and hostage situations (McNally and Solomon 1999).

Exposure to critical incidents can lead to a variety of potentially career-threatening reactions, including overreaction to perceived threats, or alternatively, underreaction to clearly dangerous situations. Officers exposed to critical incidents sometimes resign or retire prematurely. Additionally, they may have disciplinary problems or develop burnout, stress-related illnesses, posttraumatic stress disorder, or substance abuse (Decker 2002). According to one report, in the 1970s about 70% of officers who used fatal force left law enforcement within 5 years (McNally and Solomon 1999).

In the case vignette above, Ms. L, a patrol officer, had primarily been involved in minor community incidents before being called to the scene of a homicide. Many departments would have referred Officer L to their critical incident stress management program (Carlier et al. 1997). The FBI's Critical Incident Stress Management Program includes interventions such as defusing and debriefing, peer support, family outreach, manager support, referral for therapy, and post–critical incident seminars (McNally and Solomon 1999).

When intervention fails and the officer's functioning has deteriorated, the supervisor will meet with the officer. The discussion alone may result in some remediation, or the encounter may result in an agreement for voluntary assessment and treatment. In the case of Officer L, the supervisor arranged for light duty and presumably suggested referral for treatment. When these steps are unsuccessful, a fitness for duty evaluation may be requested. However, if an officer leaves on disability, the supervisor could request a fitness for duty evaluation on return if indications of ongoing difficulty are present. On occasion, the seriousness of the situation may dictate an urgent response (International Association of Chiefs of Police 1993).

A fitness for duty evaluation involving a law enforcement officer requires familiarity with the functions of the officer (Finn and Esselman-Tomz 1996) and the nature of police work. Evaluators should also be familiar with conducting independent assessments related to work functioning. The evaluator should request that the department supply information regarding the police work done by the officer and written documentation of the behavior and concerns. The Police Psychological Services Section of the International Association of Chiefs of Police recommends that the department provide information about attempts at remediation. This could include additional training, supervision, discipline, mentoring, reassignment, or referral to EAP for treatment. Collateral data may help distinguish whether the problem is indicative of a long-standing pattern of disruptive behavior or represents a recent change, perhaps in response to a specific stressor as was present in the case example (International Association of Chiefs of Police 1993). Consideration of current relationships with coworkers is important, especially given the need to work closely with colleagues and the tight social network among police.

The examiner should perform a detailed psychiatric interview. A fitness for duty examination should identify whether the officer is experiencing a psychiatric disorder that is affecting ability to function. The contribution of substance abuse needs to be explored. The examiner should note the level of impairment and offer an opinion about prognosis and the likely response to treatment. The evaluator should assess the officer's amenability to treatment intervention. The evaluating psychiatrist should consider both the effects of the underlying condition and the potential side effects of treatment on the safe use of firearms. The effects on judgment, reaction time, memory, and fine motor skills should be carefully assessed. The clinical interview may need to be supplemented by psychological or neuropsychological testing (Decker 2002).

The standards for fitness for duty of officers should be higher than the minimum level of functioning for non–law enforcement individuals because police officers must be able to carry firearms and make on-the-spot life-and-death decisions (Decker 2002). The police officer's conduct and mental state may be called into question in court. Officers may need to justify accusations of being either trigger-happy or too scared to carry out their duty. The report will need to address whether there are contraindications to the officer continuing to carry a weapon (Decker 2002).

The risk of suicide and homicide needs to be carefully assessed, given the ready access to a firearm. Although there is controversy over whether officers have a higher risk of suicide than the general population (Hem et al. 2001; Marzuk 2002), the study by Janik and Kravitz (1994) illustrates the importance of inquiring about suicidal ideation. They reviewed the records of 134 police officers at the time of their first fitness for duty evaluation. Surprisingly, 55% of officers admitted to previous suicide attempts. High-risk groups were identified. Officers reporting marital problems were 4.8 times more likely to have attempted suicide. Officers who had been suspended were 6.7 times more likely to have attempted suicide than those who had not been suspended.

Under high-risk circumstances, there would be a need for weapon removal and referral for emergency psychiatric assessment. Mohandie and Hatcher (1999) recommend that in weapon-removal situations there should be a 30- to 60-day period during which the officer is precluded from carrying a weapon. The premise is to allow time to ensure that the precipitating factors have been successfully managed.

Depending on departmental policy, the report provided to the department will become part of the confidential personnel record, although there is no real guarantee that it will remain confidential. Even if it remains in that file, the evaluator does not know who in the department (and beyond) may have access to it. Thus, the report should contain only the information necessary to document the presence or absence of job-related personality traits, characteristics, disorders, propensities, and conditions that would interfere with the performance of essential job functions. The amount of feedback given to supervisors should be limited to issues related to referral questions (International Association of Chiefs of Police 1993). The evaluator should be aware of the agency policy about the report contents (Hyams 2001).

The officer could be returned without limitation or with optional time-limited accommodations. The officer could be found temporarily fit for duty pending a proposed intervention or unfit with little likelihood of remediation. Departments are not required to create light duty positions as a form of reasonable accommodation, and the development of a light duty policy is a function of managerial discretion. However, most departments consider light duty preferable to having the officer out on sick leave, receiving benefits (McNaught and Schofield 1998).

Exceptions to the limited disclosure of the report do exist. Further information derived from the evaluation could be discovered if the officer has a pending lawsuit, arbitration, grievance, or workers' compensation claim or challenge. While many officers are eager to address problems in a fitness for duty evaluation and return to work, others may be litigious or in search of secondary gain through the fitness for duty situation (Decker 2002).

The primary functions of the evaluator are to provide a comprehensive evaluation, diagnosis, and opinion on fitness. The evaluator will make recommendations related to the officer's need for further treatment and monitoring, if appropriate. By the evaluator's noting in the opinion that specific treatment is warranted, the appropriate representatives or supervisors will be able to initiate a plan, such as referral for treatment, that makes sense for the officer. A timely referral to an appropriate source can keep an otherwise volatile situation from escalating. The evaluating psychiatrist who frequently consults to a police department may wish to consider offering, on an informal or formal level, guidance aimed at decreasing the overall level of organizational stress and at ensuring the adequacy of the mental health program offered for officers.

## Conclusion

The intersection of mental health and law enforcement is a growing area of interest for many psychiatrists. Mental health training for police, crisis negotiation, reviews of officer-assisted suicides, and police fitness for duty are aspects of the work that is often undertaken in this arena, and there is an expanding literature exploring those areas. A psychiatrist taking on this work, however, should have a sound understanding of the unique issues at play. Psychiatrists are often seen by others as having easy and ready solutions to some of the complex challenges that arise in police work, such as suicide and violence risk prediction and assessment of officers and citizens, based on little information. It can be useful to remind police of the importance of each profession working within its role, and to tolerate the unpredictable nature of some of the issues that surface. Psychiatrists who work with law enforcement should work within their expertise and training and recognize the potential risks, limitations, and benefits involved.

## Key Points

### Mental Health Training

- Community models of systematized responses to mental health crises include 1) police-based specialized mental health response, 2) mental health–based, specialized mental health response, and 3) police-based specialized police response.
- Mental health training aimed toward reducing stigma and improving communication skills is an important addition to other types of police education and can improve overall knowledge.
- Officers frequently rely on their own discretion in making dispositional decisions, so that education related to mental illness may enhance their understanding of appropriate and available options.

### Suicide by Cop

- *Suicide by cop* refers to an incident in which suicidal individuals intentionally engage in life-threatening and dangerous behavior specifically to provoke officers to kill them.
- Suicide by cop may be planned in advance or may develop in the course of a police-citizen encounter.
- Suicide by cop may be driven by a desire to accomplish certain goals through being killed and create an opportunity for self-expression.

### Crisis Negotiation

- The goal of crisis/hostage negotiation remains to provide nonviolent resolution options.
- Incidents are classified as hostage or nonhostage situations.
- The recommended role of the mental health professional is that of a consultant to the negotiation team.

### Fitness for Duty Evaluations: Law Enforcement Officers

- The evaluator should consider the suitability of officers for continued work in their normal capacity.
- If the person is not fit for duty, then the evaluator should comment on the likelihood of successful return following treatment.
- The need to carry a weapon should be an important factor in the assessment of fitness for duty.

## Practice Guidelines

### Mental Health Training for Police Officers

1. When collaborating with police, attempt a focus that provides opportunities for cross-training.
2. Develop education around priority topics that can be accomplished in allotted time.
3. Recognize and work within your limits as a psychiatrist in providing advice to officers.

### Suicide by Cop

1. When reviewing encounters with police that involve victim provocation, assess intent and planning for suicide by cop.
2. Attempt to gather information about premorbid functioning of the suicidal person in retrospective reviews of suicide by cop and attempted suicide by cop.
3. In evaluating individuals who have engaged in suicide by cop behavior, explore reasons for attempting this means of suicide.

### Crisis Negotiation

1. Be clear about the limits of your role as consultant.
2. Obtain the necessary training before acting as a consultant to the negotiation team.
3. Be clear as to the limits of your opinion and expertise.

### Fitness for Duty Evaluations: Law Enforcement Officers

1. Be aware of the legal standards in the community and departmental procedures when performing fitness for duty evaluations.
2. Consider the unique job requirements of law enforcement officers and issues related to firearm access.

## References

Appelbaum KL: Police encounters with persons with mental illness: introduction. J Am Acad Psychiatry Law 28:325, 2000

Bahn C, Louden RJ: Hostage negotiation as a team enterprise. Group 23:77–85, 1999

Becker JB: The first amendment goes tactical: news media negligence and ongoing criminal incidents. Loyola of Los Angeles Entertainment Law Journal 15:625–629, 1995

Belcher JR: Are jails replacing the mental health system for the homeless mentally ill? Community Ment Health J 24:185–195, 1988

Bonsignore v City of New York, 683 F.2d 635, 2d Cir. 1982

Boxer PA, Burnett C, Swanson N: Suicide and occupation: a review of the literature. J Occup Environ Med 37:442–452, 1995

Borum R: Improving high risk encounters between people with mental illness and police. J Am Acad Psychiatry Law 28:332–337, 2000

Borum R, Deane MW, Steadman HJ, et al: Police perspectives on responding to mentally ill people in crisis: perceptions of program effectiveness. Behav Sci Law 16:393–405, 1998

Bresler S, Scalora MJ, Elbogen EB, et al: Attempted suicide by cop: a case study of traumatic brain injury and the insanity defense. J Forensic Sci 48:190–194, 2003

Burns B, Phillips R, McGee J, et al: The role of mental health professionals in hostage negotiation. Panel presented at 32nd annual meeting of the American Academy of Psychiatry and the Law, Boston, MA, October 2001

Butler WM, Leitenber GH, Fuselier GD: The use of mental health professional consultants to police hostage negotiation teams. Behav Sci Law 11:213–21, 1993

Carlier IV, Lamberts RD, Gersons BP: Risk factors for posttraumatic stress symptomology in police officers: a prospective analysis. J Nerv Ment Dis 195:498–506, 1997

Conte v Harcher, 365 N.E.2d 567, Ill,. App. (1977)

Davey JD, Obst PL, Sheehan MC: Work demographics and officers' perception of the work environment, which add to the prediction of at risk alcohol consumption within an Australian police sample. Policing: An International Journal of Police Strategies and Management 23:69–81, 2000

Deane MW, Steadman HJ, Borum R, et al: Emerging partnerships between mental health and law enforcement. Psychiatr Serv 50:99–101, 1999

Decker KP: Fitness for duty evaluation in law enforcement personnel: theory and practice. Presentation at the 33rd annual meeting of the American Academy of Psychiatry and the Law, Newport Beach, CA, October 2002

Dupont R, Cochran S: Police response to mental health emergencies-barriers to change. J Am Acad Psychiatry Law 28:338–344, 2000

FBI Hostage Barricade Study (HOBAS) (database). Quantico, VA, Crisis Negotiation Unit, FBI Academy, 2001

Feldman TB: Psychiatric consultation to police hostage negotiation teams. American Journal of Forensic Psychiatry 19:27–44, 1998

Feldman TB: Dealing with large scale hostage and barricade incidents: Implications for negotiation and training, in Collective Violence: Effective Strategies for Assessing and Interviewing in Fatal Group and Institutional Aggression. Edited by Hall HV, Whitaker LC. Boca Raton, FL, CRC Press, 1999, pp 335–337

Finn P, Esselman-Tomz J: Developing a law enforcement stress program for officers and their families, in Issues and Practices in Criminal Justice (NCJ 163175). U.S. Dept of Justice, National Institute of Justice, 1996, pp 21–89

Finn P, Esselman-Tomz J: Using peer supporters to help address law enforcement stress. FBI Law Enforcement Bulletin 67(5):10–18, 1998

Fisher R, Ury W: Getting to Yes. New York, Penguin, 1991, pp 1–172

Forastiere F, Perucci CA, Di Pietro A, et al: Morality among urban policemen in Rome. Am J Ind Med 26:785–798, 1994

Fuselier D, Van Zandt C, Lanceley F: Hostage barricade incidents: high risk factor and the action criteria. FBI Law Enforcement Bulletin 60(1):6–12, 1991

Fyfe JJ: Policing the emotionally disturbed. J Am Acad Psychiatry Law 28:345–347, 2000

Gillig PM, Dumaine M, Stammer JW, et al: What do police officers really want from the mental health system? Hosp Community Psychiatry 41:663–665, 1990

Gilmartin KM: The lethal triad: understanding the nature of isolated extremist groups. FBI Law Enforcement Bulletin 65(9):1–5, 1996

Godschalx SM: Effect of a mental health educational program upon police officers. Res Nurs Health 7(2):111–117, 1984

Graham v Connor et al, 490 U.S. 386 (1989)

Green TM: Police as frontline mental health workers: the decision to arrest or refer to mental health agencies. Int J Law Psychiatry 20:469–486, 1997

Hatcher C, Mohandie K, Turner J, et al: The role of the psychologist in crisis/hostage negotiations. Behav Sci Law 16:455–472, 1998

Hawton K, Appleby L, Platt S, et al: The psychological autopsy approach to studying suicide: a review of methodological issues. J Affect Disord 50:269–276, 1998

Hem E, Berg AM, Ekberg O: Suicide in police—a critical review. Suicide Life Threat Behav 31:224–233, 2001

Higginbotham J: Legal issues in crisis management. FBI Law Enforcement Bulletin 60(6):27–35, 1994

Homant RJ, Kennedy DB: Suicide by police: a proposed typology of law enforcement officer-assisted suicide. Policing: An International Journal of Police Strategies and Management 23:339–355, 2000

Husted JR, Charter RA, Perrou B: California law enforcement agencies and the mentally ill offender. Bull Am Acad Psychiatry Law 23:315–329, 1995

Hutson HR, Anglin D, Yarbrough J: Suicide by cop. Ann Emerg Med 32:665–669, 1998

Hyams M: Fitness for Duty Evaluations: A Sample Policy. Sacramento, California Peace Officers' Association, 2001. Available at: http://www.cpoa.org/Publication/Sample%20Policies/fit_for_duty.shtml. Accessed November 16, 2003.

International Association of Chiefs of Police, Police Psychological Services Section: Psychological guidelines for issues in law enforcement. Alexandria, VA, International Association of Chiefs of Police, adopted 1993. Available at: http://www.theiacp.org/div_sec_com/sections/Psych.htm. Accessed November 16, 2003.

Janik J, Kravitz HM: Linking work and domestic problems with police suicide. Suicide Life Threat Behav 24:267–274, 1994

Kennedy DB, Homant RJ, Hupp RT: Suicide by cop. FBI Law Enforcement Bulletin 67(8):21–27, 1998

Kopel H, Friedman M: Posttraumatic symptoms in South African police exposed to violence. J Trauma Stress 10:307–317, 1997

Kureczka AW: Critical incident stress in law enforcement. FBI Law Enforcement Bulletin 65(3):1–10, 1996

Lamb HR, Lamb DM: Factors contributing to homelessness among the chronically and severely mentally ill. Hosp Community Psychiatry 41:301–305, 1990

Lamb HR, Weinberger LE, DeCuir WJ: The police and mental health. Psychiatr Serv 53:1266–1271, 2002

Liberman R: Police as a community mental health resource. Community Ment Health J 5:111–120, 1969

Louden RJ: The development of hostage negotiation by the NYPD, in Crime and Justice. Edited by Karmen A. New York, McGraw-Hill, 1998, pp 245–250

Marzuk PM, Nock MK, Leon AC, et al: Suicide among New York City police officers, 1977–1996. Am J Psychiatry 159:2069–2071, 2002

McNally VJ, Solomon RM: The FBI's critical incident stress management program. FBI Law Enforcement Bulletin 68(2):20–26, 1999

McNaught MC, Schofield S: Managing sick and injured employees. FBI Law Enforcement Bulletin 67(1):26–31, 1998

Mincey v Arizona, 437 U.S. 393, 1978

Mohandie K, Hatcher C: Suicide and violence risk in law enforcement: practical guidelines for risk assessment, prevention and intervention. Behav Sci Law 17:357–376, 1999

Mohandie K, Meloy JR: Clinical and forensic indicators of "suicide by cop." Journal of Forensic Sciences 45:384–389, 2000

National Council of Negotiation Associations: Recommended negotiation guidelines and principles. Quantico, VA, National Council of Negotiation Associations, adopted October 4, 2001. Available at: http://www.tahn.org/ncna%20guidelines.html. Accessed November 16, 2003.

Neylan TC, Metzler TJ, Best SR, et al: Critical incident exposure and sleep quality in police officers. Psychosom Med 64:345–352, 2002

Noesner G: Negotiation concepts for commanders. FBI Law Enforcement Bulletin 68(1):1–10, 1999

Noesner G, Webster M: Crisis intervention: using active listening skills in negotiation. FBI Law Enforcement Bulletin 66(8):1–7, 1997

Palmquist v Selvik and the Village of Bensenville, 111 F.3d 1332 (1997)

People v Ganz, 480 N.Y.S.2d 583 (N.Y. Sup. Ct. 1984)

Price M, Kelly B: Crisis/hostage negotiation. Newsl Am Acad Psychiatry Law 27(1):15–17, 2002

Pruessner D: The forgotten foundation of state-created danger claims. Rev Litig 20:357–376, 2001

Raven K, Goree W, Miller C: Hostage negotiations after the first shots are fired. The Tactical Edge, Fall 1999, pp 22–29

Richmond RL, Wodak A, Kehoe L, et al: How healthy are police? A survey of lifestyle factors. Addiction 93:1729–1737, 1998

Rivard JM, Dietz P, Martell D, et al: Acute dissociative responses in law enforcement officers involved in critical shooting incidents: the clinical and forensic implications. Journal of Forensic Sciences 47:1093–1100, 2002

Rogan RG, Hammer MR: Assessing message affect in crisis negotiations: an exploratory study. Human Communication Research 21:553–574, 1995

Romano SJ: Third party intermediaries in crisis negotiation. FBI Law Enforcement Bulletin 67(10):20–25, 1998

Sims A, Sims D: The phenomenology of posttraumatic stress disorder: a symptomatic study of 70 victims of psychological trauma. Psychopathology 31:96–112, 1998

Slatkin A: Enhancing negotiator training: therapeutic communication. FBI Law Enforcement Bulletin 65(5):1–8, 1996

State v Sands, 700 P.2d 1369 (Ariz. App. 1985)

Stephens C, Miller I: Traumatic experiences and posttraumatic stress disorder in the New Zealand police. Policing: An International Journal of Police Strategies and Management 21:178–191, 1998

Stincelli R: Suicide by cop. Available at http://www.suicidebycop.com/page2.html. Accessed March 23, 2003.

Taylor PJ: A cylindrical model of communication behavior in crisis negotiation. Human Communication Research 28:7–48, 2002

Taylor PJ: A partial order scalogram analysis of communication behavior in crisis negotiation with prediction of outcome. International Journal of Conflict Management 13:4–37, 2002

Teplin LA, Pruett NS: Police as streetcorner psychiatrist: managing the mentally ill. Int J Law Psychiatry 15:139–156, 1992

Trompetter PS, Honig AL: Risk assessment in barricade/hostage incidents. The Tactical Edge, Summer 1999, pp 30–38

Tuchsen F, Anderson O, Costa G, et al: Occupational and ischemic heart disease in the European community: a comparative study of occupations at high risk. Am J Ind Med 30:407–414, 1996

Vecchi GM: Hostage/barricade management. FBI Law Enforcement Bulletin 71(5):1–14, 2002

Violanti J, Paton D: Police trauma: Psychological aftermath of civilian combat. Policing: An International Journal of Police Strategies and Management 23:268–272, 2000

Violanti JM, Vena JE, Marshall JR, et al: Suicides, homicides and accidental deaths: a comparative risk assessment of police officer and municipal workers. Am J Ind Med 30:99–104, 1996

Wilson EF, Davis JH, Bloom JD, et al: Homicide or suicide: the killing of suicidal persons by law enforcement officers. Journal of Forensic Sciences 43:46–52, 1998

Wilson MA: Toward a model of terrorist behavior in hostage-taking incidents. Journal of Conflict Resolution 44:403–425, 2000

Wolfgang ME: Victim-precipitated criminal homicide. Journal of Criminal Law and Criminology 48:1–11, 1957

Wolfgang ME: Suicide by means of victim-precipitated homicide. J Clin Exp Psychopathol 20:335–349, 1959

Yin v State of California, 95 F.3d 864 9th Cir., 1996, cert. denied, 117 S. Ct. 955, 1997

## Suggested Readings

Borum R: Improving high risk encounters between people with mental illness and police. J Am Acad Psychiatry Law 28:332–337, 2000

Butler WM, Leitenber GH, Fuselier GD: The use of mental health professional consultants to police hostage negotiation teams. Behav Sci Law 11:213–221, 1993

Feldman TB: Psychiatric consultation to police hostage negotiation teams. American Journal of Forensic Psychiatry 19:27–44, 1998

Hatcher C, Mohandie K, Turner J, et al: The role of the psychologist in crisis/hostage negotiations. Behav Sci Law 16:455–472, 1998

Lamb HR, Weinberger LE, DeCuir WJ: The police and mental health. Psychiatr Serv 53:1266–1271, 2002

Mohandie K, Meloy JR: Clinical and forensic indicators of "suicide by cop." Journal of Forensic Sciences 45:384–389, 2000

Rivard JM, Dietz P, Martell D, et al: Acute dissociative responses in law enforcement officers involved in critical shooting incidents: the clinical and forensic implications. Journal of Forensic Sciences 47: 1093–1100, 2002

# PART IV

# Special Topics

CHAPTER 19

# Malingering

John W. Thompson Jr., M.D.

H.W. LeBourgeois III, M.D.

F. William Black, Ph.D.

## Introduction

The assessment of malingering presents a significant challenge to clinicians working in mental health settings. This challenge arises from the fact that the diagnosis of psychiatric disorders is based largely on self-reported, subjective symptoms that may be learned and feigned. The traditional clinician-patient relationship, which is based largely on trust and accurate self-report of symptoms, further complicates such assessments. Malingering represents the opposite of trust and accurate self-report: it involves deception. Accordingly, when confronted with a suspected case of malingering, clinicians, by training and experience, are biased toward believing an evaluee's report of presenting symptoms. Nevertheless, clinicians should be prepared to consider the possibility of malingering, particularly in forensic settings. They should also be prepared to engage in the detective work needed to make this diagnosis.

This chapter reviews basic knowledge of malingering, provides examples of individuals engaged in malingering, and reviews methods that have received scientific support in assessment of the condition. The difficulties clinicians face when interacting with malingering evaluees and guidelines for assessment are also discussed.

## Malingering Overview

### Historical Background

Malingering is reported to have existed since biblical times. David, fearful of a king's wrath, "feigned himself mad" (Samuel 21:1). Malingering has also appeared in mythological tales. In Homer's *Odyssey,* Ulysses feigns mental illness to avoid combat in the Trojan War (Palermo et al. 1996).

In the nineteenth century, the term *malingering* found its way into the English medical literature with Gavin's book *On Feigned and Factitious Diseases Chiefly of Soldiers and Seamen* (1843). In the late nineteenth century and early twentieth century, industrial expansion paired with the introduction of workmen's compensation led to increased concerns about the socioeconomic implications of malingering (Turner 1997). Pejorative terms such as "compensation neurosis" and "profit neurosis" began to appear to describe suspected malingered claims of mental injury following traumatic accidents (Resnick 1997b, pp. 130–131).

Today, malingering is a condition that garners attention in the medical literature as well as the lay press. Popular movies using forensic topics and psychiatric consultants portray malingerers as sly and cunning psychopaths. The film *Primal Fear* (1996), in which Edward Norton's character feigns multiple personality disorder after being arrested for murder, is an example of such a portrayal.

### Definitions and Subtypes

*Diagnostic and Statistical Manual of Mental Disorders,* 4th Edition (American Psychiatric Association 1994), and its text revision, DSM-IV-TR (American Psychiatric Association 2000, p. 739), define malingering as "the intentional production of false or grossly exaggerated physical or psychological symptoms, motivated by external incentives such as avoiding military duty, avoiding work, obtaining financial compensation, evading criminal prosecution, or obtaining drugs." DSM-IV-TR also notes that malingering is a condition not attributable to a mental disorder (p. 731).

Resnick (1997b) identified three subcategories of malingering: 1) pure malingering, 2) partial malingering, and 3) false imputation. *Pure malingering* exists when an evaluee feigns a disorder that does not exist at all. In contrast, *partial malingering* occurs when an evaluee consciously exaggerates existing symptoms. *False imputation* occurs when an evaluee intentionally attributes symptoms to an etiology that has no relationship to the development of symptoms. Such an example would be an individual treated for multiple injuries to the lower back who seeks compensation from his employer, claiming that all symptoms of back pain began after a work accident.

Clinicians should bear in mind the distinction between pure malingering, partial malingering, and false imputation during assessment and evaluation, and the settings in which each form is most commonly encountered. Pure malingering may be seen more often in criminal forensic contexts. Partial malingering and false imputation may be encountered more often in civil forensic evaluations and clinical settings.

## Base Rates

Base rates of malingering depend on the evaluation setting. A sample of 320 experienced forensic psychologists yielded estimates for malingering of 15.7% in the forensic setting and 7.4% in the nonforensic setting (Rogers et al. 1994). Rogers (1986) found that 20.8% of criminal defendants undergoing insanity evaluations engaged in definite or suspected malingering. The base rate of malingering and/or inadequate effort has been extensively studied in the civil personal injury venue, especially with respect to individuals alleging mild traumatic brain injury. A base rate ranging from approximately 8% to 33% is generally accepted in the personal injury context (Iverson and Binder 2000; Sweet 1999).

Forensic settings generally harbor higher base rates of malingering; however, estimates of malingering in particular clinical settings approach those in the forensic setting. From their analysis of Minnesota Multiphasic Personality Inventory–2 (MMPI-2) validity scales, Gold et al. (1997) estimated a 20%–30% base rate of malingering among veterans seeking compensation for PTSD. Yates et al. (1996) found that resident psychiatrists working in an urban emergency room strongly suspected or definitely diagnosed malingering in 13% of patients evaluated. A relatively high rate of malingering of 10%–12% was found among patients who were hospitalized for suicidal ideation (Rissmiller et al. 1999).

An examination of the cost of health insurance fraud in the United States reveals that malingering is not uncommon. The Coalition Against Insurance Fraud (1997), a U.S. association of consumers, government agencies, and insurers that addresses the issue of insurance fraud, estimated the total cost of health insurance fraud in 1995 at $59 billion, resulting in a cost of $1,050 in added premiums for the average American family.

## Malingered Conditions

Mental health clinicians should bear in mind the malingered conditions that they may encounter in forensic and nonforensic settings. Literature reviews demonstrate that malingered conditions include dissociative identity disorder (Labott and Wallach 2002), psychosis (Greenfield 1987), suicidality (Rissmiller et al. 1999), and posttraumatic stress disorder (PTSD) (Frueh et al. 1997). Malingered conditions that cross the spectrum of both psychiatry and neurology that have been reported include acute dystonia (Rubinstein 1978), amnesia (Bolan et al. 2002), cognitive deficits (Iverson and Binder 2000; Sweet 1999), dementia (Gittelman 1998), seizure (DeToledo 2001), and sleep disorder (Mahowald et al. 1992).

Of the above conditions, forensic mental health clinicians are most likely to encounter malingered psychosis, malingered PTSD, and malingered amnesia/cognitive deficits (see section "Clinical Vignettes" later in this chapter, where each of these malingered conditions is discussed).

## Psychiatric Disorders That May Be Mistaken for Malingering

Factitious disorders and somatoform disorders share common elements with malingering (Cunnien 1997; Eisendrath 1996). Thus, clinicians should be familiar with these conditions when examining suspected cases of malingering. Both malingering and factitious disorders involve the "intentional production of physical or psychological symptoms" (American Psychiatric Association 2000, p. 513). However, the motivation for behavior associated with factitious disorders is an unconscious desire to assume the sick role. It is presumed that individuals with factitious disorders pursue a sick role to obtain the psychological gains associated with conditions of true illness. Munchausen syndrome is the best-known example of a factitious disorder. Like patients with other factitious disorders, patients with Munchausen syndrome may inflict serious medical problems on themselves, travel widely to health care venues, and have a history of unceasing patienthood (Eisendrath 1996).

Factitious disorders may have primarily physical or psychological manifestations or a combination of both. Individuals with factitious disorders have been reported to induce illness in persons under their care in order to assume the sick role by proxy. This disorder is known as factitious disorder by proxy (also referred to as Munchausen syndrome by proxy). Usually, cases of factitious disorder by proxy involve a mother and her preschool child presenting in pediatric settings (American Psychiatric Association 2000, pp. 781–783).

**TABLE 19–1.** Symptom production and motivation in malingering, factitious disorders, and somatoform disorders

| | Symptom production | Motivation |
|---|---|---|
| Malingering | Conscious | Conscious |
| Factitious disorders | Conscious | Unconscious |
| Somatoform disorders | Unconscious | Unconscious |

Individuals with somatoform disorders present with a distinct history as well as physical symptoms suggesting a general medical condition; however, comprehensive medical workups in search of organic illness yield negative results. In contrast to malingering and factitious disorders, individuals with somatoform disorders have no conscious intention to deceive clinicians. Their physical symptoms are manifested unconsciously.

The somatoform disorders include hypochondriasis, pain disorder, body dysmorphic disorder, and conversion disorder. Conversion disorder is the somatoform disorder most likely to be mistaken for malingering. In this disorder, individuals present with pseudoneurological deficits of voluntary motor or sensory function that typically fail to follow known anatomical pathways. Other conversion symptoms include aphonia, urinary retention, blindness, deafness, hallucinations, and seizures. The somatoform disorders should be diagnosed provisionally, as a medical illness that can explain the symptoms may surface later (American Psychiatric Association 2000).

The distinction between factitious disorders, somatoform disorders, and malingering is not always clear-cut (Table 19–1). Eisendrath (1996) provides a detailed comparison between factitious disorders and malingering. The simplified flowchart in Figure 19–1 may be helpful to clinicians when they are attempting to make this distinction.

## Models of Malingering Behavior

Rogers and colleagues (Rogers 1990; Rogers et al. 1994) have outlined the primary motivations implicit in three explanatory models of malingering: 1) pathogenic, 2) criminological, and 3) adaptational. The *pathogenic model* proposes that malingering is prompted by an underlying mental disorder that eventually surfaces as the illness progresses (Rogers 1997). This model has lost support over the last several decades.

The *criminological model* focuses on multiple aspects of an individual's bad character and bad behavior, "namely, a bad person (APD [antisocial personality disorder]), in bad circumstances (legal difficulties),

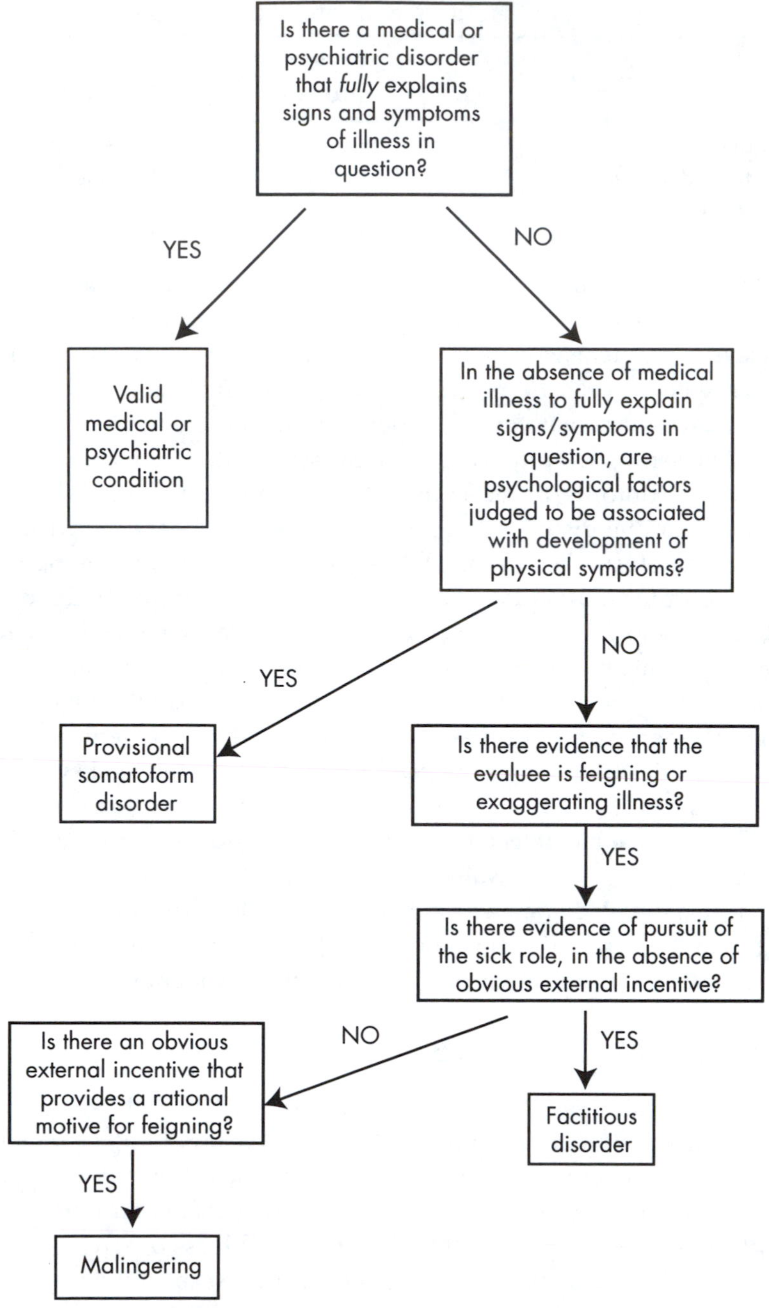


**FIGURE 19–1.** Differentiation between malingering, factitious disorders, somatoform disorders, and valid medical/psychiatric conditions.

who is performing badly (uncooperative)" (Rogers 1997, p. 7). Studies have specifically examined the relationship between psychopathy and malingering. Sierles (1984) found greater measures of psychopathy in malingering veterans as compared with medical student controls. Another study (Gacono et al. 1995) compared hospitalized insanity acquitees who had successfully malingered mental illness to insanity acquitees who were deemed to be truly insane. This study found a significantly higher number of APD diagnoses among malingerers. A study of 143 college students investigated the relationship between psychopathic personality traits and malingering, using the Psychopathic Personality Inventory (PPI). The study authors proposed that "psychopathy is somewhat predictive of a willingness to feign mental illness across various forensic/correctional settings" (Edens et al. 2000, p. 290).

The *adaptational model*, delineated by Rogers (1997), proposes that malingerers engage in a "cost-benefit analysis" (p. 8) during clinician assessment. As Rogers (1997) noted, "Malingering is more likely to occur when 1) the context of the evaluation is perceived as adversarial, 2) the personal stakes are very high, and 3) no other alternatives appear to be viable" (p. 8). In this model, individuals malinger on the basis of their estimate of success in obtaining the desired external incentive.

## Personality and Malingering

DSM-IV-TR (American Psychiatric Association 2000, p. 739) notes that malingering should be "strongly suspected if any combination of the following" is noted:

1. Medicolegal context of presentation
2. Marked discrepancy between the person's claimed stress or disability and the objective findings
3. Lack of cooperation during the diagnostic evaluation and in complying with the prescribed treatment regimen
4. The presence of antisocial personality disorder

Clark (1997) has questioned the utility of singling out evaluees with APD. He suggests that these individuals are simply more likely to be involved in adversarial situations in which it would benefit them to malinger, for example, facing criminal charges. Edens et al. (2000) endorse a contrary opinion, stating that results of their study within the forensic population "lend support to the position that the relationship between psychopathic personality features and malingering is not exclusively a function of an increased likelihood that dissimulation will occur in forensic contexts" (p. 293). Edens et al. concluded that psychopathic traits are associated with attitudes that may be conducive to engaging in malingering in forensic settings.

The psychological research in this area suggests that a wide range of individuals with and without Axis I and Axis II psychiatric disorders engage in a variety of symptom exaggeration behaviors. Limiting the consideration of malingering only to individuals with diagnosable APD will result in significant underdetection of individuals who are overendorsing or fabricating emotional and/or cognitive symptoms.

### Financial Incentive and Malingering

Individuals who are seeking some form of compensation are commonly believed to be more likely to exaggerate symptoms. Three studies published by different authors in the last decade have attempted to evaluate this belief. Frueh and colleagues (1997) found that veterans seeking compensation for PTSD, compared with non-compensation-seeking veterans, endorsed dramatically higher levels of psychopathology across psychometric measures and produced sharply elevated fake-bad validity indices. Binder and Rohling (1996) evaluated the impact of financial incentives on disability, symptoms, and objective findings after closed head injury. They found more abnormality and disability in evaluees with financial incentives despite less severe injuries. Paniak and colleagues (2002) reported that evaluees seeking compensation following mild traumatic brain injury, compared with non-compensation-seeking evaluees, reported symptoms approximately one standard deviation higher at intake, 3 months, and 12 months postinjury. These studies taken as a whole suggest that the effect of financial incentives should be considered during evaluation.

## Clinical Vignettes

### Malingered PTSD

> A 50-year-old man was found wandering through an orange grove in central Florida dressed in combat fatigues and carrying a quilt with an "Airborne" inscription. The evaluee was admitted to a VA hospital with a diagnosis of PTSD and a rule-out of psychosis NOS (not otherwise specified). He reported a history of Vietnam combat experience and gave details of the Tet Offensive. He stated that his life was in danger on many occasions during combat and told of witnessing a friend being "blown up" by grenade. He reported symptoms of reexperiencing the trauma through nightmares (a single repeating dream) and flashbacks of seeing

his friend killed. He attributed his insomnia, irritability, and difficulty concentrating directly to the trauma. He reported an inability to part with his "survivor quilt," which bore inscriptions of the names of fellow soldiers who had fallen in battle.

On the unit, staff noticed that he became noticeably enthused discussing the war. He wanted to watch war-based television programs that made other veterans anxious, and he went to the library with staff to look up information on the Vietnam War and its battles. His affect was cheerful when not speaking with the psychiatrist.

Concerned that this evaluee might be malingering PTSD, the resident psychiatrist asked for information verifying his dates of service and combat experience. The veteran was found to have served in Vietnam in a noncombat supply position. When confronted by staff, the evaluee showed staff a flier that described all of the symptoms of PTSD but mistakenly misspelled "survivor guilt" as "survivor quilt." Shortly after confrontation, the evaluee requested discharge.

### *Discussion*

This evaluee was diagnosed with malingering. He subsequently admitted to feigning of symptoms for an obvious external incentive: disability payments. Melton (1984) and Resnick (1997b) have offered clues to the presence of malingered Vietnam PTSD, some of which were displayed by the evaluee in this case. These include the observations that 1) factual data regarding military service were discrepant from the evaluee's report, 2) the evaluee seemed to relish telling others about the trauma and did not avoid situations reminiscent of the trauma, and 3) the evaluee emphasized the relationship of symptoms to trauma (evaluees with genuine combat-related PTSD tend to minimize relationship of symptoms to trauma). Additionally, this evaluee's affect and behaviors changed depending on whether the psychiatrist was present or absent, suggesting voluntary control over symptoms.

In civilians with genuine PTSD, posttraumatic nightmares usually show variations on the theme of the traumatic event. In contrast, veterans' posttraumatic nightmares may play out in an identical fashion for many years (Resnick 2003). Thus, a *single repeating nightmare* should arouse suspicion of malingering in *civilians*, but not in veterans, being evaluated for PTSD. Examiners should keep this distinction in mind when they are evaluating PTSD in different settings.

## Malingered Cognitive Deficits

A 38-year-old man presented for neuropsychological evaluation of memory deficits upon referral by his attorney. The evaluee reported that he had been struck on the vertex of the head by a "125-pound piece of metal" 1 year prior to the evaluation while working on an oil rig. Immediately following the trauma, he reported a period of disorientation but no loss of consciousness. He was evacuated to an emergency room, where he was treated for a "4-inch" laceration, given nonnarcotic pain medication, and released to his home.

He failed to return to work—citing increasing problems remembering "anything"—despite the company's attempts to accommodate him by altering his work responsibilities. He retained an attorney and was referred to a number of physicians. Upon neuropsychological evaluation, he tested within the moderate mental retardation range of general cognitive ability and demonstrated markedly impaired language, memory, abstraction ability, and overall performance on other psychological tests. He failed all four tests of symptom validity that were administered, was "unable" to read (despite demonstrating an ability to do so during the weeks after the accident), and produced personality test results reflecting a psychotic state, but he appeared to be not even vaguely psychotic during the evaluation.

The incident report from the oil rig documented that the injury occurred when the patient dove to the floor of the oil rig after a wrench fell approximately 4 feet from him. Curiously, the patient acknowledged that he was wearing a hardhat during the incident, but it was unmarked. Records from the ER visit documented that he was treated for a "small laceration." All neuroradiological (MRI [magnetic resonance imaging] and PET [positron emission tomography]) examinations were read as "normal" by radiologists. Videotapes from various times during the evaluee's period of disability showed entirely normal daily functioning.

### *Discussion*

On the basis of an analysis of the neuropsychological test results and review of collateral information, it was determined that the evaluee was frankly malingering. A marked disparity between the reported and actual history, the discrepancy between test results and demonstrated functional abilities, and the presence of financial incentive were all consistent with a diagnosis of malingering.

## Malingered Amnesia

A 48-year-old man was seen in the emergency room after being brought in by his wife 6 hours after a minor vehicle collision. "No physical injury," no loss of consciousness, no alteration in alertness, and no complaints of physical or cognitive problems were recorded in the accident report and EMT notes. However, the evaluee presented with "memory problems," including being "totally unable" to remember "anything" that occurred prior to the instant of the accident. For instance, the patient recognized his wife but reported that he could not recall their wedding, three children, or any event from the 18-year marriage. Similarly, he could not (or would not) provide information regarding his birth and childhood, schooling, work history, or residences.

The patient was admitted to the neurology service for a workup of amnesia. For the first 2 days of hospitalization, the evaluee simply responded to questions with "I can't remember." Several days into admission, the evaluee continued to profess an inability to recall his personal history but appeared to be aware of all events transpiring in the hospital, began to call staff members by name, and watched television avidly—demonstrating enthusiasm for specific players on the local National Football League team. A comprehensive medical workup for amnesia was negative.

A neuropsychologist was consulted to assist with evaluation of the amnesia. On formal memory testing, the evaluee showed an adequate ability to learn, to recall previously presented information, and to remember this information after a short delay period. However, on the binomial choice Test of Memory Malingering and the Word Memory Test, the evaluee performed below random chance. Following observation of the evaluee and his wife discussing "fooling the doctors," the evaluee was confronted about the atypical nature of his memory complaints and the inconsistency of his symptoms with both his personal medical history and the expected memory findings in evaluees with documented brain injury. The evaluee admitted to "faking" the memory disorder (he needed money "because of debts") and rapidly regained a normal memory pattern.

### *Discussion*

This patient was diagnosed with malingering because of the clear financial incentive, the highly atypical nature of his memory complaints, the inconsistency between his clinical presentation and collateral data, and the evaluation of his psychological test performance.

## Malingered Psychosis

A 30-year-old man was admitted to the psychiatric unit of a forensic hospital after being adjudicated incompetent to stand trial. He was charged with armed robbery at a convenience store. The events were captured by video surveillance. He was noted on video to rapidly enter the store, direct the store clerk to the cash register, and exit with great haste. Records revealed that he had been convicted of two previous felonies involving robbery with weapons. Upon admission to the psychiatric unit, he refused to answer questions, acting as though he were mute, while looking around the room as though he were attending to hallucinations. After the third day of admission, he began to speak with staff. When questioned about hallucinations, he reported continuous hallucinations ("day and night") of a man's voice telling him, "Rob, rob, rob." He said he had been experiencing the voice talking to him for years and that he had acted on the voice in the commission of this crime and previous crimes.

He reported that he did not understand the roles of the judge, jury, defense attorney, or district attorney and did not know how much time he could receive if convicted of the alleged offense. During staffing with the psychiatrist, he presented as bizarre and disorganized, but staff reported that he flirted with female staff and engaged in goal-directed behavior such as playing cards.

When staff confronted him with these inconsistencies, he again became mute. He became angry and aggressive on the ward. He was administered a competency test that used a forced-choice format, which demonstrated a less-than-chance response pattern. He was administered the Structured Interview of Reported Symptoms and fell in the definite malingering category on all scales.

### *Discussion*

This evaluee was returned to court with a diagnosis of malingering and a recommendation of competent to proceed. Malingering in the criminal setting may be pursued by an evaluee to obviate responsibility for a crime. In this case, a rational, nonpsychotic motive for the robbery (money) and the fact that the robbery fit a pattern established in previous crimes suggest malingering. A partner in crime would also call into question a psychotic motive for a crime, as it is unlikely that a nonpsychotic individual would collaborate with a psychotic partner (Resnick 1997a).

Individuals attempting to feign schizophrenia have the most difficulty imitating the form of thinking (derailment, neologisms, incoherence, perseveration) (Sherman et al. 1975) and the negative symptoms characteristic of schizophrenia (Resnick 1997a). Malingerers of schizophrenia may more easily report positive symptoms of schizophrenia (hallucinations and delusions), but a skilled examiner can ask detailed questions to characterize psychotic symptoms as typical or atypical. Table 19–2 lists features of atypical hallucinations, some of which were displayed by the evaluee in this case vignette.

## Malingering Assessment

Resnick (2003) has provided guidelines for the evaluation of malingering in PTSD. These guidelines, while specifically written for the evaluation of PTSD, serve as a framework for designing guidelines for the assessment of malingering in general. The following discussion reviews useful techniques in the assessment of malingering. It also suggests guidelines derived from Resnick, as well as from the authors' own experience, for the assessment of malingering across the spectrum of psychiatric disorders.

**TABLE 19–2.** Characteristics of atypical hallucinations

- Auditory hallucinations
  - Are continuous rather than intermittent (Goodwin et al. 1971).
  - Are vague or inaudible (Goodwin et al. 1971).
  - Are spoken in stilted language (Resnick 1997a).
- Evaluee has no strategies to diminish auditory hallucinations (Resnick 1997a).
- Visual hallucinations are seen in black and white (Goodwin et al. 1971).
- Hallucinations are not associated with a delusion (Lewinsohn 1970).

## Initial Interview

The initial interview is critical in the assessment of malingering. Estimates of the prevalence of malingering in mental health settings indicate that a screening process for malingering would be useful, especially in settings where prevalence estimates are higher than in the general population. Cunnien (1997, p. 45) offers a "threshold model for consideration of malingering." This model is based entirely on clinical presentation, which makes it a suitable initial screening tool. Cunnien's threshold model guides clinicians to suspect malingering when an evaluee presents with physical and psychological symptoms accompanied by any of the following:

1. Suspicion of voluntary control over symptoms as demonstrated by
   - Bizarre or absurd symptomatology
   - Atypical symptomatic fluctuations consistent with external incentives
   - Unusual symptomatic response to treatment
2. Atypical presentation in the presence of environmental incentives or noxious environmental conditions
3. Complaints grossly in excess of clinical findings
4. Substantial noncompliance with treatment

If the initial interaction with an evaluee triggers suspicion of malingering, clinicians should search for further clinical clues that will support or refute this conclusion. Many of these clues can be obtained from the initial, unstructured clinical interview and have been reviewed in the previous section ("Clinical Vignettes").

Rogers (1990) stresses the importance of examining an evaluee's self-reports during assessment of malingering. They may be able to facilitate these reports during the initial interview. Clinicians should rely on their experience and the study of the presentations of true illnesses and their characteristic symptoms in helping them recognize an abnormal pattern of self-reported symptoms. Rogers encourages clinicians to be on watch for endorsement of an unusually high number of symptoms that are rare, blatant, absurd, and preposterous and that are nonselectively endorsed. *Rare symptoms* are those that occur very infrequently among psychiatric evaluees. *Blatant symptoms* are those that are immediately recognized by nonprofessionals as indicative of severe psychopathology. For example, an individual who presents to an ER reporting he is "suicidal, homicidal, and hearing voices telling me to kill myself and other people" is displaying blatant symptoms. Improbable or absurd symptoms are almost never reported or affirmed in even severely disturbed evaluees. An individual who endorses the belief that "honeybees are involved in a plot to kill the president" is demonstrating an improbable and absurd symptom. Nonselective endorsement of symptoms refers to a self-reporting strategy used by malingerers based on the belief that the more symptoms they endorse, the more likely they are to be assessed as ill.

Clinicians should be especially mindful of their interviewing technique if malingering is suspected during the initial interview. Lees-Haley and Dunn (1994) found that a vast majority of untrained subjects were able to endorse symptoms on checklists to meet the DSM-III-R self-report criteria for major depression, generalized anxiety disorder, and PTSD. Thus, clinicians should always be cautious in their use of leading questions when interviewing evaluees suspected of malingering (Resnick 1999). Rather, clinicians who suspect malingering should consider relying at first on open-ended questions. After evaluees have been given an adequate chance to report symptoms in their own words, clinicians can ask specific, detailed questions that help to characterize symptoms as typical or atypical. For example, in the later stages of the interview, the clinician may ask an individual reporting auditory and visual hallucinations whether he or she has a strategy to diminish voices, or whether visual hallucinations only occur in black and white (Table 19–2).

After the initial interview, some clinicians may feel comfortable having ruled out the diagnosis of malingering. Others may have found clues that heighten their suspicion. The latter clinicians should consider proceeding further, utilizing specific techniques useful in establishing the diagnosis of malingering.

## Collateral Data

The review of collateral data is a crucial part of the assessment process. Any information that supports or refutes the evaluee's symptoms may be considered collateral information. Such data may include the following:

- Depositions of the evaluee and family members in civil cases
- Employment records
- Hospital and treatment records
- Insurance records (or other information gathered by the insurance agency to investigate a claim [Crane 2000])
- Military records (Form DD 214 may be especially useful in investigating malingered Vietnam PTSD [Resnick 2003])
- Personnel files
- Police reports and witness statements in criminal cases
- Surveillance tapes

Clinicians who have access to this data have information with which to compare the evaluee interview and self-report. Information that is inconsistent with the symptoms reported by the individual during the clinical interview may support a diagnosis of malingering. Conversely, collateral data that are consistent with the findings of the interview may help clinicians rule out malingering.

Some evaluators prefer to review collateral data prior to the evaluation so they can address unclear or contradictory issues during the interview. Other evaluators prefer to review collateral data after the interview. Regardless of when collateral data are reviewed, clinicians should be certain to examine this information and look for consistencies or inconsistencies in reported symptoms.

Resnick (2003) suggests also interviewing a close family member or associate who is familiar with the evaluee's daily habits and symptoms. Such interviews can validate or refute the individual's report of symptoms and should be conducted separately from the interview of the evaluee.

Once all collateral data have been collected, the clinician may wish to confront an evaluee who is suspected of malingering. This is a difficult decision and should be handled with care, as malingerers often respond to such confrontation by escalating their behavior in an attempt to justify their self-reports. Because of this phenomenon, direct confrontation of a dangerous individual or an individual with a history of acting out should be undertaken only with adequate mental health staff and security backup.

A safer approach to confrontation involves the process of *clarification.* The skilled examiner can use the evaluation process and the interview to clarify the evaluee's symptoms and behaviors. This approach can often provide useful information about the presence or lack of malingering while allowing the evaluee to save face. The clinician notes whether the evaluee's responses to questions are reasonable, exaggerated, or malingered. The evaluator can then construct a report that supports the basis for the malingered diagnosis without compromising his or her own safety or that of the evaluee.

## Psychological Assessment and Structured Clinical Interviews

Research in the area of malingering detection has become one of the major areas of psychological study during the past decade (e.g., McCaffrey et al. 1997; Reynolds 1998; Rogers 1997; Sweet 1999). Patient personality characteristics and cognitive functioning have been prime areas of study. In addition to assessing the frequency and the characteristics of malingering, this research has focused on the use of 1) clinical personality measures, 2) specific objective measures of inadequate effort, exaggeration, and malingering, and 3) methods of analyzing unusual, inconsistent, and discrepant patterns of performance on tests used in standard psychological assessment to detect malingering and other behavioral factors that interfere with valid test performance.

Psychologists routinely administer standard personality measurement tests: MMPI-2, Millon Multiaxial Inventory–3 (MCMI-3), and Personality Assessment Inventory (PAI). Each of these objective personality measures includes validity scales that enable the psychologist to assess response tendencies such as exaggeration, defensiveness, untruthfulness, consistency in responding over time, and tendency to respond excessively in either a positive (true) or negative (false) manner. Greene (1991) and Bieliauskas (1999) provide comprehensive reviews of the use of the MMPI-2 and other personality measures in clinical and forensic practice.

Observation of the individual's behavior during test performance often provides valuable information regarding the patient's style of presentation and pattern of attention, involvement, and effort. Among the factors that should be clinically assessed are 1) inadequate and/or variable levels of effort on standard psychological tests, 2) presence of atypical or implausible behavior and test responses, and 3) inconsistency in style or quality of behavior and test performance over time and across tests of similar cognitive/emotional functioning (Sweet 1999).

A comparison of performance on tests of specific emotional and cognitive functions and functioning in real-life situations can also provide evidence of malingering. Discrepancies between test results, especially on the MMPI-2 clinical scales suggesting significant emotional distress or on cognitive tests suggesting memory dysfunction, and actual functioning that are illogical suggest exaggeration or malingering rather than a genuine disorder or deficit. In addition, an analysis of test patterns can reveal test performance that is implausible or incompatible with the patient's history and/or clinical presentation.

In addition to the standard personality measures, a number of objective structured interviews and assessment procedures are available to improve the clinical evaluation of malingered psychiatric illness. These include the Miller Forensic Assessment of Symptoms Test (M-FAST), Rogers Criminal Responsibility Assessment Scales (R-CRAS), and Structured Interview of Reported Symptoms (SIRS) (see Iverson and Binder 2000 and Vickery and colleagues 2001).

Lastly, a variety of objective cognitive measures designed for the detection of symptom validity (inadequate effort, exaggeration, and frank malingering) have been developed, primarily in the field of neuropsychology. Most such instruments are based on the premise that individuals who tend to malinger or dissimulate in an attempt to magnify symptoms will perform less adequately than predicted on even simple measures of cognitive functioning. Among the more commonly employed and most useful of these tests are the Computerized Assessment of Response Bias (CARB), Victoria Symptom Validity Test (VSVT), Word Memory Test, Portland Digit Recognition Test (PDRT), and Digit Memory Test. A wide range of other procedures are also available. Iverson and Binder (2000) and Vickery and colleagues (2001) have provided comprehensive reviews of the variety of psychometric measures currently available to aid in the assessment of symptom validity/malingering.

The psychological assessment of an evaluee who is suspected of malingering should include the following procedures:

1. Use of specific, current, and valid tests of symptom validity. Both personality and forced-choice cognitive measures should be used.
2. Careful evaluation of inadequate effort (or frank malingering) across the battery of tests used.
3. Examination of illogical or unique malingering responses (e.g., Ganser-like answers).
4. Examination of excessive inconsistency in quality of performance during the course of the evaluation. In particular, differences in the adequacy of performance on tests of similar cognitive or emotional functions (e.g., abnormal memory performance on one test and normal performance on another; significant self-reported depression but minimal symptoms of depression on the MMPI-2).
5. Comparison of the difference between performance on psychological tests and the quality of functioning in real-life situations. Objective collateral data sources are very important.

6. Determination of the logical relationship between the history (medical, psychiatric, and social) and the individual's presentation within the context of the formal evaluation. Are the observed behavior and test performance reasonably consistent with the pattern expected on the basis of the history?

## Conclusion

Forensic settings provide multiple and powerful incentives for malingering clinical conditions. Clinicians providing any type of forensic evaluation must consider the possibility of partial or total malingering, and adopt a low threshold of suspicion for making this assessment. This stance differs from that adopted in purely clinical evaluations, where, in most cases, clinicians reasonably assume that individuals seeking treatment are motivated to be truthful in order to obtain accurate diagnoses and effective treatment. Nevertheless, the conclusion that an evaluee is malingering should not be made without good supporting evidence, as its implications for the claimant may be profound. A conclusion that an evaluee is malingering should be based on a variety of evidence, including clinical presentation, review of records, collateral information, and, if possible, psychological testing.

## Key Points

- Clinicians across all specialties may encounter malingering, but clinicians should be particularly aware of the potential for malingering in forensic settings.
- An atypical presentation in the presence of external incentive should trigger suspicion of malingering during assessment of an evaluee.
- Clinicians who suspect malingering may use specialized techniques to establish or rule out the diagnosis of malingering.
- A diagnosis of malingering requires evidence gathered from clinical interview, review of collateral data, and, often, psychological testing. A diagnosis of malingering should not be made on the basis of any one piece of information, such as personality testing, but rather on the basis of an integrated assessment.
- Clinicians are aware of the potential for stigmatizing of evaluees mistakenly assessed as malingering, and therefore they may avoid making the diagnosis or confronting patients suspected of malingering. Clinicians may feel more confident in their opinions regarding malingering if they follow guidelines for a thorough malingering assessment.

## Practice Guidelines

1. Consider malingering in the differential diagnosis, especially in forensic settings.
2. During the initial interview, be on the watch for endorsement of an unusually high number of symptoms that are rare, blatant, absurd, and preposterous and that are nonselectively endorsed.
3. Be cautious in the use of leading questions when interviewing evaluees suspected of malingering. Rather, use open-ended questions at the outset of the interview and later ask detailed questions that help to characterize symptoms as typical or atypical of the mental disorder in question.
4. Review collateral data for consistencies or inconsistencies that support or refute a diagnosis of malingering.
5. Obtain psychological testing when the clinical and structured interviews result in a suspicion, but inconclusive determination, of the presence of malingering.
6. Avoid directly accusing the evaluee of lying during confrontation. An approach that asks the evaluee for clarification of inconsistencies may be a more productive and safer method of confrontation.
7. Make a diagnosis of malingering on the basis of a thorough assessment that integrates many sources of information.

## References

American Psychiatric Association: Diagnostic and Statistical Manual of Mental Disorders, 4th Edition. Washington, DC, American Psychiatric Association, 1994

American Psychiatric Association: Diagnostic and Statistical Manual of Mental Disorders, 4th Edition, Text Revision. Washington, DC, American Psychiatric Association, 2000

Bieliauskas L: The measurement of personality and emotional functioning, in Forensic Neuropsychology. Edited by Sweet JJ. Lisse, the Netherlands, Swets & Zeitlinger, 1999, pp 121–143

Binder LM, Rohling ML: Money matters: a meta-analytic review of the effects of financial incentives on recovery after closed-head injury. Am J Psychiatry 153:7–10, 1996

Bolan B, Foster JK, Schmand B, et al: A comparison of three tests to detect feigned amnesia: the effects of feedback and the measurement of response latency. J Clin Exp Neuropsychol 24:154–167, 2002

Clark RC: Sociopathy, malingering, and defensiveness, in Clinical Assessment of Malingering and Deception, 2nd Edition. Edited by Rogers R. New York, Guilford, 1997, pp 68–84

Coalition Against Insurance Fraud: Insurance fraud rises to $85.3 billion (press release). Washington, DC, Coalition Against Insurance Fraud, July 18, 1997. Available at: http://www.insurancefraud.org/news_set.html. Accessed November 9, 2003.

Crane M: How high-tech private eyes catch malingering plaintiffs. Medical Economics 77(14):122–124, 130–132, 137 passim, 2000

Cunnien AJ: Psychiatric and medical syndromes associated with deception, in Clinical Assessment of Malingering and Deception, 2nd Edition. Edited by Rogers R. New York, Guilford, 1997, pp 23–46

DeToledo JC: The epilepsy of Fyodor Dostoyevsky: insights from Smerdyakov Karamazov's use of a malingered seizure as an alibi. Arch Neurol 58:1305–1306, 2001

Edens JF, Buffington JK, Tomicic TL: An investigation of the relationship between psychopathic traits and malingering on the psychopathic personality inventory. Assessment 7:281–296, 2000

Eisendrath SJ: When Munchausen becomes malingering: factitious disorders that penetrate the legal system. Bull Am Acad Psychiatry Law 24:471–481, 1996

Frueh BC, Gold PB, de Arellano MA: Symptom overreporting in combat veterans evaluated for PTSD: differentiation on the basis of compensation seeking status. J Pers Assess 68:369–384, 1997

Gacono CB, Meloy JR, Sheppard K, et al: A clinical investigation of malingering and psychopathy in hospitalized insanity acquittees. Bull Am Acad Psychiatry Law 23:387–397, 1995

Gavin H: On Feigned and Factitious Diseases Chiefly of Soldiers and Seamen. London, J Churchill, 1843

Gittelman DK: Malingered dementia associated with battered women's syndrome. Psychosomatics 39:449–452, 1998

Goodwin DW, Alderson P, Rosenthal R: Clinical significance of hallucinations in psychiatric disorders: a study of 116 hallucinatory patients. Arch Gen Psychiatry 24:756–780, 1971

Greene RL: The MMPI-2/MMPI: An Interpretative Manual. Boston, MA, Allyn & Bacon, 1991

Greenfield D: Feigned psychosis in a 14-year-old-girl. Hosp Community Psychiatry 38:73–77, 1987

Iverson GL, Binder LM: Detecting exaggeration and malingering in neuropsychological assessment. J Head Trauma Rehabil 15:829–858, 2000

Labott SM, Wallach HR: Malingering dissociative identity disorder: objective and projective assessment. Psychol Rep 90:525–538, 2002

Lees-Haley PR, Dunn JT: The ability of naive subjects to report symptoms of mild brain injury, post-traumatic stress disorder, major depression, and generalized anxiety disorder. J Clin Psychol 50:252–256, 1994

Lewinsohn PM: An empirical test of several popular notions about hallucinations in schizophrenic patients, in Origin and Mechanisms of Hallucinations. Edited by Keup W. New York, Plenum, 1970, pp 401–403

Mahowald MW, Schenck CH, Rosen GM, et al: The role of a sleep disorder center in evaluating sleep violence. Arch Neurol 49:604–607, 1992

McCaffrey RJ, Williams AD, Fisher JM, et al (eds): The Practice of Forensic Neuropsychology. New York, Plenum, 1997

Melton R: Differential diagnosis: a commonsense guide to psychological assessment. Vet Center Voice Newsletter 5:1–12, 1984

Palermo GB, Perracuti S, Palermo MT: Malingering a challenge for the forensic examiner. Med Law 15:143–160, 1996

Paniak C, Reynolds S, Toller-Lobe G, et al: A longitudinal study of the relationship between financial compensation and symptoms after treated mild traumatic brain injury. J Clin Exp Neuropsychol 24:187–193, 2002

Resnick PJ: Malingered psychosis, in Clinical Assessment of Malingering and Deception, 2nd Edition. Edited by Rogers R. New York, Guilford, 1997a, pp 47–67

Resnick PJ: Malingering of posttraumatic stress disorders, in Clinical Assessment of Malingering and Deception, 2nd Edition. Edited by Rogers R. New York, Guilford, 1997b, pp 130–152

Resnick PJ: The detection of malingered psychosis. Psychiatr Clin North Am 22: 159–172, 1999

Resnick PJ: Guidelines for evaluation of malingering in PTSD, in Posttraumatic Stress Disorder in Litigation: Guidelines for Forensic Assessment, 2nd Edition. Edited by Simon RI. Washington, DC, American Psychiatric Publishing, 2003, pp 187–205

Reynolds CR (ed): Detection of Malingering During Head Injury Litigation. New York, Plenum, 1998

Rissmiller DA, Steer RA, Friedman M, et al: Prevalence of malingering in suicidal psychiatric inpatients: a replication. Psychol Rep 84:726–730, 1999

Rogers R: Conducting Insanity Evaluations. New York, Van Nostrand Reinhold, 1986

Rogers R: Development of a new classificatory model of malingering. Bull Am Acad Psychiatry Law 18:323–333, 1990

Rogers R: Introduction, in Clinical Assessment of Malingering and Deception, 2nd Edition. Edited by Rogers R. New York, Guilford, 1997, pp 1–19

Rogers R, Sewell KW, Goldstein A: Explanatory models of malingering: a prototypical analysis. Law Hum Behav 18:543–552, 1994

Rubinstein JS: Abuse of antiparkinsonism drugs: feigning of extrapyramidal symptoms to obtain trihexyphenidyl. JAMA 239:2365–2366, 1978

Sherman M, Trief P, Strafkin R: Impression management in the psychiatric interview. J Consult Clin Psychol 43: 867–871, 1975

Sierles FS: Correlates of malingering. Behav Sci Law 2:113–118, 1984

Sweet JJ: Malingering: differential diagnosis, in Forensic Neuropsychology. Edited by Sweet JJ. Lisse, the Netherlands: Swets & Zeitlinger, 1999, pp 255–312

Turner M: Malingering. Br J Psychiatry 171:409–411, 1997

Vickery CD, Berry DTR, Inman TH, et al: Detection of inadequate effort on neuropsychological testing: a meta-analytic review of selected procedures. Archives of Clinical Neuropsychology 16:45–73, 2001

Yates BD, Nordquist CR, Schultz-Ross RA: Feigned psychiatric symptoms in the emergency room. Psychiatr Serv 47:998–1000, 1996

## Suggested Readings

Bolan B, Foster JK, Schmand B, et al: A comparison of three tests to detect feigned amnesia: the effects of feedback and the measurement of response latency. J Clin Exp Neuropsychol 24:154–167, 2002

Edens JF, Guy LS, Otto RK, et al: Factors differentiating successful versus unsuccessful malingerers. J Pers Assess 77:333–338, 2001

Eisendrath SJ: When Munchausen becomes malingering: factitious disorders that penetrate the legal system. Bull Am Acad Psychiatry Law 24:471–481, 1996

Resnick PJ: Malingering of posttraumatic stress disorders, in Clinical Assessment of Malingering and Deception, 2nd Edition. Edited by Rogers R. New York, Guilford, 1997, pp 130–152

Resnick PJ: The detection of malingered psychosis. Psychiatr Clin North Am 22(1):159–172, 1999

Rogers R (ed): Clinical Assessment of Malingering and Deception, 2nd Edition. New York, Guilford, 1997

Simon RI (ed): Posttraumatic Stress Disorder in Litigation: Guidelines for Forensic Assessment, 2nd Edition. Washington, DC, American Psychiatric Publishing, 2003

CHAPTER 20

# Children and Adolescents

Peter Ash, M.D.

## Introduction

Forensic work in child and adolescent psychiatry tends to have a different thrust from forensic work with adults. In a case involving adults, the psychiatric expert is typically retained by a party to the case (although some evaluations are court-ordered and the expert is an expert for the court). This places the expert on one side or the other of an adversarial process. Moreover, the well-being of the evaluee is not the court's prime consideration. In contrast, regardless of which adult or agency is paying the bill, the expert in both civil and criminal matters involving juveniles is often expected to evaluate and advocate for the well-being of the child. In civil cases, the child is often not even formally a party to the case. This role allows the expert to occupy a position somewhat above the fray, as the expert is not beholden to any of the parties in the case. The expert's concern with the child's interests is similar in many ways to the expert's role in a civil commitment proceeding.

The most common civil forensic questions psychiatrists are called on to answer regarding children involve cases of divorce and child abuse or neglect. In divorce cases, the issues involve child custody and the parents are the named parties. In abuse/neglect cases, issues involve child placement and the parties are the state and the parent(s). In most criminal cases involving minors, the minor is before a juvenile court. Part of the mission of such courts includes rehabilitation of the juvenile. This also leads the court to a consideration of the minor's best interest. This emphasis on the child's interests gives child forensic work a more therapeutic focus and is more familiar to clinicians who view themselves primarily as therapists.

A second obvious difference in forensic work with children and adolescents is that interviewing young persons requires different techniques from those used in evaluating adults. General psychiatrists who lack training in child and adolescent psychiatry generally shy away from work that requires interviewing preadolescents. The accreditation guidelines for forensic psychiatry training programs specifically require that fellows who have not completed a fellowship in child and adolescent psychiatry do not independently conduct forensic evaluations of children under the age of 14 (Accreditation Council for Graduate Medical Education 2003). There is, however, a national shortage of child and adolescent psychiatrists. Thus, in underserved, nonurban areas, some general psychiatrists who lack formal fellowship training but who nevertheless have considerable experience working with youths do conduct forensic evaluations involving children. Forensic work with preadolescents that requires such specialized techniques and training is beyond the scope of this chapter. The interested reader is referred to standard works on forensic child and adolescent psychiatry (Haller 2002; Nurcombe and Partlett 1994; Schetky and Benedek 2002) and the suggested readings at the end of this chapter.

Adolescents are a different matter. Many general psychiatrists who lack child psychiatry fellowship training nevertheless have had some training and experience working with adolescents and so also conduct forensic evaluations on this population. General psychiatrists who undertake forensic evaluations of adolescents should expect that their expertise in working with this age group will be the subject of cross-examination, so they should think through carefully how they will justify their expertise to the court.

Even a clinician who does not see children will have adult patients who, in their role as parents, will become involved in litigation concerning their children. Thus, the range of issues in child and adolescent forensic psychiatry that may affect the work of a general psychiatrist is very wide.

This chapter discusses general principles in child and adolescent forensic psychiatry. Examples of child and adolescent forensic work in which the general psychiatrist is most likely to become involved, primarily cases that involve evaluating a parent of a younger child and cases involving adolescents, are emphasized.

## Comparing Child and Adolescent Cases With Adult Cases

Some child and adolescent forensic cases follow the same formal legal structure as do similar cases involving adults. For example, the statutory test for civil commitment of a minor is the same as the statutory test for the commitment of an adult. Nevertheless, a commitment case involving a minor is somewhat different in the way the case actually evolves. A minor can be admitted involuntarily when a physician recommends admission and a parent consents (*Parham v. J.R. and J.L.* 1979). Commitment of a minor becomes necessary only when parents refuse voluntary admission or actively oppose admission and the youth meets commitment criteria.

Many differences in cases involving minors follow from two legal presumptions: 1) minors are less responsible for their actions than are adults, and 2) minors are less legally competent than adults. Salient differences in child and adolescent cases in which the forensic tests are formally the same as in adult cases are listed in Table 20–1.

However, cases involving minors that have no clear adult parallels are frequently referred for evaluation. This group of cases arises from the different standing of adults and children under the law. The law presumes that children are incompetent to make decisions, and their parents legally speak for them. Forensic cases involving minors without clear adult analogues arise in situations in which the parents are not in a position to speak appropriately for the child. Such situations may include circumstances in which the parents themselves disagree (custody in divorce) or have interests opposed to those of the child (abuse and neglect), or when the child acts outside the parent's control (delinquency, certain medical care issues).

Forensic evaluations focus on whether or not the individual's condition meets a forensic test specific to the matter at issue. Forensic tests in similar cases vary from state to state and in federal jurisdictions. Nevertheless, certain general principles cut across jurisdictions. Typical forensic tests used in cases involving minors that have no clear counterpart in adult forensic work are shown in Table 20–2.

## Beginning a Forensic Evaluation

### Clarification of Role

Clinicians who do not have a great deal of forensic experience may find that some consultations go awry and result in considerable hair pulling. Generally, this situation occurs when the consultant's role is not clearly defined at the beginning of his or her involvement in the case. Before beginning the evaluation, the forensic consultant should have a clear understanding of the issues, including those addressed by the following questions:

**TABLE 20–1. Key differences in cases involving minors in which the forensic test is the same as for adults**

| Issue | Difference from adult cases |
|---|---|
| **Civil cases** | |
| Malpractice | Since minors are less responsible than adults, clinicians have a greater duty to protect them from other patients, from committing suicide, and so forth. |
| Personal injury | Minors are more sympathetic plaintiffs; they are held to a lesser degree of responsibility, which tends to shift responsibility to defendants. |
| Civil commitment | Commitment is less common because in most states it is required only if parents refuse to voluntarily admit minor. |
| Civil competency | Children are presumed legally incompetent except in specific situations authorized by state law. |
| Disability | Social Security disability criteria for children are worded slightly differently. School-related issues are mostly governed by education legislation. |
| School threat assessment | Different techniques from those used in workplace violence assessment are used in assessing school threat. |
| **Criminal cases** | |
| Competency to stand trial | Only about half the states require competency to stand trial in juvenile court. Incompetence may be due to developmental immaturity. |
| Criminal responsibility | Not usually a defense in juvenile court. Very rare in adolescents who are waived to adult court. |
| Competency to waive as constitutional right (e.g., competency to confess, waive right to counsel, or plead guilty) | Developmental considerations affect whether waiver is knowing, intelligent, and voluntary. |
| Sex offenders | Since child and adolescent sex offenders are more treatable than adult sex offenders, treatment options are more relevant. |

**TABLE 20–2.** Forensic child and adolescent cases without clear adult analogues

| Issue | Typical forensic test |
|---|---|
| Custody in the context of divorce | Best interests of the child. |
| Abuse/neglect proceedings | Varies according to the stage of the proceeding:<br>Was the child abused or neglected?<br>Are the parents fit to raise the child?<br>Should protective services pursue reunification?<br>Is termination of parental rights in the best interests of the child? |
| Adoption | Is termination of parental rights in the best interests of the child?<br>If mother is a minor, is she competent to give up child for adoption? |
| Medical care | |
| Consent by minor | Varies according to state law.<br>Can minor provide consent? While the general rule is that minors cannot provide consent, state law may give some minors authority to provide consent in certain situations (such as outpatient therapy, treatment of sexually transmitted diseases, contraception) or a right to object (such as to psychiatric hospitalization). Some states allow a "mature minor" to provide consent. |
| Consent to an abortion without parental consent | Is girl a "mature minor"? |
| Participation in research that will not benefit minor | Assent required if minor can understand general nature of participation, in addition to parental consent. |
| Consent for organ donation | For donations that pose more than minimal health risk to minor, assent of minor plus judicial review. |
| Delinquency | |
| Study and report | What mental health issues are relevant in rehabilitating and planning a disposition for the delinquent? |
| Waiver to adult court | Risk of future dangerousness and amenability to rehabilitation. |
| Special education services | Is child "seriously emotionally disturbed"? If so, what special educational services are appropriate? |

- What is the forensic question that needs to be answered?
- Who is requesting the evaluation? The minor? A parent? An attorney? The court? A guardian *ad litem* (a person appointed by the judge to speak for the child's interests in the case at hand)?
- Who is to be interviewed?
- If a minor is being interviewed, who will give informed consent for the evaluation?
- What are the limits on confidentiality in the evaluation?
- To whom will the report be sent? (A related issue that must be considered is to what extent a parent will control whether the report is sent at all.)
- What are the arrangements for paying the fees?

These issues are frequently more complex in cases involving minors than in cases involving adults. First, minors have limited formal decision-making authority; whereas the minor may be the subject of a case, others will often be speaking for the minor in court. Second, in custody cases, both in divorce and in abuse/neglect proceedings, the child is typically not a formal party to the case at all. In such cases, the consultant should consider in advance and how (or if) the report will be brought to the attention of the court in the event a parent does not like the outcome. If the child is not a party to the case, the court may appoint a guardian *ad litem* to speak for the child's interests. Some particulars of defining role will be discussed in the example cases later in this chapter.

Fees should generally be paid prior to conducting the work, and in any event prior to completing the evaluation, unless the retaining agent is a corporate defendant or state agency. A parent who is disappointed in an evaluation is easily tempted to withhold payment, either to save money or to prevent distribution of the report. An evaluator who is concerned that he might not be paid his full fees may be subject to a subtle source of bias, which may be brought out on cross-examination ("Now doctor, do you really think you'll be paid for your testimony today if it's not favorable to Mr. X?").

## Forensic Evaluations of One's Own Patients

Not uncommonly, a minor or a parent in treatment will become the subject of a legal proceeding. The attorney for either the child or parent may wish to use the treating clinician as the expert on the grounds that the clinician knows the child or parent best. However, a treating clinician is best advised not to become the expert in such cases. By conducting a forensic evaluation, the clinician takes on a duty toward the court, in addition to his or her continuing his duty to the patient. This dual-role conflict is known as the *double-agent problem* (being the agent of the child, as therapist, and being an agent of the court or parent, as forensic evaluator). Conflicting duties give rise to a host of difficulties (see Chapter 2: "Introduction to the Legal System" and Chapter 3: "Starting a Forensic Practice," this volume). Even if the psychiatrist believes the double-agent problem can be surmounted, the court is likely to see the treating psychiatrist as biased toward his or her patient and partially discount the weight it gives to the expert's opinions. It is almost always preferable to refer one's patient to another clinician for forensic evaluation.

Such a referral is also advisable because the expert role usually is quite disruptive of the treatment. Conducting a forensic assessment will generally require going outside the established treatment relationship. Once the child (or parent) knows that the therapist is a route to the judge, confidentiality goes out the window, the patient has a motive to distort what he or she tells the therapist, and the parameters of the treatment change. Furthermore, the clinician may not have a well-formed opinion on the particular forensic issue. For example, if a divorcing parent wishes the clinician to give an opinion on postdivorce custody arrangements, the clinician may well not have assessed the parents' parenting capacities or compared their relationships with the child.

An attorney for a parent may nevertheless subpoena the treating psychiatrist out of a sense of efficiency or for other reasons. Such actions can sometimes be discouraged. For example, in a child custody case in which a mother's attorney threatens to subpoena the child's treating psychiatrist, the therapist may point out that such an action will disrupt the child's treatment and thus may serve as evidence that the mother is not acting in the best interest of the child.

## Consent for Evaluation

If a forensic evaluation of a minor is court-ordered, parental consent is not required. If an evaluation is requested by a parent, the evaluator should obtain the informed consent of the parent, which should include a signed release to send the report to designated recipients. In limited situations, an adolescent can provide consent for the evaluation. Such situations arise if the adolescent is emancipated (because he or she is married, in the military, or self-supporting and living independently), waived to adult criminal jurisdiction, or can consent to treatment (as when a girl is seeking to obtain an abortion without her parents' knowledge). In any event, the evaluator should explain to the child or adolescent, in developmentally appropriate terms, the nature of the evaluation and with whom information will be shared.

## Exceptions to Confidentiality

As a general rule, confidentiality is controlled by the person or agency that provides legal consent for the evaluation. In some instances, most often in order to protect a child, legal and ethical obligations compel a treating clinician to disclose forensically relevant information to outside agencies without a release from the consenting party. All psychiatrists in all states have a duty to report reasonable suspicions of child abuse to the state child protective agency, even if the information that gave rise to the concern was obtained in a confidential communication. State laws vary in some respects, for example, as to what behaviors constitute abuse and whether abuse by noncaretakers needs to be reported. All clinicians should be familiar with the reporting statute in their jurisdiction. However, they should also be aware that the duty to breach confidentiality ends with the report and the basis for it. Courts have generally held that only that information which gave rise to the report is discoverable (*People v. Stritzinger* 1983; *State v. Andring* 1984). The clinician does not generally have a duty to further investigate the abuse (although the abuse may well become a clinical issue needing attention).

Clinicians confronting the unenviable necessity of reporting their own patient as a suspected child abuser face the difficult challenge of conforming to their duty to report and attempting to maintain the therapeutic alliance. Under such circumstances, it is almost always best to discuss with the patient that one is making the report and why. Many therapists fear that the patient in such cases will become angry and either quit therapy or mistrust the therapist in the future. Generally, however, an open acknowledgment of the difficulty and an offer to help the parent resolve the difficulties that gave rise to the reported behaviors allow the patient to continue to see the therapist as an ally. A clinician who does not tell his or her patient about the report runs the risk that the patient will think the therapist is complicit with the abuse (many patients know about reporting duties) or that the patient will later find out about the report (the anonymity of reports is not all it might be) and feel betrayed.

# Child Custody Related to Divorce

Mr. J came to treatment for help with his depressed feelings arising out of an impending divorce. While in treatment, he asked his psychiatrist to write a letter to the court recommending that he have custody of his 8-year-old son. He offered to bring his son in "because he'll tell you he wants to live with me."

Child custody issues often arise when a parent who is in treatment is going through a divorce and contesting custody of his or her child, as in the case above. There are a number of reasons for the clinician not to accede to Mr. J's request for a letter to the court supporting his arguments regarding custody. First, the clinician may lack training for these specialized evaluations. Second, as discussed in the previous section, performing forensic evaluations on one's own patients is generally not advisable. Finally, current standards for conducting custody evaluations strongly recommend that all parties to a custody case (including both parents and all children) be interviewed before an opinion on child custody matters is rendered (see, e.g., guidelines of the American Academy of Child and Adolescent Psychiatry [Herman 1997] and the American Psychological Association [1994]).

In the case example above, the psychiatrist recommended that Mr. J obtain a full custody evaluation by an independent clinician. The central issue before the court in a custody dispute is a comparison of custody options and a determination of which of these is in the best interest of the child. The clinician presenting an opinion based on the assessment of only one parent is not likely to have a basis for comparing the custody options or making a well-informed recommendation regarding the child's best interest. An evaluation of the parent and parent-child relationship by an independent evaluator is usually much more helpful to the court. Parents sometimes want a letter that is essentially a clean bill of mental health. Such letters are unlikely to be of much use to the court except in rare cases, as when one parent asserts visitation should be terminated solely on the grounds that the other parent is mentally ill. In these cases, an attorney fears the judge will focus on the parent's diagnosis and not understand the importance of looking into the nature of the parent-child relationship.

In the event a patient does obtain an independent evaluation, the psychiatrist will need to consider carefully his or her role as a collateral source of information. Custody evaluators commonly request releases from parties to a custody case in order to talk to the parties' therapists. The patient may feel some pressure to provide the release, if for no other reason than to appear cooperative with the evaluation. The therapist should bear in mind that all such conversations are discoverable and that releasing information to the evaluator may have effects on the treatment.

In these circumstances, clinicians should consider the option of having a telephone discussion with the evaluator but not providing written records. Many custody evaluators are interested in talking to therapists as a means of identifying some of the patient's salient issues. However, evaluators then utilize that information in their own interviews of the parent to hone in more quickly on important issues relevant to custody. By doing so, evaluators can base their recommendations on their own findings, rather than relying solely on the conclusions of the therapist. This provides a stronger basis for the evaluator's opinions and protects the confidentiality of the treatment.

Most custody disputes reflect marital disputes that compromise one or both parents' abilities to reason about their children's best interests. However, few divorces stem from disagreements about how to raise children. A psychiatrist working with a patient who is going through a divorce and contemplating obtaining a child custody evaluation can provide assistance by helping the parent understand why he or she is having difficulty negotiating with his or her spouse regarding the post-divorce arrangements for their children. There are many types of interferences in parents' ability to reach their own resolution (Johnston et al. 1985), and understanding the impasse is important in helping parents resolve their difficulties without resorting to the aggravation and expense of a trial. Parents may be helped to settle the case themselves, to settle through mediation (Benjamin and Irving 1995; Emery 1994), or even to settle after a custody evaluation (Ash and Guyer 1986).

## Parenting Evaluations in Abuse and Neglect Cases

> Ms. G, who suffers from chronic bipolar disorder, had her infant removed at birth because of neglect. The baby tested positive for cocaine. Ms. G had not been taking her mood-stabilizing medication for many months prior to delivery and was thought to be psychotic while in the hospital. Child protective services had set out a plan for the mother, which included going into psychiatric treatment and substance abuse treatment, and remaining abstinent from street drugs. After 6 months, the juvenile court ordered the mother to obtain a psychiatric evaluation regarding her capacity to parent her infant.

Assessments of parenting capacity may be requested by courts in a wide variety of circumstances and at any stage of an abuse or neglect proceeding. Such requests most often come to general psychiatrists after a child has been removed for abuse or neglect and some practical or therapeutic intervention has occurred intended to increase the child's safety. The psychiatrist is then asked to assess whether the parent can now safely resume custody of the child. A request for such an evaluation may be initiated by a child protection agency, by a judge, or by a parent who has been instructed by the court to obtain such an evaluation and present it to the court. Evaluation may also be requested when the child protection agency has given up on reunification and is petitioning for termination of parental rights. In order for the court to terminate parental rights, the state must show, with clear and convincing evidence, that termination is necessary (*Santosky v. Kramer* 1982).

Precise legal standards describing fitness to raise one's child after a finding of abuse or neglect vary among the states. Typically, such standards require a determination that the child will be safe from further abuse and neglect and that the parent or parents are fit to raise the child. However, clear definitions of these terms are not available. Indeed, a clear professional consensus on the specifics of what parenting functions render a person a "fit parent" does not exist, and there is even less agreement on how to measure those functions.

Assessing parenting capacity after an adjudication of neglect or abuse typically involves addressing the following questions:

1. Are there specific legal tests that must be addressed in this jurisdiction or this case, and if so, what are they?
2. What were the mental health issues and other factors that gave rise to the abuse or neglect?
3. To what extent have those difficulties been treated?
4. What is the likelihood of relapse?
5. What is the likelihood of recurring abuse or neglect?
6. What are the parenting needs of this particular child?
7. Can the parent meet this child's needs? How will the parent carry out essential parenting functions, such as providing for the child's safety, basic needs, medical care, discipline, education, and emotional needs?
8. What is the nature of the relationship between the parent and child?
9. What treatment or other interventions are needed to improve or maintain the parent's functioning?

Psychiatric evaluations are commonly obtained in cases in which a parent has a severe mental illness and the court is particularly interested in the course, treatment efficacy, and prognosis of the parent. Such assessment should focus on parenting functions. While the evaluator will conduct a standard psychiatric assessment as one component of the evaluation, a parent's mental illness is important to the extent that it interferes with parenting. A "standard" psychiatric evaluation that does not make the link between mental disorder and parenting function is of very little use to the court.

If the psychiatrist evaluates only the parent(s) but not the child or the parent-child relationship, only some of the questions presented above can be answered, and the lack of data and opinions about the child should be made explicit in the report. The general psychiatrist's report will be only one piece of information. The court will take this report into consideration with other information from other sources. A more comprehensive evaluation in such cases may include the parent as well as the child and the parent-child relationship. Such an evaluation may allow the psychiatrist to reach an opinion on the ultimate question of whether the child should be returned. In either event, however, the link between mental disorder and parenting function should be made explicit.

## Delinquency Cases in Juvenile Court

Working with juvenile court cases differs from working with adult criminal cases. These differences arise from both procedural differences and from the juvenile courts' explicit mandate to provide rehabilitation for youths who come before them. The 1967 Supreme Court decision *In re* Gault and subsequent court decisions brought most adult criminal due-process requirements to juvenile procedures (except for trial by jury), but rehabilitation remains a primary mission.

When minors are arrested on criminal charges, they are typically placed under the jurisdiction of the juvenile court. In some instances, the minor may be waived to adult court. State law governs which of three types of such waivers will apply in an individual case. Waiver statutes typically take the form of "Youths over the age of X, who are charged with one of the following offenses…, may [or shall] be waived to adult court if…" *Judicial waivers* are those in which there is a hearing before a juvenile court judge, who will typically consider the nature of the crime, the likelihood of future dangerousness, and the youth's amenability to rehabilitation in deciding whether to move the case to adult court. *Direct file* or *prosecutorial waivers* allow the prosecutor to decide in certain cases (such as murder committed by a youth over a certain age) to move the case to adult court. *Mandatory* or *legislative waivers* derive from statutes that, on the basis of the defendant's age and the charge, automatically waive the youth to adult court.

Practically all states have some form of judicial waiver. The U.S. Supreme Court has held that a judge cannot waive a youth without a hearing (*Kent v. United States* 1966). In response to the upsurge in juvenile crime in the early 1990s, many states adopted direct file or mandatory waivers. In 1998, 15 states had some form of direct file waiver and 27 states had mandatory waivers for certain crimes (Griffin et al. 1998). There are no federal juvenile courts: minors arrested on a federal charge have a hearing before a federal district court judge on whether they should be prosecuted in federal court or remanded to a state juvenile court.

Waiver hearings commonly make use of mental health evaluations to assist them in making a determination. Judges have considerable discretion in what factors they consider and how they weigh each factor. The statutory criteria for waiver to federal court (18 U.S.C. § 5032) are typical and include the age and social background of the juvenile, the nature of the alleged offense, the extent and nature of the juvenile's prior delinquency record, the juvenile's present intellectual development and psychological maturity, the nature of past treatment efforts and the juvenile's response to such efforts, and the availability of programs designed to treat the juvenile's behavioral problems.

If a youth is waived to adult court, the full panoply of adult criminal process comes into play, including issues of competency to stand trial and insanity or other diminished-capacity defenses. Insanity defenses are very rare in waived youths because the incidence of psychosis is considerably lower in adolescents than in adults and because severe mental illness is a strong reason not to waive a youth to adult jurisdiction.

If a youth remains under juvenile court jurisdiction and emotional disturbance is thought to play a role in the youth's behavior, the juvenile court judge will often order a mental health evaluation. This evaluation, often referred to as a "study and report," is intended to assist in formulating a disposition. A study and report is a general psychological evaluation that often includes psychological testing and concludes with recommendations for mental health interventions. If the defendant youth was in treatment prior to arrest, the treating clinician may be contacted to provide collateral information.

## Assessments Around the Time of Arrest

> G, age 14, was brought by his father for an urgent consultation after a neighbor said that his 4 year-old daughter alleged that G had asked her to take off her pants and "touched my privates." G had had no previous history of such problems or of any other mental health problems. The father wanted to know "Did I miss something?" and was very worried G might be arrested.

A parent may bring a youth to a psychiatrist because the parent anticipates an arrest and wishes to receive guidance on how to proceed. In this case example, the clinician at this point owes a duty to G as his patient, not to the police. However, the possible impending arrest makes this evaluation different from other clinical encounters. First, although the evaluation is confidential, the psychiatrist has an obligation to notify child protective services if he or she has a reasonable suspicion that child abuse took place. Thus, the clinician should inform both the father and the patient of this duty prior to asking about material that may lead to such a report.

Second, if the parent has not obtained the services of an attorney for his son, the psychiatrist should recommend strongly that the parent do so. The psychiatrist should seriously consider deferring the evaluation until an attorney has been retained or appointed. In most cases, the psychiatrist should not ask about the circumstances of the alleged abuse (or other crimes) at all until he or she has a clear sense of what questions the attorney will ask. Following this course of action will help the psychiatrist avoid the possibility that the psychiatric evaluation will be used to incriminate the patient.

In addition, if no attorney has been obtained or appointed, the psychiatrist should discuss with the father what to do if the youth is questioned by the police. Without giving legal advice, the psychiatrist should help the father and adolescent understand their options and some of the possible consequences of cooperating with the police. As is the case for any criminal suspect, talking to the police without first consulting with an attorney is seldom in the youth's best interest. If arrested, the youth will be given a *Miranda* warning. Younger adolescents may cognitively understand what a *Miranda* warning is but are nevertheless more likely to waive their rights and confess than are older adolescents or adults (Grisso 1981). In most states, police are not allowed to question a suspect who is a minor without a parent's permission. However, parents who have raised their child to be honest and to admit mistakes may advise their child to confess to the police.

Once a youth has an attorney, the psychiatrist can be helpful to his or her patient by working with the attorney. The authorities have wide discretion in juvenile cases on questions of what charge to bring (e.g., manslaughter rather than murder) and disposition (i.e., probation with conditions rather than incarceration). This discretion includes whether to arrest the youth at all. Rapid institution of treatment may decrease the likelihood of arrest. A skilled attorney can have considerable impact on the course of a case by negotiating with the authorities without resorting to formal criminal procedures. A youth's attorney can often make effective use of mental health information and treatment plans in such negotiations.

The cautions about obtaining incriminating information discussed above become even more imperative in situations in which the youth is unaccompanied by a parent. For example, a general psychiatrist providing coverage to an emergency room may become involved in a case when the police bring a distressed, just-arrested youth to an emergency room. The psychiatrist should provide limited treatment for acute distress (assuming appropriate informed consent can be obtained). However, he or she should be acutely aware that any information obtained during evaluation and treatment may not remain confidential. A clinician unfamiliar with juvenile criminal processes, in the mistaken belief that he or she is helping, all too often will begin an interview in the emergency room by asking, "What happened?" The clinician then continues to obtain highly incriminating information that may get passed along, formally or informally, to law enforcement. Even if the information obtained remains confidential, legal consequences may follow from the fact that the youth has told his story without having a clear understanding of the implications of doing so. One of these may be the youth's own belief that he has already "confessed" and so is ready to repeat his story before obtaining the advice of counsel ("After all, I already told the doctor what happened…").

## Treatment Following Adjudication

> J, age 15, was adjudicated as delinquent on a charge of aggravated assault stemming from hitting a classmate in the head with a book bag. The court mandated treatment, and J was referred to a general psychiatrist who also treated adolescents. The youth's probation officer wanted regular progress reports.

A general psychiatrist who accepts a patient for whom psychiatric treatment is made a condition of probation may be required to share certain information that would normally be confidential. The psychiatrist should be certain to have a clear understanding with both the probation officer and the patient regarding the nature of the information that will be provided to the probation officer. Clinicians vary in how they structure such understandings. As a general rule, the clinician treating adult patients can attempt to maintain the confidentiality by making clear that he or she will advise the probation officer only about whether the patient is coming and whether the psychiatrist believes treatment is completed. The patient should also be advised that if the sessions are not paid for, the patient will not be seen and this will be reported to the probation officer as nonattendance. With adolescent patients, the psychiatrist may need to broaden this stance to some degree. A juvenile probation officer can assist the clinician in obtaining court and community services and thus can be a very useful ally. The psychiatrist will likely want to have the option of being able to release to the probation officer information that will justify additional services.

## School Threat Assessments

> A teacher in a small, rural town was told by a student that her friend, 16 year-old C, told her that she "might want to stay home from school next Tuesday because 'not everybody will be going home that day.'" The school referred C to the only psychiatrist in town for an emergency assessment of his dangerousness.

Mass school shootings generate enormous amounts of media coverage and grave concerns about school safety. The shootings in Littleton, Colorado, have come to exemplify such acts of violence. From 1992 through March 2001, there were 19 incidents, including two instances in which two students participated in shooting at classmates (for descriptions of these incidents, see Verlinden et al. 2000). As a result, schools have become highly sensitized to possible threats, such as the one presented in the case above. Statistics reassuringly demonstrate that schools are safer than media coverage may imply. A youth is far more likely to be shot away from school than at school (Kaufman et al. 2000). Nevertheless, students who are thought to pose some threat are frequently sent for psychiatric evaluation.

Detailed psychiatric information about school shooters is difficult to obtain. Some of the killers committed suicide immediately after the shootings. Others have been protected by the confidentiality of the juvenile court. Therefore, most information about individuals who commit such acts has been limited to publicly available data. Verlinden and colleagues (2000) identified a number of characteristics common to these offenders. These include prior threats of violence; having a detailed plan; blaming others for problems; a history of regression, uncontrolled anger, depression, and troubled family relationships; poor coping and social skills; alienation from peers; fascination with weapons and explosives; preoccupation with violent media and music and with attack-related behavior such as an interest in targeted violence; and social-environmental factors such as access to firearms. Meloy and colleagues (2001) identified consistent findings in a study of juvenile mass murderers. In all cases, peers failed to report threats of serious violence to others and to consider the threats seriously. This fact has led to prevention efforts that emphasize assessing all threats of school violence, even those seemingly made in jest.

In the example case above, the school sent C for emergency evaluation immediately upon being advised by his friend of his statements. The disclosure of a threat is usually the trigger to an evaluation. Most threats are not carried out, but all need to be considered seriously. However, not all threats are equal. More severe threats should prompt more intensive evaluation. Threats that are vague, implausible, or made in a context that suggests they will not be carried out call for a less intensive workup than threats that are specific or indicate active planning.

Threat evaluation research has grown largely out of law enforcement work focused on adults, but similar principles likely apply to adolescents. Many psychiatrists tend to think about the assessment of potential violence as similar to the assessment of suicidal thinking, with its emphasis on identifying risk factors, violent ideation, and plan. However, such evaluations have been recognized to be fairly ineffective in predicting planned, predatory violence. Threat evaluation has moved away from profiling the subject toward evaluating pathways that lead to violent action. Such evaluations look less at the characteristics of the subject and more at recent behavior that suggests the subject is moving on a path toward violence (Borum et al. 1999).

The FBI recommends assessment in four domains: personality characteristics, family dynamics, school dynamics, and social dynamics (O'Toole 1999). Since individuals frequently deny planning predatory violence, other indicators of violent thinking are important. A key concept in these evaluations is "leakage": fantasies of thinking and planning violence may spill out in identifiable ways. These can include talking about a fascination with weapons and assassinations with peers, diaries or other written communications, drawings, Internet chatting on violence-related themes, veiled threats expressed to peers, and so forth.

Using these principles, federal law enforcement agencies have developed threat assessment procedures for schools (O'Toole 1999; Vossekuil et al. 2002). These approaches emphasize that attack is the consequence of an understandable and discernible process of thinking and behavior. In evaluating a pathway toward violence, actions that indicate planning, such as practice with a weapon or surveillance of a victim, are especially worrisome. A youth will frequently deny planning violence in interviews. Therefore, collateral information, particularly from peers, is vital.

The best way to obtain a comprehensive picture of recent actions usually involves working as part of a team with school personnel and law enforcement. A clinician should be very cautious, once a serious threat has been made, in concluding, solely on the basis of findings from an individual interview, that the risk of violence is low. It is a mistake to think that an individual interview is likely to get at the most significant data. Nevertheless, an individual interview can identify many factors that may be significant in the overall and comprehensive assessment of risk of violence. The most important domains to assess in an individual interview appear to be the following:

1. Mental illness and/or substance abuse
2. Fascination with, and increasing interest in, weapons, attacks, and attack-related behaviors
3. Leakage and fantasy material of a violent nature
4. Talk or writings about committing violent acts
5. Alienation and narcissism
6. Specificity of details: plan, target, and so forth
7. Recent loss or prior history of suicidal thinking

Findings from a psychiatric evaluation then need to be integrated with information from other sources to develop an assessment of the level of risk and a prevention plan.

> C admitted to the evaluating psychiatrist that he had been feeling depressed and quite resentful of the "popular crowd." School personnel learned from several of C's peers that he had been making threats. With the parents' permission, the police searched C's bedroom and found directions for building a bomb and several drawings of schoolrooms with what looked like computations of blast effect. C was deemed to be at high risk and was admitted to an inpatient psychiatric facility.

## Conclusion

Legal cases involving children and adolescents often answer important questions affecting the child's future: whether the child will be with mother or father, with parents or in foster care, in special education or mainstreamed, in treatment or in jail. Such determinations have a profound effect on the child's development. While general psychiatrists will want to be careful about practicing within the limits of their competence when it comes to child and adolescent issues, helping to make these determinations in such a way as to benefit children makes forensic work with children very rewarding.

## Key Points

- Forensic evaluation of preadolescents usually requires specialized training in child and adolescent psychiatry.
- Forensic evaluations of adolescents may be done by general psychiatrists who additionally can demonstrate special training and experience with adolescent populations.
- Opinions on parenting functions should be limited if parent-child interaction is not directly assessed.

- The rehabilitative mission of the juvenile court broadens the usefulness of mental health input as compared with adult criminal procedures.
- Assessments of threats of predatory violence should focus on ascertaining whether the youth is on a behavioral path toward violence.

## Practice Guidelines

### Clarification of Role at Outset of Evaluation

1. Be clear on the forensic question being asked.
2. Clarify who is requesting evaluation, to whom the report will be sent, and issues of consent.
3. Avoid forensic evaluations of one's own patients.

### Evaluations of Parents Involved in Litigation With Their Child

1. Opinions on the best interests of a child in a custody arrangement should not be given without evaluation of both parents, the child, and the interaction of parents and child except under unusual circumstances.
2. Evaluations of parenting capacity should make a clear link between mental disorder and parenting.

### Evaluations of Youth Facing Criminal Charges

1. Only very limited evaluation should occur prior to a youth's obtaining an attorney.
2. Evaluations of whether to waive to adult jurisdiction turn on assessment of dangerousness and amenability to rehabilitation.

### Evaluations of Threats of Predatory Violence

1. Focus on moving along a path toward violence rather than on static risk factors.
2. Remember that collateral information, especially from peers, is very important.
3. Strongly consider a team approach that includes school personnel, law enforcement, and mental health evaluation as the preferred way of obtaining a comprehensive assessment of moderate to serious threats.

## References


Accreditation Council for Graduate Medical Education: Program Requirements for Residency Education in Forensic Psychiatry. Chicago, IL, Accreditation Council for Graduate Medical Education, 2003

American Psychological Association, Committee on Professional Practice and Standards (COPPS): Guidelines for child custody evaluations in divorce proceedings. Am Psychol 49:677–680, 1994

Ash P, Guyer M: The functions of psychiatric evaluations in contested child custody and visitation cases. J Am Acad Child Psychiatry 25:554–561, 1986

Benjamin M, Irving HH: Research in family mediation: review and implications. Mediation Quarterly 13:53–82, 1995

Borum R, Fein R, Vossekuil B, et al: Threat assessment: defining an approach for evaluating risk of targeted violence. Behav Sci Law 17:323–337, 1999

Emery RE: Renegotiating Family Relationships: Divorce, Child Custody, and Mediation. New York, Guilford, 1994

Griffin P, Torbet P, Szymanski L: Trying Juveniles as Adults in Criminal Court: An Analysis of State Transfer Provisions (NCJ 172836). Washington, DC, U.S. Department of Justice, Office of Justice Programs, Office of Juvenile Justice and Delinquency Prevention, 1998

Grisso T: Juveniles' Waiver of Rights. New York, Plenum, 1981

Haller LH (ed): Forensic psychiatry. Child Adolesc Psychiatr Clin N Am 11(4) (entire issue), 2002

Herman SP: American Academy of Child and Adolescent Psychiatry. Practice parameters for child custody evaluation. J Am Acad Child Adolesc Psychiatry 36 (10, suppl):57S–68S, 1997

In re Gault, 387 U.S. 1 (1967)

Johnston JR, Campbell LE, Tall MC: Impasses to the resolution of custody and visitation disputes. Am J Orthopsychiatry 55:112–129, 1985

Kaufman P, Chen X, Choy SP, et al: Indicators of School Crime and Safety, 2000 (NCES 2001-017/NCJ 184176). Washington, DC, U.S. Departments of Education and Justice, 2000

Kent v United States, 383 U.S. 541 (1966)

Meloy JR, Hempel AG, Mohandie K, et al: Offender and offense characteristics of a nonrandom sample of adolescent mass murderers. J Am Acad Child Adolesc Psychiatry 40:719–728, 2001

Nurcombe B, Partlett DF: Child Mental Health and the Law. New York, Macmillan, 1994

O'Toole ME: The School Shooter: A Threat Assessment Perspective. Washington, DC, U.S. Department of Justice, 1999

Parham v J.R. and J.L., 442 U.S. 584 (1979)

People v Stritzinger, 668 P.2d 738 (Cal. 1983)

Santosky v Kramer, 455 U.S. 745 (1982)

Schetky DH, Benedek EP (eds): Principles and Practice of Child and Adolescent Forensic Psychiatry. Washington, DC, American Psychiatric Publishing, 2002

State v Andring, 342 N.W.2d 128 (Minn. 1984)

Verlinden S, Hersen M, Thomas J: Risk factors in school shootings. Clin Psychol Rev 20:3–56, 2000

Vossekuil B, Fein R, Reddy M, et al: The Final Report and Findings of the Safe School Initiative: Implications for the Prevention of School Attacks in the United States. Washington, DC, U.S. Department of Education, Office of Elementary and Secondary Education, Safe and Drug-Free Schools Program, and U.S. Secret Service, National Threat Assessment Center, 2002

## Suggested Readings

Ash P: Malpractice in child and adolescent psychiatry. Child Adolesc Psychiatr Clin N Am 11:869–886, 2002

Ash P, Derdeyn AP: Forensic child and adolescent psychiatry: a review of the past 10 years. J Am Acad Child Adolesc Psychiatry 36:1493–1502, 1997

Barnum R: Parenting assessment in cases of neglect and abuse, in Principles and Practice of Child and Adolescent Forensic Psychiatry. Edited by Schetky DH, Benedek EP. Washington, DC, American Psychiatric Publishing, 2002, pp 81–96

Bernet W: Practice parameters for the forensic evaluation of children and adolescents who may have been physically or sexually abused. AACAP Official Action. American Academy of Child and Adolescent Psychiatry. J Am Acad Child Adolesc Psychiatry 36:423–442, 1997

Ceci SJ, Bruck M: Jeopardy in the Courtroom: A Scientific Analysis of Children's Testimony. Washington, DC, American Psychological Association, 1995

Dalton MA: Education rights and the special needs child. Child Adolesc Psychiatr Clin N Am 11:859–868, 2002

Elliott DS: Serious violent offenders: onset, developmental course, and termination. The American Society of Criminology 1993 Presidential Address. Criminology 32:1–21, 1994

Grisso T: Forensic Evaluation of Juveniles. Sarasota, FL, Professional Resource Press, 1998

Haller LH (ed): Forensic psychiatry. Child Adolesc Psychiatr Clin N Am 11(4) (entire issue), 2002

Herman SP: American Academy of Child and Adolescent Psychiatry. Practice parameters for child custody evaluation. J Am Acad Child Adolesc Psychiatry 36 (10, suppl):57S–68S, 1997

Leavitt WT, Armitage DT: The forensic role of the child psychiatrist in child abuse and neglect cases. Child Adolesc Psychiatr Clin N Am 11:767–780, 2002

Nurcombe B, Partlett DF: Child Mental Health and the Law. New York, Macmillan, 1994

O'Toole ME: The School Shooter: A Threat Assessment Perspective. Washington, DC, U.S. Department of Justice, 1999

Schetky DH, Benedek EP (eds): Principles and Practice of Child and Adolescent Forensic Psychiatry. Washington, DC, American Psychiatric Publishing, 2002

U.S. Dept. Health and Human Services: Youth Violence: A Report of the Surgeon General. Rockville, MD, U.S. Dept of Health and Human Services, Centers for Disease Control and Prevention, National Center for Injury Prevention and Control; Substance Abuse and Mental Health Services Administration, Center for Mental Health Services; and National Instititutes of Health, National Institute of Mental Health, 2001

Vossekuil B, Fein R, Reddy M, et al: The Final Report and Findings of the Safe School Initiative: Implications for the Prevention of School Attacks in the United States. Washington, DC, U.S. Department of Education, Office of Elementary and Secondary Education, Safe and Drug-Free Schools Program, and U.S. Secret Service, National Threat Assessment Center, 2002

CHAPTER 21

# Personal Violence

Alan R. Felthous, M.D.

## Introduction

Potentially violent patients are the concern of every psychiatrist and mental health professional. Assessment and treatment of clinical violence have been described in various texts and articles with which the reader is undoubtedly familiar. Here the focus is on contexts of special relevance to forensic psychiatric consultations.

Despite common themes in consultations regarding past or potential violence, contextual distinctions warrant the consultant's attention. Forensic psychiatrists are likely to be consulted in response to one of two situations involving potentially violent individuals: 1) in determining how to appropriately deal with a potentially violent person within the criminal justice system or in the community, and 2) in determining a legal duty to protect when a clinician is accused of professional negligence in failing to take reasonable action to prevent the patient from inflicting violence on others.

Forensic consultations concerning acts of personal violence can arise in the criminal justice system when the actor is charged with a criminal offense. The emphasis in this context is on risk assessment and prevention, not criminal competencies or adjudication of guilt. This chapter addresses consultation within the criminal justice system involving jail risk assessments, pretrial dispositions, dispositional determinations, not guilty by reason of insanity (NGRI) dispositions, and criminal sentencing and release decisions. Consultations regarding potentially violent individuals free in the community are also preventive in aim, designed to assess and diminish the risks. Contexts for consultations in the civil sphere include workplaces, schools, and homes, as well as other situations.

Professional negligence cases that involved the death or injury of a third person are of particular relevance to forensic consultants. Contexts to be addressed in claims of professional negligence include inpatient violence, post–hospital discharge violence, and outpatient violence.

## The Evaluation of Violence

Principles in risk assessment and approaches to preventing violence that cut across contexts include documentation, character pathology, and impulsive aggression. Any discussion of good practices and risk management appropriately emphasizes the importance of quality documentation in the medical record (Tardiff 2002). Assessment, treatment, and management of clinical violence should be supported by data and logic. Quality documentation in the evaluation and management of potentially violent patients forces clarity of thought and enhances the utility of the record as a clinical tool. Although "treatment of the chart" is certainly secondary to treatment of the patient, quality treatment must be based on data, sound clinical logic, and effective implementation, all supported by documentation. In claims of professional negligence, absence of charted information does not mean absence of care; however, establishing that appropriate care was provided becomes more difficult to demonstrate convincingly.

Character pathology presents a paradox for clinical assessment and management of future violence. Typically the most effective method for a clinician to protect the public from a patient's violence is to hospitalize the patient. Clinicians hospitalize patients for the treatment of major mental illness, including psychotic disorders. However, hospitalization for the purposes of treatment is not as universally accepted for patients whose primary pathology is that of a personality disorder absent an acute Axis I condition. Yet psychopathy, a severe form of character pathology, is a better predictor of future violence than any disorder of major mental illness (Hare 1991; Hare et al. 2000). In fact, current research indicates conventional treatments can make psychopathy worse (Hare 1991; Hare et al. 2000; Rice et al. 2002). The obvious paradox is that measurement of psychopathy will improve assessments of the risk of future violence for individuals for whom the safest short-term clinical intervention, hospitalization, may be antitherapeutic and, indeed, may enhance the future risk of violence. The consultant must confront this troublesome paradox and place appropriate emphasis on clinical issues and currently accepted standards of care.

A person's risk for violent behavior is dynamic and subject to change, sometimes dramatic change. The most violent of individuals are not violent all of the time, or even most of the time. Internal changes involving toxic or metabolic factors can lead to altered mental states with increased potential for aggressive behavior. External events that result in frustration, provocation, losses, and other acute stresses, as well as social influences such as gang activity, can also increase the potential for violence. In addition, these two categories are interactive and cannot always be separated. For example, environmental changes commonly lead to physical discomfort or autonomic arousal. Therefore, effective risk assessment is a dynamic, ongoing process, wherein an evaluator or treater looks for environmental and internal changes that promote or diminish the individual's likelihood of acting aggressively. Concurrent, ongoing assessment can also be coupled with efforts to gain a more complete and accurate history of static factors and to better understand the sensitive issues most likely to trigger an aggressive response.

Impulsive aggression (Barratt et al. 1997a, 1997b; Felthous and Barratt 2003; Stanford et al. 2001) is increasingly recognized as a treatable condition that is manifested by violent behaviors. The consultant who addresses violent individuals within and outside the criminal justice system must be prepared to identify the presence of impulsive aggression when assessing the intensity, severity, and frequency of violent acts. Impulsive aggression is a condition probably better recognized by researchers than by clinicians. Thus, its full assessment and appropriate treatment arguably are not yet mandated by standards of practice. Nonetheless, the favorable response of impulsive aggression to pharmacotherapy can result in better control of impulsive aggression among individuals with antisocial personality disorder (Barratt et al. 1997a), persons who would otherwise be considered resistant to treatment efforts.

The relevance of the concept of impulsive aggression to consulting forensic psychiatrists may not be immediately obvious. It is not a formal *Diagnostic and Statistical Manual* (DSM) disorder, and it has much in common with intermittent explosive disorder (IED), which is a DSM disorder (American Psychiatric Association 2000). However, consultants familiar with the literature on impulsive aggression and IED will be better informed about the nature of common forms of abnormal aggression. They will therefore be better able to evaluate, treat, and manage aggression and to provide opinions regarding the clinical performance of other clinicians in cases of claimed professional negligence.

In addition, useful knowledge about impulsive aggression has increased significantly in recent years, while the basic concept has remained unchanged. In contrast, the criteria for IED in DSM-IV (American Psychiatric Association 1994) changed significantly. Until this edition of DSM, IED was conceptualized as episodic dyscontrol of aggressive behavior out of character and inconsistent with the individual's baseline patterns of behavior. This feature was ensured by the exclusion criteria that specified the absence of generalized impulsiveness or aggressiveness between the episodes. Although this exclusionary criterion was eliminated in DSM-IV, the earlier concept persists. Thus, clinicians using the principle of parsimony in diagnosis attribute impulsive aggression to character pathology when, for example, a diagnosis of antisocial personality disorder or borderline personality disorder can be made.

The concept of impulsive aggression has been and continues to be more inclusive yet more precise in its description and therefore more often indicative of potentially efficacious therapeutic approaches. The importance of its familiarity to consultants is the disorder's conceptual constancy, construct validity, psychological and physiological manifestations, frequency, comorbidity with other disorders, and favorable response to treatment (Barratt et al. 1997a, 1997b; Felthous and Barratt 2003). In fact, a case has been made for recognizing impulsive aggression as a disorder (Felthous and Barratt 2003). Although the use of a non-DSM diagnosis may be problematic in testimony (see Chapter 6: "Psychiatric Diagnosis in Litigation," this volume), it is nevertheless particularly helpful in treatment consultation contexts.

Despite the commonality of such issues in the forensic assessment of violence, context will clearly be of major significance in any assessment. Space does not allow inclusion of all the contexts in which the forensic evaluation of personal violence may arise or the comprehensive treatment in any single context. This chapter does not attempt to address every possible situation but rather emphasizes issues specific to each context and encourages the reader to examine other treatises for a more complete understanding of any particular setting.

Two principles relative to any situation will determine the focus and depth of the evaluation of violence: the apparent need (e.g., the subject is threatening violence vs. the subject is showing no signs of aggression) and the clinical situation (e.g., providing anxiety reduction for people trying to give up cigarette smoking vs. treating hospitalized insanity acquittees).

## Potentially Violent Persons in the Criminal Justice System

Forensic consultations in the criminal justice system subserve the general purpose of preventing future violence. In criminal law, however, the consultant can also be called on to provide input regarding assessment of guilt and, after adjudication, of punishment. Courts may not always use or require clinical information in making their determinations. Nevertheless, many courts may use psychiatric assessments of the risk of violence in determining whether to deny bail, whether restoration of competency should take place in a secure hospital setting, or whether after conviction it is safe to release the defendant on probation. Parole boards may rely on psychiatric or psychological assessments in determining whether a prisoner is sufficiently risk-free to warrant early parole.

## Jail

### Clinical Vignette[1]

A 29-year-old jail inmate was referred for a psychiatric consultation after he assaulted another inmate. His family history and childhood behaviors were consistent with an assaultive predisposition. Mother and father fought physically when intoxicated, and mother once shot father. She left him and married a man who abused the subject. Mother also punished the subject excessively by whipping him with extension cords, coat hangers, and a water hose and slapping him in the face.

Childhood behavior consistent with conduct disorder included school truancy, behavior leading to school suspensions, fighting, destruction of property, window breaking, and recurrent, severe cruelty to animals, including many cats.

After mental status examination and further studies, diagnoses included antisocial personality disorder and mixed personality disorder with schizotypal, borderline, and paranoid features, as well as a history of alcohol and cocaine abuse.

The night before the assault that occasioned his psychiatric referral, the inmate dreamt that another inmate attempted to harm him. Though not in any other way psychotic or delusional, he was convinced by virtue of his dream that this particular inmate would seriously harm him if he did not attack the other inmate first. Careful history revealed that the same pattern had happened at least twice before. On two previous occasions, a nocturnal dream had identified someone in the subject's social environment as a threat. Both times, he attacked the other person preemptively, once with a knife.

In an attempt to favorably alter the inmate's sleep architecture and to decrease the sense of tension, the consultant prescribed doxepin, which had no effect. Though seen by the consultant with increased regularity, the violent dream–persecutory belief–violent act sequence occurred again. This time the inmate attempted to enucleate another inmate's eye. Doxepin was replaced with thiothixene concentrate 10 mg/day, which was apparently effective in treating the encapsulated persecutory

[1]Felthous 1993; condensed and printed with permission from Whurr Publishers, Ltd.

beliefs associated with violent dreams. No further troubling dreams or acts of violence occurred for the duration of the inmate's jail detainment.

*Comment.* Sometimes the pathology behind a violent act is an uncommon and unstudied but exquisitely treatable condition. In looking for commonly recognized factors in individual assessments, psychiatrists should remain alert for unusual psychological processes that can benefit from appropriate treatment (Felthous 1993). In this case, if the evaluation had concluded after the mental status exam and other studies, a critically important clinical finding would have been overlooked.

A common task for psychiatrists who consult to jails is to conduct risk assessments of inmates. Even though suicide is a more frequent risk than homicide for suspects booked into a jail, the criminal behaviors for which individuals are arrested are often aggressive. Some attempt to assess for the risk of violence is useful. Occasionally recent threats, preparatory behaviors, or recent overt acts make such an assessment imperative.

Serious assaults and homicides can occur inside jails. These acts can be impulsive and without warning or carefully planned well in advance. All inmates who are seen for the first time should be screened for homicidal ideation. When special reason for concern arises, the consultant should examine recent and past acts of violence, motivations, circumstances, methods of execution, seriousness of injuries, and other outcomes. Assaultive ideation should be evaluated for seriousness of intention and care in planning and should be probed for the degree of absolutistic (no other alternatives) and deterministic (strong and unwavering) thinking. When an identifiable victim resides in the jail and the risk is high, some physical separation may be indicated. When the identifiable victim is in the community, an attempt to warn the victim may be indicated (see "The Potentially Violent Person in the Community" section later in this chapter).

The consulting psychiatrist's initial assessment should include, at a minimum, a review of the index offense, especially if violent in nature. As in any psychiatric evaluation, a history of prior violent acts and a mental status exam that includes inquiry about current thoughts of homicide or other acts of violence should also be obtained. When the risk of violence appears to be imminent and high, the psychiatrist should make reasonable preventive recommendations. If the inmate is mentally ill as well as potentially violent, appropriate care and management should include arrangements for psychiatric treatment and follow-up care. Such planning is complicated by the fact that the consultant may not know when the inmate will be released from jail.

The assessment of the risk of violence for any individual requires that the consultant follow the two-step process of first determining the diagnosis, if one exists, and then characterizing the nature of the potential aggression. If the most likely next act of violence is expected to be impulsive and the inmate is without evidence of other mental illness or defect, the consultant should evaluate for intermittent explosive disorder (American Psychiatric Association 1994, 2000; Felthous et al. 1991) or impulsive aggression (Felthous and Barratt 2003). Therapeutic interventions in these conditions may prevent violent acts.

## Pretrial Dispositions

### Clinical Vignette

A young man arrested and jailed in connection with an apparent homicide was referred for a forensic consultation to address competency to stand trial and the need for psychiatric hospitalization. Anamnesis revealed that he did not have a significant history of assaulting people. However, he had tortured and killed cats and dogs over the years for sadistic pleasure. Close relatives confirmed his animal cruelty. He explained the homicide as an extension of his animal cruelty; motivated by pleasure, not by passion or personal gain. Diagnoses included antisocial personality disorder and malingering. On the basis of these diagnoses, hospitalization was not recommended.

During the course of the evaluation, the defendant threatened to kill the evaluator, the evaluator's secretary, and several principals in the upcoming trial once he had an opportunity to do so. He was detained in jail and could be convicted and transferred to prison. Nonetheless, the risk was substantial, within his means once released, and he had already demonstrated the capacity for such violence. In addition, hospitalization was not an option. Therefore, careful documentation and warnings to the identifiable victims were made. The court and the head of the jail were also notified, as was the defendant's attorney to ensure that his legal rights were protected. All of these measures were explained to the defendant to further enhance protection for potential victims and to benefit the defendant himself. After a short time in prison, the man was released; no one was notified, but he was reportedly soon rearrested, this time for robbery.

*Comment.* A psychiatric disposition was not indicated in this case. Nonetheless, the defendant's credible threats raised the question of what other safety measures, if any, were appropriate. Some might advise against warnings in this situation, because the risk, though substantial, was not clearly imminent. The state supreme court would later find that no duty to warn identifiable victims exists and that such warnings could violate confidentiality laws. Arguably, confidentiality in the face of a violent peril is not paramount in *forensic* evaluations performed at the request of the court. Nevertheless, the warnings and notifications in the case seemed practical, helpful, and consistent with the *Tarasoff* case (*Tarasoff v. Regents of the University of California* 1976) and other appellate decisions in the state. Perhaps the fact that this man did not follow through on his homicidal threats once released indicates the risk was short-lived. On the other hand, he may have been deterred from carrying out his threats by the warnings and notifications and the informing of the defendant about the necessity for these disclosures. The interventions may have avoided any wrongful death litigation by lessening the risk of homicide, even if, retrospectively after the state supreme court's holding, the disclosures created some risk of liability.

## Dispositional Determinations

A number of dispositional determinations may require risk assessments. These include hospitalization, placement on parole, placement on probation, and various other placements associated with special offender adjudications. In some jurisdictions the statute on competency to stand trial requires the consultant to address in a separate report the dispositional needs of the defendant, such as hospitalization or placement in a facility for the retarded. Criteria for hospitalization in order to provide treatment and restore to competency include danger to self or others. Such dispositional recommendations serve therapeutic and humanitarian rather than penal purposes. They assist the court in placing the defendant in the least restrictive and most therapeutically appropriate setting while protecting the public. Sometimes, when hospitalization is not appropriate, other protective measures are nonetheless reasonable.

## Not Guilty by Reason of Insanity Dispositions

Some offenses are inherently violent (e.g., murder vs. illegal possession of a controlled substance). However, the presence or degree of violence is not an element of a mental illness defense. Tests for insanity do not include a criterion as to whether or not the defendant acted violently at the time of the offense. A consultant addressing the defendant's mental state at the time of the offense should make every effort to remain objective and honest and to avoid any bias from the nature of the criminal act. It would obviously be improper if, for example, an expert were to offer findings in support of sanity because the charge is murder rather than a nonviolent offense.

Once a defendant is found NGRI, a consultant may be called on to conduct a diagnostic and risk assessment for appropriate placement. Options may include an outpatient setting or a nonsecure, medium secure, or maximum security hospital. A determination regarding the level of security required involves assessment of the risk of escape as well as the risk of violent behavior. After a NGRI acquittee is hospitalized, the patient should be assessed and monitored for inpatient violence potential to ensure safe management. The acquittee should be reassessed for risk of violence prior to any dispositional decision such as discharge or transfer to a less restrictive hospital setting. If the patient is in a maximum security hospital, a critical issue is when the patient can be transferred to a less restrictive hospital setting. The risk assessment for a patient found NGRI of a violent offense such as murder should be especially thorough and methodical.

The effort to separate therapy and treatment from forensic evaluations is clinically and ethically important to avoid conflicting roles vis-à-vis the patient. This does not mean, however, that all clinical assessments should be hermetically compartmentalized from clinical treatments. If the treating clinician is to be most effective, legal objectives such as restoration of competency to stand trial and restoration of sanity must be kept in mind. For example, one of the most common treatment goals in a maximum security facility is rendering the patient suitable for transfer to a less restrictive setting by increased symptom control as well as reduced risk of violence. Both accurate diagnostic assessment and effective treatment are ongoing processes. Similarly, safe management during treatment requires a dynamic process of continuous risk assessment.

Analysis of past violent acts, with studied attention given to their relationship to the perpetrator's mental state and mental disorder at the time of the act, is of special importance in treating NGRI acquittees, making discharge decisions, and planning for aftercare. Tardiff (2002) has nicely summarized the relationship between common mental disorders and violence to assist the clinician in understanding, anticipating, and minimizing the risk of future violence.

The evaluation of violence risk in the setting of insanity acquittal of an individual who committed a violent act is held to a higher standard for thoroughness and detail than the evaluation of violence risk in other settings, such as a routine civil inpatient admission. Moreover, a second-level review process, such as that conducted by a hospital transfer committee or dangerousness review board, is recommended practice before the insanity acquittee patient is placed in a less protective setting. An adequate period of inpatient observation can be useful for evaluation as well as treatment. Step-down phases can assist in ongoing risk assessment, in ensuring least restrictive treatment, and in protecting the public in cases in which mentally ill persons have committed acts of extreme violence. For example, instead of being confined in a maximum security hospital until ready for release directly into the community, patients in a maximum security hospital are first transferred to a lower-level security or behavioral unit. From there, they are transferred to a typical inpatient setting, followed by supervised grounds passes, unsupervised grounds passes, and eventually total ambulatory care in the community. More will be said about evaluating a potentially violent patient prior to hospital discharge under the appropriate subsection on professional negligence consultations (see "Postdischarge Violence").

Administrative notification of victims and/or witnesses of a violent criminal act may apply to NGRI acquittees as well as convicted prisoners. As will be explained, this is an administrative requirement, not to be confused with the *Tarasoff* protective duties of clinicians. Nonetheless, the consultant should be aware that the notification process can impact the dynamics of risk assessment and management.

## Criminal Sentencing Dispositions and Release Decisions

The American Psychiatric Association's Task Force on the Role of Psychiatry in the Sentencing Process (1984) advises psychiatrists against making dispositional recommendations but approves of disclosing factors that can increase or decrease the risk of violence. Apart from insanity verdicts, in which defendants are found guilty of an offense, psychiatric input may be requested to assist the court in decisions regarding probation. Information about diagnoses, recommended treatments, and risk assessment are useful components of presentencing evaluations. The consultant can list and attempt to weigh those factors that enhance the risk of future violence and those expected to promote rehabilitation and control over recidivistic behaviors without making a recommendation for or against probation.

Risk assessments for purposes of sentencing will be most effective from an adjudicative perspective if the psychiatrist addresses contextual issues. For example, if the offender is an alcoholic given to binge drinking on the weekends and barroom fights while intoxicated, the consultant may advise initiating rehabilitation in jail and then continuing rehabilitation efforts, including Alcoholics Anonymous (AA) and avoidance of bars, when the individual is placed on probation. If the defendant is found guilty, the judge may use the consultant's recommendations to order the defendant placed on probation with the conditions that he attend AA and substance abuse counseling and that he be prohibited from visiting bars. Although less restrictive than imprisonment, these conditions could be experienced by the offender as less lenient than total confinement (Felthous 1989d). Nonetheless, the consultant addressed appropriate risk and contextual factors without recommending a specific disposition.

Consultations regarding parole are informed by similar considerations. The Hare Psychopathy Checklist—Revised (PCL-R; Hare 1991; Hare et al. 2000) is especially useful in assessing the risk of reoffending and violent behaviors in this context. Actuarial methods provide more accurate predictions of future violence than clinical methods (Monahan et al. 2001), and static variables are more predictive than dynamic ones (Rice et al. 2002). Thus, actuarial risk assessment instruments with static predictors are especially useful for early-release decisions in which concerns for future dangerousness are more compelling than need for immediate interventions. Ironically, some of the most powerful predictors of future violence are clinical disorders: psychopathy and drug or alcohol abuse (Monahan et al. 2001). Recent research indicates that early onset of criminal behavior predicts later violence in men diagnosed with schizophrenia (Tengström et al. 2001). These findings are consistent with the association between antisocial disposition and future violent behavior.

A reasonable predictor of future violence is a history of violent behavior (Klassen and O'Connor 1988; Resnick and Scott 1997), especially an ongoing pattern of aggressive acts. A thorough risk assessment, in either a civil or criminal context, will include a detailed history of prior acts of violence. Such a review should address the nature, frequency, and severity of such acts and the contextual or other factors that seem to have exacerbated or diminished the risk. Offense records, criminal records, and records of incidents within prison can be especially useful when the subject is already within the criminal justice system.

The prisoner who is potentially violent because of mental illness and whose sentence is about to expire should be considered for transfer to an appropriate mental hospital. This disposition should be considered whether or not the victim of the violence is identifiable. Civil commitment may be necessary if the individual is unwilling to admit himself or herself. Assessing and managing situations involving verbally threatened individuals who could foreseeably be victimized by the subject if given the opportunity will be discussed in the next section.

If the prisoner does not meet criteria for hospitalization (e.g., is not mentally ill) and another person lies in foreseeable peril after appropriate threat assessment, warning the likely victim and notifying police may be prudent, and even legally required, depending on state law. In the event that the prisoner expresses a threat against a person whom he or she has already victimized and who requested notification, the consultant should be aware of the administrative notification procedure. Specifically, the consultant should be familiar with the applicable victims' rights act, which may require a victim of a violent crime to be notified of the offender's release if such notification is requested in advance and in writing by the victim (e.g., Rights of Crime Victims and Witnesses Act in Illinois). The required notification does not require a verbal threat by the prisoner, or a threat assessment, or mental health evaluation of the offender by a mental health professional. The notification is handled administratively through the appropriate state's attorney's office.

## The Potentially Violent Person in the Community

### Workplace Violence

A forensic psychiatrist may be called on to consult to corporate personnel regarding an employee who is feared to have the potential for acting violently at the workplace. Lion (1999) has provided a useful discussion of such consultations, which the reader is encouraged to reference. Here some contrasts will be made between consultations regarding violence in a more typical civil context and those in employment settings.

In workplace violence consultations, the consultant evaluates the risk of violence before it happens and addresses what can be done to prevent future violence. Documentation and audio or visual recordings of threats, if they exist, should be reviewed. However, this type of risk assessment involves interviewing people more than reading records. Interviews should be conducted with supervisors, managers, coworkers, and, if cooperative, subjects themselves. The consultant then makes specific recommendations about helpful interventions for the individual and violence prevention for the company. Although actuarial approaches to risk assessment associate violence with youth, within the workplace, the risk of violence may actually be increased with advancing age and tenure within the company (Lion 1999).

The Americans with Disabilities Act (ADA) (1990) sets some parameters for dealing with employees who are mentally disabled and who present some risk of violence at the workplace. Two questions that first must be addressed are whether the employee has a *disability* and whether the individual presents a *direct threat* (Wylonis 1999). Employers must provide reasonable accommodation for employees with qualifying psychiatric disabilities unless such efforts would cause an undue hardship for the employer or the employee presents a direct threat at the workplace. Thus, the consulting psychiatrist, in addition to addressing diagnosis and assessing the risk of violence to others, will assist in resolving the question of whether the employee in question poses "a significant risk to the health or safety of others that cannot be eliminated by reasonable accommodation" (Americans with Disabilities Act 1990, § 101-3, Title I [42 U.S.C. § 12111]).

### Other Civil Issues

Forensic consultants conduct risk assessments that address an individual's potential for violence in a variety of other civil legal contexts. Examples of such situations are domestic violence, including abuse of children, developmentally disabled persons, elderly persons, or partners (Resnick and Scott 1997); potential violence by children or adolescents at school; independent assessment for civil commitment; and fitness for inherently risky job assignments. Some of these assessments involve unique circumstances and inquiry needs, and some require assessment of other risks as well (e.g., risk of nonviolent child neglect). All such assessments should follow the two-phase process of addressing first diagnostic issues and then any psycholegal issue involving risk assessment (Felthous et al. 2000). However, the psychiatrist should bear in mind that risk assessment for violence potential is to some degree inherent in and flows from the diagnostic assessment. Such assessments should also include nondiagnostic considerations, such as circumstances that could increase or decrease risks.

## Professional Negligence and Third-Party Litigation

When a psychiatric patient injures or kills another person, the treating psychiatrist is often named in the subsequent lawsuit. In such situations, a forensic psychiatrist is typically consulted by attorneys either for the plaintiff or for the defendant clinician. Framed either as medical malpractice or as public policy, the assertion is that the clinician had a protective duty to the victim(s) and failed to conduct an adequate risk assessment or to take reasonable measures to protect the victim or both. One of the most important considerations in the determination of a legal duty to protect in such cases is the amount of control the psychiatrist had over the patient assailant. A psychiatrist is thought to have more control over an inpatient than an outpatient and more control over a court-committed patient than a voluntary inpatient. Three contexts warrant separate consideration: inpatient violence, violence following hospital discharge, and outpatient violence.

## Inpatient Violence

If an inpatient assaults and injures another patient or a staff member, the victim may sue the assailant's psychiatrist. Typically, the victim claims that the psychiatrist knew or should have known of the assailant's violent propensities and should have taken reasonable protective action. The forensic psychiatrist who receives a consultation request regarding third-party violence in a hospital should first determine whether jurisdictional law creates or circumscribes protective duties when an inpatient is the assailant. A psychiatrist, or the hospital, may have a duty to protect other hospitalized patients from assault, since they are less able to protect themselves by virtue of being confined and dependent on treaters. Whether protective duties exist at all depends on the relationship between the victim and the psychiatrist as much as that between the attacking patient and the psychiatrist.

The consultant should therefore first clarify whether case or statutory law in the jurisdiction would create, support, delimit, or bar protective duties involving inpatient violence against the particular victim. For example, a protective relationship does not necessarily pertain to hospital employees. Courts are divided on whether a psychiatrist has a duty to protect a hospital employee (Felthous and Kachigian 2001). In some cases the appellate courts have held that the lack of an exceptional relationship with the staff victim precluded the imposition of protective duties for the victim nurse (e.g., *Charleston v. Larson* 1998). In contrast, the Supreme Court of Tennessee (*Turner v. Jordan* 1997), finding the act and the victim to have been foreseeable, considered this sufficient to allow protective duties to flow directly to the victim nurse.

Third-party liability may also arise in an inpatient setting when the treating psychiatrist or another staff member is accused of deliberately harming an inpatient (e.g., *Almonte v. New York Medical College* 1994). The plaintiff will argue that the treater's therapist or supervisor should have foreseen and prevented the act. In such cases, the issue is not one of control. Rather, arguments center on whether the treater's supervisor should have foreseen the act and failed to take reasonable protective actions. A duty to protect inpatients from their treaters is actually more akin to outpatient protective duties, which will be discussed further below.

Such evaluations require an assessment of whether the standard of care was followed. The consultant should remain aware of the hospital clinician's continuous need to weigh the indications of restraining and other intrusive or coercive measures against the mandate to provide the least restrictive treatment. Thus, the consultant should recognize the need for inpatient psychiatrists to have enough flexibility to exercise clinical discretion. The consultant should examine available clinical findings and note omissions or oversights in the diagnostic and risk assessments, treatment, management, and application of protective measures. The consultant should at the same time systematically note the appropriate actions of the responsible psychiatrist. The final report may predominately support the defendant psychiatrist's case, criticize, or constitute a mixture of support and criticism.

Some attempt to assess for violence potential should be conducted on every hospital admission, even if just a question or two about aggressive behaviors and ideation. If aggressive behavior was the occasion for the admission or otherwise a prominent part of the initial presentation, a more extensive risk assessment for externally directed aggression would be expected. Patients may demonstrate no signs of abnormal aggression on admission but later make threats of harm or show excessive agitation. In these cases, the patient should have been evaluated again, with an attempt to identify precipitants and potential victims, and monitored accordingly.

Diagnosis and risk assessment go hand in hand. The consultant will look for adequacy of both assessments. Focus on risk of violence includes history with emphasis on frequency, severity, circumstances, predisposing factors and targets, behavior observed in the hospital, and mental status examination. The mental status exam should have addressed presence of irritability, impulsivity, anger, hostility, perceptions of mistreatment or delusions of persecution, and auditory hallucinations accompanied by intolerable affect or experienced as commands from familiar voices and congruent with delusions. Much like assessment for suicide, the mental status exam should also have addressed assaultive and homicidal ideation, plans, and seriousness of intent.

Beyond simply assessing the risk of violence, the competent clinician should have attempted to determine the *nature* of actual or potential aggressive behavior. For example, Barratt (1991) has classified human aggression as premeditated, impulsive, or medically related. Aggressive behavior that is medically related is the direct result of the primary medical or psychiatric disorder. This type of aggressive behavior generally improves when the symptoms of the disorder are brought under control.

Thus, the provision of the most appropriate treatment is one of the best means of preventing hospital violence (Felthous 1984). A psychiatrist who allows a patient's psychotic agitation to go unmedicated, for example, could be courting disaster. Impulsive aggression (Felthous and Barratt 2003), with intermittent, Vesuvian outbursts, may have responded to anticonvulsant, antimanic, or beta-blocker medication.

However, in many cases aggression is a shifting, fluid phenomenon, a hybrid of several types and resistant to intervention. Therefore, failure of clinical response does not necessarily mean that the clinician provided substandard care. Self-serving aggression, for instance, is least amenable to a medical approach in the course of hospitalization. Even purely medically related aggression does not always respond immediately to the first medicine or combination of medicines. Examination of the appropriateness and timeliness of treatment modalities specific to the disorder is an important task for the forensic consultant.

Consultants reviewing the pharmacotherapeutic management of an uncooperative inpatient should also consider whether emergency enforced medication should have been given. The most commonly prescribed medications for emergencies in which there is a risk of violent behaviors are antipsychotics and benzodiazepines. Indications for considering this intervention include agitation, impending violence, and a mental condition for which emergency medication is indicated. The use of emergency medication is restricted by jurisdictional law, and specific medications may have been contraindicated by the patient's medical condition or history of adverse side effects. If such medication was administered, consultants should check to ensure it was properly prescribed. They should also review whether the patient was appropriately monitored for any adverse or paradoxical effect such as intolerable akathisia or behavioral disinhibition.

Typically, use of emergency medication will have been followed by a petition for court-ordered medication. Court-ordered administration of medicine does not, however, invariably follow emergency administration. For example, the patient may have consented to take the medicine after the first forced administration and prior to the hearing. Likewise, depending on the mental health code, petitioning the court for enforced medication may have been appropriate, even essential, because of the substantial risk of violence to others without medication. This may be the case even when emergency administration was not legally justifiable because the risk, though substantial, was not yet immediate.

The consultant must consider, and look for, reasons both for and against each protective intervention that a prudent psychiatrist would have considered. The consultant should address not only whether less intrusive interventions were appropriate and attempted to prevent the violent incident but also whether the more restrictive measures of seclusion or restraint should have been implemented. Tardiff (1996) lists three indications that apply to both seclusion and restraint and two other indications that pertain only to the use of seclusion. Even with clinical indications present, the patient may have had a medical contraindication to seclusion or restraint. Alternatively, jurisdictional law and regulatory organizations may have restricted application, such that seclusion or restraint was not possible after all.

As in assessing risk for suicide, higher standards for evaluation and prevention of violence are expected in inpatient than in outpatient settings. Clinicians have more opportunity to evaluate, observe, monitor, and control patients' risky behaviors in a hospital setting. On the other hand, because they are in need of hospitalization, such severely and acutely disturbed patients can be extremely challenging. For this reason, sometimes despite everyone's best efforts, a patient acts violently, even in a hospital, and even when a thorough evaluation has been made and appropriate measures taken.

Inpatient care is likely to be provided by a treatment team or an array of professionals from different disciplines. Just as good care is the result of combined efforts, substandard care may be due to poor care from several different individuals or, not uncommonly, from poor communication between members of the treatment team. The psychiatrist may be considered to have oversight and directional accountability for other members of a treatment team. However, forensic experts may have to examine the performance of several individuals and to make independent assessments about the role of each in contributing or not contributing to a failure to protect a victim of inpatient violence.

## Postdischarge Violence

Proper risk assessment and its application to the discharge decision are important considerations for the consulting psychiatrist. Wrongful discharge may be claimed as a cause of action against the responsible psychiatrist or the hospital if a foreseeably violent inpatient is discharged, released into the community, and then seriously injures or kills someone. A number of third-party liability cases involve claims of negligent discharge or release (e.g., *Cairl v. State* 1982; *Canon v. Thumudo* 1985; *Chrite v. United States* 1983; *Davis v. Lhim* 1983; *Durflinger v. Artiles* 1981; *Holmes v. Wampler* 1982; *Paul v. Plymouth General Hospital* 1987; *Perriera v. State* 1986; *Sharpe v. S.C. Department of Mental Health* 1987).

As with third-party liability cases involving violent injury caused by inpatients, the consulting psychiatrist should first reference the jurisdictional law. The rules regarding liability are different in various states. As discussed elsewhere (Felthous 1989c), California psychiatrists enjoy statutory immunity for wrongful discharge decisions (*Karash v. County of San Diego* 1986; *Tarasoff v. Regents of the University of California* 1976).

Michigan psychiatrists who are state employees have sovereign immunity (*Canon v. Thumudo* 1985). In Kansas (*Hokansen v. United States* 1989), Texas (*Peavy v. Home Management of Texas* 1999; *Thapar v. Zezulka* 1998), and Virginia (*Nasser v. Parker* 1995), there is no liability associated with wrongful discharge unless the patient was civilly committed or under the psychiatrist's actual legal control.

Nonetheless, one would expect a reasonably prudent physician to conduct a risk assessment before discharging a patient with known violent propensities, even if the physician faces no professional liability for not doing so. At a minimum, basic questions about homicidal ideation and violent history should have been asked at admission and again prior to discharge. A specific claim such as wrongful discharge is typically accompanied by other traditional claims such as failure to properly diagnose and to provide appropriate treatment. Risk assessment may be subsumed under diagnosis, and discharge decisions and aftercare planning can be considered as aspects of treatment. The consultant should look for and note both proper and improper or insufficient diagnostic assessment and treatment, especially as such procedures pertain to the decision to discharge the patient and the timing of the discharge.

Diagnosis, risk assessment, treatment, and symptom control, including the control of violent behavior, are all interrelated efforts. Accordingly, the consulting psychiatrist should ascertain that members of the treatment team did not overly rely on a single, simple formula such as a no-harm contract in deciding when to discharge the patient. An extended period of time in the hospital without violent behavior supports discharge decisions, but this must be considered together with other clinical findings. For example, a patient who is violent as a result of psychotic agitation in the pathological context of schizophrenia, disorganized type, should be ready for discharge when violent behaviors have been brought under control with appropriate pharmacotherapy.

In contrast, a patient with delusional disorder, persecutory type, who acted violently when he had free access to weapons and victims in the community may not behave aggressively while under the supervision and structure afforded by hospital milieu. Yet the delusions that drove the patient to act violently in the community are as undiminished and compelling as they were before hospitalization. An extended period of nonviolence in the hospital is not as supportive of a release decision for this patient as it was for the schizophrenic patient whose aggressive behavior and psychotic symptoms improved concurrently as a result of effective treatment. Although most delusions are not associated with violence, some are, and the motivation for the violent act often appears congruent with or even driven by the delusions (Taylor et al. 1994). Thus, beyond comportment in the hospital, the consultant should attempt to look for a relationship between the delusion and the act and, prior to transfer of the patient to a less structured setting, ask, "What's changed?"

Managed care companies and other parties may encourage a pattern of premature discharge to contain costs. The consultant must bear in mind that such external pressures do not by themselves alter the standard of care for critically important clinical decisions such as when to discharge a patient who has demonstrated violent propensities (Felthous 1999; Simon 2001, pp. 179–214). For example, a patient may suddenly promise to control his aggression and show no aggressive behavior over 24 hours. However, over the previous week in the hospital, he acted aggressively on five separate occasions. This patient's recent improvement may therefore represent only a brief interval and does not necessarily establish the patient's readiness to be released. Similarly, the consultant should not place undue emphasis on the patient's no-harm contract when numerous other signs indicated that the patient could not have been expected to follow such a contract.

Some would advocate administration of a standardized risk assessment instrument prior to discharge. Such formal assessment instruments may increase the accuracy, limited as it is, of assessing the risk of postdischarge violence. The Psychopathy Checklist—Screening Version (PCL-SV), for example, has been shown to be a relatively strong predictor of violence among civil psychiatric patients (Skeem and Mulvey 2000).

Nevertheless, the omission of a risk assessment instrument does not in itself fall short of the present standard of care (Tardiff 2002). Although such instruments offer useful information, some contextual limitations should be appreciated. Recommended instruments tend not to focus on the nature of the mental disorder for which the patient received hospital treatment in the first place. Rather, the predictors are simply actuarial or they support a finding of some degree of psychopathology or antisocial behavior or both. For decisions whether to release prisoners on parole, as already discussed, assessment of psychopathy can be critically important. However, when the purpose of hospitalization is treatment, high scores on such instruments could favor preventive detention under the guise of treatment. Until this dilemma is more satisfactorily resolved, the consultant should hesitate to find that omission of a standardized risk assessment instrument constitutes a departure from the standard of care. Likewise, when such instruments are used, scores can be taken into account but should not form the sole basis for a decision of whether or not to discharge a patient.

## Littleton Guidelines

The Supreme Court of Ohio in *Littleton v. Good Samaritan Hospital* (1988) addressed the problem of how to determine whether a psychiatrist exercised professional judgment upon deciding to discharge a patient (Felthous 1989b; Felthous et al. 1991). In this case, the court formulated a legal standard that is sufficiently reasonable to provide general guidance in determining whether a reasonable, prudent psychiatrist standard was satisfied. The court held that a hospital psychiatrist should not be liable for the violent acts of a mental patient after discharge if the following conditions are satisfied:

> 1. [T]he patient did not manifest violent propensities while being hospitalized and there was no reason to suspect the patient would become violent after discharge, or
> 2. [A] thorough evaluation of the patient's propensity for violence was conducted, taking into account all relevant factors, and a good faith decision was made by the psychiatrist that the patient had no violent propensity, or
> 3. [T]he patient was diagnosed as having violent propensities, and after a thorough evaluation of the severity of the propensities and a balancing of the patient's interest and the interests of the potential victims, a treatment plan was formulated in good faith which included discharge of the patient. (*Littleton v. Good Samaritan Hospital* 1988)

The *Littleton* guidelines emphasize the importance of titrating the extent of assessment and intervention to the apparent need. The standard defined in this decision is not binding in other jurisdictions. However, it proffers well-reasoned parameters that can guide the forensic consultant's assessment of standard of care in cases in which violence has occurred after discharge.

## Duty to Warn

Forensic consultants may be asked to offer opinions regarding a clinician's duty to warn identifiable victims of a patient's potential for violence if a suit arises under circumstances such as those of *Tarasoff*. In that case, Prosenjit Poddar, a graduate student at the University of California at Berkeley, became infatuated with Tatiana Tarasoff, who was far less invested in their relationship. When Tatiana went to Brazil for the summer, Prosenjit felt dejected and began seeing a therapist at the university clinic. In the course of therapy Prosenjit told his therapist "that he was going to kill an unnamed girl readily identifiable as Tatiana" (*Tarasoff v. Regents of the University of California* 1976, p. 341) after her return from Brazil. Upon consultation with a clinic psychiatrist, the therapist notified the campus police and sent a letter to the chief of the campus police requesting police assistance in delivering Prosenjit to the hospital for admission. The police interviewed Prosenjit, obtained his promise not to go near Tatiana, and, without consulting his therapist, released him.

After this episode, Prosenjit dropped out of therapy. Two months later, Prosenjit went to Tatiana's place with a kitchen knife and a pellet gun. He attempted to talk with her and then stabbed her to death.

Tatiana's parent brought complaints against his treaters and the police officers. After a succession of appeals, the case reached the Supreme Court of California. The court articulated what has become known as the *Tarasoff principle,* or the therapist's duty to protect, which is most explicit about the obligation to issue *warnings:*

> When a psychotherapist determines, or pursuant to the standards of his profession should determine, that his patient presents a serious danger of violence to another, he incurs an obligation to use reasonable care to protect the intended victim against such danger. That discharge of such duty may require the therapist to take one or more of various steps, depending on the nature of the case, including warning the intended victim or others likely to apprise the victim of the danger, notify the police or taking whatever steps are reasonably necessary under the circumstances. (*Tarasoff v. Regents of the University of California* 1976, p. 340)

Traditionally, hospitalization was the most frequent and presumably the most effective intervention made by mental health professionals to prevent their patients from seriously harming others in the immediate future. In 1976 the California Supreme Court put psychiatrists and psychologists on notice that another protective intervention, warning potential victims or notifying police of the risk, existed. Failure to take these measures could result in liability.

Appelbaum (1985) recommended a three-step approach for dealing with Tarasoff duty-to-warn situations: 1) assessment of dangerousness, 2) selection of a course of action, and 3) implementation. This process applies to any clinical situation involving potential violence and is also consistent with the *Littleton* guidelines in the context of hospital discharge. Psychiatrists should not incur liability if they have documented their findings, reasoning, conclusions, and their acts of notification and warning (Felthous 1989c, pp. 108–109). The forensic consultant can use these models to come to an opinion regarding the standard of care in these situations.

Liability due to failure to warn upon discharging a patient should not be a frequent issue. Any danger to others caused by mental illness should have been brought substantially under control as a result of treatment in the hospital or the patient would not have been discharged. Nonetheless, such cases may arise and require evaluation by a forensic consultant. Several situations can occur in which warnings are prudent if not legally required by jurisdictional law. For example, even when the potential for violence is no longer present because of favorable response to treatment, clinicians who assume responsibilities for aftercare should be informed of any serious risks encountered earlier in the patient's treatment.

A patient known to be violent who escapes from the hospital should trigger concerns about warnings. The assistance of police will be required to have the patient safely returned if he or she was already involuntarily committed at the time of elopement or the psychiatrist had initiated commitment procedures. Police should be informed of specific risks presented by the patient. If the patient is targeting specific individuals who can best protect themselves if forewarned, then someone should warn them. When deciding who to warn, the clinician will have to consider which warnings are most practical and likely to be protective on the one hand and what the jurisdictional law allows on the other.

A second situation in which the duty to warn may arise is when the judicial system fails and a patient who is known to be dangerous is allowed to be lawfully discharged. An example of such a situation would be when a judge decides that a patient does not satisfy civil commitment criteria and the patient insists upon discharge but the psychiatrist has good reasons to believe the patient would seriously harm or kill an identifiable victim if he or she were to be released. A record supporting this scenario would establish the prudence of the psychiatrist's having notified the police and any identifiable victims of the specific danger. In evaluating any of these scenarios, the consultant will have to weigh prudent care against what the law permits and requires in the way of warnings.

A more difficult judgment for the clinician is whether to warn an identifiable victim when the risk is substantial but not imminent and the unwilling patient does not satisfy commitment criteria. Here the patient can be involved in the warning process, or at the very least aftercare treatment providers can be apprised so they can monitor the risk accordingly.

### *Vehicular Crashes*

An automobile is a potentially lethal machine. Litigation involving psychiatrists has resulted when a hospitalized patient, after discharge, caused a two-vehicle accident with death or injuries to one or more victims in the other car (*Cain v. Rijken* 1986; *Hasenei v. United States* 1982; *Naidu v. Laird* 1988; *Petersen v. State* 1983; *Schuster v. Altenberg* 1988). Such cases involve three different types of scenarios. One is the vehicular crash that results from medication-induced drowsiness at the wheel and the prescribing physician failed to inform the patient that the medicine could cause oversedation and impair driving (*Gooden v. Tips* 1983; *Kirk v. Michael Reese Hospital and Medical Center* 1985). The second scenario is when the crash is a true accident but is unrelated to any prescribed medication. Rather, the patient's driving is impaired by the disabling effects of mental illness and/or recent consumption of nonprescribed drugs or alcohol. The third situation is when the patient deliberately crashes into another vehicle.

A forensic consultant could be called upon to assess whether the standard of care was followed by the responsible hospital clinicians. Should the hospital psychiatrist have foreseen the patient's causing a vehicular crash and taken measures to prevent it? If the patient had a pattern of deliberate crashes or expressed crash ideation or threats, the reasonable physician should have evaluated such expressions and history as he or she would any other form of recurrent or threatened violence.

A task force of the American Psychiatric Association has stated that psychiatrists should not be responsible for determining whether their patients are safe and competent drivers (American Psychiatric Association 1993). Several authors (Godard and Bloom 1990; Pettis 1992) recommend that psychiatrists resist acknowledging responsibility for predicting and ensuring their patient's safe driving. Nonetheless, the issue has arisen in the past and is likely to occur in the future (Felthous 1989a). Appellate court decisions range from disapproval of holding psychiatrists responsible for their patients' automobile accidents (*Hasenei v. United States* 1982) to acknowledging valid claims in such litigation (*Naidu v. Laird* 1988; *Petersen v. State* 1983; *Schuster v. Altenberg* 1988). Thus, the consultant must again be aware of the appropriate jurisdictional law.

## Outpatient Violence

If the assailant who violently attacks or kills another person is an outpatient, the surviving victim or relatives of the deceased victim may claim that the psychotherapist or treating psychiatrist failed to take reasonable measures to protect the victim. Jurisdictional law defines whether protective measures, such as warning the victims and/or notifying the police, are legally required or even permissible. These laws vary widely (Felthous 1989b, 1989c; Felthous and Kachigian 2001; Simon and Sadoff

1992; Walcott et al. 2001). Even within a given state, appellate court holdings on whether therapists have a duty to take protective measures do not necessarily predict what the state's supreme court will determine (Felthous and Scarano 1999). In those states where legislatures have attempted to bring statutory clarity to the issue, the corresponding appellate courts do not necessarily follow, or in some cases even acknowledge, the protective disclosure statute (Kachigian and Felthous 2002).

If jurisdictional law establishes a legal duty for psychiatrists to make protective disclosures but none were made before the patient acted violently, the consultant should address whether such omissions would have been reasonable and within current standards of practice. Was the seriousness of the threat assessed and found insufficiently serious to warrant warning disclosures? Appelbaum's (1985) assessment, plan, and implementation approach described earlier (see "Duty to Warn" subsection) is especially appropriate in dealing with verbal threats by outpatients and is general and basic enough to be considered standard of practice. Borum and Ready (2001) offer a well-reasoned, methodical approach to assessing the seriousness of a threat. The Borum model, like other guidelines also available for threat assessment, is not widely enough used to be considered the standard of practice. Nonetheless, a data-based, reasoned decision that addresses magnitude of the threatened harm (e.g., lethality), undeterability of the intent, and the elements discussed by Borum and Ready may well have justified decisions to make or decline making protective disclosures.

Felthous (1999) has proffered an algorithm that can assist the forensic consultant beyond addressing the seriousness of the threat alone. He identified two questions critical in the assessment of the clinician's actions. The first is whether the patient should have been hospitalized. The second is whether protective disclosures should have been made to prevent harm to third persons. These two necessarily dichotomous decisions are based on four critical assessments:

1. Whether the patient was dangerous (i.e., risk for violence considered high)
2. Whether the patient's potential for violence was likely due to mental illness
3. Whether the risk of violence was imminent
4. Whether potential victims were identifiable

The consultant should describe the legal standard, including inconsistencies if any. He or she should then discuss whether the clinician's decision to issue or not to issue protective warnings was reasonable. If the law requires or permits protective disclosures and such disclosures were issued by the defendant clinician, the consultant should point out the appropriate action that was taken. Conversely, the issue from a legal point of view could be undisputed if the state supreme court prohibits disclosures. A treating clinician should not be faulted for failing to take a measure that was illegal. On the other hand, sometimes even an illegal measure can be eminently logical and even lifesaving. In some cases, the law itself is contradictory, for example, as when the statutory and judicial law are inconsistent.

The most common questions evaluated by forensic consultants regarding outpatient treatment and management of potentially violent patients tend to be more relevant to clinical issues than to protective disclosures. Was the patient appropriately diagnosed? Did the clinician perform a risk assessment? Was the patient seen with appropriate frequency? Was the treatment plan appropriate? Was hospitalization attempted when the patient's behavior demonstrated that he or she could not continue to be safely managed as an outpatient? Even in jurisdictions where no legal duty to hospitalize a dangerous patient exists, hospitalization of a patient who is manifestly dangerous to others because of an acute, serious mental illness clearly falls within the standard of practice.

## Conclusion

The discussion in this chapter has been directed toward assessing potential violence of individuals within the criminal justice system and responding to allegations of professional negligence when a psychiatric patient harms another person. These tend to be the contexts in which forensic consultants are asked to offer opinions regarding the appropriate evaluation and management of potentially violent patients. Unfortunately, despite the best efforts of clinicians and forensic consultants, the law may impose certain limitations on the ability to manage potentially violent patients. Not every patient who will foreseeably act violently and refuses voluntary hospitalization meets civil commitment criteria. Not every patient whose violence would be better controlled with medication but who refuses to give consent meets criteria for court-ordered medication. And, the law does not always permit, let alone require, the issuance of protective warnings. Whether the consult is in regard to management and treatment or to professional negligence, the forensic psychiatrist must always take into account the contours of jurisdictional law.

## Key Points

- The most common forensic consultations concerning acts of personal violence arise in the criminal justice system and in civil litigation alleging negligence against a defendant psychiatrist whose patient commits an act of violence.
- Risk assessments of violence, regardless of context, should consider diagnosis, amenability to treatment interventions, the nature of the potential aggression, history of violent behavior, and imminence of future violent behavior.
- One of the best ways to decrease the potential for violent behavior in a hospitalized patient whose aggression is causally related to mental illness is to provide adequate treatment for the underlying medical condition. This may include the administration of emergency medication on an involuntary basis.
- Jurisdictional law regarding the duty to warn potential victims of the possibility of harm varies. Clinicians should be aware of their responsibilities as defined by the law, but they should also consider taking prudent and reasonable steps to warn identifiable victims even if they are not legally required to do so.

## Practice Guidelines

1. Identify internal and external factors, including underlying character pathology, that may interact to increase or decrease potential risk of violence. Remember that risk of violent behavior is dynamic and subject to change.
2. Be sure to include in assessments of the risk of violence a review of history of prior violent acts and determination of a diagnosis and the nature of the potential aggression.
3. Consider the need for civil commitment for a prisoner who is potentially violent due to mental illness and whose sentence is about to expire.
4. In the evaluation of the standard of care in liability cases, consider the extent of the assessment and intervention relative to the apparent need.
5. In the evaluation of liability due to failure to warn, be familiar with the legal responsibilities according to jurisdiction. Remember that the duty to warn varies according to jurisdictional law. Evaluate the clinician's assessment of dangerousness, selected course of action, and implementation of that action.

## References


Almonte v New York Medical College, 851 F.Supp. 34 (D. Conn. 1994)

Americans with Disabilities Act, Public Law 101-336, stat. 327, July 26, 1990a, § 2 (42 U.S.C. §§ 12101, 12111)

American Psychiatric Association: A Report of the Task Force on the Role of Psychiatry in the Sentencing Process, in Issues in Forensic Psychiatry. Washington, DC, American Psychiatric Press, 1984, pp 181–215

American Psychiatric Association: The role of the psychiatrist in assessing driving ability (Position Statement No 930004). Washington, DC, American Psychiatric Association. Approved 1993.

American Psychiatric Association: Diagnostic and Statistical Manual of Mental Disorders, 4th Edition. Washington, DC, American Psychiatric Association, 1994

American Psychiatric Association: Diagnostic and Statistical Manual of Mental Disorders, 4th Edition, Text Revision. Washington, DC, American Psychiatric Association, 2000

Appelbaum PS: Rethinking the duty to protect, in The Potentially Violent Patient and the Tarasoff Decision in Psychiatric Practice. Edited by Beck J. Washington, DC, American Psychiatric Press, 1985, pp 110–130

Barratt ES: Measuring and predicting aggression within the context of a personality theory. Journal of Neuropsychology 3(2):535–539, 1991

Barratt ES, Stanford MS, Felthous AR, et al: The effects of phenytoin on impulsive and premeditated aggression: a controlled study. J Clin Psychopharmacol 17(5):341–349, 1997a

Barratt ES, Stanford MS, Kent TA, et al: Neurological and cognitive psychophysiological substrates of impulsive aggression. Biol Psychiatry 41:1045–1061, 1997b

Borum R, Reddy G: Assessing violence risk in *Tarasoff* situations: a fact-based model of inquiry. Behav Sci Law 19(3):375–386, 2001

Boulanger v. Pol, 900 P.2d. 823 (Kan. 1995)

Cain v Rijken, 717 P.2d. 140 (Or. 1986)

Cairl v State, 323 N.W.2d 20 (Minn. 1982)

Canon v Thumudo, 144 Mich. App. 604, 375 N.W.2d 773 (1985)

Charleston v. Larson, 297 Ill.3d 540; 696 N.E.2d 793; 231 Ill. Dec. 497 (Ill. App. Ct. 1998)

Chrite v United States, 564 F.Supp. 341 (E.D. Mich. 1983)

Davis v Lhim, 335 N.W.2d 481 (Mich. App. 1983)

Durflinger v Artiles, 563 F.Supp. 322 (D. Kan. 1981)

Felthous AR: Preventing assaults on a psychiatric inpatient ward. Hosp Community Psychiatry 35(12):1223–1226, 1984

Felthous AR: The duty to warn or protect to prevent automobile accidents, in American Psychiatric Press Annual Review of Clinical Psychiatry and the Law, Vol 1. Edited by Simon RI. Washington, DC, American Psychiatric Press, 1989a, pp 221–238

Felthous AR: The ever confusing jurisprudence of the psychiatrist's duty to protect. Journal of Psychiatry and Law 17(4):575–594, 1989b

Felthous AR: The Psychotherapist's Duty to Warn or Protect. Springfield, IL, Charles C Thomas, 1989c

Felthous AR: The use of psychiatric evaluations in the determination of sentencing, in Criminal Court Consultations. Edited by Rosner R, Harmon RB. New York, Plenum, 1989d, pp 189–208

Felthous AR: Unusual case report: do violent dreams cause violent acts? Criminal Behaviour and Mental Health 3(1):12–18, 1993

Felthous AR: The clinician's duty to protect third parties. Psychiatr Clin North Am 22(1):49–60, 1999

Felthous AR, Barratt ES: Impulsive aggression, in Aggression: Psychiatric Assessment and Treatment (Medical Psychiatry Series 22). Edited by Coccaro EF. New York, Marcel Dekker, 2003, pp 123–148

Felthous AR, Kachigian C: The fin de millénaire duty to warn or protect. Journal of Forensic Sciences 46(5):1103–1112, 2001

Felthous AR, Scarano VR: Tarasoff in Texas. J Texas Med 95(3):72–78, 1999

Felthous AR, Bryant SG, Wingerter CB, et al: The diagnosis of intermittent explosive disorder in violent men. Bull Am Acad Psychiatry Law 19(1):71–80, 1991

Felthous AR, Kröber H, Saß HL: Forensic evaluations for civil and criminal competencies and criminal responsibility in German and Anglo-American systems, in Psychiatry for Today. Edited by Henn F, Sartorius N, Helmehen H. Heidelberg, Germany, Springer-Verlag, 2000, pp 287–302

Godard SL, Bloom JD: Driving, mental illness, and the duty to protect, in Confidentiality Versus the Duty to Protect: Foreseeable Harm in the Practice of Psychiatry. Edited by Beck JC. Washington, DC, American Psychiatric Press, 1990, pp 191–204

Gooden v Tips, 651 S.W.2d 364 (Tex. App. 1983)

Hare RD: The Hare Psychopathy Checklist—Revised. Toronto, Ontario, Multi-Health Systems, 1991

Hare RD, Clark D, Grann M, et al: Psychopathy and the predictive validity of the PCL-R: an international perspective. Behav Sci Law 18(5):623–645, 2000

Hasenei v United States, 541 F.Supp. 999 (1982)

Hokansen v United States, 868 F.2d 372 (Tenth Circ. 1989)

Holmes v Wampler, 546 F.Supp. 500 (E.D. Vir. 1982)

Kachigian C, Felthous AR: Judicial responses to "Tarasoff" statutes (No 83B), in Syllabus and Proceedings Summary of the Annual Meeting of the American Psychiatric Association, Philadelphia, Pennsylvania, May 18–23, 2002, p 155

Karash v County of San Diego, Court of Appeal, Fourth Appellate District One, State of California Superior Ct (No. 420863) (1986)

Kirk v Michael Reese Hospital and Medical Center, 483 N.E.2d 906 (Ill. App. 1 Dist. 1985)

Klassen D, O'Connor WA: A prospective study of predictors of violence in adult male mental health admissions. Law Hum Behav 12:143–158, 1988

Lion JR: The clinician's role in assessing workplace violence. Psychiatr Clin North Am 22(1):101–108, 1999

Littleton v Good Samaritan Hospital, 529 N.E.2d 449 (Ohio 1988)

Monahan J, Steadman H, Silver E, et al: Rethinking Risk Assessment: The MacArthur Study of Mental Disorder and Violence. New York, Oxford University Press, 2001

Naidu v Laird, 539 A.2d 1064 (1988)

Nasser v Parker, 455 S.E.2d 502 (Va. 1995)

Paul v Plymouth General Hospital, 408 N.W.2d 492 (Mich. App. 1987)
Peavy v Home Management of Texas, 7 S.W.2d 795 (First Dist., Houston 1999)
Perriera v State, 738 P.2d 4 (Colo. App. 1986)
Petersen v State, 100 Wash.2d 421, 671 P.2d 230 (Wash. 1983)
Pettis RW: Tarasoff and the dangerous driver: a look at the driving cases. Bull Am Acad Psychiatry Law 20(4):427–437, 1992
Resnick PJ, Scott SL: Legal issues in treating perpetrators and victims of violence. Psychiatr Clin North Am 20(2):473–487, 1997
Rice ME, Harris GT, Cormier CA: An evaluation of a maximum-security therapeutic community for psychopaths and other mentally disordered offenders. Law Hum Behav 16:399–412, 1992
Rice ME, Harris GT, Quinsey VL: The appraisal of violence risk. Current Opinion in Psychiatry 15(6):589–593, 2002
Rights of Crime Victims and Witnesses Act, Illinois Compiled Statutes, ch. 725, § 120
Schuster v Altenberg, 424 N.W.2d 159 (Wis. 1988)
Sharpe v S.C. Dept of Mental Health, 354 S.E.2d 788 (S.C. App. 1987)
Simon RI: Concise Guide to Psychiatry and Law for Clinicians, 3rd Edition. Washington, DC, American Psychiatric Publishing, 2001
Simon RI, Sadoff RL: Violent behavior toward others, in Psychiatric Malpractice: Cases and Comments for Clinicians. Washington, DC, American Psychiatric Press, 1992, pp 191–232
Skeem JL, Mulvey EP: Psychopathy and community violence among civil psychiatric patients: results from the MacArthur Risk Assessment Study. J Consult Clin Psychol 69(3):358–374, 2000
Stanford MS, Houston RJ, Mathias CW, et al: A double-blind placebo-controlled crossover study of phenytoin in individuals with impulsive aggression. Psychiatry Res 103:193–203, 2001
Tarasoff v Regents of the University of California, 17 Cal.3d 425 (1976)
Tardiff K: Assessment and Management of Violent Patients, 2nd Edition. Washington, DC, American Psychiatric Press, 1996
Tardiff K: The past as prologue: assessment of future violence in individuals with a history of past violence, in Retrospective Assessment of Mental States in Litigation: Predicting the Past. Edited by Simon RI, Shuman DW. Washington, DC, American Psychiatric Publishing, 2002, pp 181–207
Taylor PJ, Garety P, Buchanan A, et al: Delusions and violence, in Violence and Mental Disorders: Developments in Risk Assessment. Edited by Monahan J, Steadman HJ. Chicago, IL, University of Chicago Press, 1994, pp 161–182
Tengström A, Hodgins S, Kullgren G: Men with schizophrenia who behave violently: the usefulness of early versus late-start offender typology. Schizophr Bull 27(2):205–218, 2001
Thapar v Zezulka, 994 S.W.2d 635 (1998)
Turner v Jordan, 957 S.W.2d 8125 (Tenn. 1997)
Walcott DM, Gerundolo P, Beck JC: Current analysis of the Tarasoff duty: an evolution towards the limitation of the duty to protect. Behav Sci Law 19(3): 325–343, 2001
Wylonis L: Psychiatric disability, employment and the Americans with Disabilities Act. Psychiatr Clin North Am 22(1):147–158, 1999

## Suggested Readings

Felthous AR: The clinician's duty to protect third parties. Psychiatr Clin North Am 22(1):49–60, 1999

Lion JR: The clinician's role in assessing workplace violence. Psychiatr Clin North Am 22(1):101–108, 1999

Resnick PJ, Scott SL: Legal issues in treating perpetrators and victims of violence. Psychiatr Clin North Am 20(2):473–487, 1997

Simon RI, Sadoff RL: Violent behavior toward others, in Psychiatric Malpractice: Cases and Comments for Clinicians. Washington, DC, American Psychiatric Press, 1992, pp 191–232

Tardiff K: Assessment and Management of Violent Patients, 2nd Edition. Washington, DC, American Psychiatric Press, 1996

Tardiff K: The past as prologue: assessment of future violence in individuals with a history of past violence, in Retrospective Assessment of Mental States in Litigation: Predicting the Past. Edited by Simon RI, Shuman DW. Washington, DC, American Psychiatric Publishing, 2002, pp 181–207

C H A P T E R 2 2

# Understanding Prediction Instruments

Douglas Mossman, M.D.

## Introduction

Psychiatrists make predictions all the time, but usually without realizing it. Prescribing medication may not seem like a prediction, but a physician's deciding to use a drug in a patient's treatment entails a belief that the drug might help. That belief, in turn, rests on an implicit prediction about what the drug will do to alleviate the patient's distress. Making a psychotherapeutic interpretation involves an implicit prediction that formulating a patient's experience in a particular way will help the patient grasp connections among feelings, perceptions, events, and actions and will thereby let the patient function better.

Although psychiatrists learn to take these everyday clinical predictions in stride, being asked explicitly to make a prediction about what persons will do often makes psychiatrists uncomfortable. And probably no type of prediction generates more anxiety than one involving a person's future "dangerousness." One reason for this—the reason for the scare quotes in the previous sentence—is that "dangerousness" is an

---

Portions of this chapter are adapted from Mossman D: "Assessing Predictions of Violence: Being Accurate About Accuracy." *Journal of Consulting and Clinical Psychology* 62:783–792, 1994; Mossman D: "Commentary: Assessing the Risk of Violence—Are "Accurate" Predictions Useful?" *Journal of the American Academy of Psychiatry and the Law* 28:272–281, 2000; and Mossman D: "Evaluating Violence Risk "by the Book": A Review of *HCR-20: Assessing Risk for Violence,* Version 2 and the *Manual for the Sexual Violence Risk–20. Behavioral Sciences and the Law* 18:781–789, 2000.

ambiguous term: it can refer to harm-causing acts, to acts with potential to cause harm, to behavior that seems threatening but does not itself cause harm, to having a high probability for acting violently, or to simply having any propensity to act violently. A second reason is that since the 1970s, the *Tarasoff* decision (*Tarasoff v. Regents of the University of California* 1976) in California and related cases in other states have declared that society expects mental health professionals to try to identify patients who pose a threat to others, and that courts may hold mental health professionals accountable if they fail to do this. A third source of anxiety comes from the magnitude and gravity of the potential consequences of being wrong about dangerousness. Wrong guesses about medication rarely amount to more than a failed treatment effort or an intolerable side effect, problems that can easily be solved with another clinical intervention. Wrong guesses about a patient's potential for violence, however, can have a devastating effect on the patient, the victim (often a family member or acquaintance of the patient), and the psychiatrist's emotional well-being.

Few, if any, psychiatrists can avoid making predictions about dangerous behavior because dozens of common clinical actions require implicit judgments about the violence potential of a patient or evaluee. Twenty-five years ago, Shah (1978) identified 15 areas of forensic decision making that require mental health professionals to assess the risk of violence. More recently, Hall and Ebert (2002, pp. 167–168) noted 27 circumstances that require dangerousness assessments; their list includes activities common to most psychiatric practices, such as releasing patients from hospitals, treating potentially violent patients in psychotherapy, and initiating emergency hospitalization or civil commitment.

Depending on their work setting and clientele, psychiatrists may have to make many other kinds of assessments of dangerousness. Fitness-for-duty determinations, sentencing recommendations, custody assessments involving previously abusive parents, intervention recommendations concerning stalkers or their victims, and planning treatment for substance abusers who commit violent crimes to support their habit all require implicit estimates of the risk of violence. For some release decisions (e.g., discharging previously violent patients or allowing insanity acquittees to leave hospitals and return to the community), preventing or minimizing potential risk to the public dwarfs all other considerations in shaping a patient's clinical management. The frequency and popularity of continuing education seminars on "assessing dangerousness" attest to the concern and anxiety mental health practitioners experience when they have to make judgments about future violence.

Until recently, mental health professionals who made decisions about dangerousness had to rely primarily on what their "gut" told them. Expressed more formally, mental health professionals relied on their "clinical judgment" to make predictions about future violence risk and to plan treatment interventions to reduce that risk. In recent years, however, researchers have developed several instruments with demonstrated accuracy in predicting violent behavior. Psychologists describe these instruments as "actuarial" tools for making "risk assessments" about individuals. The term *actuarial* refers to a type of decision making in which a clinician gathers information about a (usually small) number of factors concerning an individual who is being evaluated. The clinician then categorizes the information by using an explicit scoring system and combines the scores into an overall numerical value that summarizes the individual's risk of violence. Published manuals for these instruments explain their development and rationale, and guide clinicians through the process of assembling the data needed to make actuarially based judgments.

It is easy to underestimate both the value of actuarial instruments and the advantages they afford over the old way of doing things. It also is easy to attribute more significance to results produced by actuarial measures than the developers of these measures intended. This chapter explains how actuarial prediction instruments can probably improve clinical judgments about violence; it also explains why even fairly accurate predictions may have limited practical importance. We shall begin by examining results from a hypothetical contest about the accuracy of violence prediction.

## A Violence Prediction Contest

Once upon a time, two psychiatrists, Drs. Sybil Commitment and Lesley Faire, worked in a psychiatric emergency service at Gevalt Hospital. They respected each other's clinical talents but often disagreed about which patient needed to undergo hospitalization. Dr. Commitment hospitalized many patients because she worried about their violence potential; Dr. Faire hospitalized patients less frequently because she thought doctors should minimize the use of coercion. To see whose approach was best, the doctors had a contest. Each of them evaluated 1,000 patients whom a third colleague, Dr. Maven, had decided to admit to Gevalt Hospital. Drs. Commitment and Faire each rated these patients on a 5-point scale ("1" implying lowest risk, "5" implying highest); they also made yes-or-no predictions for each patient about whether he or she would become violent within 72 hours of admission. Because Gevalt Hospital carefully watched patients and kept good records about them,

Drs. Commitment and Faire knew that any act of violence (which they carefully and unambiguously defined for purposes of their contest) would get noticed and recorded. The doctor whose predictions were most accurate would win the contest.

Several months later, Dr. Maven had admitted 1,000 patients, 100 of whom actually became violent, and Drs. Commitment and Faire were ready to learn who had been the best predictor. Some terminology (summarized in Table 22–1) will help us understand how Drs. Commitment and Faire tried to interpret the results of their contest. If a doctor predicted violence and the patient subsequently acted violently, the doctor's prediction was a *true positive* (TP) prediction. A *false negative* (FN) prediction was one in which the doctor did not predict violence for a patient who actually was violent. A *true negative* (TN) was a prediction of nonviolence that turned out to be correct, and a *false positive* (FP) was a prediction of violence that was incorrect. By examining a doctor's predictions and the patients' actual behavior, the doctors could calculate what fraction of predictions was correct in light of subsequent events. They also could calculate the ratio of TP to FP predictions to find the odds that a prediction of violence were correct.

Imagine the doctors' discussion of their results, which are shown in Table 22–2. Dr. Commitment was right only 36% of the time, while Dr. Faire was correct for about 86% of the patients. Yet Dr. Faire was wrong about 75% of the patients who acted violently, while Dr. Commitment missed just 10% of these patients. Dr. Commitment felt her performance reflected her concern about a psychiatrist's responsibility to protect the community. But Dr. Commitment made more than seven wrong predictions of violence for every correct one. Because Dr. Faire made fewer wrong predictions of violence, she believed that her performance vindicated her favoring decision making that preserved patients' freedom.

**TABLE 22–1.** Definitions of some terms used to describe prediction accuracy

| Actual behavior | Predicted violent | Predicted not violent |
|---|---|---|
| Violent | True positive (TP) | False negative (FN) |
| Not violent | False positive (FP) | True negative (TN) |

Correct fraction (CF) = (TP+TN)/(TP+FP+FN+TN)

TP:FP ratio = TP/FP

True positive rate (TPR) = Sensitivity = TP/(TP+FN)

True negative rate (TNR) = Specificity = TN/(TN+FP)

False positive rate (FPR) = (1 – Specificity) = FP/(FP+TN)

**TABLE 22–2.** Results of the violence prediction contest

| | Dr. Commitment's predictions | | Dr. Faire's predictions | |
|---|---|---|---|---|
| **Actual behavior** | **Violent** | **Not violent** | **Violent** | **Not violent** |
| Violent | 90 | 10 | 25 | 75 |
| Not violent | 634 | 266 | 70 | 830 |
| Correct fraction | 0.356 | | 0.855 | |
| TP:FP ratio | 1:7 | | 1:2.8 | |
| Sensitivity | 0.900 | | 0.250 | |
| Specificity | 0.296 | | 0.922 | |

In fact, both psychiatrists did significantly better than chance at predicting violence, but you cannot tell this by looking at either the fraction of predictions that were correct or the ratio of TP to FP predictions. A doctor who simply had said *everybody* was not violent would have been correct 90% of the time. If half of the patients had been violent, a doctor who randomly predicted violence for half the patients would have a TP:FP ratio of about 1, despite no-better-than-chance performance.

The lower part of Table 22–1 includes accuracy indices that allow investigators to describe results in ways that do not conflate accuracy with the effects of base rates (Somoza and Mossman 1990). Medical publications often use the terms *sensitivity* and *specificity* to quantify diagnostic accuracy. If we interpret the psychiatrists' predictions as "diagnoses" of future violence, then sensitivity is the probability that a prediction of violence was made for an actually-violent patient, and specificity is the probability that a prediction of nonviolence was made for a nonviolent patient. The sensitivities and specificities for the doctors appear in Table 22–2. Notice, however, that these values still do not help much in deciding who did better.

In fact, as Table 22–3 shows, the psychiatrists made identical classifications of patients' risk of violence, but they used different decision thresholds when making the predictions. Dr. Commitment minimized false negative outcomes and avoided missing violent patients, and the result was high sensitivity but low specificity. Dr. Faire minimized false positive outcomes and predicted violence only when she had a very strong suspicion that a patient would become violent, and the result was high specificity but low sensitivity.

These observations suggest that we should measure diagnostic accuracy by using techniques that are not affected by base rates or clinicians'

**TABLE 22–3.** Future violence ratings and decision thresholds

| | | Ratings | | | | | | | | |
|---|---|---|---|---|---|---|---|---|---|---|
| **Doctor's name** | **Actual behavior** | **1** | | **2** | | **3** | | **4** | | **5** |
| Sybil Commitment | Violent | 10 | | 15 | | 30 | | 20 | | 25 |
| | Not violent | 266 | | 209 | | 252 | | 103 | | 70 |
| Lesley Faire | Violent | 10 | | 15 | | 30 | | 20 | | 25 |
| | Not violent | 266 | | 209 | | 252 | | 103 | | 70 |
| | True positive rate | | 0.90 | | 0.75 | | 0.45 | | 0.25 | |
| | False positive rate | | 0.70 | | 0.47 | | 0.19 | | 0.078 | |

*Note.* Vertical bars indicate doctor's decision threshold.

preferences for certain types of outcomes (Swets 1979). Single pairs of results from yes-or-no predictions will not tell the full picture about the accuracy of violence assessments. Ideally, we should describe accuracy in a way that reflects the trade-offs between sensitivity and specificity and that is independent of a clinician's actual cutoff or decision threshold.

As Table 22–3 shows, one can calculate four sensitivity-specificity pairs using the divisions between the clinicians' five rating categories as potential decision thresholds. At Dr. Faire's strict threshold, violence is predicted only for those patients rated 5. At this strictest threshold, the violence detection rate, or the *true positive rate* (TPR), is only 0.25, but the "false alarm" rate, or *false positive rate* (FPR), is just 0.08. (Note that TPR=sensitivity and FPR=1−specificity.) At the second strictest threshold, violence is predicted for patients rated 4 or 5; the FPR increases to 0.19 and the TPR increases to 0.45. One obtains the FPR and TPR for the two other thresholds in Table 22–3 similarly.

In the mid-1990s, several writers (Mossman 1994a, 1994b; Rice and Harris 1995; Gardner et al. 1996) recognized that adjustable thresholds are a feature of most violence prediction techniques and that the accuracy of violence prediction methods should therefore be described using *receiver operating characteristic* (ROC) analysis. This term, originally derived from radar applications (Lusted 1984), suggests that detection is characterized by the threshold at which the "receiver" (here, a clinician) operates. ROC analysis allows investigators to characterize the trade-offs between errors and correct identifications that arise from the intrinsic discrimination capacity of a detection method and to distinguish these features from the threshold or operating point that is used to make a decision (Mossman and Somoza 1991). ROC analyses typically utilize a ROC graph, which succinctly summarizes the results of a detection method as the threshold is moved throughout its range of possible values. A ROC graph customarily plots the TPR as a function of the FPR and depicts how the TPR increases as the FPR increases.

Figure 22–1 is an example of such a graph, based on the results shown in Table 22–3. Notice that the four possible thresholds lie along a *ROC curve* joining them. (To learn more about the mathematical assumptions used to fit ROC curves to data points, see Somoza and Mossman 1991 and Mossman 1994b.) The better a test or detection system, the greater the *area under the ROC curve* (AUC) that describes the performance of the test or detection system. The AUC of a test or detection system has a direct, practical interpretation (Hanley and McNeil 1982). In the context of quantifying the accuracy of violence prediction, AUC equals the probability that the detection method would rate a randomly selected, actu-

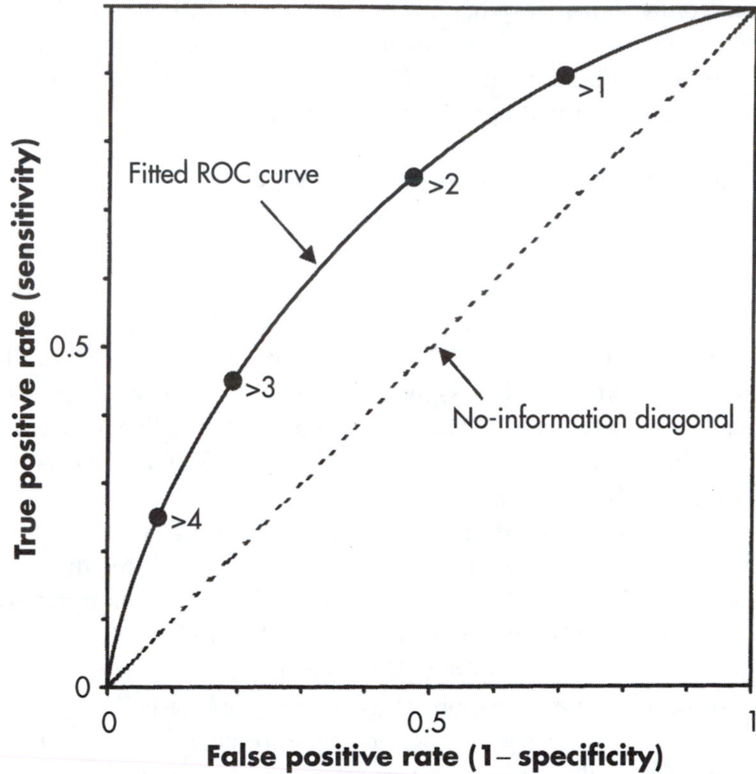


**FIGURE 22–1.** ROC graph based on the results shown in Table 22–3.
The four possible thresholds are fit to ROC curve, the area under which is 0.701. The no-information diagonal (ROC area = 0.5) is also shown.

ally violent person as more likely to be violent than a randomly selected, nonviolent person. A prediction method that always rated violent and nonviolent persons correctly would have an AUC of 1.0; a prediction method that gave no information would have an AUC of 0.5 and would be described by the diagonal line in Figure 22–1. For the hypothetical results from Table 22–3, AUC=0.701±0.028, implying an accuracy level that is significantly better than chance and is fairly typical of clinical judgments about future violence (Mossman 1994b).

These results can help us understand and lay to rest the often-voiced but mistaken (Mossman 2000) belief that predictions of violence—especially long-term predictions—are inaccurate. For the past two decades, many mental health professionals have thought that, as the U.S. Supreme Court put it, "[p]sychiatric predictions of future violent behavior by the mentally ill are inaccurate" (*Heller v. Doe* 1993, p. 324). The Court's view reflects conclusions in John Monahan's influential monograph *The Clinical Prediction of Violent Behavior* (1981), which summarized previously published studies of violence prediction in support of this conclusion. Looking at results such as those shown in Table 22–2 for Drs. Commitment and Faire, Professor Monahan correctly concluded "that psychiatrists and psychologists are accurate in no more than one out of three predictions of violent behavior" (Monahan 1981, p. 92). As we have seen, however, Drs. Commitment and Faire did much better than chance at categorizing patients according to their risk of violence. Their error pattern (the low TP:FP ratio) was a consequence of the low "base rate" of violence among the 1,000 subjects, only 10% of whom were violent during the follow-up.

ROC methods keep low base rates from fooling us. Because neither FPR nor TPR is affected by base rates, ROC methods describe the accuracy of violence predictions in a way that separates properties of the detection process from the frequency of violence in the population being studied. As Mossman (1994b, 2000) and Buchanan and Leese (2001) have pointed out, reanalyses of previously published data (including those from the studies that Monahan described) show that short-, medium-, and long-term clinical predictions of violence all have a roughly similar, modestly-better-than-chance level of accuracy.

## Clinical Versus Actuarial Prediction Methods

Our discussion of a make-believe contest looks at how well two hypothetical doctors used their "clinical judgment" to assess violence risk and make predictions about it. Most decisions about psychiatric care, and probably most decisions in medicine, are made this way. That is, doctors use facts they have gathered, their background knowledge, their specific knowledge about the person they are evaluating, their intuition, their "gut instincts," and/or whatever else they think is relevant to anticipate (predict) what will happen, and then intervene. Psychologists who study human decision making contrast predictions based on "clinical" judgments (also called "subjective" or "impressionistic" judgments) with "actuarial" predictions based on formulae, algorithms, or other "mechanical" means. As was stated earlier, actuarial tools direct the clinician's attention to specific "aspects, behavior, and other features" of the individuals they are evaluating. The clinician then uses these data to come up with a numerical value that summarizes the evaluee's risk of violence.

## HCR-20

The HCR-20 (Webster et al. 1997) provides an easy-to-understand example of this process. This instrument, whose name is an acronym for its overall structure, directs the clinician's attention toward 20 factors—10 **H**istorical items, 5 **C**linical items, and 5 **R**isk management items—that are associated with increased risk of violence (Table 22–4). The manual for the HCR-20 succinctly describes published research that supports including each item as a risk factor. To use the HCR-20, a clinician gathers the information about each of the risk factor items and then, using the manual's instructions about coding information related to each risk factor, gives each item a score of 0, 1, or 2. An individual's score on the HCR-20 thus can range from 0 to 40, with higher scores implying higher probabilities of future violence.

**TABLE 22–4.** Historical, clinical, and risk management items from the HCR-20

| |
|---|
| **Historical items** |
| H1. Previous Violence |
| H2. Young Age at First Incident |
| H3. Relationship Instability |
| H4. Employment Problems |
| H5. Substance Use Problems |
| H6. Major Mental Illness |
| H7. Psychopathy |
| H8. Early Maladjustment |
| H9. Personality Disorder |
| H10. Prior Supervision Failure |
| **Clinical items** |
| C1. Lack of Insight |
| C2. Negative Attitudes |
| C3. Active Symptoms of Major Mental Illness |
| C4. Impulsivity |
| C5. Unresponsive to Treatment |
| **Risk management items** |
| R1. Plans Lack Feasibility |
| R2. Exposure to Destabilizers |
| R3. Lack of Personal Support |
| R4. Noncompliance With Remediation Attempts |
| R5. Stress |

*Source.* Reprinted from Webster CD, Douglas KS, Eaves E, et al.: *HCR-20: Assessing Risk for Violence,* Version 2. Burnaby, British Columbia, Mental Health, Law and Policy Institute, Simon Fraser University, 1997. Used with permission.

A brief look at a few items on the HCR-20 will help readers appreciate how its creators have tried to identify a few salient risk factors for violence and have used these factors to produce a straightforward, reliable instrument for risk assessment.

An example of a historical item on the HCR-20 is H5, "Substance Use Problems." The authors justify including this item on the basis of several studies, including the finding by Swanson (1994), based on data originally obtained in the Epidemiologic Catchment Area study, that "having a substance abuse diagnosis yielded much stronger associations with violence than did having a mental disorder" (Webster et al. 1997, p. 36). One assigns a score of 0 on item H5 if the individual has "no substance use problems"; a score of 2 is assigned for "definite/serious substance use problems" that interfere with functioning; and a score of 1 is assigned for "possible/less serious substance use problems" (Webster et al. 1997, p. 37).

Item C3, "Active Symptoms of Major Mental Illness," serves as a good example of a clinical item in the HCR-20. Inclusion of this item gains support from research that associates active psychotic symptoms with violence (e.g., Swanson et al. 1996). A clinician codes this item 0 if an evaluee has "no active symptoms of major mental illness," 1 for "possible/ less serious active symptoms," or 2 for "definite/serious active symptoms" (Webster et al. 1997, p. 55).

Item R4, "Noncompliance With Remediation Attempts," asks the evaluator to score the probability that a patient will not take medication or adhere to other therapeutic regimens. A score of 0 implies a "low probability of noncompliance"; 1, a "moderate probability"; and 2, a "high probability." Again, the authors cite research available in 1997 (e.g., Bartels et al. 1991; Haywood et al. 1995) to support inclusion of this risk factor. Subsequent studies (e.g., Swartz et al. 1998) have confirmed the importance of noncompliance as a predictor of posthospitalization violence.

Figure 22–2 is based on a study of the HCR-20 by Douglas and colleagues (1999) and is presented to help readers understand the relationship between patients' actual scores on an actuarial instrument, their future violence, and the ways that ROC techniques quantify the accuracy of predictions. In their study, Douglas and colleagues used the HCR-20 assessment scheme to code information about 193 former inpatients who had been civilly committed. Patients had subsequently been released to the community for an average of almost 2 years, during which time 73 of the patients became violent. Figure 22–2 contains histograms showing the patients' HCR-20 scores (which one can figure out from data presented by the authors in their original paper). Notice that the violent

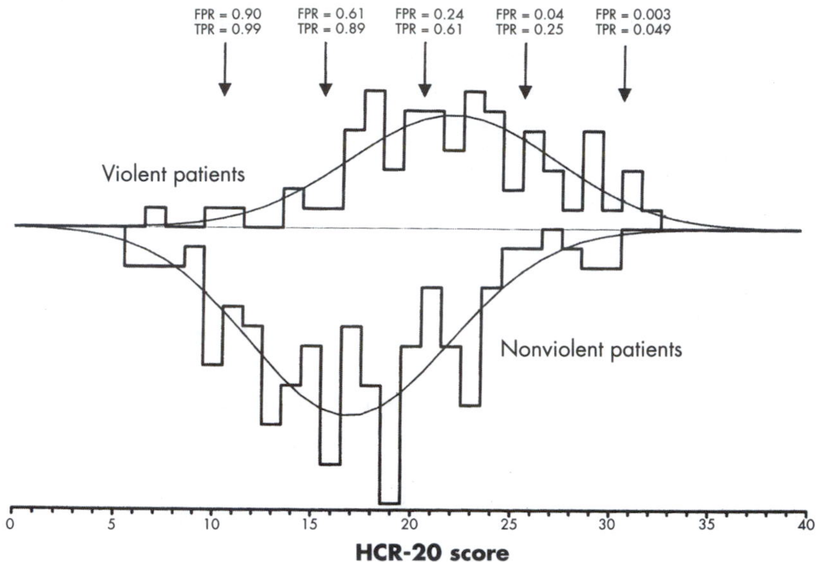


**FIGURE 22–2. Histograms showing HCR-20 scores of 73 violent patients and 120 nonviolent patients studied by Douglas et al. (1999).** Superimposed on the histograms are two "bell-shaped" (Gaussian) curves that represent a best fit of the data. Also shown are the values of FPR and TPR associated with five possible cutoffs. The bell-shaped curves imply that the effect of using the HCR-20 is to shift the distributions of violent and nonviolent patients about one standard deviation apart from each other. This is equivalent to saying that about three-quarters of the time, the HCR-20 score of a randomly chosen violent patient will be higher than the score of a randomly chosen nonviolent patient.

patients tended to score higher than did the nonviolent patients. Superimposed on the histograms are two bell-shaped (Gaussian) curves that represent a best fit of the data (produced by using maximum likelihood estimation software available from Charles E. Metz, Ph.D., of the University of Chicago Department of Radiology). What one sees from examining the bell-shaped curves is that the effect of using the HCR-20 is to shift the distributions of violent and nonviolent patients about one standard deviation apart from each other.

Also shown in Figure 22–2 are arrows representing a few possible cutoffs, and the values of the FPR and TPR associated with those cutoffs. For example, a cutoff score of 20 (i.e., patients with scores above 20 are predicted violent, and those with scores of 20 or less are predicted nonviolent) can be expected to identify 61% of the violent patients and to mislabel 24% of the nonviolent patients (i.e., specificity is 76%). For the smooth ROC curve implied by the best-fit bell-shaped curves in Figure 22–2, AUC=0.758±0.035. In other words, Douglas et al.'s study suggests that about three-quarters of the time, the HCR-20 score of a randomly chosen violent patient will be higher than the score of a randomly chosen nonviolent patient.

When committing a violent crime was the outcome criterion, Douglas et al. (1999) found that the HCR-20 did even better—it had an AUC of 0.80. Other investigators have evaluated the HCR-20 in other countries and clinical contexts and have found that violent evaluees consistently get higher scores than nonviolent evaluees (Belfrage et al. 2000; Dernevik et al. 2002; Douglas and Webster 1999; Doyle et al. 2002; Grann et al. 2000; Tengström 2001). In other words, using the HCR-20 consistently helps an evaluator make a better-than-chance guess about who has been or will become violent.

## Other Actuarial Methods

The HCR-20 is just one of several actuarial methods that have been developed recently and that are being actively evaluated by researchers. Examples of other methods are described below.

### *Violence Risk Appraisal Guide*

The Violence Risk Appraisal Guide (VRAG; Quinsey et al. 1998) was developed by using data on mentally disordered offenders who were detained in a Canadian prison psychiatric facility between 1965 and 1980. Post-incarceration follow-up data on violent behavior (ranging from assault to murder) were collected from Royal Canadian Mounted Police files. The reliability and predictive utility of the VRAG have been demonstrated for several other populations, including mentally disordered offenders in Sweden (Grann et al. 2000), previously incarcerated sex offenders (Hanson and Harris 1998; Rice and Harris 1997), and wife assaulters (Hilton et al. 2001). The VRAG directs evaluators to 12 items that are scored and then assigned weightings by using a simple procedure designed by the instrument's creators. Unlike the items in the HCR-20, items and weightings in the VRAG were empirically derived, based on what the instrument's creators found had worked in their original data sample. The instrument's creators found, for example, that having schizophrenia *decreased* the risk of future violence, so having this diagnosis was weighted so as to lower predicted risk of violence. Available research (e.g., Rice and Harris 1995) suggests accuracy levels for the VRAG that are comparable to those for the HCR-20.

"Psychopathy" appears as an element in both the HCR-20 and the VRAG. It turns out that an evaluee's psychopathy score, as measured by the Hare Psychopathy Checklist—Revised (PCL-R; Hare 1991) or the Psychopathy Checklist—Screening Version (PCL:SV; Hart et al. 1995), is itself a decent predictor of violent behavior (Grann et al. 1999), though perhaps not as accurate a predictor as are the HCR-20 and VRAG (e.g., Douglas et al. 1999; Glover et al. 2002; Hilton et al. 2001). To use the PCL-R, the evaluator takes interview information and collateral data (from clinical files, police records, etc.) to assign scores of 0, 1, or 2 to 20 items, so that a total PCL-R score ranges from 0 to 40. The PCL-R items refer to two "factors" that characterize PCL-R-defined psychopathy: 1) callous, unremorseful use of others (as reflected, e.g., in glibness, lying, manipulation of others, lack of remorse, and unwillingness to accept responsibility) and 2) a chronically unstable and antisocial lifestyle (as reflected in, e.g., early behavioral problems, stimulation seeking, impulsiveness, and multiple sexual relationships).

### *Iterative Classification Tree*

The Iterative Classification Tree (ICT) method (Monahan et al. 2000; Steadman et al. 2000) represents another potentially useful way of assessing violence risk. Using a sequence set out by the classification tree, an evaluator asks an initial question about an evaluee. Depending on the answer to the first question, the evaluator asks one of two second questions and continues with this procedure until the evaluee is classified in one of the terminal categories on the ICT's branches. Membership in particular categories allows the assignment of evaluees to subgroups with risks that are lower than, higher than, or not distinguishable from the full group's base rate of violence.

Although the authors claim a high level of accuracy for their risk assessment scheme (AUC=0.80–0.82), their ICT was designed specifically for their test sample, and their statistical analyses do not tell us how well their ICT would perform in another sample (Mossman 2000). As a result, they appropriately caution users that the accuracy of the ICT in "other types of clinical setting (e.g., forensic hospitals) is unknown" (Monahan et al. 2000, p. 318).

### *Instruments Designed to Predict Sexual Offender Recidivism*

The Sex Offender Risk Appraisal Guide (SORAG; Quinsey et al. 1998), Rapid Risk Assessment for Sexual Offense Recidivism (RRASOR; Hanson 1997), and Static-99 (Hanson and Thornton 2000) are three of the currently available actuarial instruments designed to predict recidivism in individuals convicted of sexual offenses. All appear to have modestly-better-than-chance accuracy in predicting who will reoffend over long periods (10 years or more) of community release. The SORAG is very similar to the VRAG, and the latter instrument may indeed be as good as the former at predicting sexual recidivism (Hall and Ebert 2002; Rice and Harris 1997, 2002). The RRASOR and Static-99 direct evaluators to just a few historical items about the offender—in the case of the RRASOR, number of prior sex offenses, age, sex of victim(s), and relationship to victim(s)—and yield scores that are significantly correlated with long-term likelihood of recidivism.

## Clinical Judgment or Actuarial Method?

If a psychiatrist has a choice between using clinical judgment or actuarial measures to assess violence risk, which method is better? The best current answer is "We're not sure, but probably the actuarial method." The reason is that, in a broad variety of prediction tasks, actuarial methods consistently yield better predictions than those made by unaided clinicians (Grove and Meehl 1996). For those who are not familiar with studies comparing clinical and actuarial predictions, this finding may come as a surprise. After all, clinical judgments presumably incorporate things such as detailed lessons from experience, human pattern recognition abilities, and subtle nuances that simple formulas leave out. It would seem, therefore, that clinical predictions *must* be more accurate than predictions generated by algorithms or formulas.

The psychological literature strongly suggests that the opposite is true, however. The reason may be that clinicians do not assign proper significance to the kinds of information used in actuarial prediction formulas or that clinicians may just not reliably and consistently weight the information they use. In most cases, making a prediction may be more like figuring out a grocery bill than deciding whether a portrait accurately depicts its subject. It is very difficult to program a computer to identify faces (something people do easily and well), but when it comes to calculating a grocery bill, checking prices and using a simple calculator will be much more accurate than eyeballing a shopping cart and estimating the total cost (Dawes et al. 1989).

Some authors (e.g., Gardner et al. 1996; Harris et al. 2002; Mossman 1994a; Quinsey et al. 1998) have interpreted available research as indicating that actuarial measures are superior to clinical judgments in predicting future violence. On the basis of their own research findings and the general finding that actuarial measures outperform clinical predictions, Quinsey and colleagues (1998) have argued for "the complete replacement of existing practice with actuarial methods" (p. 171).

As Litwack (2001) has pointed out, however, only a few studies have directly compared clinical and actuarial predictions of violence, and these have not demonstrated the clear superiority of either approach. Thus, although research suggests that actuarial methods are superior to clinical judgments in many prediction tasks, we cannot be sure that this general finding applies to predicting violence. "Assessments of dangerousness are inherently different from many other predictive tasks, in ways that make it very difficult to meaningfully compare clinical and actuarial assessments," argues Litwack. Moreover, "even the best studied and validated actuarial tool for assessing dangerousness, the [VRAG] . . . has not been demonstrated as suitable for practical purposes in many instances, or to be superior to clinical assessments." Given the currently available evidence, concludes Litwack, the call for replacement of clinical assessment by actuarial methods is "premature" (p. 410). Litwack believes, however, that available evidence has shown that instruments such as the PCL-R and the HCR-20 "can enhance a variety of dangerousness risk assessments," and he feels that clinicians who perform "risk assessments have a professional responsibility to be aware of the advantages and limitations of using such risk assessment tools" (p. 438).

Even if their predictive superiority is unclear, actuarial methods have other advantages over clinical judgment. When used properly, actuarial methods are impartial, systematic, and thorough. They also have the virtue of "transparency," in that they use fairly objective data and an explicitly prescribed method of combining those data. This makes actuarial methods and their results open to inspection, questioning, and, when necessary, critique. Finally, actuarial methods allow for an approach to judgments about future violence called "structured risk assessment" (Hanson and Thornton 2000) or "structured clinical judgment" (Douglas and Kropp 2002; Kropp et al. 2002). Indeed, the designers of the Static-99 and the HCR-20 believe that actuarial measures should be used only as a first step in evaluating violence risk, "as an aide-mémoire and as a research instrument" (Webster et al. 1997, p. 5). Actuarial scales force the evaluator to proceed from and give appropriate consideration to a set of known factors associated with violence risk. But the evaluator then may (and usually should) consider additional factors specific to an evaluee's situation—for example, dynamic factors not included in the risk assessment, characteristics and availability of known potential victims, the evaluee's known response to treatment, the evaluee's anticipated future situation, and the degree to which the actuarial measure fits the population from which the evaluee is drawn—to make an ultimate judgment about violence risk. Most important, the power of actuarial instruments should not lead evaluators to ignore common sense. Sometimes data that do not appear in an actuarial instrument—for example, a clearly stated intent to kill someone following an acute precipitant—put a person at high, imminent risk to act violently. As Hart (1999) has pointed out, assessors would be negligent if they ignored an individual's prior history of violence or homicidal ideation and threats, variables that have been shown to be linked to violence (Grisso et al. 2000).

## The Practical Usefulness of Predictions

The success of actuarial measures such as the HCR-20 and the VRAG in sorting violent from nonviolent individuals clearly indicates that long-term predictions of violence can be accurate. Yet clinicians should not overestimate the usefulness of these instruments. To understand why, consider two more hypothetical psychiatrists, Dr. Jones and Dr. Smith, who have created a hypothetical actuarial measure, the Violence Prediction Scale (VPS), to make decisions concerning their patients' future violence. After thorough testing, Drs. Jones and Smith have learned that the VPS performs as well as or better than other currently available instruments: its ROC curve has an AUC of 0.83. The ROC curve for the VPS passes through the point where the FPR is 0.25 and the TPR is 0.75, and Drs. Jones and Smith decide to use the VPS score corresponding to this cutoff as their decision threshold. They now plan to evaluate inpatients for whom they are responsible. From past experience, they know that one out of four of the inpatients (25%) will engage in a seriously violent act, a base rate of violence that is typical in studies of inpatients (Borum 1996).

Imagine two situations in which the doctors might put the VPS to use. In the first situation, Dr. Jones must assign 160 new, simultaneously arriving inpatients to treatment units. One hundred of the available hospital beds are in general treatment units, and 60 of the available beds are in special care units. The special care units have been specially designed and staffed, and they reduce patients' violence by 50% compared with what it would otherwise be. If Dr. Jones were to assign patients to the special and general units at random, the rate of violence for the 60 patients in the special care unit would be 1 out of 8 (i.e., half the base rate = 0.125) and 8 patients would become violent. On the general treatment units, 25 of the 100 patients would become violent. Overall, the rate of violence would be 33 out of 160 patients. But by using the VPS, Dr. Jones can divide the patients into two subgroups: a 60-member "predicted violent" group for whom the rate of violence is 0.50 (1 out of 2), and a 100-member "predicted nonviolent" group for whom the rate is 0.10 (1 out of 10). If the "predicted violent" patients are placed in special care, their rate of violence is halved from what it would otherwise be, so only 15 of them become violent. On the general units, 10 "predicted nonviolent" patients become violent. The system is imperfect, but by using the VPS, Dr. Jones has reduced the total rate of violence by one-quarter (from 33 to 25 patients out of 160).

Dr. Jones's clinical task—evaluating 160 new arrivals and assigning them to one of two types of treatment units—is not the sort of problem that most clinicians encounter. A more typical problem is the task faced by Dr. Smith. He, too, is responsible for 160 inpatients, but his patients are placed in similar treatment units. (For purposes of this illustration, it does not matter whether the patients are already present in the hospital or arrive individually over a period of time.) Like Dr. Jones, Dr. Smith can use the VPS to sort the patients into a "high risk" group, 50% of whose members will act violently, and a "low risk" group, of whom 10% will be violent. But how might Dr. Smith react to this information? He probably would be more concerned about those patients to whom the VPS assigns a 50% chance of becoming violent. But would he want to do *nothing* about the potential dangerousness of the "low-risk" patients, who have (only) a 10% risk of acting violently? If the violent behavior of one of these "low-risk" patients resulted in a *Tarasoff*-type lawsuit, Dr. Smith probably would not want to tell jurors that having a 1-in-2 chance of serious violence implied a need for special attention, but a 1-in-10 chance was too low to warrant thoughtful efforts to prevent harm to others. Under most circumstances, it would be hard to justify treating patients with a 10% risk of serious violence very differently from those with a 50% risk. For both groups of patients, Dr. Smith—and most real-life psychiatrists—would probably exercise similar precautions when formulating inpatient treatment, making follow-up plans, and completing other treatment arrangements.

## Conclusion

Two decades ago, G.E. Dix (1983) wrote, "Intuition suggests that psychiatrists' predictive ability is substantially greater when it is called into play concerning the short-term risk posed by persons whose assaultive tendencies are related to symptoms of identifiable serious mental illnesses" (p. 256). Yet research since the mid-1990s has suggested that persons' likelihood of being violent also is a function of several enduring characteristics. Psychiatric impairments affect how well a person can interpret behavior, resolve conflicts, and get along with others (Swanson et al. 1998), which may explain why having a mental illness statistically increases a person's violence risk. Other enduring individual variables that statistically influence the likelihood of violence (e.g., sex, age, level of education, and income level) provide information that helps make reasonable statements about an individual's long-term violence risk. As a result, simple "actuarial" prediction tools that focus on known risk factors can help clinicians identify patients with higher or lower probabilities of becoming violent.

Recent research suggests that actuarial tools may well let clinicians make better predictions than they would by using their unaided clinical judgment. Yet clinicians may often find that predictions made with these tools do not change how they manage patients, because for typical clinical tasks even fairly accurate prediction techniques may not sort patients into subgroups with meaningfully different levels of risk.

The practical value of violence prediction measures may inhere in the help they give psychiatrists in focusing on important aspects of clinical management. Noncompliance with treatment and substance abuse—two items found in the HCR-20—are risk factors for violent behavior following hospital discharge (Steadman et al. 1998; Swartz et al. 1998). By addressing these problems (e.g., by finding ways to improve patients' adherence to community treatment and avoidance of intoxicants), mental health professionals might reduce their patients' risk of acting violently. Of course, improving compliance and preventing substance abuse are good things for patients, whether or not these interventions reduce violence. Perhaps the greatest current value of actuarial prediction instruments rests not in their predictive powers but in their ability to translate what current research tells us about violence risk into knowledge that clinicians can use to make evidence-based decisions about treatment.

## Key Points

- Recent publications suggest that short-term and long-term predictions of violence have comparable, better-than-chance levels of accuracy.
- In recent years, researchers have developed "actuarial" instruments for conducting risk assessments.
- These actuarial instruments, which are based on established risk factors for violence, probably lead to assessments that are more accurate than assessments based solely on clinical judgment.
- Using actuarial methods may help psychiatrists improve their assessments of the risk of violence.

- Actuarial instruments also may help clinicians identify factors that can potentially be addressed in treatment and should be considered in any violence risk assessment.

## Practice Guidelines

1. When making formal assessments of the risk of violence, familiarize yourself with actuarial prediction instruments.
2. When conducting a risk assessment, focus on research-proven factors that influence an individual's risk of violence.
3. Consider using actuarial prediction tools in standard risk assessments when possible, because these tools force you to proceed from and give appropriate consideration to a set of known factors associated with violence risk.
4. Consider additional factors specific to an evaluee's situation—for example, the availability of known potential victims—when making judgments about violence risk.

## References

Bartels SJ, Drake RE, Wallach MA, et al: Characteristic hostility in schizophrenic outpatients. Schizophr Bull 17:163–171, 1991

Belfrage H, Fransson G, Strand S: Prediction of violence using the HCR-20: a prospective study in two maximum-security correctional institutions. Journal of Forensic Psychiatry 11:167–175, 2000

Borum R: Improving the clinical practice of violence risk assessment: technology, guidelines, and training. Am Psychol 51:945–956, 1996

Buchanan A, Leese M: Detection of people with dangerous severe personality disorders: a systematic review. Lancet 358:1955–1959, 2001

Dawes RM, Faust D, Meehl PE: Clinical versus actuarial judgment. Science 243: 1668–1674, 1989

Dernevik M, Grann M, Johansson S: Violent behaviour in forensic psychiatric patients: risk assessment and different risk-management levels using the HCR-20. Psychology, Crime and Law 8:93–111, 2002

Dix GE: A legal perspective on dangerousness: current status. Psychiatric Annals 13:243–256, 1983

Douglas KS, Kropp PR: A prevention-based paradigm for violence risk assessment: clinical and research applications. Criminal Justice and Behavior 29: 617–658, 2002

Douglas KS, Webster CD: The HCR-20 violence risk assessment scheme: concurrent validity in a sample of incarcerated offenders. Criminal Justice and Behavior 26:3–19, 1999

Douglas KS, Ogloff JRP, Nicholls TL, et al: Assessing risk for violence among psychiatric patients: the HCR-20 risk assessment scheme and the Psychopathy Checklist: Screening Version. J Consult Clin Psychol 67:917–930, 1999

Doyle M, Dolan M, McGovern J: The validity of North American risk assessment tools in predicting inpatient violent behaviour in England. Legal and Criminological Psychology 7:141–154, 2002

Gardner W, Lidz CW, Mulvey EP, et al: Clinical versus actuarial predictions of violence in patients with mental illness. J Consult Clin Psychol 64:602–609, 1996

Glover AJJ, Nicholson DE, Hemmati T, et al: A comparison of predictors of general and violent recidivism among high risk federal offenders. Criminal Justice and Behavior 29:235–249, 2002

Grann M, Langstrom N, Tengström A: Psychopathy (PCL-R) predicts violent recidivism among criminal offenders with personality disorders in Sweden. Law Hum Behav 23(2):205–217, 1999

Grann M, Belfrage H, Tengström A: Actuarial assessment of risk for violence: predictive validity of the VRAG and the historical part of the HCR-20. Criminal Justice and Behavior 27:97–114, 2000

Grisso T, Davis J, Vesselinov R, et al: Violent thoughts and violent behavior following hospitalization for mental disorder. J Consult Clin Psychol 68:388–398, 2000

Grove WM, Meehl PE: Comparative efficiency of informal (subjective, impressionistic) and formal (mechanical, algorithmic) prediction procedures: the clinical-statistical controversy. Psychology, Public Policy, and Law 2:293–323, 1996

Hall HV, Ebert RS: Violence Prediction: Guidelines for the Forensic Practitioner. Springfield, IL, Charles C Thomas, 2002

Hanley JA, McNeil BJ: The meaning and use of the area under a receiver operating characteristic (ROC) curve. Radiology 143:29–36, 1982

Hanson RK: The Development of a Brief Actuarial Risk Scale for Sexual Offender Recidivism (User Report 97-04). Ottawa, Ontario, Department of the Solicitor General of Canada, 1997

Hanson RK, Harris A: Dynamic Predictors of Sexual Recidivism (User Report No 1998-01). Ottawa, Ontario, Solicitor General Canada, 1998

Hanson RK, Thornton D: Improving risk assessments for sex offenders: a comparison of three actuarial scales. Law Hum Behav 24:119–136, 2000

Hanson RK, Thornton D: Improving risk assessments for sex offenders: a comparison of three actuarial scales. Law Hum Behav 24:119–136 2000

Hare RD: Manual for the Hare Psychopathy Checklist—Revised. Toronto, Ontario, Multi Health Systems, 1991

Harris GT, Rice ME, Cormier CA: Prospective replication of the Violence Risk Appraisal Guide in predicting violent recidivism among forensic patients. Law Hum Behav 26:377–394, 2002

Hart SD: Assessing violence risk: thoughts and second thought (review of *Violent Offenders: Appraising and Managing Risk*). Contemporary Psychology 44:486–488, 1999

Hart SD, Cox DN, Hare RD: The PCL:SV—Psychopathy Checklist: Screening Version. Toronto, Ontario, Multi Health Systems, 1995

Haywood TW, Kravitz HM, Grossman LS, et al: Predicting the "revolving door" phenomenon among patients with schizophrenic, schizoaffective, and affective disorders. Am J Psychiatry 152:856–861, 1995

Heller v Doe, 509 U.S. 312 (1993)

Hilton NZ, Harris GT, Rice ME: Predicting violence by serious wife assaulters. Journal of Interpersonal Violence 16:408–423, 2001

Kropp PR, Hart SD, Lyon DR: Risk assessment of stalkers: some problems and possible solutions. Criminal Justice and Behavior 29:590–616, 2002

Litwack TR: Actuarial versus clinical assessments of dangerousness. Psychology, Public Policy, and Law 7:409–443, 2001

Lusted LB: ROC recollected. Med Decis Making 4:131–135, 1984

Monahan J: The Clinical Prediction of Violent Behavior (DHHS Publ No ADM 81-921). Rockville, MD, National Institute of Mental Health, 1981

Monahan J, Steadman HJ, Appelbaum PS, et al: Developing a clinically useful actuarial tool for assessing violence risk. Br J Psychiatry 176:312–319, 2000

Mossman D: Assessing predictions of violence: being accurate about accuracy. J Consult Clin Psychol 62:783–792, 1994a

Mossman D: Further comments on portraying the accuracy of violence predictions. Law Hum Behav 18:587–593, 1994b

Mossman D: Commentary: Assessing the risk of violence—are "accurate" predictions useful? J Am Acad Psychiatry Law 28:272–281, 2000

Mossman D, Somoza E: ROC curves, test accuracy, and the description of diagnostic tests. J Neuropsychiatry Clin Neurosci 3:330–333, 1991

Quinsey VL, Harris GT, Rice ME, et al: Violent Offenders: Appraising and Managing Risk. Washington, DC, American Psychological Association, 1998

Rice ME, Harris G: Violent recidivism: assessing predictive validity. J Consult Clin Psychol 63:737–748, 1995

Rice ME, Harris GT: Cross-validation and extension of the Violence Risk Appraisal Guide for child molesters and rapists. Law Hum Behav 21:231–241, 1997

Rice ME, Harris GT: Men who molest their sexually immature daughters: is a special explanation required? J Abnorm Psychol 111:329–339, 2002

Shah SA: Dangerousness: a paradigm for exploring some issues in law and psychology. Am Psychol 33:224–238, 1978

Somoza E, Mossman D: Introduction to neuropsychiatric decision making: binary diagnostic tests. J Neuropsychiatry Clin Neurosci 2:297–300, 1990

Somoza E, Mossman D: ROC curves and the binormal assumption. J Neuropsychiatry Clin Neurosci 3:436–439, 1991

Steadman HJ, Mulvey EP, Monahan J, et al: Violence by people discharged from acute psychiatric inpatient facilities and by others in the same neighborhoods. Arch Gen Psychiatry 55:393–401, 1998

Steadman, HJ, Silver E, Monahan J, et al: A classification tree approach to the development of actuarial violence risk assessment tools. Law Hum Behav 24: 83–100, 2000

Swanson JW: Mental disorder, substance abuse, and community violence: an epidemiological approach, in Violence and Mental Disorder: Developments in Risk Assessment. Edited by Monahan J, Steadman HJ. Chicago, IL, University of Chicago Press, 1994, pp 101–136

Swanson JW, Borum R, Swartz MS, et al: Psychotic symptoms and disorders and the risk of violent behavior in the community. Criminal Behaviour and Mental Health 6:317–338, 1996

Swanson JW, Swartz M, Estroff S, et al: Psychiatric impairment, social contact, and violent behavior: evidence from a study of outpatient-committed persons with severe mental disorder. Soc Psychiatry Psychiatr Epidemiol 33 (suppl 1):S86–S94, 1998

Swartz MS, Swanson JW, Hiday VA, et al: Violence and severe mental illness: the effects of substance abuse and nonadherence to medication. Am J Psychiatry 155:226–231, 1998

Swets JA: ROC analysis applied to the evaluation of medical imaging techniques. Invest Radiol 14:109–121, 1979

Tarasoff v Regents of the University of California, 551 P.2d 334 (Calif. 1976)

Tengström A: Long-term predictive validity of historical factors in two risk assessment instruments in a group of violent offenders with schizophrenia. Nord J Psychiatry 55:243–249, 2001

Webster CD, Douglas KS, Eaves E, et al: HCR-20: Assessing Risk for Violence, Version 2. Burnaby, British Columbia, Mental Health, Law and Policy Institute, Simon Fraser University, 1997

## Suggested Readings

Douglas KS, Kropp PR: A prevention-based paradigm for violence risk assessment: clinical and research applications. Criminal Justice and Behavior 29:617–658, 2002

Grove WM, Meehl PE: Comparative efficiency of informal (subjective, impressionistic) and formal (mechanical, algorithmic) prediction procedures: the clinical-statistical controversy. Psychology, Public Policy, and Law 2:293–323, 1996

Litwack TR: Actuarial versus clinical assessments of dangerousness. Psychology, Public Policy, and Law 7:409–443, 2001

Quinsey VL, Harris GT, Rice ME, et al: Violent Offenders: Appraising and Managing Risk. Washington, DC, American Psychological Association, 1998

Swanson JW: Mental disorder, substance abuse, and community violence: an epidemiological approach, in Violence and Mental Disorder: Developments in Risk Assessment. Edited by Monahan J, Steadman HJ. Chicago, IL, University of Chicago Press, 1994, pp 101–136

Webster CD, Douglas KS, Eaves E, et al: HCR-20: Assessing Risk for Violence, Version 2. Burnaby, British Columbia, Mental Health, Law and Policy Institute, Simon Fraser University, 1997

C H A P T E R 2 3

# The Evolving Standard in Forensic Psychological Testing

Daniel Brown, Ph.D.

## Introduction

Forensic psychology has rapidly grown and come into its own as a specialty area over the past three decades. In the 1970s the first textbooks appeared on the use of psychological expert testimony for competency evaluations (McGarry 1973; Roesch and Golding 1980) and criminal responsibility (Brodsky 1973; Megargee and Bohn 1979; Shapiro 1984). In 1973, Pacht and colleagues identified a "trend toward acceptance of testimony by psychologists" (p. 410). By the 1980s, the courts had become quite familiar with expert psychologists offering testimony in a wide range of areas: dangerousness, competency to stand trial, criminal responsibility, mental status at time of offense, insanity pleadings, involuntary commitment, personal injury damages, wrongful death, and custody determination (Ackerman 1999; Blau 1984; Melton et al. 1987). "Since the late 1980s in particular," note Borum and Otto (2000, p. 2), "there has been a remarkable surge of interest and growth in forensic psychology."

This rapid proliferation of psychology expert testimony has not meant that such testimony has always been well received. Critics have pointed out that such testimony cannot claim to be truly scientific and demonstrates neither reliability nor validity (Ennis and Litwack 1974; Gass 1979; Morse 1978a, 1978b). Some have argued that "professionals often fail to reach reliable or valid conclusions . . . that the accuracy of their judgments does not necessarily surpass that of laypersons . . . and [yet such testimony] alters many lives" (Faust and Ziskin 1988, pp. 31–32). Some critics have gone as far as to call psychiatric and psychological testimony nothing more that "informed speculation" (Ziskin 1995, p. 34; see also Faust and Ziskin 1988).

In response to this minority of vocal critics, an equally vigorous defense was launched by Joseph D. Matarazzo, then president of the American Psychological Association. In a letter responding to the *Science* article by Faust and Ziskin (1988), he argued that viewpoints such as that in the article disregard "a wide body of more recent research that demonstrates acceptably high reliability for many psychological and psychiatric diagnoses." While some commentators caution that expert psychological opinions not overreach the scientific evidence is merited, arguing for a prudent approach is not the same as arguing "for the elimination of experts in the courtroom" (Fowler and Matarazzo 1988, p. 1143; Matarazzo 1990; but see Ziskin and Faust 1991). Since the appearance of *Diagnostic and Statistical Manual of Mental Disorders*, 3rd Edition (DSM-III; American Psychiatric Association 1980), an increasing number of scientific studies have shown a marked increase in both reliability and validity and meet an acceptable standard within psychiatry (Meyer et al. 2001; von Talge 1995). The overall quality of forensic psychological reports has improved (Nicholson and Norwood 2000; Petrella and Poythress 1983).

The position taken in this chapter is that science has adequately responded to this debate with an increasing number of better designed studies, so that the standard of expert psychological testimony is evolving to a higher level along a number of dimensions. The purpose of this chapter is to illustrate how this standard is evolving, so that contemporary psychological expert testimony can be measured against this evolving yardstick.

## Clinical Vignette

The plaintiff in a personal injury lawsuit, Ms. R, sued a hospital and three defendant clinicians, a psychiatrist and two psychologists, for suggestively implanting false memories of childhood sexual abuse and giving a false diagnosis of a major dissociative disorder. Ms. R was admitted to an inpatient treatment unit at age 16 for alcohol abuse, a severe eating disorder, and an impulsive suicide attempt. During the course of that 2-month hospitalization, she developed the suspicion that she had been sexually abused by her father. This was immediately followed by the emergence of dissociative symptoms and shifting self states but not the emergence of discrete alter personality states that took executive control. Although the sexual abuse was not the focus of treatment, Ms. R discussed her suspicions about her father in a family meeting. Mr. R vehemently denied ever abusing his daughter. Ms. R's eating disorder symptoms and depression were stabilized and she was discharged.

Approximately 6 years later Ms. R developed the belief that the clinicians who had treated her during her previous inpatient hospitalizations had implanted false memories of abuse. She and her parents filed a malpractice suit against the hospital and the three treating clinicians: the psychiatrist and two psychologists. Plaintiff expert was a psychiatrist who had conducted an open-ended psychiatric interview with the plaintiff but had not conducted any formal psychological testing. He concluded through his interview that plaintiff was suffering from depression, anxiety, posttraumatic stress disorder, and severe mistrust of engaging in relationships, all causally related to the alleged malpractice. He also concluded that plaintiff had histrionic features to her personality and was "highly suggestible."

Defendant expert was a psychologist who conducted extensive, videotaped psychological testing over 2 full days. The testing consisted of a variety of structured clinical psychiatric interviews, a range of psychometric tests, and psychophysiological assessment of the alleged PTSD. All administration, scoring, and interpretation of the test followed standardized procedures. The testing also included a number of psychometric instruments specifically designed to assess legally relevant issues, including the degree to which the plaintiff might be suggestible; the areas of damage, if any, causally related to the alleged negligence; and the validity of the plaintiff's report of symptoms in the context of the lawsuit.

The test findings showed that Ms. R measured extremely low in general suggestibility, and in memory suggestibility specifically. She did not have the type of personality that would be prone to implanted false memories. The structured interviews showed that she had a long-standing mixed personality disorder with borderline features. Standardized administration of the structured interview with its strict scoring rules ruled out histrionic features. Various psychometric tests on interpersonal problems, along with ample historical data, showed that her alleged mistrust in relationships was not causally related to alleged malpractice by the defendants but had been an issue throughout her life, preexisting the treatment rendered by the defendants. Psychometric tests showed that Ms. R had a dissociative coping style. However, she denied the existence of significant dissociative symptoms on a standardized structured interview for major dissociative disorders. Empirically derived instruments designed to assess the validity of self-report indicated that her failure to report significant dissociative symptoms was unlikely to be a valid report. The testing also demonstrtated that Ms. R's eating disorder, major depressive disorder, and substance abuse were in complete remission. In other words, the defendants' treatment had been successful for the issues it had addressed during her inpatient stay.

The case went to jury trial. The jury found in favor of the defendants. The psychological testing evidence was cited as being a significant factor in the jury's determination that Ms. R was not sufficiently suggestible to be likely to have false memories implanted and that the evidence for psychiatric damages was not compelling.

## The Psychiatric Interview as a Standard for Expert Opinion

A recent study of forensic reports in six states (Nicholson and Norwood 2000, p. 18) concluded that "a clinical interview and mental status examination were fundamental components of the criminal forensic evaluations examined in these studies" and that the use of psychological testing, at least in the criminal forensic context, varied considerably across states. However, the use of open-ended interviewing techniques has come under considerable criticism from inside and outside the profession of psychiatry. Such interviews, critics point out, are subject to variation, selectivity, and biases of the examiners and thus, although useful, have at best only moderate validity.

The use of psychologists as expert witnesses in the courts increased over the years because psychologists typically administered psychological tests, whereas most psychiatrists based their opinions on psychiatric interviews (Ziskin 1995). Open-ended interviews fail to control for what information is and is not collected and for how it is collected or evaluated. The potential biases that limit the accuracy of clinical judgments and expert opinions include examiner effects (Ziskin 1995), hindsight bias (Hawkins and Hastie 1990), confirmatory bias (Garb 1998), bias to perceive pathology (Garb 1998), and disregard of base rates (Ziskin 1995). Open-ended psychiatric interviews are "subject to a great deal of uncontrolled variation" as well as to the "selectivity and biases of the examiner" (Ziskin 1995, pp. 327–328). Within the psychiatric profession itself, Robins (1985) lamented that the validity of psychiatric interviews was "well below the ideal" and that, though such interviews were useful, they had only "moderate validity" (p. 923; see Matarazzo 1983). At least in theory, pychological testing promised a remedy, as Ziskin (1995) has noted:

> The desire to overcome the limitations of interviewing techniques was one of the driving forces behind the development of psychological tests. For example, tests provide a potential means for standardizing data collection and the scoring or coding of the obtained data.... (p. 660)
>
> Much like interview data, a wide range of extraneous or uncontrolled influences can greatly affect the data on psychological testing. (p. 663)

Ziskin (1995) further noted:

> One potential advantage of many psychological tests over interview is that they specify just what it is the examiner is to record, thus decreasing the likelihood of major omissions or biased practices in record keeping. . . .
>
> The expert who follows such recommendations and is diligent in recording and scoring responses has created important safeguards for himself. However, experts are not necessarily so careful. (p. 678)

## The Traditional Psychological Test Battery as a Basis for Expert Testimony

Before discussing how the standard of expert psychological testimony is evolving, it would be useful to review what standard is actually represented in testimony customarily given by expert psychologists. The traditional approach to psychological testing was first articulated in the 1940s by Rapaport, Gill, and Schafer (1968). As it evolved in the 1950s through the 1980s, the so-called standard battery of psychological tests typically included intelligence tests (e.g., the Wechsler Adult Intelligence Scale), projective tests (e.g., Rorschach Inkblot Test, Thematic Apperception Test, Sentence Completion, and/or drawings), and organic screening tests such as the Bender-Gestalt Test. Many clinical psychologists also began to use actuarial tests such as the Minnesota Multiphasic Personality Inventory (MMPI) as part of the standard battery in their clinical practice. As increasing numbers of psychologists began offering expert opinions in the courts, the reliance on this standard battery of tests was simply transferred from the clinic to the court (Borum and Otto 2000).

Studies conducted to determine the degree to which forensic psychologists have utilized psychological testing, the tests they generally use, and other sources of evidence they use in constructing expert opinions demonstrate three distinct patterns. First, the traditional psychological test battery is the norm. In an early review of the literature from 1980 through 1982, Lanyon (1984) found that the MMPI and Rorschach accounted for two-thirds of all the literature of the top 15 psychological tests used in forensic settings. However, he also noted a growing tendency to select specific tests according to the purpose of the assessment. About three-quarters of forensic psychologists conducting custody evaluations used psychological tests, most frequently the MMPI and Rorschach (Keilin and Bloom 1986). Similar studies appearing in the 1990s concurred that the majority of forensic psychologists most frequently use a traditional battery of tests, including intelligence tests, the MMPI, and projective tests, mainly the Rorschach (Ackerman and Ackerman

1997; Boccaccini and Brodsky 1999; Borum and Grisso 1995; Heilbrun and Collins 1995; Holub 1992; LaFortune 1997; Lees-Haley 1992; Skeem et al. 1998). Second, there has been a very modest trend toward the development of specialized tests specifically for forensic assessment. Borum and Grisso (1995) and Ackerman and Ackerman (1997) noted a tendency to use newer assessment instruments that are specifically designed to address legally relevant questions such as competency to stand trial, criminal responsibility, and custody determination. Borum and Grisso (1995) noted, "Only 34% of psychologists and 7% of psychiatrists sometimes or more often used forensic assessment instruments" (p. 467). Third, many forensic psychologists fail to use other important sources of information besides testing (e.g., legal filings, interrogatories, deposition and trial testimony, historical information, medical records). Heilbrun and Collins (1995) found that the majority of competency reports "were written without the evaluator having reviewed important information such as the arrest report or prior mental health evaluations" (p. 66).

With rare exceptions, expert psychological testimony based on psychological test evidence has been found admissible by the court. Meloy and colleagues (1997), for example, surveyed legal citations to the Rorschach over a half century and found that the reliability and validity of the test were challenged in only 26 of 247 cases and that only once were the test results found inadmissible. Writing from a legal perspective, Gass (1979) feared that "seemingly 'objective' psychological testimony might have a 'prejudicial effect' [on jurors]" (p. 593). Likewise, from a clinical perspective, Nemeth (1995) argued that a traditional clinical battery of psychological tests served as a better standard than psychometric tests because the seemingly more scientific "objective" tests run the risk of "creat[ing] a deceptive effect on the judiciary" (p. 47) that confers pseudo-scientific validation yet often leads to erroneous conclusions or missing important clinical facts.

## Criticisms of Traditional Psychiatric Interviews and the Standard Psychological Test Battery in the Courtroom and a Response

The use of open-ended psychiatric interviews, the standard psychiatric mental status examination, and the traditional psychological test battery became increasingly vulnerable to attack during cross-examination for two reasons. First, an increasing number of scientific studies addressed the issue of reliability and validity of assessments, with the results not always demonstrating high reliability and validity. Second, negative results became powerful weapons in cross-examination by attorneys who were increasingly informed by emerging scientific evidence (Ziskin 1995).

In essence, the criticism of traditional psychiatric and psychological expert evidence centers on three factors: 1) standardization of the inquiry, 2) reliability of the observations across observers and across time, and 3) overall validity or accuracy of the findings (Dawes 1994; Garb 1998; Grove and Barden 1999; Ziskin 1995). According to critics, these approaches are vulnerable to too many "uncontrolled or extraneous influences" (Ziskin 1995, p. 380) and biases (Bolocofsky 1989) that make it unlikely that expert opinions will meet a legal standard of *reasonable certainty* (Ziskin 1995, p. 32).

The traditional psychiatric mental status examination, for example, lacks standardization of both its administration and scoring (Rogers 1995). Some tests in the traditional battery of psychological tests, notably the Rorschach and the Draw-a-Person Test (DAP), have been particularly criticized because of their failure to follow standardized methods of administration, scoring, or interpretation. A detailed investigation of the DAP found that clinicians persisted in making very specific interpretations lacking any scientific validity (Smith and Dumont 1995). This finding justified the view that some clinicians operate according to "illusory beliefs" despite negative findings that should have corrected persistent misbeliefs (Garb 1998; Ziskin 1995, p. 690).

In addition, traditional psychiatric interviews and mental status examinations, and also the standard psychological test battery, have been criticized because they seem to lack acceptable reliability and validity. *Interrater reliability* refers to the amount of agreement different observers reach regarding a psychiatric diagnosis or test score. The kappa coefficient has become the standard over calculation of interrater agreement because it corrects for chance agreement. The current consensus is that the kappa coefficient for psychiatric diagnoses made by different interviewers is poor if under 0.40, fair if between 0.40 and 0.59, good if between 0.60 and 0.74, and excellent if above 0.75 (Garb 1998).

Strong criticism from the legal arena that psychiatric diagnoses generally are unreliable and therefore should be inadmissible as evidence in the court (Ennis and Litwack 1974; Ziskin 1995) has unfortunately been premature. A related argument that data on reliability have been "unavailable" (Campbell 1999) is misleading; although these data were not published in DSM-III or DSM-IV (American Psychiatric Association 1994) (or its text revision, DSM-IV-TR [American Psychiatric Association 2000]), they are available, albeit generally scattered through peer-reviewed journals. The increasingly sophisticated scientific studies on diagnostic reliability in the past decade have made even skeptics recently conclude that interrater reliability is now good to excellent, at least for most DSM-IV Axis I and *International Classification of Diseases,* 10th Revision (ICD-10; World Health Organization 1992) conditions (Garb 1998), provided clinicians use the available diagnostic criteria (see Ziskin 2000).

*Validity* refers to the overall accuracy of psychiatric assessments. Ziskin (1995) considered questionable validity to be the "soft spot of psychological tests" (p. 685). The issue of validity is indeed complex. It would be misleading to speak of validity as an all-or-nothing phenomenon. The correct question is, Valid for what? Investigators have moved away from evaluating psychiatric interviews or psychological tests as being either valid or invalid. They now tend to evaluate such procedures in terms of issue-specific validity. Meyer and colleagues (2001) recently made a strong conclusion about the prevailing scientific evidence regarding the validity of psychological tests, especially if interpreted in the context of other sources of data such as medical records and historical information:

> Data from more than 125 meta-analyses on test validity and 800 samples examining multi-method assessment suggest 4 general conclusions: (a) psychological test validity is strong and compelling; (b) psychological test validity is comparable to medical test validity; (c) distinct assessment methods provide unique sources of information, and (d) clinicians who rely exclusively on interviews are prone to incomplete understandings. . . . a multi-method assessment battery provides a structured means for skilled clinicians to maximize the validity of individualized assessments. (p. 128)

## Psychological Testimony in the Courtroom in the Post-*Daubert* Era

*Frye v. United States* (1923), on the admissibility of expert testimony from lie detection studies, served to exclude seemingly scientific evidence that was potentially biased, influenced by numerous extraneous factors, or lacked accuracy. Only expert testimony that was "generally acceptable" was admissible (Gass 1979). More recently, the U.S. Supreme Court set a more refined standard in *Daubert v. Merrell Dow Pharmaceuticals, Inc.* (1993). The Court held that trial judges would serve as the gatekeepers in evaluating the nature and admissibility of the scientific status of expert testimony under Rule 702 of the Federal Rules of Evidence (1975), and to do so they could use four guidelines:

1. Whether the theory is testable
2. Whether the evidence has been subjected to peer review
3. Whether there is a known or potential error rate
4. Whether the scientific method is generally accepted by the relevant scientific community

The implications of *Daubert* for the admissibility of expert testimony are not yet fully clear because they in part depend on how trial judges interpret the decision (Goodman-Delahunty 1997). Nonetheless, it is becoming increasingly clear that trial judges will adopt some sort of scientific standard when scrutinizing expert testimony.

*Daubert* has ushered in an era of empirically supported expert testimony. This new era has been characterized by three new trends:

1. A distinct shift in preference toward expert opinions informed by empirically derived psychological assessment
2. A greater sensitivity to the overall context of a forensic assessment
3. A shift toward a greater tendency to address how the expert psychological opinion is or is not relevant to the legal issues in question

Rotgers and Barrett (1996) have discussed the implications of *Daubert* for forensic psychologists. They believe that forensic psychologists are more likely to be "held to the requirements of *Daubert*" (p. 468), so that testimony based on theoretical formulations, clinical beliefs, or methods of data gathering that are not scientifically established are less likely to be found admissible. They suggest four guidelines for post-*Daubert* forensic psychologists to follow (cited in Rotgers and Barrett 1996, pp. 471–472):

1. Use theoretically and psychometrically adequate data-gathering instruments.
2. Draw conclusions on the basis of scientifically validated theoretical positions.
3. Qualify testimony on the basis of adequacy of theory and empirical research on the questions being addressed.
4. Be prepared to defend data-gathering methods.

## The Rorschach Controversy as Illustrative of the *Daubert* Debate

The history of the controversy over the use of the Rorschach in the courtroom illustrates the evolution of scientific evidence and its usefulness in forensic evaluations. Ziskin (1995), in the fifth edition of *Coping With Psychiatric and Psychological Testimony*, argues that the Rorschach inkblot test is seldom administered or scored in a standardized manner by forensic experts, and that even given the evidence of more recent attempts to develop a standardized method for administration and scoring, and an empirically driven approach to interpretation (Exner 1991), "there is enough evidence challenging the reliability and validity of the system to call the entire system into question" (p. 863). More recently, Grove and Barden (1999) virtually dismissed the use of the Rorschach in the courts on the basis of the argument that it is 'junk science.' Research psychologists also have dismissed its clinical use on the basis of similar arguments (Dawes 1994; Garb 1984).

These arguments, however, are not exactly fair to the available evidence. Since 1991 considerable research has been devoted to scientific refinement of the Exner Comprehensive System. *Psychological Assessment* has devoted two special editions to the Rorschach (1999, 2001), wherein invited experts critically evaluated its scientific status. The Rorschach chapter in the fifth edition of Ziskin's (1995) *Coping With Psychiatric and Psychological Testimony*, written by a graduate student, does not compare to these authoritative works in *Psychological Assessment*. Writing against the validity of the Rorschach in the 1999 edition of *Psychological Assessment*, Hunsley and Bailey take the skeptical position that the validity data on the Exner Standardized Comprehensive System are "insufficient," even where a number of scales demonstrate good reliability. Viglione (1999) takes the credulous position that across 446 publications from 1977 through 1997 the Rorschach shows "impressive temporal consistency and reliability" and that "accurate clinical interpretation is achievable by well-trained clinicians using the standardized Comprehensive System" (p. 252). In the 2001 special edition of *Psychological Assessment*, Viglione dismisses the critics on the grounds that a "large body of empirical evidence supports the reliability, validity, and clinical utility of the Rorschach, suggesting that the recent criticisms of the Rorschach are largely without merit" (Viglione 2001, p. 452). He reviewed a number of meta-analytic analyses of the available evidence and remarked:

> Do the meta-analytic results support the validity of the Rorschach in general terms? There are at least six recent and original meta-analyses address Rorschach validity....All concluded with empirically based statements that supported the validity of the Rorschach. Opposing these five meta-analyses is one reanalysis of the Parker et al. data (1988) by Garb and colleagues (1998). (Viglione 2001, p. 457)

Summarizing the data on reliability, Weiner (2001, p. 424) cites Meyer's (1999) assessment that the kappa coefficients "for individual segments" of the Exner Standardized Comprehensive System range "from 0.72 to 0.98, with a mean value of 0.88" (i.e., generally in the excellent range). The critics, nevertheless, have not changed their position. Hunsley and Bailey (2001) state, "Having reviewed the evidence . . . we have found little reason to alter this position. Indeed, if anything, Garb et al.'s (2001) detailed review of the evidence . . . has served to amplify our concerns about the scientific status of the Rorschach" (p. 472). They add, "[S]ignificant problems currently exist . . . there remain huge gaps in our knowledge about the reliability, validity, and norms for Rorschach scales" (p. 482). Garb et al. (2001) adds, "Rorschach advocates need to provide evidence that the Rorschach contributes something that is not already contributed by self-report measures, interviews, or behavioral observations" (p. 435). However, the preponderance of the scientific evidence across the available meta-analytic studies, including an updated meta-analysis by Hiller and colleagues included in the 1999 special edition of *Psychological Assessment,* is skewed in support of increasing reliability and validity of the standardized Exner version of the Rorschach.

Some legal scholars have argued that current scientific controversies need not necessarily be resolved for expert opinions to be found admissible in the courtroom. According to Marlowe (1995), the *Daubert* standard implies only that the psychological test is generally recognized, has professional standards and norms governing its use, has appropriate data analysis procedures, and has adequate reliability and validity. McCann (1998) says that the *Daubert* standard for admissibility "does not require that a particular rate of error be zero; it is only necessary that expert opinion be based on a foundation where the potential rate of error can be established" (p. 137). McCann summarizes, "An analysis of the current clinical and research status of the Rorschach reveals that it meets professional and legal standards for admissibility of psychometric evidence and expert testimony" (p. 140). Viglione (2001) notes that the Rorschach "may be especially useful under conditions that might induce response manipulation in self-report. These might include employment, forensic, and custody evaluations, and other settings that involve adversarial examiner-respondent relationship components" (p. 465).

On the basis of such arguments, it is reasonable to conclude that even evidence from controversial psychological tests such as the Rorschach might have a legitimate place in forming expert testimony provided that a standardized form of administration, scoring, and interpretation serves as the basis of this evidence. Similar reasoning applies to other tests in the traditional battery of psychological tests. The remarkable proliferation of empirically derived studies on the Exner Standardized Comprehensive System of the Rorschach alone, along with a comparable database of studies on the MMPI and other psychological tests, illustrates the rapidly developing movement toward empirically derived clinical and forensic practice. This trend within the Rorschach literature parallels similarly rapidly accumulating databases in other areas of mental health, notably in psychotherapy outcome research (e.g., Kendall and Chambless 1998; Nathan and Gorman 1998).

## The Era of Empirically Supported Expert Testimony

### Structured Psychiatric Interviews

The lack of standardization in methods of gathering information in forensic assessments has also been a source of criticism of psychological and psychiatric testimony (Ziskin 1995). A significant amount of research has been conducted in recent years on the merits of standardized, structured psychiatric interviews as well as standardized, comprehensive mental status examinations. The reader can find a thorough review of the most widely used structured interviews and mental status examinations in Rogers's (1995) text, *Diagnostic and Structured Interviewing*.

Rogers observes that the accuracy of diagnosis is necessarily constrained when psychologists ask different questions and impose disparate meanings on patient responses. Reducing information variance standardizes the sequence of clinical inquiries. The use of structured interviews presumes 1) standardized administration, 2) strict adherence to how the questions are worded and to the sequencing of questions, 3) a defined set of diagnostic scoring criteria, and 4) clear-cut rules for determining whether or not the interview data meet each of these criteria and whether or not sufficient criteria have been met to render a given psychiatric diagnosis.

Rogers also delineates the advantages of structured interviews over open-ended interviews. Structured interviewing attempts to maximize the reliability and validity of its measurements by systematizing the assessment process. This results in the reduction of diagnostic disagreement by exerting control over information and criteria variance (Rogers 1995, pp. 17–18). Structured interviews may vary in how extensively they evaluate reported symptoms and presenting problems. Regardless, standard and optional questions are asked verbatim. Thus, structured interviewing standardizes 1) clinical inquiries and subsequent probes, 2) sequencing of clinical inquiries, and 3) systematic ratings of patient responses. The resulting uniformity allows for direct comparisons across psychologists, clinical settings, and diagnostic groups. Structured interviewing allows the reliability of testing and its generalizability to specific populations and settings to be easily ascertained.

In addition, studies on the diagnostic decisions of clinicians consistently demonstrate that many clinicians rarely adhere strictly to specified DSM diagnostic criteria and seldom use all of the criteria for a given diagnosis before rendering the diagnosis (Blashfield and Herkov 1996; Hasin et al. 1999; Morey and Ochoa 1989). The pitfalls of idiosyncratic approaches to psychiatric diagnosis are corrected by using structured psychiatric interviews, especially those designed to follow DSM diagnostic criteria closely. The Structured Clinical Interview for Diagnosis (SCID), for example, includes a comprehensive structured interview for Axis I conditions (SCID-I; First et al. 1994), Axis II conditions (SCID-II; First et al. 1997), and dissociative disorders (SCID-D; Steinberg 1994). Studies consistently have shown that such structured interviews significantly improve the reliability and accuracy of DSM diagnoses as compared with open-ended interviews (Rogers 1995; von Talge 1995).

## Psychometric or Objective Psychological Testing

The very fact that so much research has been generated to test the traditional psychological test battery indicates that these instruments meet the spirit of *Daubert*, even where controversies persist. No doubt, some trial judges acting as *Daubert* gatekeepers would prefer that these controversies remain active in the peer-reviewed scientific literature and not within the courtroom. Nevertheless, the Rorschach has rarely been successfully challenged in court (McCann 1998; Weiner 1996). The MMPI and Minnesota Multiphasic Personality Inventory–2 (MMPI-2) likewise have a long history of use in the court, as documented in the text *The MMPI, MMPI-2, and MMPI-A in Court* (Pope et al. 1999).

In addition to the use of the traditional psychological test battery, there is a growing trend toward using a wider range and greater selectivity of psychological tests in forensic assessment in forensic evaluations and testimony. For example, while both the MMPI-2 and Rorschach have been used for the forensic assessment of posttraumatic stress disorder (PTSD) in personal injury cases, a variety of empirically sound and generally accepted psychometric instruments are now available as viable alternatives. Two textbooks have been devoted entirely to a review of state-of-the-art psychometric instruments used in the assessment of PTSD (Carlson 1997; Wilson and Keane 1997). The books review such instruments as the Impact of Events Scale, the civilian version of the Mississippi Scale for PTSD, the Penn Inventory, the Davidson Trauma Scale, and many others. An important advantage of these psychometric measures of PTSD over more traditional assessment is that normative data are available for each of these instruments. Thus, these measures allow evaluators to develop an empirically derived estimate of the probability that a given individual tested does or does not have PTSD as compared with groups of individuals independently known to have PTSD (Keane 1995, p. 105). If according to established norms the probability of correctly classifying the tested individual as having PTSD is, say, 20% or 75%, the forensic expert is able to address the legal standard of *reasonable certainty* of the diagnosis in a manner that is likely to be relevant to the trier of fact and admissible.

The evaluation of depression, traditionally assessed by the Rorschach, has also been expanded by the use of new instruments. The depression index (DEPI) on the Comprehensive System of Rorschach interpretation is one of the few clinical scales that repeatedly has been shown to have questionable validity (Hunsley and Bailey 1999). In contrast, SCID-I contains a section of its standardized interview designed to detect a major depressive or dysthymic disorder with good-to-excellent reliability and validity. A variety of generally accepted psychometric tests, each with acceptable reliability and validity, also are designed to assess very specific dimensions of depression. A well-thought-out combination of psychometric tests such as the ones recommended below for assessing depression allows for very precise, normative measures of important dimensions of depression. Use of such tests allows expert opinions about depression to be more likely to meet the standard of reasonable certainty, defined in terms of being "conclusory" in a way that assists the triers of fact (Ennis and Litwack 1974, p. 698).

The Beck Depression Inventory assesses a range of depressive symptoms and can detect the presence of clinically significant depressive symptoms. The Hamilton Rating Scale for Depression is a widely used method to assess severity of depression. The Automatic Thought Questionnaire (ATQ) and Dysfunctional Attitudes Questionnaire (DAQ) assess different kinds of cognitive distortions that typically accompany depression, such as moment-by-moment negative self-talk and more stable irrational beliefs, respectively. Instruments such as the Profile of Mood States can identify the exact quality of the mood state, while instruments such as the Index of Self-Esteem assess the low self-esteem associated with depression.

Corcoran and Fischer's *Measures for Clinical Practice: A Sourcebook* (2000) and Strupp, Horowitz, and Lambert's *Measuring Patient Changes in Mood, Anxiety, and Personality Disorders* (1997) are excellent single-source collections of a wide variety of available psychometric tests, such as those described above and many more.

An expert must be prepared to justify the reasons for selecting tests, particularly as the issue of bias in test selection may be raised. Bias can be minimized by using "more than one variable for assessment and more than one test for each variable being considered" (Blau 1998, pp. 72–77). A strong advantage of the more-than-one-variable, more-than-one-test-per-variable standard is that errors are minimized. Errors that are addressed by this approach include those commonly associated with test selection biases and blind spots, as well as errors associated with the way any variable is being measured or limits of the assessment procedure. In *Daubert* terms this method of assessment is likely to reduce the overall error rate, so that the expert can render opinions meeting the criteria of reasonable certainty.

Consider the assessment of alleged PTSD in a personal injury case. Combining self-report psychometric measures such as the Impact of Events Scale or the Civilian Mississippi Scale for PTSD with actuarial scales such as the F/SC or PK subscales of the MMPI-2 meets the standard of "more than one test for each variable." Actuarial scales complement other instruments in that the questions asked are not about target symptoms. Questions are assigned to the actuarial scales on the basis of the fact that different samples of subjects known, for example, to have PTSD answer the given question or group of questions in a manner unique to PTSD groups. Thus, if individuals across samples known to have PTSD are likely to interpret the statement "I like the color blue" as "true," then that statement would become an item on an actuarial PTSD subscale, even though the content of the question has no obvious (or face-valid) relation to PTSD. Since actuarial scales are harder to fake, the use of both face-valid and actuarial methods of assessment serves as a partial correction for distortion of self-report. Heilbrun (1992, p. 267), for example, recommends a combination of objective self-report and actuarial tests specifically for forensic examinations.

Furthermore, psychophysiological assessment of the degree of physiological reactivity to trauma-specific stimuli (Orr and Kaloupek 1997) along with the self-report inventories meets the standard of "more than one variable for assessment."

As another example, the forensic psychologist might use a combination of the MMPI-2, Millon Clinical Multiaxial Inventory–II (MCMI-2), and SCID-II to assess whether or not a personality disorder is present.

The MCMI-2 yields fewer false negatives, while the MMPI-2 yields fewer false positives. The SCID-II allows a determination of whether the given individual meets sufficient criteria for a given personality disorder diagnosis. When all three tests are combined, the expert psychologist is able to form an opinion with confidence that the diagnosis has been rendered in a consensual manner, according to specified diagnostic rules, and in a way that achieves the highest sensitivity and specificity (Hills 1995; Ziskin 1995).

The standard of "more than one variable, more than one test per variable" is not without its critics. Uninformed combinations of testing instruments may simply be "combining less valid data with more valid data" in a way that could decrease the overall accuracy of the assessment (Ziskin 1995, p. 864). The incremental validity of combining evidence from a number of assessment instruments has not yet been established through research. A small number of studies addressing the incremental validity of test combinations have found that certain combinations of tests either fail to increase the overall accuracy of the findings or, in some cases, decrease it (Brody et al. 1990; Golden 1964; Wildman and Wildman 1975). However, such views represent only a minority opinion.

Most psychologists have adopted the position that multimethod assessment optimizes the validity of the conclusions. Multidimensional test batteries have been the preferred approach to testing in clinical settings for years (L'Abate 1964). Similarly, combinations of various tests (Heilbrun 1992) and comprehensive, multidimensional assessment (von Talge 1995) are rapidly becoming the standard of forensic psychological testing. In an authoritative position paper in *American Psychologist*, Meyer and colleagues (2001) concluded, after reviewing "more than 125 meta-analyses on test validity and 800 samples examining multimethod assessment," that "a multi-method assessment battery provides a structured means for skilled clinicians to maximize the validity of individualized assessments" (p. 128). Meyer et al. believe that "psychological assessment" (in which multiple test scores are combined with historical data and/or behavioral observations) is far superior to "psychological testing" (in which one test is given to yield a specific score). They described such combinations as the "optimal methodology" to enhance the validity of the conclusions: "Although there are many places in this process for errors to develop, the careful consideration of multi-method assessment data can provide a powerful antidote to the normal judgment biases that are inherent in clinical work" (Meyer et al. 2001, p. 150).

## Sensitivity to the Context of Forensic Testing

Psychologists, like psychiatrists, are becoming increasingly sensitive to the differences between conducting assessments in a forensic setting versus a clinical context. For one thing, informed consent is more problematic in the forensic setting. Research has shown that the great majority of clinicians fail to implement comprehensive, written informed consent procedures across a variety of clinical settings, even though most states have laws requiring informed consent (Lidz et al. 1984). Such results may be somewhat misleading, as some experts have argued that most clinicians appropriately integrate informed consent into ongoing discussions as part of the unfolding treatment relationship (Appelbaum et al. 1987; Gutheil 1989). Nevertheless, these findings raise concerns regarding the adequacy of procedures for obtaining informed consent in clinical settings.

Research also suggests that although there is a growing trend to use better informed consent procedures in forensic assessments, forensic psychologists generally do not address informed consent adequately (Nicholson and Norwood 2000). Informed consent is even more problematic in forensic contexts, where the adversarial context precludes the standards of confidentiality normally operable in a clinical setting. Therefore, the issue of informed consent takes on even greater ethical and practical importance.

Some forensic psychologists have also developed greater sensitivity to the issue of examiner biases, such as hindsight bias and confirmatory bias. *Hindsight bias* occurs, for example, in personal injury evaluations when the examiner shows a significantly greater likelihood of diagnosing PTSD *after* learning that a personal injury has been alleged (e.g., a car accident or sexual abuse). *Confirmatory bias* occurs when the examiner mainly selects assessment instruments or asks questions consistent with a presumptive diagnosis or theory and does not include tests or questions pertaining to alternative or disconfirming hypotheses. Some forensic psychologists in personal injury cases, for example, fail to adequately evaluate preexisting conditions or to adequately consider base rates (Ziskin 1995). Other biases, such as the phenomena of forensic identification, are also problematic. *Forensic identification* occurs when an expert opinion is based more on which side of the adversarial system the expert represents than on the available evidence (Zusman and Simon 1983). Seasoned forensic psychologists, who have withstood enough cross-examinations, generally learn to address the issues of biases in their very selection of testing instruments and interview questions.

Some experienced forensic psychologists have learned to routinely assess potential self-report distortions on the part of the examinee. Such distortions occur frequently in a forensic context (Heilbrun 1992). Motivations for initiating a lawsuit are complex, and the stress of the lawsuit itself often brings out behaviors or psychopathology that is not readily apparent in other contexts (Lees-Haley 1997). Seasoned forensic psychologists generally include empirically derived methods for assessing the reliability and validity of the self-report. The MMPI-2, for example, has a number of scales designed to assess the validity of self-reported symptoms. MMPI-2 scales such as the L, F, Fback, K, VRIN, and TRIN have been used extensively in the courts. The meaning and use of these actuarial validity scales have been thoroughly reviewed by Pope et al. (1999). The scales allow the forensic expert to render an opinion about the probability that the client's self-report of symptoms is or is not accurate and, more specifically, about whether the client is trying to exaggerate (fake bad) or minimize (fake good) psychiatric symptoms in the context of a lawsuit.

A number of other empirically derived instruments for assessing self-report validity and/or malingering, all of which have a tradition of general acceptance and usage and published reliability and validity data to support their use, are currently available. Since clinicians and forensic examiners alike generally do not do a good job detecting malingering (Rogers and Bagby 2002) or factitious behavior (Brown and Scheflin 1999), using such empirically supported instruments to assess response bias and distortion raises the standard of the forensic examination. The Malingering Probability Scale (Silverton and Gruber 1998) is a way to assess the probability of malingering psychiatric symptoms in a forensic context. The Test of Memory Malingering (Tombaugh 1996) is specifically designed to test malingering memory problems in a forensic context. The Structured Interview of Reported Symptoms (Rogers 1997) is a structured interview also designed to detect malingering.

Each of these instruments would likely meet the *Daubert* standards of testability, a known error rate, peer review, and general acceptance. Each has the advantage of allowing the forensic examiner to render empirically derived, evidentiary-informed opinions with reasonable certainty about the probability that malingering or another form of serious self-report distortion is or is not occurring.

Finally, some seasoned forensic examiners have learned not to administer narrowly focused interviews or psychological tests but rather to conduct a very comprehensive examination that includes multiple sources of evidence. The evolving standard is for the forensic psychologist to use multiple data sources (Keane 1995, p. 113), at least in personal injury cases, although the research has shown that the majority of criminal competency evaluations still fail to meet this standard (Heilbrun and Collins 1995; Nicholson and Norwood 2000; Skeem et al. 1998). According to Garb (1984, pp. 641–642), "A set of information possesses incremental validity if validity increases when the set of information is added to other data." Studies on incremental validity (e.g., Garb 1984, 1998) have consistently shown that the evaluation of extensive biographical and historical data, as compared with more limited data, in conjunction with psychological testing significantly increases the validity of the findings.

A recent survey reported a growing trend for experienced forensic psychologists to conduct more comprehensive assessments that include multiple sources of information (Nicholson and Norwood 2000). More experienced forensic examiners request significantly more information than less experienced ones (O'Byrne and Goodyear 1997). Nicholson and Norwood (2000) consider the "collection of third-party information" to be "a central characteristic of forensic assessment that distinguishes it from traditional therapeutic assessment" (p. 21). Therefore, the reasonably prudent forensic psychologist is advised to evaluate carefully all the collateral evidence, say, in a personal injury case, including the personal and family history of the client, all medical and psychiatric records; all existing interviews and psychiatric assessments; school, occupational, and disability records; military records; and all interrogatories, depositions, and trial testimony.

Forensic opinions rendered about psychological assessments that ignore important life history data and medical records are becoming increasingly harder to justify (Heilbrun 1992; Joseph et al. 2000; Matarazzo 1990). Such well-prepared experts are likely to be viewed by jurors as carefully informed, knowing the evidence, and capable of establishing reasonable conceptual links between specific findings on given psychological tests and the evidence from medical records, testimony, and other sources of information.

## The Evolving Standard of Legal Relevance

An ongoing criticism of forensic psychological assessment made by legal theorists revolves around the legal concept of relevancy. Consider for example, a forensic psychologist addressing the question of competency solely by rendering a psychiatric diagnosis, which is meant to indirectly imply incompetence. Legal competency constructs focus on an individual's functional abilities: what an individual can do or accomplish, as well as specific knowledge, understanding, or beliefs that may be necessary for the accomplishment. Functioning is related to, but distinct from, psychiatric diagnoses or conclusions about general intellectual abilities and personality traits (Grisso 1986, p. 15). The principal objective of an assessment related to legal competency should be the description of an examinee's functional abilities that are relevant conceptually to the legal competency in question. The evaluator should observe, measure, or otherwise document by reliable means the abilities themselves, rather than relying solely on diagnoses of psychopathology, psychiatric symptoms, or assessment of personality traits and general intelligence to infer the examinee's functional abilities (Grisso 1986, p. 29).

Self-report data from psychological tests may be minimally related to everyday functioning (Ziskin 1995, p. 947). For example, in the case of custody evaluations, psychologists routinely offer opinions about custody and visitation matters based to a great extent, and sometimes exclusively, on the results of psychological testing (Brodzinsky 1993, p. 214). Administering a standard battery of tests to parents or children may yield information about their intellectual competence, level of academic achievement, personality characteristics, and emotional stability. However, these data are only indirectly tied to the substantive issues involved in custody and visitation disputes. The standard psychological tests used in custody evaluations were not developed for forensic purposes. Since such testing was not designed to address directly either everyday functioning or parental competence, opinions on such issues rendered on the basis of that evidence overreach the knowledge such tests provide.

A common complaint of the court is that forensic experts fail to link their opinions to *legally* relevant determinations. Research studies have concurred that somewhere between 41% and 75% of forensic reports fail to address the ultimate legal question (Nicholson and Norwood 2000; Skeem and Golding 1998). Expert testimony that fails to establish legal relevancy runs the risk of being inadmissible to the court (Heilbrun 1992). Scores on intelligence and personality tests alone only mildly correlate with competence (Nicholson and Kugler 1991). Even a diagnosis per se does not convey anything meaningful about legally relevant questions (Melton et al. 1987; see also Chapter 6: "Psychiatric Diagnosis in Litigation," this volume). Some forensic experts are too quick to offer testimony about diagnoses without rendering any opinion about competence or to simply infer from the diagnosis alone that the client is incompetent. Even "insane" patients diagnosed as having schizophrenia often behave in *legally* competent ways, and such a diagnosis only indirectly (and sometimes inaccurately) is associated with the legal concept of competence.

Traditionally, experts were prohibited from rendering opinions about ultimate legal questions on the basis of the argument that such opinions usurped the task of the jury (Morse 1978b). Melton and colleagues believe that ultimate legal issues "involve questions of morality and justice that lie outside the mental health professional's domain of expertise" (Nicholson and Norwood 2000, p. 12), but others have argued the opposite. A balanced view is that the forensic psychologist's role is to render opinions that are directly relevant to the ultimate legal question(s), along with detailed testimony about the basis of those opinions. These opinions should be given in such a way that they *assist* the fact finders in answering the ultimate legal questions rather than usurp their role. For example, empirically supported psychometric testing of malingering might serve as the basis of exert opinions about the probability of malingering self-reported symptoms, insofar as these opinions are given in a way that do not imply a direct opinion regarding witness credibility. The expert who provides such evidence presumably assists the fact finders in determining the credibility of the witness, while not co-opting the fact finders in making the ultimate determination.

The development of highly specific, empirically derived forensic assessment instruments (FAIs) is a promising trend in forensic psychology that can assist psychiatrists and psychologists in providing testimony that is relevant to the legal issue in question (Grisso 1987; Lanyon 1986; Nicholson and Norwood 2000). Many of these FAIs meet an acceptable level of reliability and validity and therefore offer the forensic examiner a reasonably certain way to assess very specific questions that are legally relevant to the triers of fact. Examples of these FAIs include tests of competency (Competency Screening Test [Lipsitt et al. 1973], Competency to Stand Trial Assessment Instrument [McGarry 1973], Interdisciplinary Fitness Interview [Golding and Roesch 1984], Georgia Court Competency Test [Wildman et al. 1979]); criminal responsibility (Rogers Criminal Responsibility Assessment Scales [Rogers 1984]); malingering (Malingering Probability Scale [Silverton and Gruber 1998], Structured Interview of Reported Symptoms [Rogers 1997]); and suggestibility (Gudjonsson Suggestibility Scale [Gudjonsson 1984]). *Evaluating Competencies* (Grisso 1986) is a single-source collection of FAIs.

One of the main complaints about the irrelevancy of expert testimony pertains to the question of proximate cause. In personal injury cases the plaintiff must establish not only that there has been damages but also that the said damages are directly and proximately caused by the defendant's negligent or injurious actions. Consider, for example, a plaintiff alleging a personal injury from a motor vehicle accident. The forensic examiner must establish not only that the plaintiff does or does not have psychiatric conditions such as PTSD or depression but also that such conditions, if present, were proximately caused by the alleged accident and were not primarily caused by other factors. Ebaugh and Benjamin (1937) were the first to establish a list of causal possibilities, namely, that the alleged accident was 1) the sole cause of the injury; 2) a major precipitating factor without which the injury would not have become manifest at that time; 3) an aggravating factor that made a preexisting condition worse; or 4) not related to the injury. Other possibilities include that the alleged accident was one of a number of multiple, contributing causes and that the injury reactivated a preexisting condition that was in remission. Clearly, any expert assessment of proximate causality is complex.

Psychologists have learned to estimate effect sizes and to apportion the variance among competing variables from statistics training. They are therefore likely to appreciate the complexity of assessing causal relationships and to make modest claims about causal relationships in a research or clinical context. The problem, however, is that in a forensic context experts often go far beyond the evidence and render stronger opinions about causality than are entirely justified by the facts (Melton et al. 1987; Morse 1978b). Some critics have argued that "cause and effect relationships in psychiatry are more a product of speculation than scientific accuracy" that cannot meet the standard of reasonable certainty (Marcus 1983, p. 428). Such extreme opinions are not necessarily accompanied by an explicit account of the reasoning behind the causal opinion. Yet, when causal relationships are reasonably established through an examination of the evidence, and when they are supported by careful documentation of the expert's reasoning to justify those relationships, such opinions offer the promise of being relevant to the triers of fact.

## Practice Guidelines for Forensic Psychological Testing

Guidelines for the practice of forensic psychology have been clearly articulated since the early 1990s (Committee on Ethical Guidelines for Forensic Psychologists 1991; Heilbrun 1992; Marlowe 1995). These guidelines specify that psychological testing be done by clinicians with specialized training and demonstrated competence in the administration, scoring, and interpretation of test results. The use of psychological testing by untrained professionals violates existing ethical standards. While most psychologists get highly specialized training in psychological testing as part of their graduate education, most psychiatrists do not, just as most psychiatrists get highly specialized training in psychiatric medication as part of their medical education and psychologists do not.

More recently, however, the boundaries between psychology and psychiatry have become less rigidly defined. Both psychologists and psychiatrists alike have taken specialized training in the administration of structured psychiatric interviews such as SCID. Some psychiatrists have received specialized training in the use of psychometric tests through continuing education or through their ongoing research. Nevertheless, psychiatrists who have not received specialized training in psychometric testing should consider developing a solid referral base with psychologists who have specialty training and competence in the use of complex and valuable forensic psychological testing.

## Conclusion

This fourth decade of forensic psychology is characterized by a rapidly evolving standard along several fronts:

1. A trend toward the use of empirically supported structured interviews and psychometric tests
2. A greater sensitivity to the considerations of testing in a forensic context
3. An attempt to reduce the gap between psychological assessment and legally relevant questions

The post-*Daubert* era does not require error-free science. It does require that expert psychiatric and psychological opinion be based on empirically supported assessment instruments for which the reliability and validity are known and found to meet a reasonable standard. The post-*Daubert* court, and the available practice guidelines for forensic psychologists within the profession, require that the selection of instruments and interview topics be guided by an attempt to minimize biases, to be comprehensive, and to offer opinions directly relevant to the legal question(s) at hand. Psychiatrists who understand the advantages and appropriate uses of psychological testing and testimony will be better able to prepare and defend their opinions.

## Key Points

- Empirically derived forensic psychological testing can assist forensic clinicians in addressing some of the biases and extraneous influences that may arise in open-ended psychiatric interviews and traditional mental status examinations.
- In this post-*Daubert* era, even the standard battery of psychological tests, including controversial instruments such as the Rorschach, has its place, provided a standardized form of administration, scoring, and interpretation serves as the basis of this evidence.
- The error rate and biases associated with forensic psychological testing are greatly reduced and the comprehensiveness of the testing is increased when a multidimensional approach is taken to forensic testing. This multidimensional approach should include the use of
  - Structured psychiatric interviews.
  - A battery of empirically derived psychometric tests that address a range of relevant variables with more than one test per variable.
  - Specific forensic assessment instruments (in some cases).
- Testing alone does not provide enough data on which to base expert opinions. All relevant documentation and evidence should be considered.
- The selection of psychological tests and the conclusions drawn from them better assist the court when they address legally relevant issues.

## Practice Guidelines

The following guidelines are recommended whether a psychiatrist obtains specialized training in forensic psychological testing and the use of structured psychiatric interviews or has this testing performed by an experienced psychologist who understands the differences between forensic and clinical contexts.

1. Use appropriate forensic informed consent procedures.
2. Select generally accepted assessment instruments that are readily available and reasonably relied on by experts in the relevant scientific community and that have reasonable reliability and validity data.
3. Use procedures that standardize administration, scoring, and interpretation of assessment instruments.
4. Assess a wide range of relevant variables with at least several tests per variable as a way to meet the criterion of comprehensiveness and to reduce the error rate.

5. Use a battery of tests that combines different methods of assessment, such as self-report inventories, actuarial tests, forensic assessment instruments, empirically derived behavioral assessments, and psychophysiological testing.
6. Use empirically supported instruments to assess response style and other factors that might affect the validity of self-reports, such as malingering.
7. Evaluate other relevant sources of data in addition to psychological testing, such as medical records, deposition and trial testimony, and so forth.
8. Render opinions that assist the court in answering legally relevant questions.
9. Disclose the limits of the evidence and how such limits might affect the certainty of the expert opinions as well as disclosure of reasonable alternative explanations for the evidence.

## References

Ackerman MJ: Essentials of Forensic Psychological Assessment. New York, Wiley, 1999

Ackerman MJ, Ackerman MC: Custody evaluation practices: a survey of experienced professionals (revisited). Professional Psychology 28:137–145, 1997

American Psychiatric Association: Diagnostic and Statistical Manual of Mental Disorders, 3rd Edition. Washington, DC, American Psychiatric Association, 1980

American Psychiatric Association: Diagnostic and Statistical Manual of Mental Disorders, 4th Edition. Washington, DC, American Psychiatric Association, 1994

American Psychiatric Association: Diagnostic and Statistical Manual of Mental Disorders, 4th Edition, Text Revision. Washington, DC, American Psychiatric Association, 2000

Appelbaum PS, Lidz CW, Meisel A: Informed Consent: Legal Theory and Clinical Practice. New York, Oxford University Press, 1987

Blashfield RK, Herkov MJ: Investigating clinician adherence to diagnosis by criteria: a replication of Morey and Ochoa (1989). J Personal Disord 10:219–228, 1996

Blau TH: Psychological tests in the courtroom. Professional Psychology 15:176–186, 1984

Blau TH: The Psychologist as Expert Witness. New York, Wiley, 1998

Boccaccini MT, Brodsky SL: Diagnostic test use by forensic psychologists in emotional injury cases. Professional Psychology 30:253–259, 1999

Bolocofsky DN: Use and abuse of mental health experts in child custody determinations. Behav Sci Law 7:197–213, 1989

Borum R, Grisso T: Psychological test use in criminal forensic evaluations. Professional Psychology: Research and Practice 26:465–473, 1995

Borum R, Otto R: Advances in forensic assessment and treatment: an overview and introduction to the special issue. Law Hum Behav 24:1–7, 2000

Brodsky S: Psychologists in the Criminal Justice System. Urbana, University of Illinois Press, 1973

Brody GH, Stoneman Z, Millar M, et al: Assessing individual difference: effects of responding to prior questionnaires on the substantive and psychometric properties of self-esteem and depression assessments. J Pers Assess 54:401–411, 1990

Brodzinsky DM: On the use and misuse of psychological tests in child custody evaluations. Professional Psychology 24:213–219, 1993

Brown D, Scheflin AW: Factitious disorders and trauma-related diagnoses. J Psychiatry Law 27:373–422, 1999

Campbell, TW: Challenging the evidentiary reliability of DSM-IV. American Journal of Forensic Psychology 1:47–68, 1999

Carlson E: Trauma Assessments: A Clinician's Guide. New York, Guilford, 1997

Committee on Ethical Guidelines for Forensic Psychologists: Specialty guidelines for forensic psychologists. Law Hum Behav 15:655–665, 1991

Corcoran K, Fischer J: Measures for Clinical Practice: A Sourcebook, 3rd Edition. New York, Free Press, 2000

Daubert v Merrell Dow Pharmaceuticals, Inc, 113 S. Ct. 2786 (1993)

Dawes RM: House of Cards: Psychology and Psychotherapy Built on Myth. New York, Free Press, 1994

Ebaugh FG, Benjamin JD: Trauma and mental disorder, in Trauma and Disease. Edited by Bradhy L, Kahn S. Philadelphia, PA, Lea & Febiger, 1937, pp 231–272

Ennis BJ, Litwack TR: Psychiatry and the presumption of expertise: flipping coins in the courtroom. California Law Review 62:693–752, 1974

Exner JE: The Rorschach: A Comprehensive System, 2nd Edition. New York, Wiley, 1991

Faust D, Ziskin J: The expert witness in psychology and psychiatry. Science 241: 31–35, 1988

Federal Rules of Evidence for United States Courts and Magistrates. St Paul, MN, West Publishing, 1975

First MB, Spitzer RL, Gibbon M, et al: Structured Clinical Interview for DSM-IV Axis I Disorders. Washington, DC, American Psychiatric Press, 1994

First MB, Gibbon M, Spitzer RL, et al: Structured Clinical Interview for DSM-IV Axis II Personality Disorders. Washington, DC, American Psychiatric Press, 1997

Fowler RD, Matarazzo JD: Psychologists and psychiatrists as expert witnesses. Science 241:1143–1144, 1988

Frye v United States, D.C. Cir. 293 F. 1013 (1923)

Garb HN: The incremental validity of information used in personality assessment. Clin Psychol Rev 4:641–655, 1984

Garb HN: Studying the Clinician: Judgment Research and Psychological Assessment. Washington, DC, American Psychological Association, 1998

Garb HN, Florio CM, Grove WM: The validity of the Rorschach and the Minnesota Multiphasic Personality Inventory: results from meta-analyses. Psychol Science 9:402–404, 1998

Garb HN, Wood JM, Nezworski MT, et al: Toward a resolution of the Rorschach controversy. Psychol Assess 13:433–448, 2001

Gass CS: The psychologist as expert witness: science in the courtroom. Maryland Law Review 38:539–621, 1979

Golden M: Some effects of combining psychological tests on clinical inferences J Consult Clin Psychol 28:440–446, 1964

Golding S, Roesch R: Assessment and conceptualization of competency to stand trial: preliminary data on the Interdisciplinary Fitness Interview. Law Hum Behav 8:321–334, 1984

Goodman-Delahunty J: Forensic psychological expertise in the wake of *Daubert.* Law Hum Behav 21:121–140, 1997

Grisso T: Evaluating Competencies: Forensic Assessments and Instruments. New York, Plenum, 1986

Grisso T: The economic and scientific future of forensic psychological assessment. Am Psychol 42:831–839, 1987

Grove WM, Barden RC: Protecting the integrity of the legal system: the admissibility of testimony from mental health experts under *Daubert/Kumho* analysis. Psychology, Public Policy, and Law 5:224–242, 1999

Gudjonsson G: A new scale of interrogative suggestibility. Personality and Individual Differences 5:303–314, 1984

Gutheil TG: Legal issues in psychiatry, in Comprehensive Textbook in Psychiatry/V, 5th Edition. Edited by Kaplan HI, Sadock BJ. Baltimore, MD, Williams & Wilkins, 1989, pp 2107–2124

Hasin D, Paykin A, Endicott J, et al: The validity of DSM-IV alcohol abuse: drunk drivers versus all others. J Stud Alcohol 60:746–755, 1999

Hawkins SA, Hastie R: Hindsight: biased judgments of past events after the outcomes are known. Psychol Bull 107:311–327, 1990

Heilbrun K: The role of psychological testing in forensic assessment. Law Hum Behav 16:257–272, 1992

Heilbrun K, Collins S: Evaluations of trial competency and mental state at time of offense: report characteristics. Professional Psychology: Research and Practice 26:61–67, 1995

Hiller JB, Rosenthal R, Bornstein RF, et al: A comparative meta-analysis of Rorschach and MMPI validity. Psychol Assess 11:278–296, 1999

Hills HA: Diagnosing personality disorders: an examination of the MMPI-2 and MCMI-II. J Pers Assess 65:21–34, 1995

Holub RJ: Forensic psychological testing: a survey of practices and beliefs. Unpublished manuscript, Minnesota School of Professional Psychology, Bloomington, 1992

Hunsley J, Bailey JM: The clinical utility of the Rorschach: unfulfilled promises and an uncertain future. Psychol Assess 11:266–277, 1999

Hunsley J, Bailey JM: Whither the Rorschach? An analysis of the evidence. Psychol Assess 13:472–485, 2001

Joseph GW, Atkins EL, Flaks DK: Admissibility of expert psychological testimony in the era of *Daubert:* the case of hedonic damages. American Journal of Forensic Psychology 18:3–33, 2000

Keane TM: Guidelines for the forensic psychological assessment of posttraumatic stress disorder claimants, in Posttraumatic Stress Disorder in Litigation: Guidelines for Forensic Assessment. Edited by Simon RI. Washington, DC, American Psychiatric Press, 1995, pp 99–115

Keilin WG, Bloom LJ: Child custody evaluation practices: a survey of experienced professionals. Professional Psychology 17:338–346, 1986

Kendall PC, Chambless DL (guest eds): Empirically supported psychological therapies (special issue). J Consult Clin Psychol 66:3–167, 1998

L'Abate L: Principles of Clinical Psychology. New York, Grune & Stratton, 1964

LaFortune KA: An investigation of mental health and legal professionals' activities, beliefs, and experiences in domestic court: an interdisciplinary survey. Unpublished doctoral dissertation. University of Tulsa, Tulsa, OK, 1997

Lanyon RI: Personality assessment. Annu Rev Psychol 35:667–701, 1984

Lanyon, RI: Psychological assessment procedures in court-related settings. Professional Psychology: Research and Practice 17:260–268, 1986

Lees-Haley PR: Psychodiagnostic test usage by forensic psychologists. American Journal of Forensic Psychology 10:25–30, 1992

Lees-Haley PR: MMPI-2 base rates for 492 personal injury plaintiffs: implications and challenges for forensic assessment. J Clin Psychol 53:745–755, 1997

Lidz CW, Meisel A, Zerubavel E, et al: Informed Consent: A Study of Decision Making in Psychiatry. New York, Guilford, 1984

Lipsitt P, Lelos D, McGarry AL: Competency to Stand Trial and Mental Illness (DHEW Publ No ADM 77-103). Rockville, MD, National Institute of Mental Health, 1973

Marcus EH: Causation in psychiatry: realities and speculations. Medical Trial Technique Quarterly 28:424–433, 1983

Marlowe DB: A hybrid decision framework for evaluating psychometric evidence. Behav Sci Law 13:207–228, 1995

Matarazzo JD: The reliability of psychiatric and psychological diagnosis. Psychol Rev 3:103–145, 1983

Matarazzo JD: Psychological assessment versus psychological testing: validation from Binet to the school, clinic, and courtroom. Am Psychol 45:999–1017, 1990

McCann JT: Defending the Rorschach in court: an analysis of admissibility using legal and professional standards. J Pers Assess 70:125–144, 1998

McGarry AL: Competency to stand trial and mental illness (DHEW Publ No ADM 77-103). Rockville, MD, National Institute of Mental Health, 1973

Megargee E, Bohn M: Classifying Criminal Offenders: A New System Based on the MMPI. Beverly Hills, CA, Sage, 1979

Meloy JR, Hansen TL, Weiner IB: Authority of the Rorschach: legal citations during the past 50 years. J Pers Assess 69:53–62, 1997

Melton GB, Petrila J, Poythress NG, et al: Psychological Evaluations for the Courts: A Handbook for Mental Health Professionals and Lawyers, 2nd Edition. New York, Guilford, 1987

Meyer GJ: Introduction to the special series on the utility of the Rorschach for clinical assessment. Psychol Assess 11:235–239, 1999

Meyer GJ, Finn SE, Eyde LD, et al: Psychological testing and psychological assessment. Am Psychol 56:128–165, 2001

Morey LC, Ochoa ES: An investigation of clinical adherence to diagnostic criteria: clinical diagnosis of DSM-III personality disorders. J Personal Disord 3: 180–192, 1989

Morse SJ: Crazy behavior, morals, and science: an analysis of mental health law. Southern California Law Review 51:527–654, 1978a

Morse SJ: Law and mental health professionals: the limits of expertise. Professional Psychology 9:389–398, 1978b

Nathan PE, Gorman JM: A Guide to Treatments That Work. New York, Oxford University Press, 1998

Nemeth AJ: Ambiguities caused by forensic psychology's dual identity: how to deal with the prevailing quantitative bias and "scientific" posture. American Journal of Forensic Psychology 13:47–66, 1995

Nicholson RA, Kugler KE: Competent and incompetent criminal defendants: a quantitative review of comparative research. Psychol Bull 109:355–370, 1991

Nicholson RA, Norwood S: The quality of forensic psychological assessments, reports, and testimony: acknowledging the gap between promise and practice. Law Hum Behav 24:9–44, 2000

O'Byrne KR, Goodyear RK: Client assessment by novice and expert psychologists: a comparison of strategies. Educational Psychology Review 9:267–278, 1997

Orr SP, Kaloupek DG, Psychophysiological assessment of posttraumatic stress disorder, in Assessing Psychological Trauma and PTSD. Edited by Wilson JP, Keane TM. New York, Guilford, 1997, pp 69–97

Pacht AR, Kuehn JK, Bassett HT, et al: The current status of the psychologist as an expert witness. Professional Psychology: Research and Practice 4:409–412, 1973

Parker KCH, Hanson RK, Hunsley J: MMPI, Rorschach, and WAIS: a meta-analytic comparison of reliability, stability, and validity. Psychol Bull 103: 367–373, 1988

Petrella RC, Poythress NG: The quality of forensic evaluations: an interdisciplinary study. J Consult Clin Psychol 51:76–85, 1983

Pope KS, Butcher JN, Seelen J: The MMPI, MMPI-2, MMPI-A in Court: A Practical Guide for Expert Witnesses and Attorneys, 2nd Edition. Washington, DC, American Psychological Association, 1999

Rapaport D, Gill MM, Schafer R: Diagnostic Psychological Testing, Revised Edition. Edited by Holt RR. New York, International Universities Press, 1968

Robins LN: Epidemiology: reflections on testing the validity of psychiatric interviews. Arch Gen Psychiatry 42:918–924, 1985

Roesch R, Golding S: Competency to Stand Trial. Urbana-Champaign, University of Illinois Press, 1980

Rogers R: Rogers Criminal Responsibility Assessment Scales. Odessa, FL, Psychological Assessment Resources, 1984

Rogers R: Diagnostic and Structured Interviewing: A Handbook for Psychologists. Odessa, FL, Psychological Assessment Resources, 1995

Rogers R: Clinical Assessment of Malingering and Deception, 2nd Edition. New York, Guilford, 1997

Rogers R, Bagby M, Dickens SE: Structured Interview of Reported Symptoms. Lutz, FL, Psychological Assessment Resources, 2002

Rotgers F, Barrett D: *Daubert v Merrell Dow* and expert testimony by clinical psychologists: implications and recommendations for practice. Professional Psychology 27:467–474, 1996

Shapiro DL: Psychological Evaluation and Expert Testimony: A Practical Guide to Forensic Work. New York, Van Nostrand Reinhold, 1984

Silverton L, Gruber C: Malingering Probablity Scale (MPS). Los Angeles, CA, Western Psychological Services, 1998

Skeem JL, Golding SL: Community examiners' evaluations of competence to stand trial: common problems and suggestions for improvement. Professional Psychology: Research and Practice 29:357–367, 1998

Skeem JL, Golding SL, Cohn NB, et al: Logic and reliability of evaluations of competence to stand trial. Law Hum Behav 22:519–547, 1998

Smith D, Dumont F: A cautionary study: unwarranted interpretations of the Draw-a-Person Test. Professional Psychology 26:298–303, 1995

Steinberg M: Structured Clinical Interview for DSM-IV Dissociative Disorders, Revised Edition. Washington, DC, American Psychiatric Press, 1994

Strupp HH, Horowitz LM, Lambert MJ: Measuring Patient Changes in Mood, Anxiety, and Personality Disorders: Toward a Core Battery. Washington, DC, American Psychological Association, 1997

Tombaugh TN: TOMM Test of Memory Malingering. North Tonawanda, NY, Multi-Health Systems, 1996

Viglione DJ: A review of recent research addressing the utility of the Rorschach. Psychological Assessment 11:251–265, 1999

Viglione DJ, Hilsenroth MJ: The Rorschach: facts, fictions, and future. Psychol Assess 13:452–471, 2001

von Talge J: Overcoming courtroom challenges to the DSM-IV, Part II: preparing for and overcoming courtroom challenges to DSM-IV. American Journal of Forensic Psychology 13:49–54, 1995

Weiner IB: Some observations on the validity of the Rorschach Inkblot Method. Psychol Assess 8:206–213, 1996

Weiner IB: Advancing the science of psychological assessment: the Rorschach Inkblot Method as exemplar. Psychol Assess 13:423–432, 2001

Wildman RW, Wildman RW: An investigation into the comparative validity of several diagnostic tests and test batteries. J Clin Psychol 31:455–458, 1975

Wildman R, Batchelor E, Thompson L, et al: Georgia Court Competency Test. Newsletter of the American Association of Correctional Psychologists 11(2):4, 1979

Wilson JP, Keane TM: Assessing Psychological Trauma and PTSD. New York, Guilford, 1997

World Health Organization: International Classification of Diseases, 10th Revision. Geneva, World Health Organization, 1992

Ziskin J: Coping With Psychiatric and Psychological Testimony, 5th Edition, Vols 1–3. Los Angeles, CA, Law & Psychology Press, 1995

Ziskin J: Coping With Psychiatric and Psychological Testimony, 5th Edition, 1997 Supplement. Edited by Dunn JT. Los Angeles, CA, Law & Psychology Press, 1997

Ziskin J: Coping With Psychiatric and Psychological Testimony, 5th Edition, 2000 Supplement. Edited by Bersoff DN, Anderer SJ, Dodds LD, et al. Los Angeles, CA, Law & Psychology Press, 2000

Ziskin J, Faust D: Reply to Matarazzo. Am Psychol 46:881–882, 1991

Zusman J, Simon J: Differences in repeated psychiatric examinations of litigants to a lawsuit. Am J Psychiatry 140:1300–1304, 1983

## Suggested Readings

Blau TH: Psychological tests in the courtroom. Professional Psychology 15:176–186, 1984

Borum R, Grisso T: Psychological test use in criminal forensic evaluations. Professional Psychology 26:465–473, 1995

Grisso T: Evaluating Competencies: Forensic Assessments and Instruments. New York, Plenum, 1986

Heilbrun K: The role of psychological testing in forensic assessment. Law Hum Behav 16:257–272, 1992

Melton GB, Petrila J, Poythress NG, et al: Psychological Evaluations for the Courts: A Handbook for Mental Health Professionals and Lawyers, 2nd Edition. New York, Guilford, 1987

Meyer GJ, Finn SE, Eyde LD, et al: Psychological testing and psychological assessment. Am Psychol 56:128–165, 2001

Nicholson RA, Norwood S: The quality of forensic psychological assessments, reports, and testimony: acknowledging the gap between promise and practice. Law Hum Behav 24:9–44, 2000

Pope KS, Butcher JN, Seelen J: The MMPI, MMPI-2, MMPI-A in Court: A Practical Guide for Expert Witnesses and Attorneys, 2nd Edition. Washington, DC, American Psychological Association, 1999

Rogers R: Clinical Assessment of Malingering and Deception, 2nd Edition. New York, Guilford, 1997.

Rogers R, Bagby M, Dickens SE: Structured Interview of Reported Symptoms. Lutz, FL, Psychological Assessment Resources, 2002

Ziskin J: Coping With Psychiatric and Psychological Testimony, 5th Edition, Vols 1–3. Los Angeles, CA, Law & Psychology Press, 1995

Ziskin J: Coping With Psychiatric and Psychological Testimony, 5th Edition, 1997 Supplement. Edited by Dunn JT. Los Angeles, CA, Law & Psychology Press, 1997

Ziskin J: Coping With Psychiatric and Psychological Testimony, 5th Edition, 2000 Supplement. Edited by Bersoff DN, Anderer SJ, Dodds LD, et al. Los Angeles, CA, Law & Psychology Press, 2000

# Appendix

## *Glossary of Legal Terms*

**action** A civil or criminal judicial proceeding. See CIVIL ACTION.

***actus reus*** The wrongful deed that comprises the physical components of a crime and that generally must be coupled with MENS REA to establish criminal LIABILITY.

**adjudication** The formal pronouncement of a JUDGMENT or decree in a CAUSE OF ACTION.

**administrative law** The law governing the organization and operation of the executive branch of government (including independent agencies) and the relations of the executive with the legislature, the judiciary, and the public.

**advance directive** A method for individuals while competent to appoint PROXY health care decision makers in the event of future incompetency. See DURABLE POWER OF ATTORNEY; HEALTH CARE PROXY; LIVING WILL.

**adversary system** A procedural system involving active and unhindered parties contesting with each other to put forth a case before an independent decision-maker.

**affidavit** A voluntary declaration of facts written down and sworn to by the declarant before an officer authorized to administer oaths.

---

Most terms and definitions reprinted from Shahrokh NC, Hales RE: *American Psychiatric Glossary,* 8th Edition. Washington, DC, American Psychiatric Publishing, 2003, pp. 233–240. Copyright 2003, American Psychiatric Publishing, Inc. Used with permission. SMALL CAPS type indicates terms defined as main entries elsewhere in this glossary.

**appeal** The submission of a lower court's or agency's decision to a higher court for review and possible reversal.

**assault** Any willful attempt or threat to inflict injury.

**battery** Intentional and wrongful physical contact with an individual without consent that causes some injury or offensive touching.

**best interests of the child** General standard applied by courts to determine the "care and custody of minor children." Different states consider different factors relevant in defining what constitutes a "child's best interests." Some of the more common factors include the mental and physical health of all individuals involved (e.g., child, parents); the wishes of the child as to his or her choice of custodian; and the interaction and degree of "psychological connectedness" between the child and the proposed custodian.

**beyond a reasonable doubt** The level of proof required to convict a person in a criminal trial. Of the three legal standards of proof, this is the highest level (90%–95% range of certainty) and the one required to establish the guilt of someone accused of a crime. See also CLEAR AND CONVINCING EVIDENCE; PREPONDERANCE OF THE EVIDENCE.

**breach of contract** A violation of or failure to perform any or all of the terms of an agreement.

**brief** A written statement prepared by legal counsel arguing a case.

**burden of proof** The legal obligation to prove affirmatively a disputed fact related to an issue that is raised by the parties in a case.

**capacity** The status or attributes necessary for a person so that his or her acts may be legally allowed and recognized.

**case law** The aggregate of reported cases as forming a body of law on a particular subject.

**cause of action** The grounds of an ACTION; that is, those facts that, if alleged and proved in a suit, would enable the PLAINTIFF to attain a JUDGMENT.

**civil action** A lawsuit brought by a private individual or group to recover money or property, to enforce or protect a civil RIGHT, or to prevent or redress a civil wrong.

**clear and convincing evidence** The second-highest standard applied to determining whether alleged facts have been proven (75% range of certainty). This is the standard applied to civil commitment matters and similar circumstances in which there is the chance that valued civil liberty interests and freedoms are at stake. See also BEYOND A REASONABLE DOUBT; PREPONDERANCE OF THE EVIDENCE.

**commitment** A legal process for admitting, usually involuntarily, a mentally ill person to a psychiatric treatment program. Although the legal definition and procedure vary from state to state, commitment usually requires a court or judicial procedure. Commitment also may be voluntary.

**common law** A system of law based on customs, traditional usage, and prior CASE LAW rather than on codified written laws (STATUTES).

**compensatory damages** DAMAGES awarded to a person as compensation, indemnity, or restitution for harm sustained.

**competency** Having the mental CAPACITY to understand the nature of an act. See also COMPETENCY TO STAND TRIAL; INFORMED CONSENT; TESTAMENTARY CAPACITY.

**competency to stand trial** Legal test applied to all criminal DEFENDANTS regarding their cognitive ability at the time of trial to participate in the proceedings against them. As held in *Dusky v. United States* (1960), a defendant is competent to stand trial if 1) he or she possesses a factual understanding of the proceedings against him or her, and 2) he or she has sufficient present ability to consult with his or her lawyer with a reasonable degree of rational understanding.

**complaint** The initial pleading that starts a civil action and states the basis for the court's jurisdiction, the basis for the plaintiff's claim, and the demand for relief.

**confidentiality** The situation in which certain communications between persons who are in a FIDUCIARY or trust relationship to each other (e.g., physician-patient) are generally not legally permitted to be disclosed and are not admissible as evidence in court during a trial. See also PRIVILEGED COMMUNICATION.

**conflict of interest** A real or seeming incompatibility between one's private interests and one's public or fiduciary duties.

**consent decree** Agreement by a DEFENDANT to cease activities asserted as illegal by the government.

**conservatorship** The appointment of a person to manage and make decisions on behalf of an incompetent person regarding the latter's estate (e.g., authority to make CONTRACTS or sell property). See also GUARDIANSHIP; INCOMPETENCE.

**consortium** The RIGHT of a husband or wife to the care, affection, company, and cooperation of the other spouse in every aspect of the marital relationship.

**contingent fee** A fee charged for services only if the lawsuit is successful or is favorably settled out of court.

**contract** A legally enforceable agreement between two or more parties to do or not do a particular thing on sufficient consideration.

**criminal law** The branch of the law that defines crimes and provides for their punishment. Unlike civil law, penalties include imprisonment.

**damages** A sum of money awarded to a person injured by the unlawful act or NEGLIGENCE of another.

***Daubert* hearing** A hearing conducted by federal district courts, usually before trial, to determine whether proposed expert TESTIMONY meets the federal requirements for relevance and reliability as clarified by the Supreme Court in *Daubert v. Merrell Dow Pharmaceuticals, Inc.* (1993).

***Daubert* test** A method that federal district courts use to determine whether expert testimony is admissible under Federal Rule of Evidence 702, which generally requires that expert testimony consists of scientific, technical, or other specialized knowledge that will assist the fact-finder in understanding the evidence or determining a fact in issue. Suggested criteria for admissibility were set forth in the Supreme Court decision in *Daubert v. Merrell Dow Pharmaceuticals, Inc.* (1993).

**de facto** Something that is in fact, in deed, or actually in effect, especially without authority of law. Compare with DE JURE.

**defendant** A person or legal entity against whom a claim or charge is brought.

**de jure** Something that is considered "lawful," "rightful," "legitimate," or "just." Compare with DE FACTO.

**diminished capacity** Refers to insufficient cognitive ability to achieve the state of mind (MENS REA) requisite for the commission of a crime. Sometimes referred to as "partial INSANITY," this doctrine permits a court to consider the impaired mental state of the DEFENDANT for purposes of reducing punishment or lowering the degree of the offense being charged.

**due process (of law)** The constitutional guarantee protecting individuals from arbitrary and unreasonable actions by the government that would deprive them of their basic RIGHTS to life, liberty, or property.

**durable power of attorney** A person designated by another to act as his or her attorney-in-fact regardless of whether the principal eventually becomes incompetent. This is prescribed statutorily in all 50 states. See also ADVANCE DIRECTIVE; HEALTH CARE PROXY; LIVING WILL.

**duress** Compulsion or constraint, as by force or threat, exercised to make a person do or say something against his or her will.

**duty** Legal obligation that one person owes another. Whenever one person has a RIGHT, another person has a corresponding duty to preserve or not interfere with that right.

**eggshell skull rule** In tort law, the principle that a defendant is liable for a plaintiff's unforeseeable and uncommon reactions to the defendant's negligent or intentional act.

**emancipated minor** A person younger than 18 years who is considered totally self-supporting. Legal RIGHTS afforded at adulthood are typically extended to an emancipated minor.

**entitlement program** In health law, legislatively defined rights to health care, such as Medicare and Medicaid programs.

**expert witness** One who by reason of specialized education, experience, and/or training possesses superior knowledge about a subject that is beyond the understanding of an average or ordinary layperson. Expert witnesses are permitted to offer opinions about matters relevant to their expertise that will assist a jury in comprehending evidence that they would otherwise not understand or fully appreciate.

**false imprisonment** The unlawful restraint or detention of one person by another.

**felony** A serious crime, such as murder, rape, arson, or burglary, usually punishable by imprisonment for more than 1 year or by death.

**fiduciary** A person who acts for another in a capacity that involves a confidence or trust.

**fiduciary relationship** A relationship in which one person is under a duty to act for the benefit of the other on matters within the scope of the relationship

**forensic psychiatry** A subspecialty of psychiatry in which scientific and clinical expertise is applied to legal issues in legal contexts embracing civil, criminal, correctional, or legislative matters.

**fraud** Any act of trickery, deceit, or misrepresentation designed to deprive someone of property or to do harm.

***Frye* test** The defunct federal common-law rule of evidence on the admissibility of scientific evidence that required that the tests or procedures must have gained general acceptance in their particular field.

***Gault* decision** A landmark Supreme Court decision in 1967 that found that juveniles were entitled to the same DUE PROCESS RIGHTS as adults—that is, the right to counsel, the right to notice of specific charges of the offense, the right to confront and cross-examine a witness, the right to remain silent, and the right to SUBPOENA witnesses in defense. The right to trial by jury was not included.

**guardian *ad litem*** A guardian, usually a lawyer, appointed by the court to appear in a lawsuit on behalf of an incompetent or minor party.

**guardianship** The delegation, by the state, of authority over an individual's person or estate to another party. For example, a personal guardian for a mentally ill patient would have the legal RIGHT to make medical decisions on behalf of the patient.

**habeas corpus** (Latin, "you have the body") An order to bring a party before a judge or court; specifically, in regard to a person who is being retained within a hospital, to give the court the opportunity to examine that person and decide on the appropriateness of such retention.

**health care proxy** A legal instrument akin to the DURABLE POWER OF ATTORNEY but specifically created for health care decision making. See also ADVANCE DIRECTIVE; LIVING WILL.

**immunity** Freedom from DUTY or penalty.

**incompetence** A lack of ability or fitness for some legal qualification necessary for the performance of an act (e.g., by being a minor, or by mental incompetence).

**informed consent** A competent person's voluntary agreement to allow something to happen that is based on full disclosure of facts needed to make a knowing decision.

**injury** Harm or damage, or the violation of another's legal right, for which the law provides a remedy.

**insanity** In law, the term denotes that degree of mental illness that negates an individual's legal responsibility or CAPACITY.

**insanity defense** A legal concept that holds that a person cannot be held criminally responsible for his or her actions when, due to a mental illness, the person was unable to form the requisite intent for the crime he or she is charged with at the time the crime was committed. Historically, several standards or tests have been devised to define criminal INSANITY. Some of these include the following:

**American Law Institute (ALI)/Model Penal Code test** A DEFENDANT would not be responsible for his or her criminal conduct if, as a result of mental disease or defect, he or she "lacked substantial CAPACITY either to appreciate the criminality of his or her conduct or to conform his or her conduct to the requirements of law."

**Comprehensive Crime Control Act (CCCA) of 1984 standard** In 1984, as part of sweeping federal legislation, the CCCA altered the test for INSANITY in federal courts by holding that it was an affirmative defense to all federal crimes that at the time of the offense, "the DEFENDANT, as a result of a severe mental disease or defect, was unable to appreciate the nature and quality or the wrongfulness of his acts. Mental disease or defect does not otherwise constitute a defense."

***Durham* rule** A ruling by the U.S. Court of Appeals for the District of Columbia Circuit in 1954 that held that an accused person is not criminally responsible if his or her "unlawful act was the product of mental disease or mental defect." This decision was quite controversial, and within several years it was modified and then replaced altogether by the same court that originally formulated it.

**irresistible impulse test** Acquittal of criminal responsibility is allowed if a DEFENDANT'S mental disorder caused him or her to experience an "irresistible and uncontrollable impulse to commit the offense, even if he remained able to understand the nature of the offense and its wrongfulness."

***M'Naghten* rule** In 1843, the English House of Lords ruled that a person was not responsible for a crime if the accused "was laboring under such a defect of reason from a disease of mind as not to know the nature and quality of the act; or, if he knew it, that he did not know he was doing what was wrong." This rule, or some derivation of it, is still applied in many states today.

**intentional tort** A TORT in which the actor is expressly or implicitly judged to have possessed an intent or a purpose to cause INJURY.

**judgment** The final determination or ADJUDICATION by a court of the claims of parties in an ACTION.

**jurisdiction** Widely used to denote the legal RIGHT by which courts or judicial officers exercise their authority.

**liability** The quality or state of being legally obligated or accountable, or legally responsible to another or to society, enforceable by civil remedy or criminal punishment.

**strict liability** Liability that does not depend on actual negligence or intent to harm, but that is based on the breach of an absolute duty to make something safety.

**vicarious liability** Indirect legal responsibility for the actions or conduct of those over whom the principal has control. For example, a private physician is generally vicariously liable for the negligence of any assisting employees.

**lien** A legal right or interest that a creditor has in another's property, usually lasting until a debt that it secures has been satisfied.

**living will** Procedure by which competent persons can, under certain situations, direct their doctors to treat them in a prescribed way if they become incompetent (e.g., withdraw lifesaving medical care if in a vegetative state). See also ADVANCE DIRECTIVE; DURABLE POWER OF ATTORNEY; HEALTH CARE PROXY.

**medical malpractice** Generally defined as "the failure to exercise the degree of skill in diagnosis or treatment that reasonably can be expected from one licensed and holding oneself out as a physician under the circumstances of a particular case" that directly causes harm to a patient. See also NEGLIGENCE; STANDARD OF CARE; TORT.

**mens rea** Literally, "guilty mind." One of two fundamental aspects of any crime. The other aspect is the act, or ACTUS REUS.

***Miranda* warning** Refers to the *Miranda v. Arizona* decision (1966) that requires a four-part warning to be given prior to any custodial interrogation.

**misdemeanor** A crime that is less serious than a FELONY and is usually punishable by fine, penalty, forfeiture, or confinement, usually for a brief term, in a place other than a prison, such as a county jail.

**motion** A written or oral application requesting a court to make a specified ruling or order.

**negligence** In MEDICAL MALPRACTICE law, generally described as the failure to do something that a reasonable practitioner would have done (omission) or as doing something that a reasonable practitioner would not have done (commission) under particular circumstances. See also STANDARD OF CARE; TORT.

**nominal damages** Generally, DAMAGES of a small monetary amount indicating a violation of a legal RIGHT without any important loss or damage to the PLAINTIFF.

**parens patriae** The authority of the state to exercise sovereignty and GUARDIANSHIP of a person of legal disability so as to act on his or her behalf in protecting health, comfort, and welfare interests.

**plaintiff** The complaining party in an ACTION; the person who brings a CAUSE OF ACTION.

**police power** The power of government to make and enforce all laws and regulations necessary for the welfare of the state and its citizens.

**preponderance of the evidence** The lowest of three levels or standards applied to determining whether alleged facts have been proven (51% range of certainty); more likely than not. This is the standard applied to civil lawsuits.

**privilege** A statutorily based RIGHT of the patient to restrict or bar the disclosure of confidential information in a court of law in most circumstances. See also CONFIDENTIALITY.

**privileged communication** Those statements made by certain persons within a protected relationship (e.g., doctor-patient) that the law protects from forced disclosure. See also CONFIDENTIALITY.

**proximate cause** The direct, immediate cause to which an injury or loss can be attributed and without which the injury or loss would not have occurred.

**proxy** A person empowered by another to represent, act, or vote for him or her.

**punitive damages** DAMAGES awarded over and above those to which the PLAINTIFF is entitled, generally given to punish or make an example of the DEFENDANT.

**reasonable medical certainty** In proving the cause of an injury, a standard requiring a showing that the injury was more likely than not caused by a particular stimulus, based on the general consensus of recognized medical thought.

**reasonable person** A hypothetical person used as a legal standard to determine whether someone acted with negligence.

**respondeat superior** The doctrine whereby the master (i.e., the employer) is liable in certain cases for the wrongful acts of his or her servants (i.e., the employees).

**right** A power, privilege, demand, or claim possessed by a particular person by virtue of law. Every legal right that one person has imposes corresponding legal DUTIES on other persons.

**sovereign immunity** The IMMUNITY of a government from being sued in court except with its consent.

**standard of care** In the law of medical negligence, that degree of care that a reasonably prudent medical practitioner having ordinary skill, training, and learning would exercise under the same or similar circumstances. Unless the practitioner is considered an expert or a specialist, the requisite degree of care is held to be only "ordinary" and "reasonable" care. If a physician's conduct falls below the standard of care, he or she may be liable in DAMAGES for any injuries resulting from such conduct.

**standard of proof** The degree or level of proof demanded in a specific case, such as "beyond a reasonable doubt" or "by a preponderance of evidence."

**stare decisis** To adhere to precedents and not to unsettle principles of law that are established.

**statute** An act of the legislature declaring, commanding, or prohibiting something.

**strict liability** See LIABILITY.

**subpoena** A command, typically at the request of a litigating party, to appear at a certain time and place to give TESTIMONY on a certain matter. Unless signed by a judge, a subpoena is not a court order compelling testimony but merely a court-issued order to show up.

**subpoena ad testificandum** A writ commanding a person to appear in court to give TESTIMONY.

**subpoena duces tecum** A writ commanding a person to produce specified records or documents at a certain time and place at trial.

***Tarasoff* rule** Based on the 1976 California decision *Tarasoff v. the Regents of the University of California*, this landmark opinion held that when a patient presents a serious, imminent danger of violence to a foreseeable victim, the psychotherapist of that patient has a DUTY to use reasonable care to protect the intended victim against such danger. A number of JURISDICTIONS have issued a ruling or STATUTE involving some variation of the *Tarasoff* "duty to protect" doctrine.

**testamentary capacity** Pertains to the state of mind of an individual at the time he or she writes or executes his or her will. Generally, to have sufficient testamentary capacity, testators must possess a certain level of understanding of the nature and extent of their property, of the persons who are the natural objects of their bounty, and of the disposition that they are making of their property and must appreciate these elements in relation to one another and form an orderly desire as to the disposition of their property.

**testimony** Evidence that a competent witness under oath or affirmation gives at trial or in an AFFIDAVIT or deposition.

**Title VII of the Civil Rights Act of 1964** A law that prohibits employment discrimination on the basis of race, sex, pregnancy, religion, and national origin, often referred to simply as Title VII.

**tort** A civil wrong subject to lawsuit by private individuals, as distinguished from a criminal offense, which is only brought or prosecuted by the state on behalf of its citizens. See also CIVIL ACTION.

**tortfeasor** One who commits a tort; a wrongdoer.

**United States Code (U.S.C.)** The compilation of laws derived from federal legislation.

**vicarious liability** See LIABILITY.

**voir dire** A preliminary examination by a judge or lawyer to test the competence of a witness.

# Legal Case Index

**Boldface** *type indicates pages of this textbook on which cases are cited or discussed.*

# Subject Index

*Page numbers printed in* **boldface** *type refer to tables or figures.*